Surgical Treatment of Parkinson's Disease and Other Movement Disorders

CURRENT CLINICAL NEUROLOGY

Daniel Tarsy, MD, SERIES EDITORS

The Visual Field: A Perimetric Atlas, edited by ***Jason J. S. Barton and Michael Benatar****, 2003*

Surgical Treatment of Parkinson's Disease and Other Movement Disorders, edited by ***Daniel Tarsy, Jerrold L. Vitek, and Andres M. Lozano****, 2003*

Myasthenia Gravis and Related Disorders, edited by ***Henry J. Kaminski****, 2003*

Seizures: Medical Causes and Management, edited by ***Norman Delanty****, 2002*

Clinical Evaluation and Management of Spasticity, edited by ***David A. Gelber and Douglas R. Jeffery****, 2002*

Early Diagnosis of Alzheimer's Disease, edited by ***Leonard F. M. Scinto and Kirk R. Daffner****, 2000*

Sexual and Reproductive Neurorehabilitation, edited by ***Mindy Aisen****, 1997*

Surgical Treatment of Parkinson's Disease

and Other Movement Disorders

Edited by

***Daniel Tarsy,* MD**

Beth Israel Deaconess Medical Center, Harvard Medical School, Boston, MA

***Jerrold L. Vitek,* MD, PhD**

Emory University School of Medicine, Atlanta, GA

and

***Andres M. Lozano,* MD, PhD**

Toronto Western Hospital, Toronto, ON, Canada

Humana Press
Totowa, New Jersey

999 Riverview Drive, Suite 208
Totowa, New Jersey 07512

humanapress.com

This publication is printed on acid-free paper. ∞
ANSI Z39.48-1984 (American Standards Institute) Permanence of Paper for Printed Library Materials.

Cover illustration: T2-weighted coronal image for direct targeting of the subthalamic nuclei bilaterally. *See* Fig. 4 on page 90.

Cover design by Patricia F. Cleary.

Production Editor: Mark J. Breaugh.

For additional copies, pricing for bulk purchases, and/or information about other Humana titles, contact Humana at the above address or at any of the following numbers: Tel.: 973-256-1699; Fax: 973-256-8314; E-mail: humana@humanapr.com, or visit our Website: http://humanapress.com

Printed in the United States of America. 10 9 8 7 6 5 4 3 2 1

Library of Congress Cataloging in Publication Data

Surgical treatment of Parkinson's disease and other movement disorders / edited by
Daniel Tarsy, Jerrold L. Vitek and Andres M. Lozano.
p. ; cm.
Includes bibliographical references and index.
ISBN 0-89603-921-8 (alk. paper)
1. Parkinson's disease--Surgery. 2. Movement disorders--Surgery. I. Lozano, A. M. (Andres M.), 1959– II. Tarsy, Daniel. III. Vitek, Jerrold Lee.
[DNLM: 1. Parkinson Disease--surgery. 2. Movement Disorders--surgery. 3. Neurosurgical Procedures. 4. Stereotaxic Techniques. WL 359 S9528 2003]
RC382.S875 2003
617.4'81--dc21

2002068476

Preface

There has been a major resurgence in stereotactic neurosurgery for the treatment of Parkinson's disease and tremor in the past several years. More recently, interest has also been rekindled in stereotactic neurosurgery for the treatment of dystonia and other movement disorders. This is based on a large number of factors, which include recognized limitations of pharmacologic therapies for these conditions, better understanding of the functional neuroanatomy and neurophysiology of the basal ganglia, use of microelectrode recording techniques for lesion localization, improved brain imaging, improved brain lesioning techniques, the rapid emergence of deep brain stimulation technology, progress in neurotransplantation, better patient selection, and improved objective methods for the evaluation of surgical results. These changes have led to increased collaboration between neurosurgeons, neurologists, clinical neurophysiologists, and neuropsychologists, all of which appear to be resulting in a better therapeutic result for patients afflicted with these disorders.

The aim of *Surgical Treatment of Parkinson's Disease and Other Movement Disorders* is to create a reference handbook that describes the methodologies we believe are necessary to carry out neurosurgical procedures for the treatment of Parkinson's disease and other movement disorders. It is directed toward neurologists who participate in these procedures or are referring patients to have them done, to neurosurgeons who are already carrying out these procedures or contemplating becoming involved, and to other health care professionals including neuropsychologists and general medical physicians seeking better familiarity with this rapidly evolving area of therapeutics. Several books concerning this subject currently exist, most of which have emerged from symposia on surgical treatment of movement disorders. We have tried here to provide a systematic and comprehensive review of the subject, which (where possible) takes a "horizontal" view of the approaches and methodologies common to more than one surgical procedure, including patient selection, patient assessment, target localization, postoperative programming methods, and positron emission tomography.

We have gathered a group of experienced and recognized authorities in the field who have provided authoritative reviews that define the current state of the art of surgical treatment of Parkinson's disease and related movement disorders. We greatly appreciate their excellent contributions as well as the work of Paul Dolgert, Craig Adams, and Mark Breaugh at Humana Press who made this work a reality. We especially thank our very patient and understanding families whose love and support helped to make this book possible. Finally we dedicate this book to our patients whose courage and persistence in the face of great adversity have allowed the work described in this book to progress toward some measure of relief of their difficult conditions.

Daniel Tarsy, MD
Jerrold L. Vitek, MD, PhD
Andres M. Lozano, MD, PhD

Contents

Contributors

AVIVA ABOSCH, MD, PhD • Division of Neurosurgery, Toronto Western Hospital, Toronto, Ontario, Canada

J. ERIC AHLSKOG, MD, PhD • Department of Neurology, Mayo Clinic, Rochester, MN

TIPU Z. AZIZ, MD • Department of Neurosurgery, The Radcliffe Infirmary, Oxford, UK

ROY A. E. BAKAY, MD • Department of Neurosurgery, Rush Medical College, Chicago, IL

GUY BOUVIER, MD • Hôpital Notre-Dame, University of Montreal, Montreal, Quebec, Canada

JIN WOO CHANG, MD, PhD • Department of Neurosurgery, Yonsei University College of Medicine, Seoul, South Korea

ALI CHARARA, PhD • Yerkes Primate Research Center, Emory University, Atlanta, GA

ESTHER CUBO, MD • Department of Neurological Sciences, Rush Medical College, Chicago, IL

DUDLEY H. DAVIS, MD • Department of Neurosurgery, Mayo Clinic, Rochester, MN

CHRISTINE EDWARDS, MA • Center for Neurosciences, North Shore-Long Island Jewish Research Institute, Manhasset, NY

DAVID EIDELBERG, MD • Center for Neurosciences, North Shore-Long Island Jewish Research Institute, Manhasset, NY

STANLEY FAHN, MD • Neurological Institute, Columbia-Presbyterian Medical Center, New York, NY

JULIE A. FIELDS, BA • Department of Psychiatry and Behavioral Sciences, University of Washington School of Medicine, Seattle, WA

BLAIR FORD, MD • Neurological Institute, Columbia-Presbyterian Medical Center, New York, NY

MASAFUMI FUKUDA, MD • Center for Neurosciences, North Shore-Long Island Jewish Research Institute, Manhasset, NY

IRA M. GARONZIK, MD • Department of Neurosurgery, Johns Hopkins Hospital, Baltimore, MD

STEVEN S. GILL, MS • Department of Neurosurgery, Frenchay Hospital, Bristol, UK

CHRISTOPHER G. GOETZ, MD • Department of Neurological Sciences, Rush Medical College, Chicago, IL

PAUL GREENE, MD • Neurological Institute, Columbia-Presbyterian Medical Center, New York, NY

PETER HEYWOOD, PhD • Department of Neurosurgery, Frenchay Hospital, Bristol, UK

SHERWIN E. HUA, MD, PhD • Department of Neurosurgery, Johns Hopkins Hospital, Baltimore, MD

JEAN HUBBLE, MD • Department of Neurology, The Ohio State University, Columbus, OH

WILLIAM D. HUTCHISON, PhD • Division of Neurosurgery, Toronto Western Hospital, Toronto, Ontario, Canada

CAROLE JOINT, RGN • Department of Neurosurgery, The Radcliffe Infirmary, Oxford, UK
UN JUNG KANG, MD • Department of Neurology, The University of Chicago, Chicago, IL
MICHAEL KAPLITT, MD, PhD • Department of Neurosurgery, Weill Medical College of Cornell University, New York, NY
WILLIAM C. KOLLER, MD, PhD • Department of Neurology, University of Miami School of Medicine, Miami, FL
RAJEEV KUMAR, MD • Colorado Neurological Institute, Englewood, CO
ANTHONY E. LANG, MD • Department of Neurology, Toronto Western Hospital, Toronto, Ontario, Canada
JUNG-IL LEE, MD • Department of Neurosurgery, Johns Hopkins Hospital, Baltimore, MD
WON YONG LEE, MD, PhD • Department of Neurology, Samsung Medical Center, Seoul, Korea
FREDERICK A. LENZ, MD, PhD • Department of Neurosurgery, Johns Hopkins Hospital, Baltimore, MD
ANDRES M. LOZANO, MD, PhD • Division of Neurosurgery, Toronto Western Hospital, Toronto, Ontario, Canada
KELLY E. LYONS, PhD • Department of Neurology, University of Miami School of Medicine, Miami, FL
JOSEPH Y. MATSUMOTO, MD • Department of Neurology, Mayo Clinic, Rochester, MN
ALIREZA MINAGAR, MD • Department of Neurology, University of Miami School of Medicine, Miami, FL
PEDRO MOLINA-NEGRO, MD, PhD • Hôpital Notre-Dame, University of Montreal, Montreal, Quebec, Canada
THORKILD NORREGAARD, MD • Division of Neurosurgery, Beth Israel Deaconess Medical Center, Boston, MA
RAJESH PAHWA, MD • Department of Neurology, University of Kansas Medical Center, Kansas City, KS
NORA PAPASIAN, PhD • Department of Neurology, The University of Chicago, Chicago, IL
SIMON PARKIN, MRCP • Department of Neurology, The Radcliffe Infirmary, Oxford, UK
NIKUNJ K. PATEL, BS • Department of Neurosurgery, Frenchay Hospital, Bristol, UK
RICHARD SCOTT, PhD • Department of Neurosurgery, The Radcliffe Infirmary, Oxford, UK
MAMADOU SIDIBÉ, PhD • Yerkes Primate Research Center, Emory University, Atlanta, GA
DIANE K. SIERENS, MD • Department of Neurosurgery, Rush Medical College, Chicago, IL
YOLAND SMITH, PhD • Yerkes Primate Research Center, Emory University, Atlanta, GA
VOLKER STURM, MD, PhD • Department of Stereotactic and Functional Neurosurgery, University of Cologne, Cologne, Germany
DANIEL TARSY, MD • Department of Neurology, Beth Israel Deaconess Medical Center, Boston, MA

RONALD R. TASKER, MD • Department of Neurosurgery, Toronto Western Hospital, Toronto, Ontario, Canada

ALEXANDER I. TRÖSTER, PhD • Department of Psychiatry and Behavioral Sciences and Department of Neurological Surgery, University of Washington School of Medicine, Seattle, WA

JERROLD L. VITEK, MD, PhD • Department of Neurology, Emory University Medical Center, Atlanta, GA

JENS VOLKMANN, MD, PhD • Department of Neurology, University of Christian-Albrechts University, Kiel, Germany

THOMAS WICHMANN, MD • Department of Neurology, Emory University Medical Center, Atlanta, GA

I Rationale for Surgical Therapy

1

Physiology of the Basal Ganglia and Pathophysiology of Movement Disorders

Thomas Wichmann and Jerrold L. Vitek

1. INTRODUCTION

Insights into the structure and function of the basal ganglia and their role in the pathophysiology of movement disorders resulted in the 1980s in the development of testable models of hypokinetic and hyperkinetic movement disorders. Further refinement in the 1990s resulted from continued research in animal models and the addition of physiological recordings of neuronal activity in humans undergoing functional neurosurgical procedures *(1–7)*. These models have gained considerable practical value, guiding the development of new pharmacologic and surgical treatments, but, in their current form, more and more insufficiencies of these simplified schemes are becoming apparent. In the following chapter we discuss both models, as well as some of the most important criticisms.

2. NORMAL ANATOMY AND FUNCTION OF THE BASAL GANGLIA

The basal ganglia are components of circuits that include the cerebral cortex and thalamus *(8)*. These circuits originate in specific cortical areas, pass through separate portions of the basal ganglia and thalamus, and project back to the frontal cortical area from which they took origin. The cortical sites of origin of these circuits define their presumed function and include "motor," "oculomotor," "associative," and "limbic." In each of these circuits, the striatum and subthalamic nucleus (STN) serve as the input stage of the basal ganglia, and globus pallidus interna (GPi) and substantia nigra, pars reticulata (SNr) serve as output stations. This anatomic organization is consistent with the clinical evidence for motor and nonmotor functions and the development of cognitive and emotional/behavioral disturbances in diseases of the basal ganglia.

The motor circuit is particularly important in the pathophysiology of movement disorders. This circuit originates in pre- and postcentral sensorimotor fields, which project to the putamen. These projections either are direct connections to the putamen from the cortex, or reach the putamen via the intercalated centromedian nucleus (CM) of the thalamus *(9–15)*. Putamenal output reaches GPi/SNr via two pathways, a "direct" monosynaptic route, and an "indirect" polysynaptic route that passes through the external pallidal segment (GPe) to GPi directly or via GPe projections to the STN *(16,17)*. Although the main neurotransmitter of all striatal output neurons is GABA, one difference between the source neurons in the direct and indirect pathways is that neurons in the indirect pathway contain the neuropeptide substance P, whereas source neurons of the indirect pathway carry the neuropeptides enkephalin and dynorphin.

From: Current Clinical Neurology: Surgical Treatment of Parkinson's Disease and Other Movement Disorders
Edited by: D. Tarsy, J. L. Vitek, and A. M. Lozano © Humana Press Inc., Totowa, NJ

In addition to changes in the cortico-striatal pathway, the cortico-subthalamic pathway *(18–20)* may also influence basal ganglia activity *(14,21)*. The importance of this pathway is underscored by the fact that neuronal responses to sensorimotor examination in GPe and GPi are greatly reduced after lesions of the STN, suggesting that this pathway is largely responsible for relaying sensory input to the basal ganglia *(22)*. The close relationship between neuronal activity in the cerebral cortex and the STN is suggested by the fact that oscillatory activity in the STN and the pallidum is closely correlated to oscillatory activity in the cortex *(23)*. Furthermore, cortical stimulation results in a complex pattern of excitation-inhibition in GPi, which is likely mediated by the STN and its connection to both pallidal segments *(24)*.

Basal ganglia output is directed toward the thalamic ventral anterior, ventral lateral, and intralaminar nuclei (ventralis anterioris [VA], ventralis lateralis pars oralis [VLo], centromedian and parafascicular nucleus CM/Pf) *(25–34)*, and to the brainstem, in particular to portions of the pedunculopontine nucleus (PPN), which may serve to connect the basal ganglia to spinal centers *(35–39)*. Portions of the PPN also project back to the basal ganglia, and may modulate basal ganglia output. Basal ganglia output to the thalamus remains segregated into "motor" and "nonmotor" functions. Even within the movement-related circuitry, there may be a certain degree of specialization. Output from the motor portion of GPi reaches predominately VA and VLo, which, in turn, project to cortical motor areas that are closely related to the sequencing and execution of movements *(34)*. Motor output from SNr, on the other hand, reaches premotor areas that are more closely related to the planning of movement *(34)*. In addition, output from the SNr reaches areas closely related to eye movements, such as the frontal eye fields *(34)*, and the superior colliculus. The latter is the phylogenetically oldest basal ganglia connection, whose more general relevance may lie in a contribution to the control of orienting behaviors *(40–45)*. STN, PPN, thalamus, and cortical projection neurons are excitatory (glutamatergic), whereas other neurons intrinsic to the basal ganglia are inhibitory (GABAergic).

The neurotransmitter dopamine plays a central role in striatal function. The net effect of striatal dopamine is to reduce basal ganglia output, leading to disinhibition of thalamocortical projection neurons. This may occur, however, via a number of different mechanisms, including a "fast" synaptic and a slower modulatory mode. The fast synaptic mode modulates transmission along the spines of striatal neurons, which are the major targets of cortical and thalamic inputs to the striatum *(46)*. By this mechanism, dopamine may be important in motor learning or in the selection of contextually appropriate movements *(47–49)*. The slower mode may modulate striatal activity on a slower time scale via a broad neuromodulatory mechanism. Changes in this neuromodulatory control of striatal outflow may underlie some of the behavioral alterations seen in movement disorders *(5)*. Although under considerable debate *(50,51)*, it appears that dopamine predominately facilitates transmission over the direct pathway and inhibits transmission over the indirect pathway via dopamine D_1 and D_2 receptors, respectively *(52,53)*.

By virtue of being part of the aforementioned cortico-subcortical re-entrant loops that terminate in the frontal lobes, the basal ganglia have a major impact on cortical function and on the control of behavior. Both GPi and SNr output neurons exhibit a high tonic discharge rate in intact animals *(54–57)*. Modulation of this discharge by alteration in phasic and tonic activity over multiple afferent pathways occurs with voluntary movement, as well as involuntary movements. Details of the basal ganglia mechanisms involved in the control of voluntary movements are still far from clear, but it is thought that motor commands generated at the cortical level are transmitted to the putamen directly and via the CM. Stated in the most simple terms, phasic activation of the direct striato-pallidal pathway may result in reduction of tonic-inhibitory basal ganglia output, resulting in disinhibition of thalamocortical neurons, and facilitation of movement. By contrast, phasic activation of the indirect pathway may lead to increased basal ganglia output *(18)* and to suppression of movement.

The combination of information traveling via the direct and the indirect pathways of the motor circuit may serve basic motor control functions such as "scaling" or "focusing" of movements *(8,58–60)*.

Scaling or termination of movements would be achieved if in an orderly temporal sequence striatal output would first inhibit GPi/SNr neurons via the direct pathway (facilitating a movement in progress), followed by disinhibition of the same GPi/SNr neuron via the indirect pathway (terminating the movement). By contrast, focusing would be achieved if separate target populations of neurons in GPi/SNr would receive simultaneous input via the direct and indirect pathways in a center-surround (facilitating/inhibiting) manner *(58–60)*. In this manner, increased activity along the direct pathway would lead to inhibition of some GPi/SNr neurons, allowing intended movements to proceed, while increased activity along the indirect pathway would activate other GPi/SNr neurons, acting to inhibit unintended movements. Similar models have been proposed for the generation of saccades in the oculomotor circuit *(61)*.

Direct anatomical support for either of these functions is lacking, because it is uncertain whether the direct and indirect pathways (emanating from neurons that are concerned with the same movement) converge on the same, or on separate neurons in GPi/SNr *(17,62–64)*, and thus, whether focusing or scaling would be anatomically possible. In addition to the anatomic uncertainty, it is not clear whether cortico-striatal neurons carry information that would be consistent with a focusing or scaling function of the basal ganglia.

The lack of effect of STN lesions on voluntary movement is difficult to reconcile with either hypothesis. Such lesions induce dyskinesias (hemiballism), but voluntary movements can still be carried out. Lack of focusing would be expected to result in inappropriate activation of antagonistic muscle groups (dystonia), and lack of scaling would be expected to result in hypo- or hypermetric movements. Neither effect is observed after STN lesions.

In general, movement-related changes in neuronal discharge occur too late in the basal ganglia to influence the initiation of movement. However, such changes in discharge could still influence the amplitude or limit the overall extent of ongoing movements *(24,65,66)*. Conceivably, neurons with shorter onset latencies or with "preparatory" activity may indeed play such a role *(31,67–75)*. Recent PET studies have reported that basal ganglia activity is modulated in relation to low-level parameters of movement, such as force or movement speed *(76,77)*, supporting a scaling function of the basal ganglia.

The basal ganglia may also serve more global functions such as the planning, initiation, sequencing, and execution of movements *(78,79)*. Most recently, an involvement of these structures in the performance of learned movements, and in motor learning itself has been proposed *(80–83)*. For instance, both dopaminergic nigrostriatal neurons and tonically active neurons in the striatum have been shown to develop transient responses to sensory conditioning stimuli during behavioral training in classical conditioning tasks *(48,80,84,85)*. In addition, shifts in the response properties of striatal output neurons during a procedural motor learning task have been demonstrated *(86)*.

A problem with all schemes that attribute a significant indispensable motor function to the basal ganglia, however, is the fact that lesions of the basal ganglia output nuclei do not lead to obvious motor deficits in humans or experimental animals. Most studies have found either no effect or only subtle short-lived effects on skilled fine movements after such lesions (*87–90*; *see* also *58,60*). Given the paucity of motor side-effects in animals and humans with lesions in the pallidal or thalamic motor regions, one would conclude that basal ganglia output does not play a significant role in the initiation or execution of most movements *(78)*. One explanation for this apparent discrepancy is the notion that motor functions of the basal ganglia could be readily compensated for by actions in other areas of the circuitry or even by other cortical areas not directly related to the motor portion of the basal ganglia.

3. MOVEMENT DISORDERS

Although the precise role of the basal ganglia in normal motor control remains unclear, alterations in basal ganglia function clearly underlie the development of a variety of movement disorders. These diseases are conventionally categorized into either hypokinetic disorders, such as Parkinson's disease, or hyperkinetic disorders such as hemiballism or drug-induced dyskinesias. This classification is clinically useful, but is of limited relevance for pathophysiologic interpretations of the different movement disorders, because of the existence of movement disorders such as Huntington's disease (HD) or dystonia, which seem to cross the boundary between these diseases. Another common misconception is that movement disorders are basal ganglia diseases. Given the anatomic facts previously mentioned, it is now clear that even the most straightforward pathophysiologic models of these disorders have to take into account that all movement disorders are *network* dysfunctions, affecting the activity of related cortical and thalamic neurons as much as that of basal ganglia neurons. Reports of movement disorders secondary to extrastriatal pathology should therefore come as no surprise.

3.1. Parkinson's Disease

Early idiopathic Parkinson's disease (PD) is a well-circumscribed pathologic entity whose pathologic hallmark is loss of dopaminergic nigrostriatal projection neurons. The resulting motor problems such as tremor, rigidity, akinesia, and bradykinesia can be treated with dopaminergic replacement strategies. In later stages of the disease the dopamine loss is accompanied by additional anatomic deficits outside of the basal ganglia-thalamocortical circuitry, such as the loss of brainstem *(91)* and cortical neurons, resulting in abnormalities that are generally not amenable to dopaminergic replacement therapy, such as autonomic dysfunction, postural instability, and cognitive dysfunction.

The dopaminergic deficit in the basal ganglia circuitry of early Parkinson's disease results in a number of fairly well-circumscribed changes in neuronal discharge, which in turn result in the development of the cardinal motor abnormalities of the disease. According to the model proposed by Albin et al. *(1)* and Delong et al. *(5)*, dopamine loss results in increased activity along the indirect pathway, and reduced activity along the direct pathway. Both effects together will lead to increased excitation of GPi and SNr neurons, and to inhibition of thalamocortical cells, and reduced excitation of cortex, clinically manifest in the development of the aforementioned cardinal motor signs of Parkinson's disease *(6)*. Descending basal ganglia output to the PPN may also play a role in the development of parkinsonism. The PPN region was shown to be metabolically overactive in parkinsonian animals, consistent with a major increase of input to this region *(92,93)*, and it has been shown that inactivation of this nucleus alone is sufficient to induce a form of akinesia in experimental animals *(94,95)*, although it is not certain how the poverty of movement after PPN inactivation relates to that present in parkinsonism.

Activity at the cortical level have been explored with PET studies. These experiments have indicated that parkinsonism is associated with relatively selective underactivity of the supplementary motor area, dorsal prefrontal cortex, and frontal association areas that receive subcortical input principally from the basal ganglia. At the same time there appears to be compensatory overactivity of the lateral premotor and parietal cortex, areas that have a primary role in facilitating motor responses to visual and auditory cues *(96)*.

The realization that increased basal ganglia output may be a major pathophysiologic step in the development of parkinsonian motor signs has stimulated attempts to reduce this output pharmacologically and surgically. The demonstration that lesions of the STN in MPTP-treated primates reverses all of the cardinal motor signs of parkinsonism by reducing GPi activity has contributed to these efforts *(87,97)*. Stereotactic lesions of the motor portion of GPi (GPi pallidotomy), which has been reintroduced in human patients, has been shown to be effective against all the major motor signs of Parkinson's disease *(89,90,98–103)*. PET studies have shown that frontal motor areas whose metabolic activity was reduced in the parkinsonian state were again active following pallidotomy *(98,104–108)*.

The latest addition to the neurosurgical armamentarium used in the treatment of parkinsonism is deep brain stimulation (DBS). DBS of the STN and of GPi has been shown to be highly effective against parkinsonism *(109–114)*. Although the exact mechanism of action remains uncertain, the clinical and neuroimaging effect of DBS closely mimics that of ablation, suggesting a net inhibitory action *(115–117)*. A variety of mechanisms have been proposed, including depolarization block, activation of inhibitory pathways, "jamming" of abnormal activity along output pathways, and depletion of neuro-

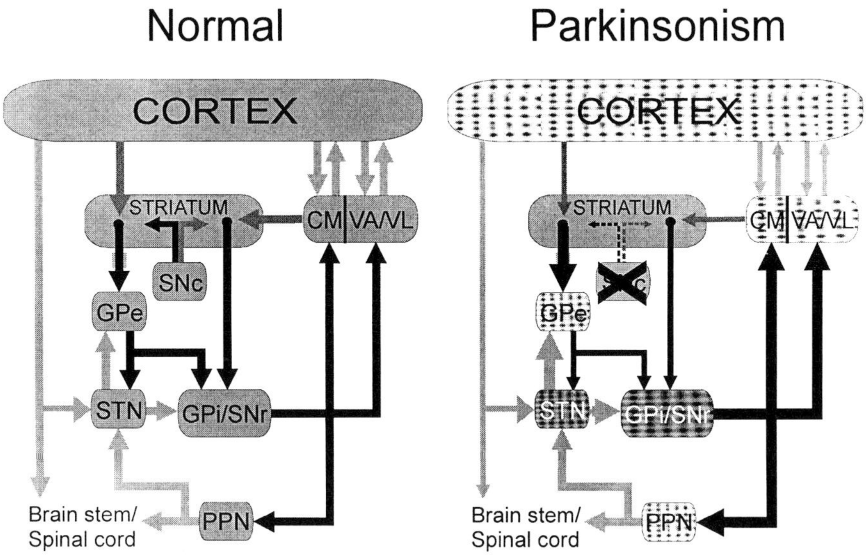

Fig. 1. Basal ganglia-thalamorcortical circuitry under normal (left) and parkinsonian conditions (right). The basal ganglia circuitry involves striatum, Gpe, Gpi, SNr, STN, and SNc. Basal ganglia output is directed toward the centromedian (CM) and ventral anterior/ventral lateral nucleus of the thalamus (VA/VL), as well as PPN. Excitatory connections are shown in gray, inhibitory pathways in black. Changes in the mean discharge rate are reflected by the width of the lines. Wider lines reflect increased rates, narrower lines decreased rates. Known or presumed changes in discharge patterns are indicated by the pattern of individual nuclei.

transmitters. Several more recent studies, however, have suggested that DBS may, in fact, activate the stimulated area, perhaps leading to a normalization in the pattern of neuronal activity *(118,119)*.

The pathophysiologic model outlined below (*see* Fig. 1) may account for changes in discharge rates and global metabolic activity in the basal ganglia, but fails to explain several key findings in animals and humans with such disorders. The most serious shortcoming of the aforementioned scheme of parkinsonian pathophysiology is, perhaps, that changes in the spontaneous discharge patterns, and the responses of basal ganglia neurons to external stimuli is significantly different in the parkinsonian state when compared to the normal state *(120–125)*. Thus, the neuronal responses to passive limb manipulations in STN, GPi, and thalamus are increased *(120–122,126)*, suggesting an increased "gain" by the subcortical portions of the circuit as compared to the normal state. In addition to changes in the response to peripheral inputs, there is also a marked increase in the synchronization of discharge between neurons in the basal ganglia under parkinsonian conditions, as demonstrated in primates through crosscorrelation studies of the neuronal discharge in GPi and STN *(122)*. This is in contrast to the virtual absence of synchronized discharge of these neurons in normal monkeys *(65)*. In addition, a very prominent abnormality in the pattern of basal ganglia discharge in parkinsonian primates and humans is an increase in the proportion of cells in STN, GPi, and SNr with oscillatory discharge characteristics *(121,122,125,127–129)*. Increased oscillatory activity and synchronization have also been demonstrated in the basal ganglia-receiving areas of the cerebral cortex in parkinsonian individuals *(130–134)*. In patients with unilateral parkinsonian tremor, EMG and contralateral EEG were found to be coherent at the tremor frequency (or its first harmonic), particularly over cortical motor areas *(135)*. Dopaminergic therapy has been shown to desynchronize cortical activity in parkinsonian subjects *(136–141)*. There is also some evidence that basal ganglia activity may be synchronized in parkinson ian subjects, at least during episodes of tremor *(142–145)*. Conceivably, reductions in synchronization and oscillatory activity could be related to the improvements in motor function seen with dopaminergic therapy or neurosurgical interventions, although direct proof of this is lacking.

The mechanisms underlying increased synchronization and oscillations in the basal ganglia-thalamocortical circuitry are not clear. Attempts have been made to link these changes to the dopaminergic deficit in the striatum. For instance, it has been shown that the predominant oscillation frequency in many basal ganglia neurons is influenced by the presence or absence of dopamine. Thus, low-frequency oscillations appear to be enhanced in the presence of dopamine receptor agonists *(146)*. On the other hand, oscillatory discharge with predominant frequencies >3 Hz are present in only a small percentage of neurons in GPe, STN, GPi, and SNr in the normal state, but are strikingly enhanced in the parkinsonian state *(54,122,147–152)*.

The most obvious consequence of increased synchronized oscillatory discharge in the basal ganglia-thalamo-cortical loops may be tremor *(122,142,143,150,153–155)*. For instance, parkinsonian African green monkeys show prominent 5 Hz tremor, along with 5-Hz oscillations in STN and GPi *(122)*. Oscillatory discharge at higher dominant frequencies (8–15 Hz), is seen in the basal ganglia of parkinsonian Rhesus monkeys, which typically do not exhibit tremor *(54,151)*. It seems obvious that strong oscillations in the basal ganglia could be very disruptive with regard to the transfer and processing of information in these nuclei, and in the basal ganglia-thalamocortical circuitry as a whole.

Via their widespread influence on the frontal cortex, synchronized oscillatory basal ganglia activity may adversely influence cortical activity in a large part of the frontal cortex, and could therefore (in a rather nonspecific manner) contribute to the cortical dysfunction, which underlies the development of parkinsonian motor signs such as akinesia or bradykinesia. Positron emission tomography (PET) studies in parkinsonian subjects indicate reduced activation of frontal and prefrontal recipient areas of basal ganglia output, perhaps as a result of a functional impairment of cortical activation through reduced activity in thalamocortical projections or through thalamocortical transmission of nonsense patterns (subcortical "noise," e.g., oscillatory activity, synchronization, and other abnormal neuronal discharge patterns). These changes may induce plastic changes in the cortex, which in turn may disrupt normal motor function *(156,157)*. The development of parkinsonian motor abnormalities such as akinesia or bradykinesia may to some extent depend on the inefficiencies of partial redistribution of the impaired premotor activities at the cortical level.

The view that the pathophysiology of movement disorders may be far more complicated than suggested by the "rate" model introduced earlier is further supported by the observation that pallidotomy and DBS, not only ameliorate *parkinsonian* abnormalities, but also most of the major *hyperkinetic* syndromes, including drug-induced dyskinesias *(100,158,159)*, hemiballism *(160)*, and dystonia *(160–162)*, which, according to the earlier pathophysiologic scheme, should be worsened by lesions of GPi. Furthermore, these hyperkinetic disorders can also be treated with lesions of the thalamus without producing parkinsonism. These findings suggest that pallidotomy, thalamotomy, and DBS may act by removing abnormal disruptive signals or reducing the amount of "noise" in cortical motor areas, rendering functional previously dysfunctional cortical areas (Fig. 1B; see also refs. *6,78,163*). This view would be consistent with the proposal that deep brain stimulation improves parkinsonian motor signs by changing the pattern of neuronal activity from an irregular, "noisy" pattern to a more tonic one *(118)*.

Another significant area of discussion with regard to the models introduced above relates to the role of GPe in the development of parkinsonism. For instance, on the basis of metabolic and biochemical studies, it has been questioned whether reduced GPe activity is indeed important in the development of parkinsonism as stated by the traditional models *(3,164–168)*. In addition, the view that GPe activity is increased in drug-induced dyskinesias, as postulated by the traditional model has been challenged by studies such as those by Bedard et al., in which excitotoxic lesions of GPe did not resolve levodopa-induced dyskinesias in parkinsonian primates *(169)*.

Finally, although the anatomy and function of the intrinsic basal ganglia circuitry is known in considerable detail, the anatomy and function of several key portions of the circuit models outside of the basal ganglia have been far less explored. Among others, this includes the interaction of the basal ganglia with brainstem nuclei such as the PPN, as well as input and output connections between the basal ganglia and the intralaminar thalamic nuclei CM and Pf. The connection with CM and Pf may form potentially important (positive) feedback circuits that may exaggerate changes in basal ganglia output, and may therefore have an important role in the pathophysiology of movement disorders. Furthermore, the processing of basal ganglia output at the thalamic level is not well understood. The input and output interactions between the basal ganglia and related areas of cortex also remain also largely unexplored at this time.

3.2. Dyskinetic Disorders

In disorders associated with dyskinesias, basal ganglia output is thought to be reduced, resulting in disinhibition of thalamocortical systems and dyskinesias *(1,5)*. This is best documented for hemiballism, a disorder that follows discrete lesions of the STN, which result in reduced activity in GPi in both experimental primates and in humans *(22,160)*. The mechanisms underlying chorea in Huntington's disease are thought to be similar to those in hemiballism in that degeneration of striatal neurons projecting to GPe (indirect pathway) leads to disinhibition of GPe, followed by increased inhibition of the STN and thus reduced output from GPi *(2,170)*. Thus, whereas in hemiballism there is a distinct lesion in the STN, in early Huntington's disease the nucleus is functionally underactive. Drug-induced dyskinesias may also result from a similar reduction in STN and GPi activity. Support for the validity of these models comes from direct recording of neuronal activity *(121,122,125,128,171–173)* as well as metabolic studies in primates, and a number of PET studies investigating cortical and subcortical metabolism in humans with movement disorders *(4,174)*. For instance, in animals with drug-induced dyskinesias, STN and GPi activity was found to be greatly reduced, concomitant to the expression of dyskinetic movements.

The experience with pallidal and nigral lesions *(58,175,176)* suggests that dyskinesias do not result from reduced basal ganglia output alone (*see* ref. *177*). Such lesions, when done in humans and animals, do *not* result in significant dyskinesias, despite presumably complete cessation of activity of the lesioned areas, although brief episodes of dyskinesias can occasionally be seen immediately after pallidal lesions in parkinsonian patients (Vitek et al., unpublished observations). In experiments in primates, we have not seen the development of dyskinesias after transient inactivation of small areas of the pallidum with the GABAergic agonist muscimol *(178)*, over a wide range of injected concentrations and volumes of the drug. These findings suggest that subtle rather than total reduction of pallidal output to the thalamus results in dyskinesias and that specific alterations in discharge patterns rather than global reduction of pallidal output may be particularly conducive to dyskinetic movements, although such specific alterations remain elusive. Compensatory mechanisms at the thalamic or cortical level may also be at work to prevent the development of dyskinesias after reduction of pallidal or nigral output. The importance of these mechanisms is most strikingly evident in animals and humans with hemiballism. In many cases, the dyskinetic movements are transient *(179)*, despite the continued presence of reduced and abnormal neuronal discharge in GPi *(22)*. Last, the induction of synchronized activity across a large population of neurons in an uncontrolled fashion may play a role in the development of dyskinetic movements *(180)*.

Similar to the earlier discussion of parkinsonism, the specific role of some of the recently discovered connections of the basal ganglia with brainstem centers and thalamus also remain undetermined. In particular, the PPN and the CM/Pf nuclei of the thalamus may have important roles in the development of (some forms of) dyskinesia.

3.3. Dystonia

Dystonia is a disorder characterized by slow, sustained abnormal movements and postures with co-contraction of agonist-antagonist muscle groups, and overflow phenomena. Preliminary pathophysiologic evidence indicates that dystonia may be a hybrid disorder with features common to both

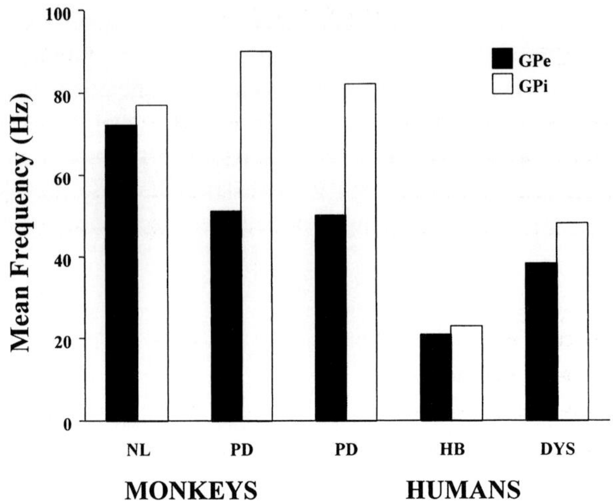

Fig. 2. Mean discharge rates (Hz) of spontaneous neuronal activity in the external and internal segments of the globus pallidus (Gpe and Gpi, respectively) for normal (NL) and parkinsonian (PD) monkeys, and for human patients with Parkinson's disease (PD), Hemiballismus (HB), and dystonia (DYS).

hypo- and hyperkinetic disorders. Dystonia is not a homogeneous entity; it may result from genetic disorders, from focal lesions of the basal ganglia or other structures, and from disorders of dopamine metabolism *(181–189)*. It appears likely, however, that most of these conditions eventually affect the functioning of the basal ganglia-thalamocortical network.

There are no universally accepted animal models available for this condition. The available animal models of dystonia, such as the genetically dystonic hamster, or models of drug-induced dystonia in rodents and monkeys are not satisfactory, because they are either associated with unusual phenotypic features or are too transient and unreliable to permit thorough study of the condition. Most of the current pathophysiologic evidence regarding this condition is based on the results of intraoperative recording in a small number of human patients undergoing neurosurgical procedures for treatment of dystonia. This is a fairly select group of patients that probably does not represent the full range of dystonic conditions. Based on these recordings, it appears that the activity along both the direct and indirect pathways may be increased in dystonia. Thus, recent recording studies in dystonic patients undergoing pallidotomy revealed low average discharge rates in both pallidal segments (Fig. 2), *(160,162,190–192)*. The reduction of discharge in GPe in these dystonic patients attest to increased activity along the indirect pathway, which by itself would have led to increased GPi discharge. The fact that discharge rates in GPi were actually reduced, argues therefore in favor of additional overactivity along the direct pathway.

The fact that in both dystonia and ballism GPi output appears to be reduced indicates that factors other than changes in discharge rates are playing a significant role in their development. Most likely, a major part of the pathophysiology of dystonia is abnormally patterned activity (Fig. 3), or increased synchronization of basal ganglia output neurons, which is not accounted for by the model (*see* below, and refs. *160,180,190*). Changes suggestive of a reorganization of the activity of the basal ganglia-thalamocortical circuits in dystonia have also been shown, where abnormal receptive field have been described in both the pallidum and thalamus *(160,193,194)*. At the cortical level, a degradation of the discrete cortical representation of individual body parts has been demonstrated in dystonic patients *(195–197)*. Thus, altered somatosensory responses have been demonstrated at multiple stages in the basal ganglia thalamocortical circuit, consistent with previous suggestions that sensory dysfunction may play a significant role in the development of dystonia *(162,195,196,198,199)*.

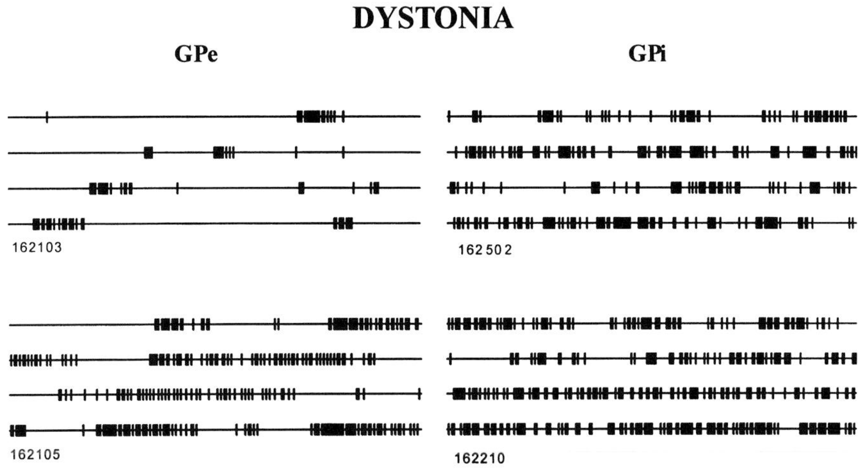

Fig. 3. Raster diagrams of spontaneous neuronal activity in the external and internal segments of the globus pallidus, GPe (left column) and GPi (right column), in patients with dystonia.

4. CONCLUSIONS

There has been significant progress in the understanding of basal ganglia anatomy and physiology over the last years, but the functions of these nuclei remain unclear. Current models of basal ganglia function have been of tremendous value in stimulating basal ganglia research and providing a rationale for neurosurgical interventions. At the same time, the scientific shortcomings of these models have become increasingly obvious, particularly with regard to the fact that the models are predominantly based on anatomic data, do not account for the ameliorating effect of basal ganglia lesions in patient with already reduced levels of pallidal activity and do not take into account the multiple dynamic changes that take place in the basal ganglia in individuals with movement disorders. Alternative models have been proposed to account for these observations based on new information, but important information concerning the relationship between the basal ganglia and related areas of cortex as well as thalamic and brainstem structures is lacking. These data will greatly help us to better understand the normal function of the basal ganglia and the pathophysiology of movement disorders and will, in turn, promote the improvement of current and the development of new therapeutic approaches to the treatment of these disorders.

REFERENCES

1. Albin, R. L., Young, A. B., and Penney, J. B. (1989) The functional anatomy of basal ganglia disorders. *Trends Neurosci.* **12,** 366–375.
2. Albin, R. L. (1995) The pathophysiology of chorea/ballism and parkinsonism. *Parkinson. Rel. Disord.* **1,** 3–11.
3. Chesselet, M. F. and Delfs, J. M. (1996) Basal ganglia and movement disorders: an update. *Trends Neurosci.* **19,** 417–422.
4. Brooks, D. J. (1995) The role of the basal ganglia in motor control: contributions from PET. *J. Neurol. Sci.* **128,** 1–13.
5. DeLong, M. R. (1990) Primate models of movement disorders of basal ganglia origin. *Trends Neurosci.* **13,** 281–285.
6. Wichmann, T. and DeLong, M. R. (1996) Functional and pathophysiological models of the basal ganglia. *Curr. Opin. Neurobiol.* **6,** 751–758.
7. Vitek, J. L., Chockkan, V., Zhang, J. Y., Kaneoke, Y., Evatt, M., DeLong, M. R., et al. (1999) Neuronal activity in the basal ganglia in patients with generalized dystonia and hemiballismus. *Ann. Neurol.* **46,** 22–35.
8. Alexander, G. E., Crutcher, M. D., and DeLong, M. R. (1990) Basal ganglia-thalamocortical circuits: parallel substrates for motor, oculomotor, 'prefrontal' and 'limbic' functions. *Prog. Brain. Res.* **85,** 119–146.

9. Kemp, J. M. and Powell, T. P. S. (1971) The connections of the striatum and globus pallidus: synthesis and speculation. *Phil. Trans. R. Soc. Lond.* **262,** 441–457.
10. Wilson, C. J., Chang, H. T., and Kitai, S. T. (1983) Origins of post synaptic potentials evoked in spiny neostriatal projection neurons by thalamic stimulation in the rat. *Exp. Brain Res.* **51,** 217–226.
11. Dube, L., Smith, A. D., and Bolam, J. P. (1988) Identification of synaptic terminals of thalamic or cortical origin in contact with distinct medium-size spiny neurons in the rat neostriatum. *J. Comp. Neurol.* **267,** 455–471.
12. Sadikot, A. F., Parent, A., Smith, Y., and Bolam, J. P. (1992) Efferent conncetions of the centromedian and parafascicular thalamic nuclei in the squirrell monkey: a light and electron microscopic study of the thalamostriatal projection in relation to striatal heterogeneity. *J. Comp. Neurol.* **320,** 228–242.
13. Sadikot, A. F., Parent, A., and Francois, C. (1992) Efferent connections of the centromedian and parafascicular thalamic nuclei in the squirrel monkey: a PHA-L study of subcortical projections. *J. Comparat. Neurol.* **315,** 137–159.
14. Smith, Y. and Parent, A. (1986) Differential connections of caudate nucleus and putamen in the squirrel monkey (Saimiri Sciureus). *Neuroscience* **18,** 347–371.
15. Nakano, K., Hasegawa, Y., Tokushige, A., Nakagawa, S., Kayahara, T., and Mizuno, N. (1990) Topographical projections from the thalamus, subthalamic nucleus and pedunculopontine tegmental nucleus to the striatum in the Japanese monkey, Macaca fuscata. *Brain Res.* **537,** 54–68.
16. Hazrati, L. N., Parent, A., Mitchell, S., and Haber, S. N. (1990) Evidence for interconnections between the two segments of the globus pallidus in primates: a PHA-L anterograde tracing study. *Brain Res.* **533,** 171–175.
17. Parent, A. and Hazrati, L.-N. (1995) Functional anatomy of the basal ganglia. I. The cortico-basal ganglia-thalamo-cortical loop. *Brain Res. Rev.* **20,** 91–127.
18. Kita, H. (1994) Physiology of two disynaptic pathways from the sensorimotor cortex to the basal ganglia output nuclei. In: *The Basal Ganglia IV. New Ideas and Data on Structure and Function* (Percheron, G., McKenzie, J. S., and Feger, J., eds.), Plenum Press, New York, pp. 263–276.
19. Nambu, A., Takada, M., Inase, M., and Tokuno, H. (1996) Dual somatotopical representations in the primate subthalamic nucleus: evidence for ordered but reversed body-map transformations from the primary motor cortex and the supplementary motor area. *J. Neurosci.* **16,** 2671–2683.
20. Hartmann-von Monakow, K., Akert, K., and Kunzle, H. (1978) Projections of the precentral motor cortex and other cortical areas of the frontal lobe to the subthalamic nucleus in the monkey. *Exp. Brain Res.* **33,** 395–403.
21. Smith, Y., Hazrati, L. N., and Parent, A. (1990) Efferent projections of the subthalamic nucleus in the squirrel monkey as studied by PHA-L anterograde tracing method. *J. Comp. Neurol.* **294,** 306–323.
22. Hamada, I. and DeLong, M. R. (1992) Excitotoxic acid lesions of the primate subthalamic nucleus result in reduced pallidal neuronal activity during active holding. *J. Neurophysiol.* **68,** 1859–1866.
23. Magill, P. J., Bolam, J. P., and Bevan, M. D. (2000) Relationship of activity in the subthalamic nucleus-globus pallidus network to cortical electroencephalogram. *J. Neurosci.* **20,** 820–833.
24. Nambu, A., Tokuno, H., Hamada, I., Kita, H., Imanishi, M., Akazawa, T., et al. (2000) Excitatory cortical inputs to pallidal neurons via the subthalamic nucleus in the monkey. *J. Neurophysiol.* **84,** 289–300.
25. Goldman-Rakic, P. S. and Porrino, L. J. (1985) The primate mediodorsal (MD) nucleus and its projection to the frontal lobe. *J. Comp. Neurol.* **242,** 535–560.
26. Schell, G. R. and Strick, P. L. (1984) The origin of thalamic inputs to the arcuate premotor and supplementary motor areas. *J. Neurosci.* **4,** 539–560.
27. Strick, P. L. (1985) How do the basal ganglia and cerebellum gain access to the cortical motor areas? *Behav. Brain Res.* **18,** 107–123.
28. Inase, M. and Tanji, J. (1995) Thalamic distribution of projection neurons to the primary motor cortex relative to afferent terminal fields from the globus pallidus in the macaque monkey. *J. Comp. Neurol.* **353,** 415–426.
29. Nambu, A., Yoshida, S., and Jinnai, K. (1988) Projection on the motor cortex of thalamic neurons with pallidal input in the monkey. *Exp. Brain Res.* **71,** 658–662.
30. Hoover, J. E. and Strick, P. L. (1993) Multiple output channels in the basal ganglia. *Science* **259,** 819–821.
31. Jinnai, K., Nambu, A., Yoshida, S., and Tanibuchi, I. (1993) The two separate neuron circuits through the basal ganglia concerning the preparatory or execution proceses of motor control. In: *Role of the Cerebellum and Basal Ganglia in Voluntary Movement* (Mamo, N., Hamada, I., and DeLong, M. R., eds.), Elsevier Science, pp. 153–161.
32. Sidibe, M., Bevan, M. D., Bolam, J. P., and Smith, Y. (1997) Efferent connections of the internal globus pallidus in the squirrel monkey: I. Topography and synaptic organization of the pallidothalamic projection. *J. Comp. Neurol.* **382,** 323–347.
33. Middleton, F. A. and Strick, P. L. (1994) Anatomical evidence for cerebellar and basal ganglia involvement in higher cognitive function. *Science* **266,** 458–461.
34. Ilinsky, I. A., Jouandet, M. L., and Goldman-Rakic, P. S. (1985) Organization of the nigrothalamocortical system in the rhesus monkey. *J. Comp. Neurol.* **236,** 315–330.
35. Bevan, M. D. and Bolam, J. P. (1995) Cholinergic, GABAergic, and glutamate-enriched inputs from the mesopontine tegmentum to the subthalamic nucleus in the rat. *J. Neurosci.* **15,** 7105–7120.
36. Jaffer, A., van der Spuy, G. D., Russell, V. A., Mintz, M., and Taljaard, J. J. (1995) Activation of the subthalamic nucleus and pedunculopontine tegmentum: does it affect dopamine levels in the substantia nigra, nucleus accumbens and striatum? *Neurodegeneration* **4,** 139–145.
37. Lavoie, B. and Parent, A. (1994) Pedunculopontine nucleus in the squirrel monkey: projections to the basal ganglia as revealed by anterograde tract-tracing methods. *J. Comp. Neurol.* **344,** 210–231.

38. Rye, D. B., Lee, H. J., Saper, C. B., and Wainer, B. H. (1988) Medullary and spinal efferents of the pedunculopontine tegmental nucleus and adjacent mesopontine tegmentum in the rat. *J. Comp. Neurol.* **269,** 315–341.
39. Steininger, T. L., Wainer, B. H., and Rye, D. B. (1997) Ultrastructural study of cholinergic and noncholinergic neurons in the pars compacta of the rat pedunculopontine tegmental nucleus. *J. Comp. Neurol.* **382,** 285–301.
40. Hikosaka, O. and Wurtz, R. H. (1983) Visual and oculomotor functions of monkey substantia nigra pars reticulata. IV. Relation of substantia nigra to superior colliculus. *J. Neurophysiol.* **49,** 1285–1301.
41. Anderson, M. and Yoshida, M. (1977) Electrophysiological evidence for branching nigral projections to the thalamus and the superior colliculus. *Brain Res.* **137,** 361–364.
42. Lynch, J. C., Hoover, J. E., and Strick, P. L. (1994) Input to the primate frontal eye field from the substantia nigra, superior colliculus, and dentate nucleus demonstrated by transneuronal transport. *Exp. Brain Res.* **100,** 181–186.
43. Deniau, J. M., Hammond, C., Riszk, A., and Feger, J. (1978) Electrophysiological properties of identified output neurons of the rat substantia nigra (pars compacta and pars reticulata): evidences for the existence of branched neurons. *Exp. Brain Res.* **32,** 409–422.
44. Parent, A., Mackey, A., Smith, Y., and Boucher, R. (1983) The output organization of the substantia nigra in primate as revealed by a retrograde double labeling method. *Brain Res. Bull.* **10,** 529–537.
45. Wurtz, R. H. and Hikosaka, O. (1986) Role of the basal ganglia in the initiation of saccadic eye movements. *Progr. Brain Res.* **64,** 175–190.
46. Gerfen, C. R. (1988) Synaptic organization of the striatum. *J. Electron Microsc. Techn.* **10,** 265–281.
47. Waelti, P., Dickinson, A., and Schultz, W. (2001) Dopamine responses comply with basic assumptions of formal learning theory. *Nature* **412,** 43–48.
48. Schultz, W. (1998) The phasic reward signal of primate dopamine neurons. *Adv. Pharmacol.* **42,** 686–690.
49. Schultz, W. (1994) Behavior-related activity of primate dopamine neurons. *Revue Neurologique* **150,** 634–639.
50. Aizman, O., Brismar, H., Uhlen, P., Zettergren, E., Levey, A. I., Forssberg, H., et al. (2000) Anatomical and physiological evidence for D1 and D2 dopamine receptor colocalization in neostriatal neurons. *Nature Neurosci.* **3,** 226–230.
51. Surmeier, D. J., Reiner, A., Levine, M. S., and Ariano, M. A. (1993) Are neostriatal dopamine receptors co-localized? [see comments]. *Trends Neurosci.* **16,** 299–305.
52. Gerfen, C. R. (1995) Dopamine receptor function in the basal ganglia. *Clin. Neuropharmacol.* **18,** S162–S177.
53. Gerfen, C. R., Engber, T. M., Mahan, L. C., Susel, Z., Chase, T. N., Monsma, F. J. Jr., and Sibley, D. R. (1990) D1 and D2 dopamine receptor-regulated gene expression of striatonigral and striatopallidal neurons. *Science* **250,** 1429–1432.
54. Wichmann, T., Bergman, H., Starr, P. A., Subramanian, T., Watts, R. L., and DeLong, M. R. (1999) Comparison of MPTP-induced changes in spontaneous neuronal discharge in the internal pallidal segment and in the substantia nigra pars reticulata in primates. *Exp. Brain Res.* **125,** 397–409.
55. DeLong, M. R., Crutcher, M. D., and Georgopoulos, A. P. (1983) Relations between movement and single cell discharge in the substantia nigra of the behaving monkey. *J. Neurosci.* **3,** 1599–1606.
56. Rodriguez, M. C., Gorospe, A., Mozo, A., Guridi, J., Ramos, E., Linazasoro, G., et al. (1997) Characteristics of neuronal activity in the subthalamic nucleus (STN) and substantia nigra pars reticulata (SNr) in Parkinson's disease (PD). *Soc. Neurosci. Abstr.* **23,** 470.
57. DeLong, M. R. (1971) Activity of pallidal neurons during movement. *J. Neurophysiol.* **34,** 414–427.
58. Mink, J. W. and Thach, W. T. (1991) Basal ganglia motor control. III. Pallidal ablation: normal reaction time, muscle cocontraction, and slow movement. *J. Neurophysiol.* **65,** 330–351.
59. Mink, J. W. (1996) The basal ganglia: focused selection and inhibition of competing motor programs. *Progr. Neurobiol.* **50,** 381–425.
60. Wenger, K. K., Musch, K. L., and Mink, J. W. (1999) Impaired reaching and grasping after focal inactivation of globus pallidus pars interna in the monkey. *J. Neurophysiol.* **82,** 2049–2060.
61. Hikosaka, O., Matsumara, M., Kojima, J., and Gardiner, T. W. (1993) Role of basal ganglia in initiation and suppression of saccadic eye movements. In: *Role of the Cerebellum and Basal Ganglia in Voluntary Movement* (Mano, N., Hamada, I., and DeLong, M. R., eds.), Elsevier, Amsterdam, pp. 213–220.
62. Bevan, M. D., Bolam, J. P., and Crossman, A. R. (1994) Convergent synaptic input from the neostriatum and the subthalamus onto identified nigrothalamic neurons in the rat. *Euro. J. Neurosci.* **6,** 320–334.
63. Bolam, J. P. and Smith, Y. (1992) The striatum and the globus pallidus send convergent synaptic inputs onto single cells in the entopeduncular nucleus of the rat: a double anterograde labelling study combined with postembedding immunocytochemistry for GABA. *J. Comp. Neurol.* **321,** 456–476.
64. Hazrati, L. and Parent, A. (1992) Convergence of subthalamic and striatal efferents at pallidal level in primates: an anterograde double-labeling study with biocytin and PHA-L. *Brain Res.* **569,** 336–340.
65. Wichmann, T., Bergman, H., and DeLong, M. R. (1994) The primate subthalamic nucleus. I. Functional properties in intact animals. *J. Neurophysiol.* **72,** 494–506.
66. Jaeger, D., Gilman, S., and Aldridge, J. W. (1995) Neuronal activity in the striatum and pallidum of primates related to the execution of externally cued reaching movements. *Brain Res.* **694,** 111–127.
67. Jaeger, D., Gilman, S., and Aldridge, J. W. (1993) Primate basal ganglia activity in a precued reaching task: preparation for movement. *Exp. Brain Res.* **95,** 51–64.
68. Alexander, G. E. and Crutcher, M. D. (1987) Preparatory activity in primate motor cortex and putamen coded in spatial rather than limb coordinates. *Soc. Neurosci. Abstr.* **13,** 245.

69. Alexander, G. E. and Crutcher, M. D. (1989) Coding in spatial rather than joint coordinates of putamen and motor cortex preparatory activity preceding planned limb movements. In: *Neural Mechanisms in Disorders of Movement* (Sambrook, M. A. and Crossman, A. R., eds.), Blackwell, London, pp. 55–62.
70. Anderson, M., Inase, M., Buford, J., and Turner, R. (1992) Movement and preparatory activity of neurons in pallidal-receiving areas of the monkey thalamus. Role of Cerebellum and Basal Ganglia in Voluntary Movement 39.
71. Apicella, P., Scarnati, E., and Schultz, W. (1991) Tonically discharging neurons of monkey striatum respond to preparatory and rewarding stimuli. *Exp. Brain Res.* **84,** 672–675.
72. Boussaoud, D. and Kermadi, I. (1997) The primate striatum: neuronal activity in relation to spatial attention versus motor preparation. *Euro. J. Neurosci.* **9,** 2152–2168.
73. Crutcher, M. D. and Alexander, G. E. (1988) Supplementary motor area (SMA): coding of both preparatory and movement-related neural activity in spatial rather than joint coordinates. *Soc. Neurosci. Abstr.* **14,** 342.
74. Kubota, K. and Hamada, I. (1979) Preparatory activity of monkey pyramidal tract neurons related to quick movement onset during visual tracking performance. *Brain Res.* **168,** 435–439.
75. Schultz, W. and Romo, R. (1992) Role of primate basal ganglia and frontal cortex in the internal generation of movement. I. Preparatory activity in the anterior striatum. *Exp. Brain Res.* **91,** 363–384.
76. Dettmers, C., Fink, G. R., Lemon, R. N., Stephan, K. M., Passingham, R. E., Silbersweig, D., et al. (1995) Relation between cerebral activity and force in the motor areas of the human brain. *J. Neurophysiol.* **74,** 802–815.
77. Turner, R. S., Grafton, S. T., Votaw, J. R., Delong, M. R., and Hoffman, J. M. (1998) Motor subcircuits mediating the control of movement velocity: a PET study. *J. Neurophysiol.* **80,** 2162–2176.
78. Marsden, C. D. and Obeso, J. A. (1994) The functions of the basal ganglia and the paradox of stereotaxic surgery in Parkinson's disease. *Brain* **117,** 877–897.
79. Martin, K. E., Phillips, J. G., Iansek, R., and Bradshaw, J. L. (1994) Inaccuracy and instability of sequential movements in Parkinson's disease. *Exp. Brain Res.* **102,** 131–140.
80. Graybiel, A. M. (1995) Building action repertoires: memory and learning functions of the basal ganglia. *Curr. Opin. Neurobiol.* **5,** 733–741.
81. Watanabe, K. and Kimura, M. (1998) Dopamine receptor-mediated mechanisms involved in the expression of learned activity of primate striatal neurons. *J. Neurophysiol.* **79,** 2568–2580.
82. Kimura, M., Kato, M., Shimazaki, H., Watanabe, K., and Matsumoto, N. (1996) Neural information transferred from the putamen to the globus pallidus during learned movement in the monkey. *J. Neurophysiol.* **76,** 3771–3786.
83. Kimura, M. (1995) Role of basal ganglia in behavioral learning. *Neurosci. Res.* **22,** 353–358.
84. Aosaki, T., Kimura, M., and Graybiel, A. M. (1995) Temporal and spatial characteristics of tonically active neurons of the primate striatum. *J. Neurophysiol.* **73,** 1234–1252.
85. Aosaki, T., Tsubokawa, H., Watanabe, K., Graybiel, A. M., and Kimura, M. (1994) Responses of tonically active neurons in the primate's striatum undergo systematic changes during behavioral sensory-motor conditioning. *J. Neurosci.* **14,** 3969–3984.
86. Jog, M. S., Kubota, Y., Connolly, C. I., Hillegaart, V., and Graybiel, A. M. (1999) Building neural representations of habits. *Science* **286,** 1745–1749.
87. Aziz, T. Z., Peggs, D., Sambrook, M. A., and Crossman, A. R. (1991) Lesion of the subthalamic nucleus for the alleviation of 1-methyl-4-phenyl-1,2,3,6-tetrahydropyridine (MPTP)-induced parkinsonism in the primate. *Mov. Disord.* **6,** 288–292.
88. DeLong, M. R. and Georgopoulos, A. P. (1981) Motor functions of the basal ganglia. In: *Handbook of Physiology. The Nervous System. Motor Control. Sect. 1, Vol. II, Pt. 2* (Brookhart, J. M., Mountcastle, V. B., Brooks, V. B., and Geiger, S. R., eds.), American Physiological Society, Bethesda, MD, pp. 1017–1061.
89. Laitinen, L. V. (1995) Pallidotomy for Parkinson's diesease. *Neurosurg. Clin. North Am.* **6,** 105–112.
90. Baron, M. S., Vitek, J. L., Bakay, R. A. E., Green, J., Kaneoke, Y., Hashimoto, T., et al. (1996) Treatment of advanced Parkinson's disease by GPi pallidotomy: 1 year pilot-study results. *Ann. Neurol.* **40,** 355–366.
91. Zweig, R. M., Cardillo, J. E., Cohen, M., Giere, S., and Hedreen, J. C. (1993) The locus ceruleus and dementia in Parkinson's disease. *Neurology* **5,** 986–991.
92. Palombo, E., Porrino, L. J., Bankiewicz, K. S., Crane, A. M., Sokoloff, L., and Kopin, I. J. (1990) Local cerebral glucose utilization in monkeys with hemiparkinsonism induced by intracarotid infusion of the neurotoxin MPTP. *J. Neurosci.* **10,** 860–869.
93. Mitchell, I. J., Clarke, C. E., Boyce, S., Robertson, R. G., Peggs, D., Sambrook, M. A., and Crossman, A. R. (1989) Neural mechanisms underlying parkinsonian symptoms based upon regional uptake of 2-deoxyglucose in monkeys exposed to 1-methyl-4-phenyl-1,2,3,6-tetrahydropyridine. *Neuroscience* **32,** 213–226.
94. Kojima, J., Yamaji, Y., Matsumura, M., Nambu, A., Inase, M., Tokuno, H., et al. (1997) Excitotoxic lesions of the pedunculopontine tegmental nucleus produce contralateral hemiparkinsonism in the monkey. *Neurosci. Lett.* **226,** 111–114.
95. Munro-Davies, L. E., Winter, J., Aziz, T. Z., and Stein, J. F. (1999) The role of the pedunculopontine region in basal-ganglia mechanisms of akinesia. *Exp. Brain Res.* **129,** 511–517.
96. Brooks, D. J. (1999) Functional imaging of Parkinson's disease: is it possible to detect brain areas for specific symptoms? *J. Neural Transm. (Suppl.)* **56,** 139–153.
97. Bergman, H., Wichmann, T., and DeLong, M. R. (1990) Reversal of experimental parkinsonism by lesions of the subthalamic nucleus. *Science* **249,** 1436–1438.
98. Dogali, M., Fazzini, E., Kolodny, E., Eidelberg, D., Sterio, D., Devinsky, O., and Beric, A. (1995) Stereotactic ventral pallidotomy for Parkinson's disease. *Neurology* **45,** 753–761.

99. Laitinen, L. V., Bergenheim, A. T., and Hariz, M. I. (1992) Leksell's posteroventral pallidotomy in the treatment of Parkinson's disease. *J. Neurosurg.* **76,** 53–61.
100. Lozano, A. M., Lang, A. E., Galvez-Jimenez, N., Miyasaki, J., Duff, J., Hutchinson, W. D., and Dostrovsky, J. O. (1995) Effect of GPi pallidotomy on motor function in Parkinson's disease. *Lancet* **346,** 1383–1387.
101. Lozano, A. M., Lang, A. E., Hutchison, W. D., and Dostrovsky, J. O. (1997) Microelectrode recording-guided posteroventral pallidotomy in patients with Parkinson's disease. *Adv. Neurol.* **74,** 167–174.
102. Lang, A., Lozano, A., Montgomery, E., Duff, J., Tasker, R., and Hutchinson, W. (1997) Posteroventral medial pallidotomy in advanced Parkinson's disease. *N. Engl. J. Med.* **337,** 1036–1042.
103. Starr, P. A., Vitek, J. L., and Bakay, R. A. E. (1998) Pallidotomy: clinical results. In: *Neurosurgical Treatment of Movement Disorders* (Germano, I. M., ed.), American Association of Neurological Surgeons, Park Ridge, IL, pp. 143–156.
104. Ceballos-Bauman, A. O., Obeso, J. A., Vitek, J. L., DeLong, M. R., Bakay, R., Linaasoro, G., and Brooks, D. J. (1994) Restoration of thalamocortical activity after posteroventrolateral pallidotomy in Parkinson's disease. *Lancet* **344,** 814.
105. Samuel, M., Ceballos-Baumann, A. O., Turjanski, N., Boecker, H., Gorospe, A., Linazasoro, G., et al. (1997) Pallidotomy in Parkinson's disease increases supplementary motor area and prefrontal activation during performance of volitional movements an H2(15)O PET study. *Brain* **120,** 1301–1313.
106. Brooks, D. J. (1997) Motor disturbance and brain functional imaging in Parkinson's disease. *Euro. Neurol.* **38(Suppl. 2),** 26–32.
107. Grafton, S. T., Waters, C., Sutton, J., Lew, M. F., and Couldwell, W. (1995) Pallidotomy increases activity of motor association cortex in Parkinson's disease: a positron emission tomographic study. *Ann. Neurol.* **37,** 776–783.
108. Henselmans, J. M., de Jong, B. M., Pruim, J., Staal, M. J., Rutgers, A. W., and Haaxma, R. (2000) Acute effects of thalamotomy and pallidotomy on regional cerebral metabolism, evaluated by PET. *Clin. Neurol. Neurosurg.* **102,** 84–90.
109. Limousin-Dowsey, P., Pollak, P., Van Blercom, N., Krack, P., Benazzouz, A., and Benabid, A. (1999) Thalamic, subthalamic nucleus and internal pallidum stimulation in Parkinson's disease. *J. Neurol.* **246(Suppl. 2),** II42–II45.
110. Volkmann, J., Allert, N., Voges, J., Weiss, P. H., Freund, H. J., and Sturm, V. (2001) Safety and efficacy of pallidal or subthalamic nucleus stimulation in advanced PD. *Neurology* **56,** 548–551.
111. Benabid, A. L., Krack, P. P., Benazzouz, A., Limousin, P., Koudsie, A., and Pollak, P. (2000) Deep brain stimulation of the subthalamic nucleus for Parkinson's disease: methodologic aspects and clinical criteria. *Neurology* **55,** S40–S44.
112. Kumar, R., Lang, A. E., Rodriguez-Oroz, M. C., Lozano, A. M., Limousin, P., Pollak, P., et al. (2000) Deep brain stimulation of the globus pallidus pars interna in advanced Parkinson's disease. *Neurology* **55,** S34–S39.
113. Jahanshahi, M., Ardouin, C. M., Brown, R. G., Rothwell, J. C., Obeso, J., Albanese, A., et al. (2000) The impact of deep brain stimulation on executive function in Parkinson's disease. *Brain* **123,** 1142–1154.
114. Ardouin, C., Pillon, B., Peiffer, E., Bejjani, P., Limousin, P., Damier, P., et al. (1999) Bilateral subthalamic or pallidal stimulation for Parkinson's disease affects neither memory nor executive functions: a consecutive series of 62 patients. *Ann. Neurol.* **46,** 217–223.
115. Benazzouz, A., Piallat, B., Pollak, P., and Benabid, A. L. (1995) Responses of substantia nigra pars reticulata and globus pallidus complex to high frequency stimulation of the subthalamic nucleus in rats: electrophysiological data. *Neurosci. Lett.* **189,** 77–80.
116. Limousin, P., Greene, J., Pollak, P., Rothwell, J., Benabid, A. L., and Frackowiak, R. (1997) Changes in cerebral activity pattern due to subthalamic nucleus or internal pallidum stimulation in Parkinson's disease. *Ann. Neurol.* **42,** 283–291.
117. Davis, K. D., Taub, E., Houle, S., Lang, A. E., Dostrovsky, J. O., Tasker, R. R., and Lozano, A. M. (1997) Globus pallidus stimulation activates the cortical motor system during alleviation of parkinsonian symptoms. *Nature Med.* **3,** 671–674.
118. Hashimoto, T. M., Elder, C. R., DeLong, M., and Vitek, J. L. (2000) Responses of pallidal neurons to electrical stimulation of the subthalamic nucleus in experimental parkinsonism. *Mov. Disord.* (Abstract Volume) 277.
119. Windels, F., Bruet, N., Poupard, A., Urbain, N., Chouvet, G., Feuerstein, C., and Savasta, M. (2000) Effects of high frequency stimulation of subthalamic nucleus on extracellular glutamate and GABA in substantia nigra and globus pallidus in the normal rat. *Euro. J. Neurosci.* **12,** 4141–4146.
120. Filion, M., Tremblay, L., and Bedard, P. J. (1988) Abnormal influences of passive limb movement on the activity of globus pallidus neurons in parkinsonian monkeys. *Brain Res.* **444,** 165–176.
121. Miller, W. C. and DeLong, M. R. (1987) Altered tonic activity of neurons in the globus pallidus and subthalamic nucleus in the primate MPTP model of parkinsonism. In: *The Basal Ganglia II* (Carpenter, M. B. and Jayaraman, A., eds.), Plenum Press, New York, pp. 415–427.
122. Bergman, H., Wichmann, T., Karmon, B., and DeLong, M. R. (1994) The primate subthalamic nucleus. II. Neuronal activity in the MPTP model of parkinsonism. *J. Neurophysiol.* **72,** 507–520.
123. Vitek, J. L., Ashe, J., DeLong, M. R., and Alexander, G. E. (1990) Altered somatosensory response properties of neurons in the 'motor' thalamus of MPTP treated parkinsonian monkeys. *Soc. Neurosci. Abstr.* **16,** 425.
124. Raz, A., Feingold, A., Zelanskaya, V., and Bergman, H. (1996) Neuronal synchronization of tonically active neurons in the striatum of normal and parkinsonian primates. *J. Neurophysiol.*, in press.
125. Filion, M. and Tremblay, L. (1991) Abnormal spontaneous activity of globus pallidus neurons in monkeys with MPTP-induced parkinsonism. *Brain Res.* **547,** 142–151.

126. Vitek, J. L., Ashe, J., DeLong, M. R., and Alexander, G. E. (1990) Altered somatosensory response properties of neurons in the 'motor' thalamus of MPTP treated parkinsonian monkeys. *Soc. Neurosci. Abstr.* **16,** 425.
127. Vitek, J. L., Ashe, J., DeLong, M. R., and Alexander, G. E. (1994) Physiologic properties and somatotopic organization of the primate motor thalamus. *J. Neurophysiol.* **71,** 1498–1513.
128. Vitek, J. L., Kaneoke, Y., Turner, R., Baron, M., Bakay, R., and DeLong, M. (1993) Neuronal activity in the internal (GPi) and external (GPe) segments of the globus pallidus (GP) of parkinsonian patients is similar to that in the MPTP-treated primate model of parkinsonism. *Soc. Neurosci. Abstr.* **19,** 1584.
129. Wichmann, T., Bergman, H., and DeLong, M. R. (1996) Comparison of the effects of experimental parkinsonism on neuronal discharge in motor and non-motor portions of the basal ganglia output nuclei in primates. *Soc. Neurosci. Abstr.* **22,** 415.
130. Neufeld, M. Y., Inzelberg, R., and Korczyn, A. D. (1988) EEG in demented and non-demented parkinsonian patients. *Acta Neurolog. Scand.* **78,** 1–5.
131. Zijlmans, J. C., Pasman, J. W., Horstink, M. W., Stegeman, D. F., van't Hof, M. A., Poortvliet, D. J., et al. (1998) EEG findings in patients with vascular parkinsonism. *Acta Neurolog. Scand.* **98,** 243–247.
132. Primavera, A. and Novello, P. (1992) Quantitative electroencephalography in Parkinson's disease, dementia, depression and normal aging. *Neuropsychobiology* **25,** 102–105.
133. Soikkeli, R., Partanen, J., Soininen, H., Paakkonen, A., and Riekkinen, P. Sr. (1991) Slowing of EEG in Parkinson's disease. *Electroencephalogr. Clin. Neurophysiol.* **79,** 159–165.
134. Jelles, B., Achtereekte, H. A., Slaets, J. P., and Stam, C. J. (1995) Specific patterns of cortical dysfunction in dementia and Parkinson's disease demonstrated by the acceleration spectrum entropy of the EEG. *Clin. Electroencephalogr.* **26,** 188–192.
135. Hellwig, B., Haussler, S., Lauk, M., Guschlbauer, B., Koster, B., Kristeva-Feige, R., et al. (2000) Tremor-correlated cortical activity detected by electroencephalography. *Clin. Neurophysiol.* **111,** 806–809.
136. Boulton, A. A. and Marjerrison, G. L. (1972) Effect of L-dopa therapy on urinary p-tyramine excretion and EEG changes in Parkinson's disease. *Nature* **236,** 76–78.
137. Marjerrison, G., Boulton, A. A., and Rajput, A. (1971) Dopa therapy in parkinsonism effects on the EEG and amine metabolism. *Internationale Zeitschrift fur Klinische Pharmakologie, Therapie und Toxikologie* **4,** 263–266.
138. Marjerrison, G., Boulton, A. A., and Rajput, A. H. (1972) EEG and urinary non-catecholic amine changes during L-dopa therapy of Parkinson's disease. *Diseases of the Nervous System* **33,** 164–169.
139. Yaar, I. (1977) EEG power spectral changes secondary to L-DOPA treatment in parkinsonian patients: a pilot study. *Electroencephalogr. Clin. Neurophysiol.* **43,** 111–118.
140. Brown, P. and Marsden, C. D. (1999) Bradykinesia and impairment of EEG desynchronization in Parkinson's disease. *Mov. Disord.* **14,** 423–429.
141. Wang, H. C., Lees, A. J., and Brown, P. (1999) Impairment of EEG desynchronisation before and during movement and its relation to bradykinesia in Parkinson's disease. *J. Neurol. Neurosurg. Psychiatry* **66,** 442–446.
142. Nini, A., Feingold, A., Slovin, H., and Bergman, H. (1995) Neurons in the globus pallidus do not show correlated activity in the normal monkey, but phase-locked oscillations appear in the MPTP model of parkinsonism. *J. Neurophysiol.* **74,** 1800–1805.
143. Bergman, H., Raz, A., Feingold, A., Nini, A., Nelken, I., Hansel, D., et al. (1998) Physiology of MPTP tremor. *Mov. Disord.* **13(Suppl. 3),** 29–34.
144. Raz, A., Frechter-Mazar, V., Feingold, A., Abeles, M., Vaadia, E., and Bergman, H. (2001) Activity of pallidal and striatal tonically active neurons is correlated in mptp-treated monkeys but not in normal monkeys. *J. Neurosci.* **21,** RC128.
145. Brown, P., Oliviero, A., Mazzone, P., Insola, A., Tonali, P., and Di Lazzaro, V. (2001) Dopamine dependency of oscillations between subthalamic nucleus and pallidum in Parkinson's disease. *J. Neurosci.* **21,** 1033–1038.
146. Ruskin, D. N., Bergstrom, D. A., Kaneoke, Y., Patel, B. N., Twery, M. J., and Walters, J. R. (1999) Multisecond oscillations in firing rate in the basal ganglia: robust modulation by dopamine receptor activation and anesthesia. *J. Neurophysiol.* **81,** 2046–2055.
147. Karmon, B. and Bergman, H. (1993) Detection of neuronal periodic oscillations in the basal ganglia of normal and parkinsonian monkeys. *Israeli J. Med. Sci.* **29,** 570–579.
148. Hutchison, W. D., Lozano, A. M., Tasker, R. R., Lang, A. E., and Dostrovsky, J. O. (1997) Identification and characterization of neurons with tremor-frequency activity in human globus pallidus. *Exp. Brain Res.* **113,** 557–563.
149. Hurtado, J. M., Gray, C. M., Tamas, L. B., and Sigvardt, K. A. (1999) Dynamics of tremor-related oscillations in the human globus pallidus: a single case study. *Proc. Nat. Acad. Sci. USA* **96,** 1674–1679.
150. Hua, S., Reich, S. G., Zirh, A. T., Perry, V., Dougherty, P. M., and Lenz, F. A. (1998) The role of the thalamus and basal ganglia in parkinsonian tremor. *Mov. Disord.* **13(Suppl. 3),** 40–42.
151. Bergman, H., Feingold, A., Nini, A., Raz, A., Slovin, H., Abeles, M., and Vaadia, E. (1998) Physiological aspects of information processing in the basal ganglia of normal and parkinsonian primates. *Trends Neurosci.* **21,** 32–38.
152. Wichmann, T., Kliem, M. A., and Long, S. B. (2000) Changes in oscillatory discharge in the primate basal ganglia associated with parkinsonism and light sleep. *Mov. Disord.* (Abstract Volume) P303.
153. Hallett, M. (1998) Overview of human tremor physiology. *Mov. Disord.* **13,** 43–48.
154. Rothwell, J. C. (1998) Physiology and anatomy of possible oscillators in the central nervous system. *Mov. Disord.* **13(Suppl. 3),** 24–28.
155. Elble, R. J. (1996) Central mechanisms of tremor. *J. Clin. Neurophysiol.* **13,** 133–144.
156. Hallett, M. (1999) Motor cortex plasticity. *Electroencephalogr. Clin. Neurophysiol. (Suppl.)* **50,** 85–91.

157. Hallett, M. (1995) The plastic brain [editorial] [see comments]. *Ann. Neurol.* **38,** 4–5.
158. Johansson, F., Malm, J., Nordh, E., and Hariz, M. (1997) Usefulness of pallidotomy in advanced Parkinson's disease. *J. Neurol. Neurosurg. Psychiatry* **62,** 125–132.
159. Samuel, M., Caputo, E., Brooks, D. J., Schrag, A., Scaravilli, T., Branston, N. M., et al. (1998) A study of medial pallidotomy for Parkinson's disease: clinical outcome, MRI location and complications. *Brain* **121,** 59–75.
160. Vitek, J. L., Chockkan, V., Zhang, J. Y., Kaneoke, Y., Evatt, M., DeLong, M. R., et al. (1999) Neuronal activity in the basal ganglia in patients with generalized dystonia and hemiballismus. *Ann. Neurol.* **46,** 22–35.
161. Lozano, A. M., Kumar, R., Gross, R. E., Giladi, N., Hutchison, W. D., Dostrovsky, J. O., and Lang, A. E. (1997) Globus pallidus internus pallidotomy for generalized dystonia. *Mov. Disord.* **12,** 865–870.
162. Lenz, F. A., Suarez, J. I., Metman, L. V., Reich, S. G., Karp, B. I., Hallett, M., et al. (1998) Pallidal activity durping dystonia: somatosensory reorganisation and changes with severity. *J. Neurol. Neurosurg. Psychiatry* **65,** 767–770.
163. Wichmann, T. and DeLong, M. R. (1998) Models of basal ganglia function and pathophysiology of movement disorders. *Neurosurg. Clin. North Am.* **9,** 223–236.
164. Soghomonian, J. J., Pedneault, S., Audet, G., and Parent, A. (1994) Increased glutamate decarboxylase mRNA levels in the striatum and pallidum of MPTP-treated primates. *J. Neurosci.* **14,** 6256–6265.
165. Herrero, M. T., Levy, R., Ruberg, M., Javoy-Agid, F., Luquin, M. R., Agid, Y., et al. (1996) Glutamic acid decarboxylase mRNA expression in medial and lateral pallidal neurons in the MPTP-treated monkeys and patients with Parkinson's disease. *Adv. Neurol.* **69,** 209–216.
166. Herrero, M. T., Levy, R., Ruberg, M., Luquin, M. R., Villares, J., Guillen, J., et al. (1996) Consequence of nigrostriatal denervation and L-dopa therapy on the expression of glutamic acid decarboxylase messenger RNA in the pallidum. *Neurology* **47,** 219–224.
167. Soghomonian, J. J. and Chesselet, M. F. (1992) Effects of nigrostriatal lesions on the levels of messenger RNAs encoding two isoforms of glutamate decarboxylase in the globus pallidus and entopeduncular nucleus of the rat. *Synapse* **11,** 124–133.
168. Delfs, J. M., Anegawa, N. J., and Chesselet, M. F. (1995) Glutamate decarboxylase messenger RNA in rat pallidum: comparison of the effects of haloperidol, clozapine and combined haloperidol-scopolamine treatments. *Neuroscience* **66,** 67–80.
169. Blanchet, P. J., Boucher, R., and Bedard, P. J. (1994) Excitotoxic lateral pallidotomy does not relieve L-dopa-induced dyskinesia in MPTP parkinsonian monkeys. *Brain Res.* **650,** 32–39.
170. Albin, R. L., Reiner, A., Anderson, K. D., Penney, J. B., and Young, A. B. (1990) Striatal and nigral neuron subpopulations in rigid Huntington's disease: implications for the functional anatomy of chorea and rigidity-akinesia. *Ann. Neurol.* **27,** 357–365.
171. Papa, S. M., Desimone, R., Fiorani, M., and Oldfield, E. H. (1999) Internal globus pallidus discharge is nearly suppressed during levodopa-induced dyskinesias. *Ann. Neurol.* **46,** 732–738.
172. Lozano, A. M., Lang, A. E., Levy, R., Hutchison, W., and Dostrovsky, J. (2000) Neuronal recordings in Parkinson's disease patients with dyskinesias induced by apomorphine. *Ann. Neurol.* **47,** S141–S146.
173. Merello, M., Balej, J., Delfino, M., Cammarota, A., Betti, O., and Leiguarda, R. (1999) Apomorphine induces changes in GPi spontaneous outflow in patients with Parkinson's disease. *Mov. Disord.* **14,** 45–49.
174. Brooks, D. J. (1993) Functional imaging in relation to parkinsonian syndromes. *J. Neurol. Sci.* **115,** 1–17.
175. Horak, F. B. and Anderson, M. E. (1984) Influence of globus pallidus on arm movements in monkeys. I. Effects of kainic-induced lesions. *J. Neurophysiol.* **52,** 290–304.
176. Wichmann, T., Kliem, M. A., and DeLong, M. R. (2001) Antiparkinsonian and behavioral effects of inactivation of the substantia nigra pars reticulata in hemiparkinsonian primates. *Exp. Neurol.* In press.
177. Burbaud, P., Bonnet, B., Guehl, D., Lagueny, A., and Bioulac, B. (1998) Movement disorders induced by gamma-aminobutyric agonist and antagonist injections into the internal globus pallidus and substantia nigra pars reticulata of the monkey. *Brain Res.* **780,** 102–107.
178. Baron, M. S., Wichmann, T., Ma, D., and DeLong, M. R. (2001) The effects of transient focal inactivation of the basal ganglia in parkinsonian primates. *J. Neurosci.* Submitted.
179. Hamada, I. and DeLong, M. R. (1992) Excitotoxic acid lesions of the primate subthalamic nucleus result in transient dyskinesias of the contralateral limbs. *J. Neurophysiol.* **68,** 1850–1858.
180. Vitek, J. L. and Giroux, M. (2000) Physiology of hypokinetic and hyperkinetic movement disorders: model for dyskinesia. *Ann. Neurol.* **47,** S131–S140.
181. Gille, M., Jacquemin, C., Kiame, G., Delbecq, J., Guilmot, D., and Depre, A. (1993) Myelinolyse centropontine avec ataxie cerebelleuse et dystonie. *Rev. Neurol.* **149,** 344–346.
182. Tranchant, C., Maquet, J., Eber, A. M., Dietemann, J. L., Franck, P., and Warter, J. M. (1991) Angiome caverneux cerebelleux, dystonie cervicale et diaschisis cortical croise. *Rev. Neurol.* **147,** 599–602.
183. Janati, A., Metzer, W. S., Archer, R. L., Nickols, J., and Raval, J. (1989) Blepharospasm associated with olivopontocerebellar atrophy. *J. Clin. Neuro-Ophthalmol.* **9,** 281–284.
184. Ozelius, L. J., Hewett, J., Kramer, P., Bressman, S. B., Shalish, C., deLeon, D., et al. (1997) Fine localization of the torsion dystonia gene (DYT1) on human chromosome 9q34: YAC map and linkage disequilibrium. *Genome Res.* **7,** 483–494.
185. Risch, N., deLeon, D., Ozelius, L., Kramer, P., Almassy, L., Singer, B., Fahn, S., Breakefield, X., and Bressman, S. (1995) Genetic analysis of idiopathic torsion dystonia in Ashkenazi Jews and their recent descent from a small founder population. *Nature Genet.* **9,** 152–159.

186. Hutchison, W. D., Lozano, A. M., Davis, K., Saint-Cyr, J. A., Lang, A. E., and Dostrovsky, J. O. (1994) Differential neuronal activity in segments of globus pallidus in Parkinson's disease patients. *Neuroreport* **5,** 1533–1537.
187. Patel, K., Roskrow, T., Davis, J. S., and Heckmatt, J. Z. (1995) Dopa responsive dystonia. *Arch. Dis. Childhood* **73,** 256–257.
188. Nygaard, T. G. (1995) Dopa-responsive dystonia. *Curr. Opin. Neurol.* **8,** 310–313.
189. Ichinose, H., Ohye, T., Takayashi, E., Seki, N., Hori, T., Segawa, M., et al. (1994) Hereditary progressive dystonia with marked diurnal fluctuation caused by mutations in the GTP cyclohydrolase I gene. *Nature Genet.* **8,** 236–242.
190. Vitek, J., Evatt, M., Zhang, J., Hashimoto, T., DeLong, M., Triche, S., et al. (1997) Pallidotomy as a treatment for medically intractable dystonia. *Ann. Neurol.* **42,** 409.
191. Cardoso, F., Jankovic, J., Grossman, R. G., and Hamilton, W. J. (1995) Outcome after stereotactic thalamotomy for dystonia and hemiballismus. *Neurosurgery* **36,** 501–508.
192. Lozano, A. M., Kumar, R., Gross, R. E., Giladi, N., Hutchison, W. D., Dostrovsky, J. O., and Lang, A. E. (1997) Globus pallidus internus pallidotomy for generalized dystonia. [see comments]. *Mov. Disord.* **12,** 865–870.
193. Lenz, F. A. and Byl, N. N. (1999) Reorganization in the cutaneous core of the human thalamic principal somatic sensory nucleus (Ventral caudal) in patients with dystonia. *J. Neurophysiol.* **82,** 3204–3212.
194. Lenz, F. A., Jaeger, C. J., Seike, M. S., Lin, Y. C., Reich, S. G., DeLong, M. R., and Vitek, J. L. (1999) Thalamic single neuron activity in patients with dystonia: dystonia-related activity and somatic sensory reorganization. *J. Neurophysiol.* **82,** 2372–2392.
195. Bara-Jimenez, W., Catalan, M. J., Hallett, M., and Gerloff, C. (1998) Abnormal somatosensory homunculus in dystonia of the hand. *Ann. Neurol.* **44,** 828–831.
196. Hallett, M. and Toro, C. (1996) Dystonia and the supplementary sensorimotor area. *Adv. Neurol.* **70,** 471–476.
197. Ikoma, K., Samii, A., Mercuri, B., Wassermann, E. M., and Hallett, M. (1996) Abnormal cortical motor excitability in dystonia. *Neurology* **46,** 1371–1376.
198. Berardelli, A., Rothwell, J. C., Hallett, M., Thompson, P. D., Manfredi, M., and Marsden, C. D. (1998) The pathophysiology of primary dystonia. *Brain* **121,** 1195–1212.
199. Hallett, M. (1998) The neurophysiology of dystonia. *Arch. Neurol.* **55,** 601–603.

2

Basal Ganglia Circuitry and Synaptic Connectivity

Ali Charara, Mamadou Sidibé, and Yoland Smith

1. OVERALL ORGANIZATION OF THE BASAL GANGLIA

The basal ganglia are several synaptically interconnected subcortical structures that play important roles in regulating various aspects of psychomotor behaviors, and are central to the pathophysiology of common human movement disorders such as Parkinson's and Huntington's diseases (PD/HD). These structures classically include: 1) the striatum, which comprises the caudate nucleus (CD), putamen (PUT), and nucleus accumbens (Acc); 2) the globus pallidus, which includes the external (GPe; globus pallidus in nonprimates) and internal (GPi; entopeduncular nucleus [EPN] in nonprimates) segments; 3) the subthalamic nucleus (STN); and 4) the substantia nigra, which comprises the pars compacta (SNc) and pars reticulata (SNr) (Fig. 1).

The striatum, and to a lesser extent, the STN are the major receptive components of the basal ganglia. They both receive excitatory glutamatergic projections from the cerebral cortex and the thalamus. They also receive modulatory dopaminergic inputs from the SNc and ventral tegmental area (VTA) as well as serotonergic inputs from the dorsal raphe nucleus (DR). The striatum projects directly, and indirectly via the GPe and STN, to the output nuclei of the basal ganglia, the GPi, and SNr *(1–3)*. The direct and indirect striatal projections as well as the GPe projection to the STN use the inhibitory amino acid, γ-aminobutyric acid (GABA), as neurotransmitter. In contrast, the pathways from the STN to the GPi and SNr are excitatory and glutamatergic *(3)*. Thus, the basal ganglia output nuclei, GPi and SNr, receive opposite inhibitory and excitatory signals from the direct and indirect pathways. The GPi and SNr projections to the thalamus are GABAergic and tend to inhibit thalamocortical feedback which, in turn, is excitatory and glutamatergic. Furthermore, the output neurons of the GPi and SNr project to specific brainstem structures that provide descending projections to motor nuclei in the medulla and spinal cord (Fig. 1). Therefore, the major circuitry of the basal ganglia is from the cortex, through its component structures, which then convey the information to the thalamus and brainstem. The thalamus projects back upon frontal cortical areas whereas the brainstem sends feedback ascending projections to the basal ganglia or descending projections to medullary motor nuclei interconnected with the spinal cord (Fig.1).

In addition to these main basal ganglia circuits, there are additional loops and connections that may play important roles in basal ganglia functions. These include projections from the GPe to the striatum, the substantia nigra, and the reticular thalamic nucleus; projections from the STN to the GPe, tegmental pedunculopontine nucleus (PPN), striatum, and SNc; and projections from the thalamus to the striatum, the pallidum, and the STN *(3,4)* (Fig. 1). In dealing with such a complex circuitry, and because of space limitations, this review will not cover every aspects of the basal ganglia connectivity, but will

From: Contemporary Clinical Neurology:
Surgical Treatment of Parkinson's Disease and Other Movement Disorders
Edited by: D. Tarsy, J. L. Vitek, and A. M. Lozano © Humana Press Inc., Totowa, NJ

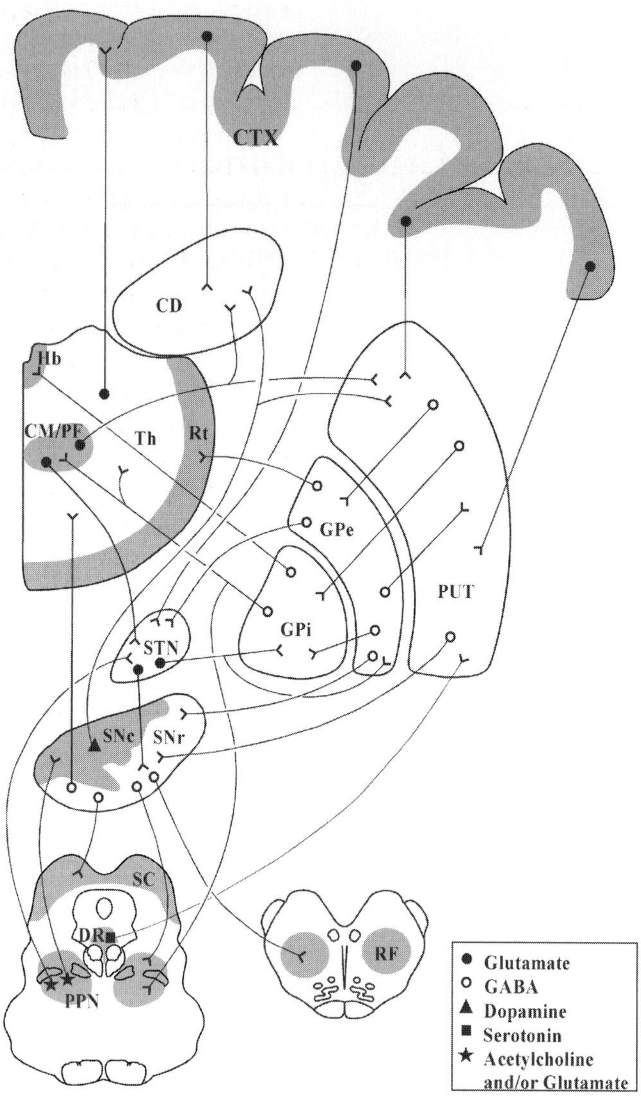

Fig. 1. Schematic diagram of major basal ganglia connections in primates. For simplification, some connections have been omitted. The main neurotransmitters are indicated by different symbols that labeled the cell bodies.

rather focus on the overall direction of information flow and highlight some recent anatomical findings that underlie novel concepts of basal ganglia organization.

2. THE STRIATUM: A MAJOR ENTRANCE TO THE BASAL GANGLIA CIRCUITRY

2.1. The Corticostriatal Projection

Nearly all regions of the cerebral cortex send topographic projections to the striatum, at varying degrees, making the cerebral cortex, by far, the strongest input to the basal ganglia; afferents from sensorimotor and associative cortices are particularly extensive, whereas those from the primary visual and auditory cortices being much less so *(4)*. There is evidence that the striatum is subdivided into different functional territories according to its cortical inputs. In monkeys, the premotor, motor, and somatosensory cortices in the frontal lobe project mostly to the postcommissural putamen where a somatotopic representation of the leg, arm, and face occurs in the form of obliquely arranged strips *(5)*. The caudate nucleus and precommissural putamen receive projections, mostly unilateral, from association areas of the prefrontal, temporal, parietal, and cingulate cortices, and motor areas in the frontal lobe that control eye movements. The afferents from limbic cortical areas as well as from the amygdala and the hippocampus terminate preferentially in the ventral portion of the striatum *(3–8)*.

Although there is a general topographic relationship between the cerebral cortex and striatum, the integration of information from several different cortical areas is governed by convergence and divergence of corticostriatal inputs. The sensorimotor cortical areas that are functionally interconnected via corticocortical connections tend to give rise to extensively overlapping projections in the ipsilateral putamen, whereas contralateral projections from M1, except those from the face area, interdigitate with ipsilateral M1/S1 overlapping regions *(9,10)*. A similar pattern of convergence exists for the striatal projections from frontal and supplementary eye fields *(11)*. However, it appears that striatal projections from reciprocally linked areas of the association cortices are either completely segregated or interdigitated within zones of overlap in the monkey striatum *(12)*. These projections occupy longitudinal sectors that are aligned along the mediolateral axis of the striatum *(12)*.

Corticostriatal neurons are divided into at least three types, as revealed by studies using double retrograde or intracellular staining techniques in rats *(13)*. The first type, which gives rise to a relatively small component of the corticostriatal pathway, includes large pyramidal cells located in deep layer V. These cells have extensive intracortical axon arborizations, contribute to the pyramidal tract, and emit fine collaterals with very restricted arborizations in the ipsilateral striatum. The focal nature of these arborizations suggests a relatively simple and highly convergent organization of the corticostriatal pathway. A second, more common, type is located in the superficial layer V and deep layer III. These neurons give rise to bilateral corticocortical and corticostriatal projections. The axons of those cells form diffuse complexes of axon terminals that occupy a large volume of the ipsilateral and contralateral striatum. Within that volume, the density of axonal arborization is very sparse, leaving large areas uninnervated, which indicates that individual axonal branches cross the dendritic field of many striatal neurons and form mostly "en passant" synapses *(6,7,14,15)*. This pattern implies a much more complex and divergent organization of the corticostriatal pathway. A third type of corticostriatal neurons is located in the superficial layer V. These neurons project mainly to the thalamus with a collateral projection to the striatum *(6,16,17)*.

Ninety percent of neurons in the striatum are medium-sized GABAergic projection neurons, which have their distal dendrites densely covered with spines *(6,7,18)*. The remaining neurons are aspiny and comprise four main populations of chemically characterized interneurons: 1) the cholinergic neurons which partly co-express calretinin; 2) the parvalbumin-containing neurons that also contain GABA; 3) the somatostatin-immunoreactive neurons that also express neuropeptide Y, nitric oxide, and GABA; and 4) the calretinin-containing neurons that partly co-localize with choline acetyltransferase *(19,20)*. A small subset of calbindin-immunoreactive neurons also display ultrastructural features and morphological characteristics of interneurons, but the majority of calbindin-positive cells in the striatum are projection neurons *(20,21)*.

The corticostriatal afferents form asymmetric synapses principally on the head of dendritic spines of projection neurons and less frequently with dendritic shafts of projection neurons and interneurons *(18)*. The density of cortical innervation of striatal interneurons is variable depending on their chemical phenotype. For instance, parvalbumin-containing interneurons receive strong cortical inputs at the level of cell bodies and proximal dendrites *(22)*, whereas cholinergic interneurons are almost completely devoid of cortical afferents except for sparse inputs on their distal dendrites and spine-like appendages *(23–25)*. On the other hand, despite this light cortical innervation, stimulation of the cerebral cortex evokes monosynaptic excitatory postsynaptic potentials in cholinergic interneurons *(26)*.

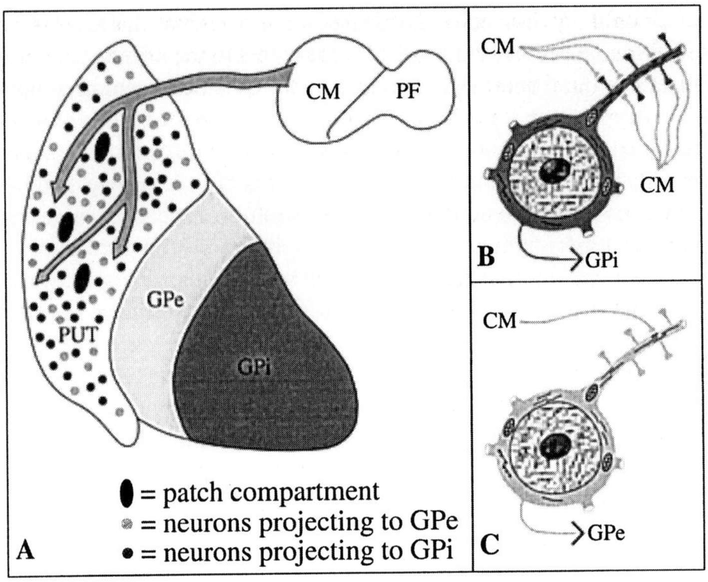

Fig. 2. Compartmental (**A**) and synaptic (**B,C**) relationships between striatopallidal neurons and thalamic afferents from the centromedian nucleus (CM) in monkeys. These data were obtained after simultaneous injections of anterograde tracers in CM and retrograde tracers in either segment of the globus pallidus. (**A**) CM inputs project mainly to the matrix striatal compartment that contains neurons projecting to GPe (light gray circles) or GPi (dark gray circles). Thalamic afferents form asymmetric synapses, frequently with striato-GPi neurons (**B**) but rarely with striato-GPe cells (**C**). (Modified with permission from ref. *29*.)

2.2. *The Thalamostriatal Projection*

The thalamostriatal projection, originating mostly from the centromedian (CM) and parafasicular (PF) intralaminar nuclei, is the second most prominent source of glutamatergic inputs to the striatum. Anterograde tracing studies in rats and monkeys revealed that the thalamostriatal projection is topographically organized *(8,27,28)*. In monkeys, the CM projects mainly to the sensorimotor territory of the striatum where it terminates in the form of elongated bands, whereas the PF innervates predominantly the associative territory and, to a lesser extent, the limbic territory, where it terminates in a patchy-like manner *(28,29)*. In all striatal territories, fibers from both CM and PF arborize preferentially in the matrix compartment *(28,29)* (Fig. 2). Recent evidence indicates that the precommissural putamen receives inputs from an area called dorsolateral PF (PFdl), a group of fusiform neurons that extend mediolaterally along the dorsal border of CM *(30)*. In rats and monkeys, thalamic inputs to the limbic territory arise largely from midline and rostral intralaminar nuclei *(31,32)*. Specific relay or association thalamic nuclei also project to the striatum, but to a lesser extent than intralaminar nuclei *(33–34a)*. A recent study demonstrated convergent projections from various interconnected ventral thalamic motor relay nuclei and frontal cortical motor areas to broad territories of the postcommissural putamen *(35)*. Together, these anatomical data indicate that thalamostriatal projections from intralaminar and relay nuclei are more massive and much better organized than previously thought.

Earlier electrophysiological and retrograde tracing studies suggested that thalamostriatal fibers emit collaterals to the cerebral cortex *(36–39)*. The existence of such collaterals was recently confirmed by single-cell labeling in rats *(40)*. These branched neurons were found in the parafascicular, ethmoid nucleus, posterior thalamic group, lateral posterior nucleus, mediodorsal nucleus, and anterior ventral nucleus. Collaterals of thalamostriatal fibers project to broad cortical areas and mostly arborize in layers

III, V, and VI *(40)*. It is unlikely that such collateralization is a general characteristic of thalamostriatal neurons in primates. For instance, neurons in CM that project to the primary motor cortex are largely segre-gated from thalamostriatal neurons that project to the putamen in squirrel monkeys *(33,41)*.

Both medium spiny projection neurons and aspiny interneurons are targeted by thalamostriatal afferents. In contrast to cortical boutons, that predominantly terminate on the head of dendritic spines *(18)*, thalamic terminals from caudal intralaminar nuclei form asymmetric synapses principally on dendritic shafts of medium-sized projection neurons *(28,29,42)*. However, studies in rat indicate that striatal inputs from rostral intralaminar nuclei target preferentially dendritic spines *(43)*. Thalamic inputs from CM form synapses more frequently with direct than indirect striatofugal neurons in monkeys, which indicates that the thalamus modulates differently the two major output pathways of the basal ganglia in primates *(29)* (Fig. 2). Striatal interneurons immunoreactive for choline acetyltransferase, parvalbumin and somatostatin, but not those containing calretinin, also receive substantial inputs from CM in monkeys *(44)*. In rats, cholinergic neurons are a major target of thalamic inputs from PF *(23,24)* whereas parvalbumin-containing neurons are much less innervated by thalamic afferents *(45)*. Whether this represents a species difference between primates and nonprimates regarding thalamic innervation of parvalbumin-containing interneurons or a difference in the postsynaptic targets of CM and PF inputs to the striatum remains to be established.

2.3. *The Nigrostriatal Projection*

The striatum receives a massive projection from midbrain dopaminergic neurons located in the SNc (cell group A9), VTA (cell group A10), and retrorubral field (RRF; cell group A8). It is largely accepted that neurons in the VTA give rise to the mesolimbocortical system, whose fibers terminate principally in the ventral striatum and frontal cortex, whereas neurons in the SNc and RRA project via the nigrostriatal pathway to the putamen and caudate nucleus. A small proportion of nigrostriatal fibers are nondopaminergic and use GABA as neurotransmitter *(46–48)*. Similarly, a GABAergic projection from the VTA to the frontal cortex has been described *(49)*. In vitro data also suggest that midbrain dopaminergic neurons may release glutamate as neurotransmitter *(50,51)*.

Various neuroanatomic studies indicate that the nigrostriatal projection is topographically organized. For instance, in rats, the sensorimotor striatum receives its main dopaminergic input from the lateral part of the SNc and dopaminergic cells in the SNr, whereas the associative striatum is mainly innervated by the medial SNc and VTA. On the other hand, the limbic striatum receives inputs from the VTA, whereas the RRA projects to all striatal territories *(52,53)*. In monkeys, attempts to outline the topographic organization of the nigrostriatal projection led to controversial results *(52)*. Some data indicate that the rostral two-thirds of the substantia nigra is connected with the head of the caudate nucleus, whereas nigral neurons projecting to the putamen are more caudally located, and display a rostrocaudal topography *(33)*. An inverse mediolateral and dorsoventral topography between the SNc and the striatum has also been proposed in monkeys *(54)*. Retrograde fluorescent double-labeling studies revealed that nigro-caudate and nigro-putamen neurons are organized in the form of interdigitated, closely intermingled clusters of various sizes distributed throughout the entire SNc in squirrel monkeys *(55)*. More recently, the organization of the nigrostriatal projection was examined in relation to the functional territories of the striatum in rhesus monkeys *(56,57)*. These studies demonstrated that the sensorimotor-related striatum receives its main input from the cell columns in the ventral tier of the SNc, whereas the limbic-related striatum is innervated preferentially by the VTA and dorsal tier of the SNc. On the other hand, the associative-related striatum receives inputs from a wide range of dopamine neurons largely localized in the densocellular part of the ventral SNc *(56,57)*.

Although some immunohistochemical data showed that the striosomes are rather poorly innervated by dopaminergic afferents compared to the extrastriosomal matrix in the striatum of adult monkeys and humans *(58,59)* most studies found that tyrosine hydroxylase- and dopamine containing fibers terminate homogenously throughout the rat striatum *(60)*. In rats, the dopaminergic projections from the dorsal tier of the SNc terminate mainly in the matrix compartment, whereas projections from the ventral tier of the SNc innervate preferentially the patch compartment *(47,47a)*. Dopaminergic cells of the VTA and RRA project only to the matrix *(47)*. However, attempts to delineate groups of DA neurons projecting to the matrix and/or striosomes have been less successful and failed to establish simple relations between striatal compartments and different subdivisions of the SNc in nonhuman primates *(52,53,56)*.

Ultrastructural studies revealed that dopaminergic terminals make symmetric synapses with dendritic shafts and spines of projection neurons *(18,53,61)*. In rats, the pattern of synaptic organization of dopaminergic terminals is similar in the matrix and striosomes *(48)*. In rodents, most dopaminergic synapses occur on the neck of spines whose head receives asymmetric contacts from corticostriatal fibers *(18,61)*, whereas, in monkeys, the majority of dopamine terminals form axodendritic synapses *(62)*. In contrast to cortical and dopamine terminals that often converge onto common postsynaptic targets, thalamic and dopaminergic afferents are not found in close proximity to each other in the monkey striatum *(62)*. Together, these data indicate that the dopaminergic afferents are positioned to exert a more direct and powerful modulation of cortical inputs than thalamic afferents in the striatum. Indeed, pre- and postsynaptic interactions between dopamine and cortical afferents have been shown, though the anatomical substrates for presynaptic interactions are still controversial *(63,64)*. It is worth noting that dopamine may also influence the activity of striatal projection neurons through nonjunctional appositions *(65)*, which is consistent with receptor localization studies that D1 and D2 receptors are mostly expressed extrasynaptically onto the plasma membranes of striatal neurons *(66,67)*.

It is important to keep in mind that dopamine may also influence basal ganglia functions via extrastriatal projections. Direct dopaminergic inputs to the pallidum and the subthalamic nucleus have, indeed, been described anatomically and electrophysiologically in various species *(47a,53,53a)*. The dopaminergic innervation of the thalamus is decreased in hemiparkinsonian monkeys, which suggests that this innervation largely arises from axon collaterals of the massive nigrostriatal pathway *(53a)*. Intrastriatal dopaminergic neurons also provide another route by which dopamine may influence striatal functions. These neurons are likely to be particularly important in Parkinson's disease since their number increases dramatically in 1-methyl-4-phenyl-1,2,3,6-tetrahydropyridine (MPTP)-treated monkeys *(53,68)*.

2.4. *Other Striatal Afferents*

The striatum receives many other afferent projections that, due to space limitation, will not be discussed in details in the present review. These include the serotonergic projection from the dorsal and median raphe nuclei as well as the subthalamostriatal projection. Serotonergic fibers arborize profusely throughout the entire striatum, but slightly more heavily in the ventral region *(69)*. In rats, dorsal raphe neurons projecting to the striatum send axon collaterals to the substantia nigra *(70)*. Although some serotonergic terminals form asymmetric axospinous and axodendritic synapses *(71)*, only a minor proportion of serotonergic fibers exhibit typical synaptic junctions in the rat striatum *(72)*.

In primates, subthalamic neurons that innervate the putamen are located in the sensorimotor-related dorsolateral two-thirds of the STN, whereas those projecting to the caudate nucleus are found ventrolaterally in the associative territory *(33,73)*. Other inputs to the striatum arise from the globus pallidus, pedunculopontine nucleus, and locus coeruleus *(33,74,75)*.

3. THE DIRECT AND INDIRECT STRIATOFUGAL PROJECTIONS

3.1. *Original Concept*

The information sent to the striatum is integrated by medium spiny projection neurons and transmitted to the output nuclei of the basal ganglia (GPi and SNr) via two pathways so-called direct and indirect pathways *(1,76)*. The direct pathway originates from a population of striatal neurons that project directly to the GPi and SNr whereas the indirect pathway arises from striatal neurons that project to GPe. In turn, the GPe conveys the information to the STN, which then relays it to the output nuclei of the basal ganglia, the GPi, and the SNr (Fig. 1). Striatal neurons that give rise to the direct and indirect pathways are further distinguished by their expression of neuroactive peptides and dopamine receptor subtypes. Although all striatal projection neurons use GABA as their main transmitter, neurons projecting to the GPe contain enkephalin and express preferentially D2 dopamine receptors, whereas those projecting to the GPi and SNr are enriched with substance P and dynorphin and express mainly D1 dopamine receptors *(6)*.

According to functional models of basal ganglia circuits, normal basal ganglia functions require a balance between the activity of the direct and indirect pathways *(77)*. This balance is maintained, in part, by dopaminergic modulation of striatal neurons. Release of dopamine facilitates transmission through the direct pathway but reduces transmission through the indirect pathway. During normal movement, the overall effect of striatal dopamine release is to reduce the GPi/SNr inhibition of the thalamus, leading to increased activity of thalamocortical projections, which is necessary for the speed and guidance of movements. However, an imbalance of activity of these two pathways can perturb the normal degree of GPi/SNr inhibition of thalamocortical activity producing hypo- or hyperkinetic disorders *(77)*. Since the introduction of the model of direct and indirect pathways, there have been many anatomical, biochemical, and molecular studies that increased our knowledge of the organization of the basal ganglia and led to reconsider some aspects of the functional circuitry of the basal ganglia. In the following account we summarize some of these data and discuss their relevance for basal ganglia pathophysiology.

3.2. *Collateralization of Striatofugal Neurons and Co-localization of Dopamine Receptors*

One of the important series of data that challenged the concept of segregated direct and indirect striatofugal pathways is the demonstration that "direct" striatofugal neurons are much more collateralized than previously thought. Based on single cell filling studies, striatofugal neurons are divided into three types in rats *(78)*: 1) a first population projecting only and extensively to the GP; 2) a second type projecting to both GP and SNr; and 3) a third type projecting to GP, EP, and SNr. Similar findings were recently found in monkeys *(79)*. Although these data provide evidence for the existence of the indirect pathway, they suggest that the so-called direct striatofugal neurons display a high degree of collateralization and that none of the striatofugal neurons examined project exclusively to the GPi (or EPN) or SNr.

Another controversial issue that has been raised by various investigators over the past few years is the differential expression of D1 and D2 dopamine receptors in direct and indirect striatofugal neurons *(6)*. Although many *in situ* hybridization studies and immunohistochemical data showed that D1 and D2 receptors are largely segregated in the rat striatum, reverse transcriptase polymerase chain reaction (RT-PCR) experiments in isolated striatal neurons *(80)* and a recent double immunofluorescence study *(81)* revealed a higher level of co-localization. Furthermore, it was found that most striatal spiny neurons respond to both D1 and D2 receptor agonists, in vitro *(80,81)*. It is now apparent that this controversy is due to the differential sensitivity of RT-PCR and *in situ* hybridization methods to detect mRNAs because the relative abundance of the two receptor subtypes in direct and indirect striatofugal neurons is strikingly different. Neurons of the indirect pathway that contain enkephalin express high levels of D2 mRNA and low level of D1 mRNA, whereas direct striatofugal neurons that contain substance P express high levels of D1 mRNA but also contain low levels of D2 mRNA *(80)*. The only striatal projection neurons that express a high level of D1 and D2 receptor subtypes are a small population that contains both enkephalin and substance P *(80,82)*. Similar findings were obtained by double immunofluorescence *(81)*. These findings must be kept in mind while considering the functional significance of the direct and indirect striatofugal pathways.

3.3. *Multiple Indirect Pathways*

In addition to the classical indirect pathway through the GPe and STN, there is a variety of other indirect pathways and loops that process the flow of information through the basal ganglia. For instance, the GPe gives rise to GABAergic projections to basal ganglia output structures (GPi, SNr) and the reticular thalamic nucleus *(3,4,8)*. Another projection from the GPe to the striatum, which targets preferentially subpopulations of interneurons, has also been identified *(83)*. The STN projections to the GPe, SNc, striatum, and PPN *(3)* are additional indirect pathways through which cortical information flows to reach basal ganglia output structures (*see* below). Although the exact functions of these connections remain unknown, it should be kept in mind that the circuitry of the basal ganglia outlined in the original model of direct and indirect pathways is, by necessity, an oversimplification *(3)*.

3.4. *Parallel Pathways through Pallido-Subthalamo-Pallidal Loops*

The connections between the GPe and the STN as well as the relationships between these structures and the GPi have been the subject of many studies that aimed at elucidating how the indirect pathways influence neurons of the output structures of the basal ganglia. The GPe gives rise to a massive, topographically organized projection, which terminates throughout the entire extent of the STN in monkeys *(3,84)*. The main projection sites of the STN are the GPe, GPi, and SNr *(3,73)*. Like most other basal ganglia components, the STN comprises segregated sensorimotor, associative, and limbic territories *(85)*. However, double anterograde tracing experiments showed that there are significant zones of overlap of inputs from functionally diverse regions of the pallidal complex in rats *(86)*. In contrast to GPi/SNr neurons where GPe terminals are confined to their proximal part, the pallidosubthalamic boutons form symmetric synapses with all parts of STN neurons (Fig. 3). In many cases, the receiving STN neurons project back to the GPe indicating the reciprocal relationships between the GPe and STN *(3,8,84)*.

New insights into the connections between the GPe and the STN as well as the relationships between these structures and the GPi have recently been provided *(84)*. On one hand, the neuronal network connecting the STN, GPe, and GPi has been examined using the anterograde and retrograde transport of biotinylated dextran amine *(84)*. The findings of this study demonstrated that interconnected neurons of the GPe and the STN innervate, via axon collaterals, functionally related neurons in the GPi *(84)*. Thus, populations of neurons within the sensorimotor, cognitive, and limbic territories in the GPe are reciprocally connected with populations of neurons in the same functional territories of the STN. In turn, neurons in each of these regions innervate the same functional territory of the GPi. Additional organizational principles that do not respect the functional topography of the direct and indirect network, but rather underlie a system for integration of functionally diverse information was also reported in this and other studies *(3,8,86,87)*. It is also important to keep in mind that all GPe neurons do not project only to the STN and vice-versa. Recent single axon-tracing studies, indeed, revealed the presence of different types of neurons in GPe and STN based on their axonal projections *(88)*. GPe neurons were found to project to: 1) GPi, STN, and SNr; 2) GPi and STN; 3) STN and SNr; and 4) striatum. None of the neurons examined projects to the STN only. Similarly, five types of STN neurons have been identified: 1) neurons projecting to GPe, GPi, and SNr; 2) neurons projecting to GPe and GPi; 3) neurons projecting to GPe and SNr; 4) neurons projecting only to GPe; and 5) neurons projecting to the striatum *(88)*. Altogether, these data highlight the heterogeneity and complex patterns of projections of the GPe and STN in primates.

4. THE SUBTHALAMIC NUCLEUS: ANOTHER ENTRANCE TO THE BASAL GANGLIA CIRCUITRY

4.1. *Intrinsic Organization*

The STN is particularly well-developed in primates. It is a highly vascularized and densely populated structure, encapsulated by major myelinated fiber bundles, the zona incerta, and the cerebral

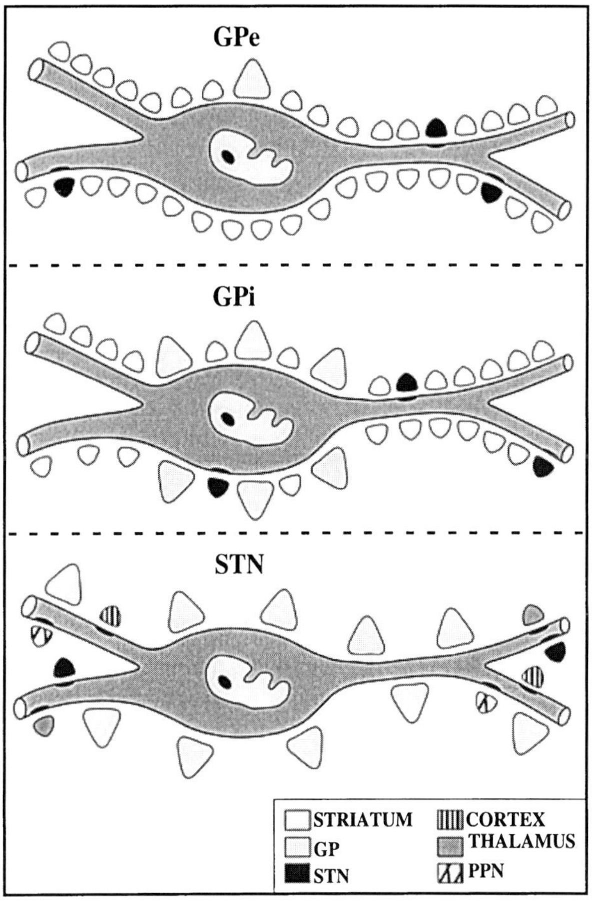

Fig. 3. Schematic drawings of the pattern of innervation of neurons in both segments of the globus pallidus and subthalamic nucleus based on data obtained in monkeys using anterograde tracers and postembedding immunogold for GABA and glutamate. The relative size and proportion of each category of terminals are represented. The major difference between GPe and GPi is that GPi neurons receive strong somatic inputs from GPe, whereas striatal and subthalamic terminals are evenly distributed on GPe and GPi neurons. (Modified with permission from ref. *3*.)

peduncle. It is noteworthy that a large number of myelinated axons, which likely convey ascending and descending information, also travel through the STN *(89,90)*. Most neurons of the STN belong to a single population of cells with spindle-shaped, pyramidal, or round perikarya *(91)*. Its principal elements are projection neurons whose dendrites can extend for more than 750 µm *(92)*. Each STN neuron gives rise to six or seven stem dendrites that branch in an ellipsoidal domain parallel to the rostrocaudal axis of the nucleus *(91)*. The existence of interneurons in the STN is controversial *(91–93)*. Although Rafols and Fox originally proposed that the monkey STN contained a population of small interneurons *(92)*, subsequent Golgi studies in cats, monkeys, and humans concluded that the STN was a relatively homogeneous structure largely composed of projection neurons *(91)*. These early findings were later supported by intracellular labeling experiments showing that the axons of all labeled STN neurons could be traced beyond the boundaries of the nucleus in rats *(94)*. Interestingly, more than half of these projection neurons had intranuclear axon collaterals that extended outside the dendritic domains of the parent neurons suggesting that they may serve as a feedforward circuit in the STN *(94)*. Such intrinsic axon collateral systems do not seem to be as extensive in primates *(91,95)*.

4.2. *The Corticosubthalamic Projection*

As is the case for the striatum, the STN also receives excitatory glutamatergic projections from the cerebral cortex *(3,8,85)*. In primates, the cortico-subthalamic projection is exclusively ipsilateral and arises principally from the primary motor cortex (area 4), with a minor contribution of prefrontal and premotor cortices. The somatosensory and visual cortical areas do not project to the STN, whereas they project quite substantially to the striatum *(3,8)*. In rats, the cortico-subthalamic projection originates mainly from pyramidal layer V neurons that also project to the striatum *(96)*. In both rats and monkeys, the cortico-subthalamic projection is topographically organized: 1) afferents from the primary motor cortex (M1) are confined to the dorsolateral part of the STN; 2) the premotor (areas 8, 9, and 6), the supplementary motor area (SMA), the presupplementary motor area, and adjacent frontal cortical areas innervate mainly the medial third of the nucleus *(97)*; and 3) the prefrontal-limbic cortices project to the medialmost tip of the nucleus *(3,85)*. By virtue of its cortical inputs, the dorsolateral sector of the STN is more specifically involved in the control of skeletomotor behavior, whereas the ventromedial part is more concerned with oculomotor and associative functions *(3,85)*. Like cortical afferents to the striatum, the cortico-subthalamic projection from M1 is somatotopically organized; the face area projects laterally, the arm area centrally, and the leg area medially *(98,99)*. Interestingly, the arrangement of somatotopical representations from the SMA to the medial STN is reversed against the ordering from the M1 to the lateral STN in macaque monkeys *(98)*. Therefore, the cerebral cortex imposes a specific functional segregation not only on the striatum, but also at the level of the STN *(99)*. However, it is worth noting that STN neurons have long dendrites that may cross boundaries of functional territories imposed by cortical projections in rats *(86)*. This anatomical arrangement opens up the possibility for some functionally segregated information at the level of the cerebral cortex to converge on individual STN neurons in rodents.

4.3. *The Thalamosubthalamic Projection*

Another major source of excitatory inputs to the STN are the caudal intralaminar thalamic nuclei *(100)*. The thalamosubthalamic projection respects the functional organization of the STN, i.e., sensorimotor neurons in CM terminate preferentially in the dorsolateral part of the nucleus whereas limbic- and associative-related neurons in PF project almost exclusively to the medial STN *(41,100)*. In rats, the thalamosubthalamic projection is excitatory and tonically drives the activity of STN neurons *(100)*. The degree of collateralization of thalamostriatal and thalamosubthalamic neurons is controversial. A retrograde double-labeling study indicated that the thalamosubthalamic and thalamostriatal projections arise largely from segregated sets of PF neurons in rats *(96)*, whereas single-cell labeling data showed that some PF neurons that project to the striatum send axon collaterals to the STN *(101)*.

Even if cortical and thalamic inputs are relatively sparse and terminate exclusively on the distal dendrites and spines of STN neurons *(102)*, electrophysiological experiments showed that activation of these inputs results in very strong short latency monosynaptic excitatory postsynaptic potentials (EPSP) with multiple spikes in STN neurons, which in turn transmit their information to basal ganglia output structures much faster than striatofugal pathways *(103–106)*.

These observations emphasize the importance of the STN in the functional organization of the basal ganglia and strongly suggest that it may serve as another entrance for extrinsic inputs to basal ganglia circuitry. Although the exact role of these projections remains to be established, electrophysiological evidence indicates that they might be important in the formation of a center-surround organization in GPi and SNr to help focusing pertinent information during voluntary movements *(107)*.

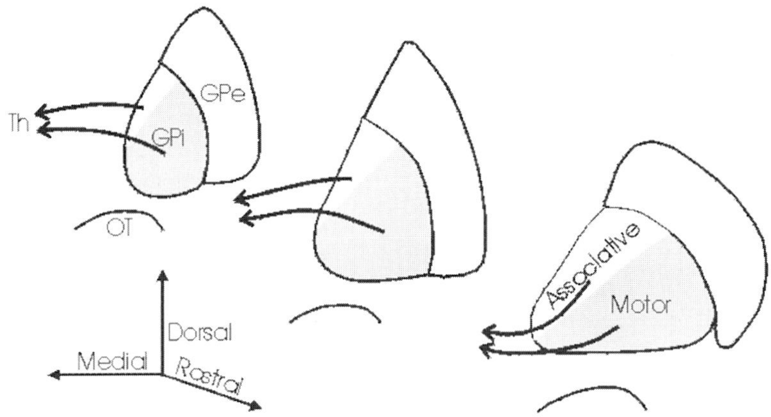

Fig. 4. Schematic diagram illustrating the course of motor and associative pallidothalamic projections originating in the caudal two-thirds of GPi (Modified with permission from ref. *110*.)

5. THE BASAL GANGLIA OUTFLOW

5.1. Pallidofugal Projections

5.1.1. The Pallidothalamic Projection

The pallidothalamic projection is topographically organized and its fibers arborize largely in the ventral anterior/ventral lateral (VA/VL) nuclei *(4,108)*. Earlier investigations of the origin of pallidothalamic fibers in the monkey, using degenerative methods, indicate that pallidothalamic fibers that travel via the ansa lenticularis and the lenticular fasciculus arise from specific portions of the GPi *(109,109a)*. According to the generally accepted scheme of pallidothalamic outflow, fibers of the ansa lenticularis arise predominantly from GPi cells located lateral to the accessory medullary laminae, which course rostrally, ventrally, and medially in the GPi. On the other hand, fibers of the lenticular fasciculus are thought to arise largely from cells in the inner part of GPi, which course dorsally and medially across the internal capsule to reach the thalamus *(109,109a)*. This scheme was recently challenged by new anatomical data obtained after injections of anterograde tracers in specific functional parts of the squirrel monkey GPi *(110)*. According to these data, the pallidothalamic fibers originating form the caudal portion of the GPi, including the motor territory, do not course ventromedially to form the ansa lenticularis, but rather, travel predominantly medially through the lenticular fasciculus en route to the thalamus. Fibers coursing below the ventral border of the pallidum in the so-called ansa lenticularis originates mostly from cells located in the rostral half of GPi *(110)* (Fig. 4). This scheme is much simpler than that currently accepted, which implies that fibers coursing through the ansa lenticularis frequently follow lengthy courses through the GPi to reach the thalamus. Therefore, the separate designation of the pallidothalamic pathways into ansa lenticularis and fasciculus lenticularis based on the location of GPi cells relative to the accessory medullary laminae is misleading and should be used with caution. This delineation is critical toward effective surgical treatment of various movement disorders *(110)*.

Efferent projections from the sensorimotor GPi remain largely segregated from the associative and limbic projections at the level of the thalamus. In squirrel monkeys, the sensorimotor GPi outputs are directed towards the posterior VL (VLp), whereas the associative and limbic GPi innervate preferentially the parvocellular VA (VApc) and the dorsal VL (VLd). The ventromedial nucleus receives inputs from the limbic GPi only *(108)*. These findings, therefore, reveal that some associative and limbic cortical information, which is largely processed in segregated cortico-striatopallidal channels,

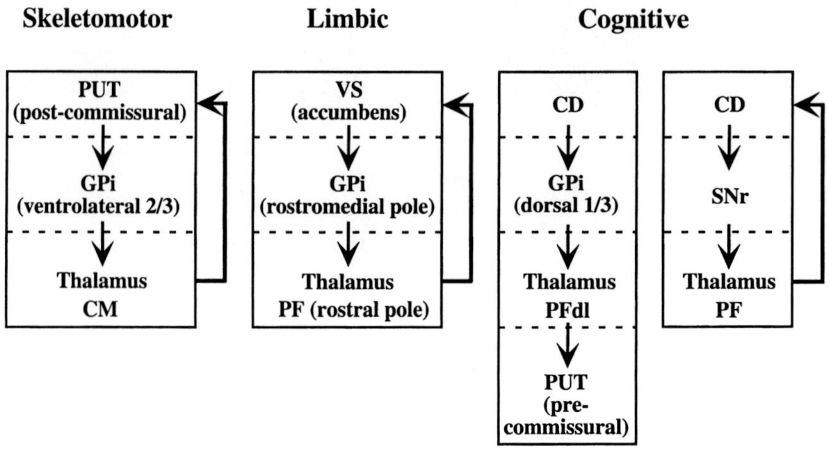

Fig. 5. Schematic diagram illustrating the synaptic interactions between basal ganglia and thalamostriatal neurons in monkeys. These data were obtained following simultaneous injections of retrograde tracers in different functional territories of the striatum and anterograde tracers in the corresponding functional regions of GPi or SNr. Note that the caudal intralaminar thalamic nuclei and the basal ganglia are interconnected by both open and closed loops.

converge to common thalamic nuclei in monkeys. It is noteworthy that about 10–20% of pallidothalamic neurons in the monkey GPi project to the contralateral VA/VL *(4,111,112)*.

Most pallidal neurons that project to thalamic motor nuclei send axon collaterals to the caudal intralaminar nuclei *(4,112,112a)*. These branched neurons are located in the central portion of GPi *(112)*. Pallidal axons arising from the sensorimotor GPi terminate in CM where they form synapses with thalamostriatal neurons projecting back to the sensorimotor territory of the striatum *(30,108)* (Fig. 5). In contrast, associative inputs from the GPi terminate massively in the dorsolateral extension of PF (PFdl), which does not project back to the caudate nucleus but rather innervates preferentially the precommissural region of the putamen (Fig. 5). Finally, the limbic GPi innervates selectively the rostrodorsal part of PF, which in turn projects back to the nucleus accumbens *(28,32)*. Therefore it appears that CM/PF is part of closed and open functional loops with the striatopallidal complex (Fig. 5).

5.1.2. The Pallidotegmental Projection

The pallidotegmental fibers terminate in the PPN, which is composed of two major subdivisions, the pars compacta and the pars diffusa *(114,118)*. Studies in monkeys indicate that more than 80% of GPi neurons projecting to the PPN send axon collaterals to the ventral thalamus *(112)*. The PPN gives rise to descending projections to the pons, medulla, and spinal cord as well as ascending projections to the thalamus and basal ganglia *(115–117)*. Thus, the pallidotegmental projection may be a route by which cortical information can reach lower motor and autonomic centers. Another possibility could be that PPN acts as an important interface between different functional territories of the GPi and sends back the processed information to the basal ganglia *(118)* (Fig. 6).

The pattern of distribution of functionally segregated pallidofugal information in the PPN has been investigated in monkeys *(118)*. The results of this study are summarized in Fig. 6. Injections of anterograde tracers in different functional territories of the GPi led to anterograde labeling, which largely converges to common regions of the pars diffusa of the PPN. The fibers that arise from the associative and limbic territories of the GPi are more widely spread than the afferents from the sensorimotor territory. Another major finding of this study was that pallidal fibers largely avoid cholinergic neurons in the pars compacta of the PPN *(118)*. These anatomical data suggest that the pars diffusa of the

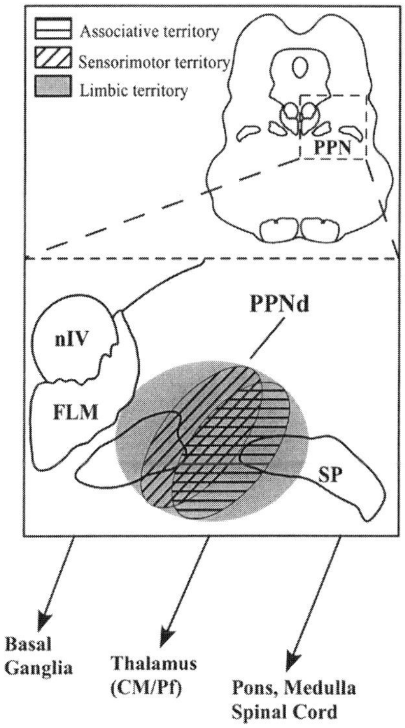

Fig. 6. Schematic drawing showing the location of anterogradely labeled fibers in the pedunculopontine tegmental nucleus (PPN) after injections of anterograde tracers in the associative, sensorimotor, and limbic terr-itories of the internal segment of the globus pallidus (GPi). Note that projections from the different functional territories of GPi largely overlap in the PPN. FLM: Medial longitudinal fasciculus; SP: Superior cerebellar peduncle. (Modified with permission from ref. *118*.)

PPN is the potential site for the integration of information arising from different functional territories of the GPi in primates (Fig. 6).

5.1.3. The Pallidohabenular Projection

In contrast to the pallidothalamic and pallidotegmental projections, which are largely collateralized, the pallidohabenular projection arises from a distinct population of neurons in the monkey GPi *(112)*. In rats, pallidohebenular neurons are located in the rostral part of the entopeduncular nucleus, whereas pallidothalamic and pallidotegmental projections arise preferentially from the caudal half of the nucleus *(119–121)*. Interestingly, pallidohabenular cells receive afferents from striatofugal neurons in the patch compartment, whereas pallidothalamic and pallidotegmental neurons are innervated by striatal neurons in the matrix compartment *(120)*. The ventral pallidum also contributes to the pallidohabenular projection in rats and cats *(122,123)*. In primates, retrograde labeling studies showed that pallidohabenular neurons are far less numerous than pallidothalamic cells and are mainly confined to a peri-GPi region, which extends medially in the lateral hypothalamus *(112,124)*. More recent studies in squirrel monkeys using sensitive anterograde labeling methods demonstrated that the pallidohabenular projection is functionally organized and more massive than previously thought *(125, 126)*. The sensorimotor GPi innervates preferentially the centrolateral part of the lateral habenular nucleus, whereas the limbic and associative GPi project massively to the medial part of the nucleus *(125)*. The pallidohabenular projection is mainly GABAergic though cholinergic neurons in the entopeduncular nucleus also contribute to this projection in rats *(125,127,128)*. Because of its prominent connections with various limbic structures, the lateral habenula is considered as a functional interface between the limbic system and basal ganglia.

5.2. Nigrofugal Projections

5.2.1. The Nigrothalamic Projection

The GPi and SNr are considered as the two main output nuclei of the basal ganglia that project massively to the ventral thalamus and brainstem nuclei. Overall, SNr and GPi afferents to the ventral thalamus are largely segregated, but in nonprimates, the ventromedial nucleus receives convergent inputs from both basal ganglia output structures and the cerebellum *(130)*. In monkeys, the nigrothalamic cells are distributed throughout the mediolateral extent of the SNr and form the largest population of nigrofugal neurons *(131)*. Inputs from the medial part of the SNr terminate mostly in the medial magnocellular division of the VA (VAmc) and the mediodorsal nucleus (MDmc) that, in turn, innervate anterior regions of the frontal lobe including the principal sulcus and the orbital cortex *(132)*. Neurons in the lateral part of the SNr project preferentially to the lateral posterior region of the VAmc and to different parts of MD mostly related to posterior regions of the frontal lobe, including the frontal eye field areas of the premotor cortex *(132)*. In rats, a lamellar organization of nigrofugal neurons has been proposed as the main constituent for the parallel processing of information flow through the SNr *(133,133a)*. According to this model, functionally segregated striatal neurons project to different lamella of SNr neurons, which in turn convey the information to different thalamic nuclei *(133,133a)*. The dendrites of individual SNr neurons largely conform to the geometry of striatonigral projections, which strongly supports the concept of a parallel architecture of striatonigral circuits *(133a)*.

SNr neurons also project to rostral and caudal intralaminar thalamic nuclei *(132–134)*. In monkeys, the nigro-intralaminar thalamic projection terminates exclusively in PF where nigral boutons form GABAergic synapses with thalamostriatal neurons that project to the caudate nucleus *(132,134)*.

5.2.2. The Nigrotegmental Projection

The nigrotegmental projection displays a dorsoventral topography and terminates preferentially on noncholinergic neurons in the medial twothirds of the PPN pars diffusa in rats *(133,135,136)*. A much smaller number of nigral fibers innervate cholinergic neurons in the PPN pars compacta *(136)*. In monkeys, the cells that give rise to the nigrotegmental projection are found throughout the mediolateral extent of the SNr and form the second largest population of SNr nigrofugal neurons *(131)*. Most nigrotegmental cells send axon collaterals to the ventral anterior thalamic nucleus *(131,133)* and receive direct inputs from the striatum *(137)*. The pattern of distribution and postsynaptic targets of nigrotegmental neurons remains to be established in primates.

5.2.3. The Nigrocollicular Projection

The SNr sends a massive and topographically organized GABAergic projection to the intermediate layer of the superior colliculus *(131,133,138)*. The nigral terminals form distinctive clusters in the deep and intermediate layers of the superior colliculus where they innervate neurons that project to the spinal cord, medulla, and periabducens area *(138–140)*. This projection plays an important role in a variety of visual and auditory responses that control saccadic eye movements toward a stimulus. This is consistent with the fact that SNr receiving neurons of the intermediate layer of the superior colliculus are targeted by visual inputs from the cortex and project to brainstem regions that control eye movements *(141)*.

5.2.4. The Nigroreticular Projection

The SNr also sends projections to the medullary reticular formation *(142,143)*. In rats, this projection arises from a population of neurons in the dorsolateral SNr and terminates in the parvicellular reticular formation *(143)*. Identified nigroreticular neurons receive GABAergic inputs from the striatum and the globus pallidus *(144)*. This projection is thought to play a role in orofacial movements because the SNr-receiving neurons of the reticular formation are directly connected with orofacial motor nuclei *(145,146)*.

6. THE PEDUNCULOPONTINE NUCLEUS: AN INTEGRAL PART OF THE BASAL GANGLIA CIRCUITRY

Many lines of anatomical and electrophysiological evidence indicate that the PPN is reciprocally connected with the basal ganglia *(155–157)*. As discussed earlier, the PPN receives substantial projections from the GPi and SNr *(118,135,136)*. An input from the STN has also been demonstrated *(73, 74)*. In turn, the PPN sends ascending projections to all basal ganglia nuclei. In rats and primates, the SNc and the STN are, by far, the most densely innervated basal ganglia structures by PPN efferents *(75,147–150)*. Both glutamate and acetylcholine are used as neurotransmitter by these projections *(150–153)*. The PPN innervation of the pallidal complex is not as dense as that of the STN and SNc, arborizes preferentially in the GPi and uses both glutamate and acetylcholine as neurotransmitters *(75,152–154)*. A light pedunculostriatal projection has also been described in rats *(147)* and monkeys *(75)*, but the chemical nature of this projection is still unknown. Taken into consideration these tight interconnections with basal ganglia structures combined with prominent descending projections to pontine, medullary, and spinal structures, the PPN is considered as a possible relay station where the striatum meets the reticular formation and the spinal cord *(115–117)*.

The PPN also sends massive cholinergic and noncholinergic projections to various thalamic nuclei *(155–158)*. These projections play a major role in mediating cortical desynchronization during waking and rapid eye movement (REM) sleep *(116,159,160)*. Cholinergic and glutamatergic PPN inputs to thalamostriatal neurons have been demonstrated *(134,161,162)*. It is interesting to note that a subpopulation of PPN neurons innervate simultaneously the basal ganglia and thalamic regions via axon collaterals *(163)*. These findings suggest that the PPN conveys information to the basal ganglia not only directly, but also indirectly via thalamostriatal neurons. Therefore, the PPN occupies a strategic position that allows modulation of neuronal activity in functional basal ganglia-thalamocortical and thalamostriatal loops. The fact that there is a significant loss of PPN neurons in parkinsonians, and that lesion of PPN results in akinesia and postural instabilities are further evidence that the PPN plays a major role in basal ganglia circuitry in both normal and pathological conditions *(117)*.

7. CONCLUDING REMARKS

Our knowledge of the basal ganglia anatomy has increased tremendously over the past 10 years, mainly owing to the introduction of highly sophisticated and sensitive tract-tracing and immunocytochemical methods suitable for light and electron microscope analysis. In this review, we highlighted recent anatomical data that has led us to reconsider some aspects of the functional circuitry of the basal ganglia.

For instance, the thalamostriatal projection, which is largely neglected in functional models of the basal ganglia connections, deserves more attention. This projection is massive and follows a highly specific pattern of functional connectivity with the striatopallidal complex. The fact that thalamic inputs are directed preferentially towards specific populations of striatal projection neurons and interneurons strongly suggests that these inputs may play a major role in the basal ganglia circuitry. The recent demonstration that thalamostriatal projections from CM/PF supply striatal neurons with information about behaviorally significant sensory events *(164)* further emphasize the importance of this projection in the functional circuitry of the basal ganglia.

Another important concern raised over the past few years relates to the validity of the direct and indirect pathways of the basal ganglia. The evidence that subpopulations of striatofugal neurons express both D1 and D2 dopamine receptors combined with the fact that striatofugal neurons are more collateralized than previously thought led to reconsider the concept that direct and indirect striatofugal pathways arise from segregated populations of striatal projection neurons. However, despite these anatomical complexities of the basal ganglia circuitry, it is clear that the "relatively simple" functional model of direct and indirect pathways still remains the most appropriate working framework for understanding changes in the basal ganglia circuitry and develop novel therapeutic strategies for movement disorders.

Another critical aspect that should deserve attention in the future is the relative importance of the STN and the striatum as major entrances of cortical information to the basal ganglia. Although the striatum receives much more massive inputs from the cerebral cortex and thalamus than the STN, the fact that the information flowing through the corticosubthalamic projection reach the output structures of the basal ganglia faster than that traveling through the striatum deserves consideration.

Finally, more attention should definitely be paid at the PPN as an integral component of the basal ganglia and a potential target for the development of new therapies for Parkinson's disease.

ACKNOWLEDGMENTS

The authors acknowledge Jean-François Paré for his skilfull technical assistance. This work was supported by NIH grants R01-37423, R01-37948 and RR 00165.

REFERENCES

1. Albin, R. L., Young, A. B., and Penney, J. B. (1989) The functional anatomy of basal ganglia disorders. *Trends Neurosci.* **12,** 366–375.
2. DeLong, M. R. (1990) Primate models of movement disorders of basal ganglia origin. *Trends Neurosci.* **13,** 281–285.
3. Smith, Y., Bevan, M. D., Shink, E., and Bolam, J. P. (1998) Microcircuitry of the direct and indirect pathways of the basal ganglia. *Neuroscience* **86,** 353–387.
4. Parent, A. and Hazrati, L.-N. (1995) Functional anatomy of the basal ganglia. I. The cortico-basal ganglia-thalamo-cortical loop. *Brain Res. Rev.* **20,** 91–127.
5. Alexander, G. E. and DeLong, M. R. (1985) Microstimulation of the primate neostriatum. II. Somatotopic of striatal microexcitable zones and their relations to neuronal response properties. *J. Neurophysiol.* **53,** 1417–1430.
6. Gerfen, C. R. and Wilson, C. J. (1996) The basal ganglia. In: *Handbook of Chemical Neuroanatomy, Integrated Systems of the CNS, Part III* (Björklund, A., Hökfelt, T., and Swanson, L., eds.), Elsevier, Amsterdam, pp. 369–466.
7. Wilson, C. J. (1998) Basal Ganglia. In: *The Synaptic Organization of the Brain* (Shepherd, G. M., ed.), Oxford University Press, New York, NY, pp. 329–375.
8. Smith, Y., Shink E., and Sidibé M. (1998) Neuronal circuitry and synaptic connectivity of the basal ganglia. In: *Neurosurgery Clinics of North America* (Bakay, A. E., ed.), W.B. Saunders, Philadelphia, PA, pp. 203–222.
9. Flaherty, A. W. and Graybiel, A. M. (1991) Corticostriatal transformation in the primate somatosensory system. Projections from physiologically mapped body-part representations. *J. Neurophysiol.* **66,** 1249–1263.
10. Flaherty, A. W. and Graybiel, A. M. (1993) Two input systems for body representations in the primate striatal matrix: experimental evidence in the squirrel monkey. *J. Neurosci.* **13,** 1120–1137.
11. Parthasarathy, H. B., Schall, J. D., and Graybiel, A. M. (1992) Distributed but convergent ordering of corticostriatal projections: analysis of the frontal eye field and the supplementary eye field in the macaque monkey. *J. Neurosci.* **12,** 4468–4488.
12. Selemon, L. D. and Goldman-Rakic, P. S. (1990) Longitudinal topography and interdigitation of corticostriatal projections in the rhesus monkey. *J. Neurosci.* **5,** 776–794.
13. Cowan, R. L. and Wilson, C.J. (1994) Spontaneous firing patterns and axonal projections of single corticostriatal neurons in the rat medial agranular cortex. *J. Neurophysiol.* **71,** 17–32.
14. Kincaid, A. E., Zheng, T., and Wilson, C. J. (1998) Connectivity and convergence of single corticostriatal axons. *J. Neurosci.* **18,** 4722–4731.
15. Wilson, C. J. (1995) The contribution of cortical neurons to the firing pattern of striatal spiny neurons. In: *Models of Information Processing in the Basal Ganglia* (Houk, J. C., Davis, J. L., and Beiser, D. G., eds.), The MIT Press, Cambridge, MA, pp. 29–50.
16. Paré, D. and Smith, Y. (1996) Thalamic collaterals of corticostriatal axons: their termination field and synaptic targets in cats. *J. Comp. Neurol.* **372,** 551–567.
17. Lévesque, M., Gagnon, S., Parent, A., and Deschênes, M. (1996) Axonal arborizations of corticostriatal and cortico-thalamic fibers arising from the second somatosensory area in the rat. *Cereb. Cortex* **6,** 759–770.
18. Smith, A. D. and Bolam, J. P. (1990) The neural network of the basal ganglia as revealed by the study of synaptic connections of identified neurons. *Trends Neurosci.* **13,** 259–265.
19. Kawaguchi, Y., Wilson, C. J., Augood, S. J., and Emson, P. C. (1995) Striatal interneurons: chemical, physiological and morphological characterization. *Trends Neurosci.* **18,** 527–535.
20. Cicchetti, F., Prensa, L., Wu, Y., and Parent, A. (2001) Chemical anatomy of striatal interneurons in normal individuals and in patients with Huntington's disease. *Brain Res. Rev.* **34,** 80–101.
21. Bennett, B. D. and Bolam, J. P. (1993) Two populations of calbindin D28k-immunoreactive neurons in the striatum of the rat. *Brain Res.* **610,** 305–310.

22. Lapper, S. R., Smith, Y., Sadikot, A. F., Parent, A., and Bolam, J. P. (1992) Cortical input to parvalbumin-immunoreactive neurons in the putamen of the squirrel monkey. *Brain Res.* **580,** 215–224.
23. Lapper, S. R. and Bolam, J. P. (1992) Input from the frontal cortex and the parafascicular nucleus to cholinergic interneurons in the dorsal striatum of the rat. *Neuroscience* **51,** 533–545.
24. Meredith, G. E. and Wouterlood, F. G. (1990) Hippocampal and midline thalamic fibers and terminals in relation to the choline acetyltransferase-immunoreactive neurons in nucleus accumbens of the rat: a light and electron microscopic study. *J. Comp. Neurol.* **296,** 204–221.
25. Thomas, T. M, Smith, Y., Levey, A. I., and Hersch, S. M. (2000) Cortical inputs to m2-immunoreactive striatal interneurons in rat and monkey. *Synapse* **37,** 252–261.
26. Wilson, C. J., Chang, H. T., and Kitai, S. T. (1990) Firing patterns and synaptic potentials of identified giant aspiny interneurons in the rat neostriatum. *J. Neurosci.* **10,** 508–519.
27. Groenewegen, H. J. and Berendse, H. W. (1994) The specificity of the nonspecific midline and intralaminar thalamic nuclei. *Trends Neurosci.* **17,** 52–57.
28. Sadikot, A. F., Parent, A., Smith, Y., and Bolam, J. P. (1992) Efferent connections of the centromedian and parafascicular nuclei in the squirrel monkey: a light and electron microscopic study of the thalamostriatal projection in relation to striatal heterogeneity. *J. Comp. Neurol.* **320,** 228–242.
29. Sidibé, M. and Smith, Y. (1996) Differential synaptic innervation of striatofugal neurons projecting to the internal or external segments of the globus pallidus by thalamic afferents in the squirrel monkey. *J. Comp. Neurol.* **365,** 445–465.
30. Sidibé, M., Paré, J.-L., and Smith, Y. (2002) Nigral and pallidal inputs to functionally segregated thalamostriatal neurons in the centromedian/parafascicular intralaminar nuclear complex in monkey. *J. Comp Neurol.* **447(3),** 286–299.
31. Groenewegen, H. J. and Berendse, H. W. (1994) The specificity of the nonspecific midline and intralaminar thalamic nuclei. *Trends Neurosci.* **17,** 52–57.
32. Giménez-Amaya, J. M., McFarland, N. R., De Las Heras, S., and Haber, S. N. (1995) Organization of thalamic projections to the ventral striatum in the primate. *J. Comp. Neurol.* **354,** 127–149.
33. Smith, Y. and Parent, A. (1986) Differential connections of the caudate nucleus and putamen in squirrel monkeys (*Saimiri sciureus*). *Neuroscience* **18,** 347–371.
34. McFarland, N. R. and Haber, S. N. (2001) Organization of thalamostriatal terminals from the ventral motor nuclei in the macaque. *J. Comp. Neurol.* **429,** 321–336.

34a. Lin, C.-S., May, P. J., and Hall, W. C. (1984) Nonintralaminar thalamostriatal projection sin the gray squirrel (*Sciureus carolinensis*) and tree shrew (*Tupaia glis*). *J. Comp. Neurol.* **230,** 33–46.

35. McFarland, N. R. and Haber, S. N. (2000) Convergent inputs from thalamic motor nuclei and frontal cortical areas to the dorsal striatum in the primate. *J. Neurosci.* **20,** 3798–3813.
36. Rasminsky, M., Mauro, A., and Albe-fessard, D. (1973) Projections of medial thalamic nuclei to the putamen and frontal cerebral cortex in the cat. *Brain Res.* **61,** 69–77.
37. Jinnai, K. and Matsuda, Y. (1979) Neurons of the motor cortex projecting commonly on the caudate nucleus and the lower brain stem in the cat. *Neurosci. Lett.* **26,** 95–99.
38. Royce, G. J. (1983) Single thalamic neurons which project to both the rostral cortex and caudate nucleus studied with the fluorescent double labeling method. *Exp. Neurol.* **79,** 773–784.
39. Macchi, G., Bentivoglio, M., Molinari, M., and Minciacchi, D. (1984) The thalamo-caudate versus thalamo-cortical projections as studied in the cat with fluorescent retrograde double labeling. *Exp. Brain Res.* **54,** 225–239.
40. Deschênes, M., Bourassa, J., and Parent, A. (1996) Striatal and cortical projections of single neurons from the central lateral thalamic nucleus in the rat. *Neuroscience* **72,** 679–687.
41. Sadikot, A. F., Parent, A., and François, C. (1992) Efferent connections of the centromedian and parafascicular thalamic nuclei in the squirrel monkey: a PHA-L study of subcortical projections. *J. Comp. Neurol.* **315,** 137–159.
42. Dubé, L., Smith, A. D., and Bolam, J. P. (1988) Identification of synaptic terminals of thalamic and cortical origin in contact with distinct medium-sized spiny neurons in the rat neostriatum. *J Comp. Neurol.* **267,** 455–471.
43. Xu, Z. C., Wilson, C. J., and Emson, P. C. (1991) Restoration of thalamostriatal projections in rat neostriatal grafts: an electron microscopic analysis. *J. Comp. Neurol.* **303,** 22–34.
44. Sidibé, M. and Smith, Y. (1999) Thalamic inputs to striatal interneurons in monkeys: synaptic organization and co-localization of calcium binding proteins. *Neuroscience* **89,** 1189–1208.
45. Rudkin, T. M. and Sadikot, A. F. (1999) Thalamic inputs to parvalbumin-immunoreactive GABAergic interneurons: Organization in normal striatum and effect of neonatal decortication. *Neuroscience* **88,** 1165–1175.
46. Rodríguez, M. and González-Hernández, T. (1999) Electrophysiological and morphological evidence for a GABAergic projection nigrostriatal pathway. *J. Neurosci.* **19,** 4682–4694.
47. Gerfen, C. R., Herkenham, M., and Thibault, J. (1987) The neostriatal mosaic: II. Patch- and matrix-directed mesostriatal dopaminergic and non-dopaminergic systems. *J. Neurosci.* **7,** 3915–3934.

47a. Prensa, L. and Parent, A. (2001) The nigrostriatal pathway in the rat: a single-axon study of the relationship between dorsal and ventral tier nigral neurons and the striosome/matrix striatal compartments. *J. Neurosci.* **21,** 7247–7260.

48. Hanley, J. J. and Bolam, J. P. (1997) Synaptology of the nigrostriatal projection in relation to the compartmental organization of the neostriatum in the rat. *Neuroscience* **81,** 353–370.
49. Steffensen, S. C., Svingos, A. L., Pickel, V. M., and Henriksen, S. J. (1998) Electrophysiological characterization of GABAergic neurons in the ventral tegmental area. *J. Neurosci.* **18,** 8003–8013.
50. Sulzer, D., Joyce, M. P., Lin, L., Geldwert, D., Haber, S. N., Hattori, T., and Rayport, S. (1998) Dopamine neurons make glutamatergic synapses in vitro. *J. Neurosci.* **18,** 4588–4602.

51. Joyce, M. P. and Rayport, S. (2000) Mesoaccumbens dopamine neuron synapses reconstructed in vitro are glutamatergic. *Neuroscience* **99,** 445–456.
52. Joel, D. and Weiner, I. (2000) The connections of the dopaminergic system with the striatum in rats and primates: an analysis with respect to the functional and compartmental organization of the striatum. *Neuroscience* **96,** 451–474.
53. Smith, Y. and Kieval, J. Z. (2000) Anatomy of the dopamine system in the basal ganglia. *Trends Neurosci.* **23,** S28–S33.
53a. Freeman, A., Ciliax, B., Bakay, R., Daley, J., Miller, R. D., Keating, G., Levey, A., and Rye, D. (2001) Nigrostriatal collaterals to thalamus degenerate in parkinsonian animal models. *Ann. Neurol.* **50,** 321–329.
54. Szabo, J. (1980) Organization of the ascending striatal afferents in monkeys. *J. Comp. Neurol.* **189,** 307–321.
55. Parent, A., Mackey, A., and De Bellefeuille, L. (1983) The subcortical afferents to caudate nucleus and putamen in primate: a fluorescence retrograde double labeling study. *Neuroscience* **10,** 1137–1150.
56. Lynd-Balta, E. and Haber, S. N. (1994) The organization of midbrain projections to the striatum in the primate: sensorimotor-related striatum versus ventral striatum. *Neuroscience* **59,** 625–640.
57. Lynd-Balta, E. and Haber, S. N. (1994) The organization of midbrain projections to the ventral striatum in the primate. *Neuroscience* **59,** 609–623.
58. Lavoie, B., Smith, Y., and Parent, A. (1989) Dopaminergic innervation of the basal ganglia in the squirrel monkey as revealed by tyrosine hydroxylase immunohistochemistry *J. Comp. Neurol.* **289,** 36–52.
59. Graybiel, A. M., Hirsch, E. C., and Agid, Y. A. (1987) Differences in tyrosine hydroxylase-like immunoreactivity characterize the mesostriatal innervation of striosomes and extrastriosomal matrix at maturity. *Proc. Natl. Acad. Sci. USA* **84,** 303–307.
60. Hökfelt, T., Martensson, R., Björklund, A., Kleinau, S., and Goldstein M. (1984) Distributional maps of tyrosine hydroxylase-immunoreactive neurons in the rat brain. In: *Handbook of Chemical Neuroanatomy. Vol. 2. Classical Transmitters in the CNS Part 1,* (Björklund, A. and Hökfelt T., eds.), Elsevier, Amsterdam, Netherlands, pp. 277–379.
61. Freund, T. F., Powell, J. F., and Smith, A. D. (1984) Tyrosine hydroxylase-immunoreactive boutons in synaptic contact with identified striatonigral neurons, with particular reference to dendritic spines. *Neuroscience* **13,** 1189–1215.
62. Smith, Y., Bennett, B. D., Bolam, J. P., Parent, A., and Sadikot, A. F. (1994) Synaptic relationships between dopaminergic afferents and cortical or thalamic input in the sensorimotor territory of the striatum in monkey. *J. Comp. Neurol.* **344,** 1–19.
63. Calabresi, P., Pisani, A., Mercuri, N. B., and Bernardi, G. (1996) The corticostriatal projection: from synaptic plasticity to dysfunctions of the basal ganglia. *Trends Neurosci.* **19,** 19–24.
64. Calabresi, P., De Murtas, M., and Bernardi, G. (1997) The neostriatum beyond the motor function: experimental and clinical evidence. *Neuroscience* **78,** 39–60.
65. Descarries, L., Watkins, K. C., Garcia, S., Bosler, O., and Doucet, G. (1996) Dual character, asynaptic and synaptic, of the dopamine innervation in adult rat neostriatum: a quantitative autoradiographic and immunocytochemical analysis. *J. Comp. Neurol.* **375,** 167–186.
66. Yung, K. K. L., Bolam, J. P., Smith, A. D., Hersch, S. M., Ciliax, B. J., and Levey, A. I. (1995) Immunocytochemical localization of D1 and D2 dopamine receptors in the basal ganglia of the rat: light and electron microscopy. *Neuroscience* **65,** 709–730.
67. Caillé, I., Dumartin, B., and Bloch, B. (1996) Ultrastructural localization of D1 dopamine receptor immunoreactivity in rat striatonigral neurons and its relation with dopaminergic innervation. *Brain Res.* **730,** 17–31.
68. Betarbet, R., Turner, R., Chockkan, V., DeLong, M. R., Allers, K. A., Walters, J., Levey, A. I., and Greenamyre, J. T. (1997) Dopaminergic neurons intrinsic to the primate striatum. *J. Neurosci.* **17,** 6761–6768.
69. Lavoie, B. and Parent, A. (1990) Immunohistochemical study of the serotoninergic innervation of the basal ganglia in the squirrel monkey. *J. Comp. Neurol.* **299,** 1–16.
70. Van der Kooy, D. and Hattori, T. (1980) Dorsal raphe cells with collateral projections to the caudate-putamen and substantia nigra: a fluorescent retrograde double labeling study in the rat. *Brain Res.* **186,** 1–7.
71. Pasik, P., Pasik, T., Holstein, G. R., and Pecci-Saavedra, J. (1984) Serotoninergic innervation of the monkey basal ganglia: an immunocytochemical study. In: *The Basal Ganglia: Structures and Function* (McKenzie, J. S., Kemm, R. E., and Wilcock, L.N., eds.), Plenum Press, New York, pp. 115–129.
72. Soghomonian, J. J., Descarries, L., and Watkins, K. C. (1989) Serotonin innervation in adult rat neostriatum. II. Ultrastructural features: a radioautographic and immunocytochemical study. *Brain Res.* **481,** 67–86.
73. Parent, A. and Smith, Y. (1987) Organization of efferent projections of the subthalamic nucleus in the squirrel monkey as revealed by retrograde labeling methods. *Brain Res.* **436,** 296–310.
74. Jackson, A. and Crossman, A. R. (1983) Nucleus tegmenti pedunculopontinus: Efferent connections with special reference to the basal ganglia, studied in the rat by anterograde and retrograde transport of horseradish peroxidase. *Neuroscience* **10,** 725–765.
75. Lavoie, B. and Parent, A. (1994) Pedunculopontine nucleus in the squirrel monkey: projections to the basal ganglia as revealed by anterograde tract-tracing methods. *J. Comp. Neurol.* **344,** 210–231.
76. Bergman, H., Wichmann, T., and DeLong, M. R. (1990) Reversal of experimental parkinsonism by lesions of the subthalamic nucleus. *Science* **249,** 1436–1438.
77. DeLong, M. R. (1990) Primate models of movement disorders of basal ganglia origin. *Trends Neurosci.* **13,** 281–285.
78. Kawaguchi, Y., Wilson, C. J., and Emson, P. C. (1990) Projection subtypes of rat neostriatal matrix cells revealed by intracellular injection of biocytin. *J. Neurosci.* **10,** 3421–3438.
79. Parent, A., Charara, A., and Pinault, D. (1995) Single striatofugal axons arborizing in both pallidal segments and in the substantia nigra in primate. *Brain Res.* **698,** 280–284.

80. Surmeier, D. J., Eberwine, J., Wilson, C. J., Cao, Y., Stefani, A., and Kitai, S. T. (1992) Dopamine receptor subtypes colocalize in rat striatonigral neurons. *Proc. Natl. Acad. Sci. USA* **89,** 10,178–10,182.
81. Aizman, O., Brismar, H., Uhlen, P., Zettergren, E., Levey, A. I., Forssberg, H., et al. (2000) Anatomical and physiological evidence for D1 and D2 dopamine receptor colocalization in neostriatal neurons. *Nat. Neurosci.* **3,** 226–230.
82. Surmeier, D. J., Song, W. J., and Yan, Z. (1996) Coordinated expression of dopamine receptors in neostriatal medium spiny neurons. *J. Neurosci.* **16,** 6579–6591.
83. Bevan, M. D., Booth, P. A., Eaton, S. A., and Bolam J. P. (1998) Selective innervation of neostriatal interneurons by a subclass of neurons in the globus pallidus of the rat. *J. Neurosci.* **18,** 9438–9452.
84. Shink, E., Bevan, M. D., Bolam, J. P., and Smith, Y. (1996) The subthalamic nucleus and the external pallidum: two tightly interconnected structures that control the output of the basal ganglia in the monkey. *Neuroscience* **73,** 335–357.
85. Parent, A. (1990) Extrinsic connections of the basal ganglia. *Trends Neurosci.* **13,** 254–258.
86. Bevan, M. D., Clarke, N. P., and Bolam, J. P. (1997) Synaptic integration of functionally diverse pallidal information in the entopeduncular nucleus and subthalamic nucleus in the rat. *J. Neurosci.* **17,** 308–324.
87. Joel, D. and Weiner, I. (1997) The connections of the primate subthalamic nucleus: indirect pathways and the open-interconnected scheme of basal ganglia-thalamocortical circuitry. *Brain Res. Rev.* **23,** 62–78.
88. Parent, A., Sato, F., Wu, Y., Gauthier, J., Lévesque, M., and Parent M. (2000) Organization of the basal ganglia: the importance of axonal collateralization. *Trends Neurosci.* **23,** S20–S27.
89. Hassler, R., Usunoff, K. G., Romansky, K. V., and Christ, J. F. (1982) Electron microscopy of the subthalamic nucleus in the baboon. I. Synaptic organization of the subthalamic nucleus in the baboon. *J. Hirnforsch.* **23,** 597–611.
90. Smith, Y., Bolam, J. P., and Von Krosigk, M. (1990) Topographical and synaptic organization of the GABA-containing pallidosubthalamic projection in the rat. *Eur. J. Neurosci.* **2,** 500–511.
91. Yelnik, J. and Percheron, G. (1979) Subthalamic neurons in primates: a quantitative and comparative analysis. *Neuroscience* **4,** 1717–1773.
92. Rafols, J. A. and Fox, C. A. (1976) The neurons in the primate subthalamic nucleus: a Golgi and electron microscopic study. *J. Comp. Neurol.* **168,** 75–111.
93. Iwahori, N. (1978) A Golgi study on the subthalamic nucleus of the cat. *J. Comp. Neurol.* **182,** 383–397.
94. Kita, H., Chang, H. T., and Kitai, S. T. (1983) The morphology of intracellularly labeled rat subthalamic neurons: a light microscopic analysis. *J. Comp. Neurol.* **215,** 245–257.
95. Sato, F., Parent, M., Levesque, M., and Parent, A. (2000) Axonal branching pattern of neurons of the subthalamic nucleus in primates. *J. Comp. Neurol.* **424,** 142–152.
96. Féger, J., Bevan, M., and Crossman, A. R. (1994) The projections from the parafascicular thalamic nucleus to the subthalamic nucleus and the striatum arise from separate neuronal populations: a comparison with the corticostriatal and corticosubthalamic efferents in a retrograde fluorescent double-labelling study. *Neuroscience* **60,** 125–132.
97. Inase, M., Tokuno, H., Nambu, A., Akazawa, T., and Takada, M. (1999) Corticostriatal and corticosubthalamic input zones from the presupplementary area in the macaque monkey: comparison with the input zones from the supplementary motor area. *Brain Res.* **833,** 191–201.
98. Nambu, A., Takada, M., Inase, M., and Tokuno, H. (1996) Dual somatotopical representations of the primate subthalamic nucleus: Evidence for ordered but reversed body-map transformations from the primary motor cortex and the supplementary motor area. *J. Neurosci.* **16,** 2671–2683.
99. Wichmann, T., Bergman, H., and DeLong, M. R. (1994) The primate subthalamic nucleus. I. Functional properties in intact animals. *J. Neurophysiol.* **72,** 494–506.
100. Féger, J., Hassani, O. K., and Mouroux, M. (1997) The subthalamic nucleus and its connections: New electrophysiological and pharmacological data. *Adv. Neurol.* **74,** 31–43.
101. Deschênes, M., Bourassa, J., Doan, V. D., and Parent, A. (1996) A single-cell study of the axonal projections arising from the posterior intralaminar nuclei in the rat. *Eur. J. Neurosci.* **8,** 329–343.
102. Bevan, M. D., Francis, C. M., and Bolam, J. P. (1995) The glutamate-enriched cortical and thalamic input to neurons in the subthalamic nucleus of the rat: convergence with GABA-positive terminals. *J. Comp. Neurol.* **361,** 491–511.
103. Kita, H. (1994) Physiology of two disynaptic pathways from the sensorimotor cortex to the basal ganglia output nuclei. In: *The Basal Ganglia IV, New Ideas and Data on Structure and Function* (Percheron, G., Mckenzie, J. S., and Féger, J., eds.), Plenum Press, New York, pp. 263–276.
104. Maurice, N., Deniau, J. M., Glowinski, J., and Thierry, A. M. (1998) Relationships between the prefrontal cortex and the basal ganglia in the rat: physiology of the corticosubthalamic circuits. *J. Neurosci.* **18,** 9539–9546.
105. Mouroux, M. and Féger, J. (1993) Evidence that the parafascicular projection to the subthalamic nucleus is glutamatergic. *Neuroreport* **4,** 613–615.
106. Nambu, A., Tokuno, H., Hamada, I., Kita, H., Imanishi, M., Akazawa, T., et al. (2000) Excitatory cortical inputs to pallidal neurons via the subthalamic nucleus in the monkey. *J. Neurophysiol.* **84,** 289–300.
107. Mink, J. W. (1996) The basal ganglia: focused selection and inhibition of competing programs. *Prog, Neurobiol.* **50,** 381–425.
108. Sidibé, M., Bevan, M. D., Bolam, J. P., and Smith Y. (1997) Efferent connections of the internal globus pallidus in the squirrel monkey: I. Topography and synaptic organization of the pallidothalamic projection. *J. Comp. Neurol.* **382,** 323–347.
109. Kuo, J. S. and Carpenter, M. B. (1973) Organization of pallidothalamic projections in the rhesus monkey. *J. Comp. Neurol.* **151,** 201–236.

109a. Parent, A. (1996) *Carpenter's Human Neuroanatomy*, 9th ed. Williams and Wilkins, Philadelphia, PA.
110. Baron, M. S., Sidibé, M., DeLong, M. R., and Smith, Y. (2001) Course of motor and associative pallidothalamic projections in monkeys. *J. Comp. Neurol.* **429,** 490–501.
111. Hazrati, L.-N. and Parent, A. (1991) Contralateral pallidothalamic and pallidotegmental projections in primates: an anterograde and retrograde labeling study. *Brain Res.* **567,** 212–223.
112. Parent, M., Lévesque, M., and Parent, A. (1999) The pallidofugal projection system in primates: evidence for neurons branching ipsilaterally and contralaterally to the thalamus and brainstem. *J. Chem. Neuroanat.* **16,** 153–165.
112a. Parent, M., Levesque, M., and Parent, A. (2001). Two types of projection neurons in the internal pallidum of primates: single-axon tracing and three-dimensional reconstruction. *J. Comp. Neurol.* **439(2),** 162–175.
113. Spann, B. M. and Grofova, I. (1992) Cholinergic and non-cholinergic neurons in the rat pedunculopontine tegmental nucleus. *Anat. Embryol.* **186,** 215–227.
114. Lavoie, B. and Parent, A. (1994b) Pedunculopontine nucleus in the squirrel monkey: distribution of cholinergic and monoaminergic neurons in the mesopontine tegmentum with evidence for the presence of glutamate in cholinergic neurons. *J. Comp. Neurol.* **344,** 190–209.
115. Inglis, W. L. and Winn, P. (1995) The pedunculopontine tegmental nucleus: where the striatum meets the reticular formation. *Prog. Neurobiol.* **47,** 1–29.
116. Rye, D. B. (1997) Contributions of the pedunculopontine region to normal and altered REM sleep. *Sleep* **20,** 757–788.
117. Pahapill, P. A. and Lozano, A. M. (2000) The pedunculopontine nucleus and Parkinson's disease. *Brain* **123,** 1767–1783.
118. Shink E, Sidibé, M., and Smith, Y. (1997) Efferent connections of the internal globus pallidus in the squirrel monkey: I. Topography and synaptic organization of the pallidal efferents to the pedunculopontine nucleus. *J. Comp. Neurol.* **382,** 348–363.
119. Larsen, K. D. and McBride, R. L. (1979) The organization of feline entopeduncular nucleus projections: anatomical studies. *J. Comp. Neurol.* **184,** 293–308.
120. Rajakumar, N., Elisevich, K., and Flumerfelt, B. A. (1993) Compartmental origin of the striato-entopeduncular projection in the rat. *J. Comp. Neurol.* **331,** 286–296.
121. Van der Kooy, D. and Carter, D. A. (1981) The organization of the efferent projections and striatal afferents of the entopeduncular nucleus and adjacent areas in the rat. *Brain Res.* **211,** 15–36.
122. Groenewegen, H. J., Berendse, H. W., and Haber, S. N. (1993) Organization of the output of the ventral striatopallidal system in the rat: ventral pallidal efferents. *Neuroscience* **57,** 113–142.
123. Spooren, W. P. M. J., Haber, S. N., Veening, J. G., and Cools, A. R. (1995) Descending efferent connections of the sub-pallidal areas in the cat: projections to the lateral habenula. *Neuroreport* **6,** 977–980.
124. Parent, A. and DeBellefeuille, L. (1982) Organization of efferent projections from the internal segment of the globus pallidus in primates as revealed by fluorescence retrograde labeling method. *Brain Res.* **245,** 201–213.
125. Shink, E., Sidibé, M., Bouffard, J.-F., and Smith, Y. (1996) Efferent projections of different functional territories of the internal pallidum in monleys. *Soc. Neurosci.* **22,** 411.
126. Parent, M., Lévesque, M., and Parent, A. (2000) Single-axon tracing study of the internal pallidum. *Soc. Neurosci.* **26,** 964.
127. Araki, M., McGeer, P. L., and McGeer, E. G. (1984) Retrograde HRP tracing combined with a pharmacohistochemical method for GABA transaminase for the identification of presumptive GABAergic projections to the habenula. *Brain Res.* **304,** 271–277.
128. Moriizumi, T. and Hattori, T. (1992) Choline acetyltransferase-immunoreactive neurons in the rat entopeduncular nucleus. *Neuroscience* **46,** 721–728.
129. Ilinsky, I. A., Tourtelotte, W. G., and Kultas-Ilinsky, K. (1993) Anatomical distinctions between the two basal ganglia afferent territories in the primate motor thalamus. *Stereotact. Funct. Neurosurg.* **60,** 62–69.
130. Sakai, S. T. and Patton, K. (1993) Distribution of cerebellothalamic and nigrothalamic projections in the dog: A double anterograde tracing study. *J. Comp. Neurol.* **330,** 183–194.
131. Parent, A., Mackey, A., Smith, Y., and Boucher R. (1983) The output organization of the substantia nigra in primate as revealed by a retrograde double labeling method. *Brain Res. Bull.* **10,** 529–537.
132. Ilinsky, I. A., Jouandet, M. L., and Goldman-Rakic, P. S. (1985) Organization of the nigrothalamocortical system in the rhesus monkey. *J. Comp. Neurol.* **236,** 315–330.
133. Deniau, J.-M. and Thierry, A.-M. (1997) Anatomical segregation processing in the rat substantia nigra pars reticulata. In: *Adv. Neurol. The Basal Ganglia and New Surgical Approaches for Parkinson's Disease* (Obeso, J. A., DeLong, M. R., Ohye, C., and Marsden, C. D., eds.), Lippinscott-Raven Publishers, Philadelphia, PA, pp. 83–96.
133a. Mailly, P., Charpier, S., Mahon, S., Menetrey, A., Thierry, A. M., Glowinsky, J., and Deniau, J.-M. (2001) Dendritic arborizations of the rat substantia nigra pars reticulata neurons: spatial organization and relation to the lamellar compartmentation of straito-nigral projections. *J. Neurosci.* **21,** 6874–6888.
134. Smith, Y., Sidibé, M., and Paré, J.-F. (2000) Synaptic inputs from the substantia nigra and the pedunculopontine nucleus to thalamostriatal neurons in monkeys. *Soc. Neurosci. Abstr.* **26,** 965.
135. Spann, B. M. and Grofova, I. (1991) Nigropedunculopontine projection in the rat: an anterograde tracing study with *phaseolus vulgaris-leucoagglutinin* (PHA-L). *J. Comp. Neurol.* **311,** 375–388.
136. Grofova, I. and Zhou, M. (1998) Nigral innervation of cholinergic and glutamatergic cells in the rat mesopontine tegmentum: light and electron microscopic anterograde tracing and immunohistochemical studies. *J. Comp. Neurol.* **395,** 359–379.

137. Tokuno, H., Moriizumi, T., Kudo, M., Kitao, Y., and Nakamura, Y. (1989) Monosynaptic striatal inputs to the nigrotegmental neurons: an electron microscopic study in the cat. *Brain Res.* **485,** 189–192.
138. Redgrave, P., Marrow, L., and Dean, P. (1992) Topographical organization of the nigrotectal projection in rat: Evidence for segregated channels. *Neuroscience* **50,** 571–595.
139. Tokuno, H. and Nakamura Y. (1987) Organization of the nigrotectospinal pathway in the cat: a light and electron microscopic study. *Brain Res.* **436,** 76–84.
140. Williams, M. N. and Faull, R. L. M. (1988) The nigrotectal projection and tectospinal neurons in the rat. A light and electron microscopic study demonstrating a monosynaptic nigral input to identified tectospinal neurons. *Neuroscience* **25,** 533–562.
141. Hikosaka, O., Takikawa, Y., and Kawagoe, R. (2000) Role of basal ganglia in the control of purposive saccadic eye movements. *Physiol. Rev.* **80,** 953–978.
142. Chronister, R. B., Walding, J. S., Aldes, L. D., and Marco, L. A. (1988) Interconnections between substantia nigra reticulata and medullary reticular formation. *Brain Res. Bull.* **21,** 313–317.
143. von Krosigk, M. and Smith, A. D. (1990) Descending projections from the substantia nigra and retrorubral field to the medullary and pontomedullary reticular formation. *Eur. J. Neurosci.* **3,** 260–273.
144. Von Krosigk, M., Smith, Y., Bolam, J. P., and Smith, A. D. (1992) Synaptic organization of GABAergic inputs from the striatum and the globus pallidus onto neurons in the substantia nigra and retrorubral field which project to the medullary reticular formation. *Neuroscience* **50,** 531–549.
145. Chandler, S. H., Turman, J. Jr., Salem, L., and Goldberg, L. J. (1990) The effects of nanoliter ejections of lidocaine into the pontomedullary reticular formation on cortically induced rhythmical jaw movements in the guinea pig. *Brain Res.* **526,** 54–64.
146. Travers, J. B. and Norgren, R. (1983) Afferent projections to the oral motor nuclei in the rat. *J. Comp. Neurol.* **220,** 280–298.
147. Rye, D. B., Saper, C. B., Lee, H. J., and Wainer, B. H. (1987) Pedunculopontine tegmental nucleus of the rat: cytoarchitecture, cytochemistry, and some extrapyramidal connections of the mesopontine tegmentum. *J. Comp. Neurol.* **259,** 483–528.
148. Moon Edley, S. and Graybiel, A. M. (1983) The afferent and efferent connections of the feline nucleus tegmenti pedunculopontinus, pars compacta. *J. Comp. Neurol.* **217,** 187–215.
149. Lee, H. J., Rye, D. B., Hallanger, A. E., Levey, A. I., and Wainer, B. H. (1988) Cholinergic vs noncholinergic efferents from the mesopontine tegmentum to the extrapyramidal motor system nuclei. *J. Comp. Neurol.* **275,** 469–492.
150. Charara, A., Smith, Y., and Parent, A. (1996) Glutamatergic inputs from the pedunculopontine nucleus to midbrain dopaminergic neurons in primates: *Phaseolus vulgaris*-leucoagglutinin anterograde labeling combined with postembedding glutamate and GABA immunohistochemistry. *J. Comp. Neurol.* **364,** 254–266.
151. Bevan, M. D. and Bolam, J. P. (1995) Cholinergic, GABAergic, and glutamate-enriched inputs from the mesopontine tegmentum to the subthalamic nucleus in the rat. *J. Neurosci.* **15,** 7105–7120.
152. Clarke, N. P., Bevan, M. D., Cozzari, C., Hartman, B. K., and Bolam, J. P. (1997) Glutamate-enriched cholinergic synaptic terminals in the entopeduncular nucleus and subthalamic nucleus of the rat. *Neuroscience* **81,** 371–385.
153. Clarke, N. P., Bolam, J. P., and Bevan, M. D. (1996) Glutamate-enriched inputs from the mesopontine tegmentum to the entopeduncular nucleus in the rat. *Eur. J. Neurosci.* **8,** 1363–1376.
154. Charara, A. and Parent, A. (1994) Brainstem dopaminergic, cholinergic and serotoninergic afferents to the pallidum in the squirrel monkey. *Brain Res.* **640,** 155–170.
155. Woolf, N. J. and Butcher, L. L. (1986) Cholinergic systems in the rat brain: III. Projections from the pontomesencephalic tegmentum to the thalamus, tectum, basal ganglia, and basal forebrain. *Brain Res. Bull.* **16,** 603–637.
156. Hallanger, A. E., Levey, A. I., Lee, H. J., Rye, D. B., and Wainer, B. H. (1987) The origins of cholinergic and other subcortical afferents to the thalamus in the rat. *J. Comp. Neurol.* **262,** 105–124.
157. Paré, D., Smith, Y., Parent, A., and Stériade, M. (1988) Projections of brainstem core cholinergic and non-cholinergic neurons of cat to intralaminar and reticular thalamic nuclei. *Neuroscience* **25,** 69–86.
158. Stériade, M., Paré, D., Parent, A., and Smith, Y. (1988) Projections of cholinergic and non-cholinergic neurons of the brainstem core to relay and associational thalamic nuclei in the cat and macaque monkey. *Neuroscience* **25,** 47–67.
159. Steriade, M., Datta, S., Paré, D., Oakson, G., and Curro Dossi, R. C. (1990) Neuronal activities in brain-stem cholinergic nuclei related to tonic activation processes in thalamocortical systems. *J. Neurosci.* **10,** 2541–2559.
160. Reese, N. B., Garcia-Rill, E., and Skinner, R. D. (1995) The pedunculopontine nucleus-auditory input, arousal and pathophysiology. *Prog. Neurobiol.* **47,** 105–133.
161. Erro, E., Lanciego, J. L., and Giménez-Amaya, J. M. (1999) Relationships between thalamostriatal neurons and pedunculopontine projections to the thalamus: a neuroanatomical tract-tracing study in the rat. *Exp. Brain Res.* **127,** 162–170.
162. Isaacson, L. G. and Tanaka, D. Jr. (1988) Cholinergic innervation of canine thalamostriatal projection neurons: an ultrastructural study combining choline acetyltransferase immunocytochemistry and WGA-HRP retrograde labeling. *J. Comp. Neurol.* **277,** 529–540.
163. Takakusaki, K., Shiroyama, T., Yamamoto, T., and Kitai S. T. (1996) Cholinergic and noncholinergic tegmental pedunculopontine projection neurons in rats revealed by intracellular labeling. *J. Comp. Neurol.* **371,** 345–361.
164. Matsumoto, N., Minamimoto, T., Graybiel, A. M., and Kimura, M. (2001) Neurons in the thalamic CM-Pf complex supply striatal neurons with information about behaviorally significant sensory events. *J. Neurophysiol.* **85,** 960–976.

3

Surgical Treatment of Parkinson's Disease

Past, Present, and Future

William C. Koller, Alireza Minagar, Kelly E. Lyons, and Rajesh Pahwa

1. PAST

Neurosurgical procedures for the management of movement disorders began prior to the introduction of stereotactic surgery. Lessons learned from these pioneering procedures established the basis for the use of stereotactic techniques in the treatment of movement disorders.

The first destructive surgical procedure on the brain to control hyperkinetic movement disorders was performed by Horsely and colleagues at the end of 19th century *(1,2)*. They excised all or part of the motor cortex for treatment of athetosis and their work became a milestone in our understanding of scientific concepts of motor neuroanatomy and physiology. This procedure was emulated by Nazaroff, who in 1927 reported on the injection of alcohol into the same area of the cortex with variable results *(3)*. The first surgical treatment of Parkinson's disease (PD) was performed in 1912 by the French physician Leriche, who did posterior cervical rhizotomy for control of parkinsonian tremor *(4)*.

A few decades passed before there was a resurgence of interest in scientific neurosurgical approaches in the management of movement disorders. Bucy and Buchanan *(5)* extirpated the motor cortex for the treatment of athetosis in 1931, for tremor control in PD in 1932, and for cerebellar tremor in 1937 *(6)*. Bucy and Case in 1939 and Kleme in 1940, excised parts of the cerebral cortex as a treatment for parkinsonian tremor and dystonia. Although the patients' symptoms improved, this type of ablative surgery caused significant motor disability such as spastic hemiparesis.

Putnam performed the first ablative surgical procedures directed to the spinal cord. In 1933, he reported successful relief of choreoathetosis by incising the spinal cord at C4-5 below the exit of the respiratory fibers in the anterolateral quadrant just anterior to the pyramidal tract and in 1938, his method of incising the corticospinal tract in the upper cervical cord, produced relief of dyskinesia at the cost of ipsilateral hemiplegia *(7–9)*. This procedure was ineffective in controlling parkinsonian tremor.

1.1. *Basal Ganglia Surgery for Movement Disorders*

Basal ganglia surgery for the treatment of movement disorders was pioneered by the American neurosurgeon Russell Meyers during the 1940s *(10,11)*. Earlier, it was generally conceived that such a surgical approach would be impossible because it might result in disorders of consciousness; a conclusion based on observations made following anterior cerebral artery strokes. In addition, Dandy had hypothesized that vegetative centers and the center for consciousness were located in the basal ganglia *(12)*. In 1939, through an open craniotomy, transventricular approach, Meyers extirpated two-thirds

From: Contemporary Clinical Neurology:
Surgical Treatment of Parkinson's Disease and Other Movement Disorders
Edited by: D. Tarsy, J. L. Vitek, and A. M. Lozano © Humana Press Inc., Totowa, NJ

of the caudate nucleus in a patient with postencephalitic parkinsonism. Meyers' procedure improved the patient's tremor; however, his result was not reproducible in subsequent surgeries. His further investigations revealed that sectioning of pallidofugal fibers was the most successful procedure. Meyers further refined his technique and focused on the putamen, the ansa lenticularis, the pallidum, and in a few cases, the internal capsule. By 1949, he had operated on 58 patients with parkinsonian syndromes, choreoathetosis, hemiballism, and cervical dystonia. Postoperative improvement was observed in 60% of his patients, but the operative mortality was as high as 12%.

1.2. *Stereotactic Surgery*

In 1908, Horsely and Clark described the first animal stereotactic apparatus *(13)*. However, several decades passed until Spiegel and his colleagues performed the first stereotactic pallidotomy in a patient with Huntington's disease (HD) to obtain a reduction of choreic movements. Their new technique employed intracerebral ventricular landmarks rather than bony landmarks to position the target. The operative procedure was safe and practical and they called it "stereoencephalotomy," meaning a three-dimensional technique using landmarks inside the brain *(14,15)*. Lesions were originally induced with an electrolytic direct current, the same that Horsely and Clark had used 40 years before. Later, other techniques such as injection of oil-procaine or alcohol were applied to coagulate the globus pallidus and its efferent fibers for the relief of tremor and rigidity in PD.

1.3. *Thalamotomy*

Hassler, based on his anatomic and physiological research, considered the ventrolateral (VL) thalamus a target for the treatment of movement disorders. In 1952, Mundinger performed the first VL thalamotomy on a patient with PD. These results were published two years later by Hassler and Riechert *(16)*.

In 1963, Albe-Fessard *(17)* performed microelectrode recordings in the cerebral hemispheres and later others such as Narabayashi in Tokyo employed this semi-microelectrode recording to localize the target area before performing an ablation *(18)*. Through this line of research, the ventral intermediate (Vim) nucleus of the thalamus was identified as the most specific target for controlling various tremors including parkinsonian, essential, cerebellar, and post-stroke *(19)*.

2. PRESENT

2.1. *Thalamotomy*

Basal ganglia stereotactic surgery initially targeted the globus pallidus and the ansa lenticularis until Hassler and Reichert selected the ventral lateral nucleus of the thalamus and its surrounding area as the favored site for tremor reduction *(16)*. Improvement in tremor and rigidity of the limbs contralateral to the side of the lesion occurs in greater than 90% of PD patients *(20–22)*. Although the assessments in the earlier studies were often qualitative rather than quantitative, these reported studies and the clinical anecdotal experience indicate that unilateral thalamotomies are an effective treatment for parkinsonian tremor.

Similarly, long-term follow-up studies have shown that thalamotomy has a lasting beneficial effect. After a mean follow-up of 33 mo, Kelly et al. *(23)* reported continued improvement of tremor in 86% of the patients. Linhares and Tasker *(24)* reported outcomes in 40 thalamotomy patients after 35.8 mo. They found that 75% of the patients had no upper extremity tremor; however, the procedure had to be repeated approx 30% of the time for tremor improvement. In another series, Nagaseki et al. *(25)* found minimal recurrence of tremor in 27 parkinsonian patients who received thalamotomies after a mean of 6.6 yr of follow-up. Jankovic et al. *(26)* reported complete abolition of tremor in 72% of patients with thalamotomies and significant improvement in tremor and functional ability in six patients after a mean follow-up of 52 mo. Kelly and Gillingham *(21)* reported that 57% of the PD patients had tremor control after 10 yr. Diedereich et al. *(27)* examined 17 PD patients with a mean follow-up of

10.9 yr and used videotapes for blinded evaluations. They reported surgery improved the absolute magnitude of tremor or ameliorated its rate of progression. Although patients had long-term improvement of the tremor, other parkinsonian symptoms like bradykinesia, rigidity, and the tremor ipsilateral to the surgery were noted to progress.

The mortality rate for thalamotomy in PD is estimated to be less than 0.3% *(28)*. Death is usually the result of basal ganglia hemorrhage or indirect postoperative complications such as pulmonary embolism or infection. Transient postoperative adverse events include headaches, seizures, confusion, dysarthria, ataxia, hemiparesis, and expressive aphasia. Persistent morbidity is uncommon, consisting mainly of dysarthria, dysphagia, and mild paresis. One of the complications not routinely reported is the number of patients who require repeat surgery after failure of the initial lesion or due to loss of benefit from the initial surgery. Complications from bilateral thalamotomy were common with greater than 25% of patients experiencing speech impairment and mental changes. Although we do not recommend bilateral thalamotomies, some investigators believe that with advances in stereotactic techniques, bilateral operations can be performed with reduced morbidity.

2.2. Deep Brain Stimulation (DBS)

The Activa Tremor Control therapy is approved by the FDA for use in thalamic stimulation for the treatment of essential tremor and PD tremor. The Activa Control therapy consists of a Deep Brain Stimulation (DBS) lead, the extension that connects the DBS lead to an Implantable Pulse Generator (IPG). There are two kinds of DBS leads available. The intracranial end of both leads has four platinum-iridium contacts. One of these leads has contacts that are separated by 1.5 mm (3387) whereas in the second lead the contacts are separated by 0.5 mm (3389). The DBS leads are connected to the IPG device by an extension lead tunneled under the skin. The IPG is usually implanted subcutaneously in the infraclavicular area. The IPG can be programmed for monopolar stimulation or bipolar stimulation. Adjustable parameters include pulse width, amplitude, stimulation frequency, and the choice of active contacts. The patient can turn the stimulator on or off using a hand-held magnet. The usual stimulation parameters are stimulation frequency of 135–185 Hz, pulse width of 60–120 microseconds and amplitude of 1–3 V. The mechanism of action of DBS is unknown. Persistent depolarization, stimulation of inhibitory systems, and neuronal jamming have been proposed as possible mechanisms of action *(37)*.

2.3. Thalamic Stimulation

Chronic thalamic stimulation is increasingly replacing thalamotomy as the preferred surgical technique for the treatment of medication-resistant disabling PD tremor. Although tremor is markedly improved in PD, there is sometimes no significant improvement in activities of daily living (ADL). This is related to the lack of improvement in bradykinesia, rigidity, and gait. Hence, thalamic stimulation should be restricted to PD patients whose major disability is tremor with minimal bradykinesia, rigidity, and gait problems.

The majority of studies that have evaluated the efficacy of unilateral thalamic stimulation have reported that approx 90% of patients report some improvement in tremor in the contralateral limb *(29–35)*. Results of bilateral thalamic stimulation in PD have not been widely reported. Koller et al. *(35)* reported the results of a double-blind multicenter study in 24 PD patients who had undergone unilateral thalamic stimulation. At 1-yr, there was significant tremor improvement, although activities of daily living as measured by the Unified Parkinson's Disease Rating Scale (UPDRS) showed no significant change. In another multicenter trial, Limousin et al. *(34)* reported 57 PD patients who had undergone unilateral implantation and 16 PD patients who had undergone bilateral implantation. At 12-mo, tremor was significantly reduced by stimulation. Although symptoms other than tremor were very mild, they observed significant reduction in contralateral akinesia and rigidity scores, a finding that has not been replicated in other studies.

There are few long-term studies regarding the use of thalamic stimulation in PD. Pollack et al. *(36)* reported their experience in 80 PD patients with a mean age of 58 yr. After a mean follow-up of 3 yr, the patients continued to have good control of their tremor without a dramatic effect on other symptoms like akinesia, rigidity, or levodopa-induced dyskinesias. The morbidity and mortality associated with thalamic stimulation is low. Complications of surgery include intracerebral hemorrhage, seizures, and confusion *(32)*. Complications related to the device include wire erosion, IPG infection, malfunction of the IPG, electrical shocking, and lead migration. Side effects directly related to stimulation are reversible with stimulation adjustments and are usually well-tolerated. Other adverse effects due to stimulation include dysarthria, disequilibrium, paresis, and gait disorder. As mentioned earlier, benefit following thalamic DBS is limited to tremor reduction with no improvement in other features of PD or levodopa-induced dyskinesias.

A double-blind study compared the efficacy and tolerability of thalamotomy vs thalamic stimulation *(38)*. Tremor was completely or almost completely suppressed in 27 of 34 PD patients in the thalamotomy group and in 30 of 33 patients in the thalamic stimulation group. At 6-mo both procedures were equally effective for the suppression of drug-resistant tremor, but thalamic DBS had fewer adverse effects and resulted in greater improvement in function. The recent introduction of DBS of the subthalamic nucleus (STN) for PD has profound impact on the indications for thalamic surgery.

2.4. *Pallidotomy*

Pallidotomies were initially used in the 1950s with inconsistent results that were believed to be due to inappropriate target selection and the surgical techniques. With the discovery of levodopa in the 1960s, the use of pallidotomy for PD waned. However, due to the long-term complications of levodopa, which were occasionally disabling and could not be improved by medications, Laitinen and his colleagues *(39)* re-explored posteroventral pallidotomy in 38 PD patients. They reported significant improvement in bradykinesia, rigidity, tremor, ambulation, speech, and drug-induced dyskinesias. Their study was criticized due to lack of standardized clinical examinations and the absence of radiological evaluations regarding precise lesion placement. Since then, there have been multiple other studies using standardized clinical rating scales that have also reported significant improvement in parkinsonian symptoms with unilateral pallidotomy.

Favre et al. *(40)* reported 44 patients who underwent pallidotomy with a median follow-up of 7 mo. Of these patients, 22 underwent unilateral pallidotomy and 17 had bilateral simultaneous pallidotomy. Using a visual analog scale, they reported that unilateral and simultaneous bilateral pallidotomy could reduce all key symptoms of PD (i.e., akinesia, tremor, rigidity) and the side effects of levodopa therapy (i.e., dyskinesias). Bilateral pallidotomy was more effective than unilateral pallidotomy in improving the cardinal symptoms of PD; however it had a higher risk of postoperative speech impairment. Severe dyskinesias and younger age were positive prognostic factors for a successful outcome.

Baron et al. *(41)* had reported the results of a 1-yr pilot study regarding the effects of GPi pallidotomy in 15 advanced PD patients. The mean total UPDRS score improved by 30%, mean ADL "off" subscale scores improved by 34% and the motor examination "off" score improved by 25%. There was a dramatic improvement in contralateral drug-induced dyskinesias and tremor. There were no significant changes in the neuropsychological assessments. Two of the patients in this study developed dementia and did not improve, suggesting that patients with moderate to severe dementia may have a poor surgical outcome. Persistent complications included superior quadrantanopia in one patient. To examine the long-term results, they reassessed 10 of the 15 patients *(42)*. Although the UPDRS motor scores returned to baseline levels in 3–4 yr, most of the patients continued to have sustained improvements in contralateral tremor, akinesia, and drug-induced dyskinesias, which were improved by 64% at 4 yr.

Fine et al. *(43)* reported follow-up results after 52 mo in 20 of their 40 patients who had undergone unilateral pallidotomy. Off period UPDRS scores were improved by 18% compared to baseline. Significant improvements were also evident in the off-period scores for contralateral tremor (65% improvement), rigidity (43% improvement), and bradykinesia (18% improvement). Dyskinesias on the contralateral side were 71% improved.

In a 10-yr follow-up review of 13 patients who had undergone unilateral pallidotomy and were originally reported in 1992, Hariz and Bergenheim *(44)* found that five patients had undergone a total of seven subsequent surgeries for their PD. The mean Hoehn and Yahr stage worsened from 3.0 to 3.7 at the last review. Although dosages of levodopa and dopamine agonists were increased in all patients, there was no appearance or recurrence of dyskinesias contralateral to pallidotomy. Although most patients exhibited a gradual recurrence of akinesia and an increase in gait freezing, contralateral tremor continued to be improved.

Alkhani and Lozano *(45)* conducted an evidence-based review of contemporary published articles on pallidotomy between 1992 and 1999. In 85 articles identified for critical review, 1959 patients with PD underwent pallidotomies at 40 centers in 12 countries. Eighty-nine percent underwent unilateral pallidotomy and 11% underwent bilateral pallidotomy. Mean patient age was 61 yr with a disease duration of 12 yr. UPDRS scores were used to document outcome in 26% of the cases at 6 mo and 11% of the cases at 12 mo. At 1 yr, mean improvement in UPDRS motor scores during the off period was 45% and improvement in contralateral dyskinesias was 86%. Overall mortality was 0.4%, with persistent adverse effects in 14% of the patients. Major adverse effects included intracerebral hemorrhage, contralateral weakness, and visual field defects in 5% of the reported patients.

2.5. Pallidal Stimulation

Based on the success of DBS for tremor and of pallidotomy for parkinsonian symptoms, Siegfried and Lippitz *(46)* used the technology of DBS for continuous stimulation of the ventroposterolateral pallidum. They implanted bilateral GPi electrodes in three PD patients. The investigators reported improvement in the Webster Rating Scale scores and on-off motor fluctuations.

Preliminary reports from other centers have confirmed those findings *(47–50)*. Pahwa et al. reported five PD patients who underwent pallidal stimulation and were followed for 3 mo *(47)*. UPDRS motor scores improved by 24% and ADL scores by 19% in the "off" state and by 21 and 42%, respectively, in the "on" state. Patient diaries demonstrated an increase in "on" time with a decrease in both "off" time and "on" time with dyskinesias. Volkmann et al. *(47a)* reported on nine patients who underwent GPi stimulation who were also followed for 3 mo. Mean improvement in UPDRS motor scores was 56%. Gross et al. *(48)* reported on seven patients who underwent GPi stimulation and were followed for 12–24 mo. Improvement in UPDRS motor scores off medication ranged between 11 and 61% at 12 mo, which was maintained at 24 mo. Stimulation and L-dopa produced similar effects but combined stimulation and L-dopa was superior to either alone. Kumar et al. *(50)* reported 22 PD patients who were treated with either unilateral ($n = 5$) or bilateral ($n = 17$) GPi stimulation. At 6 mo there was a 32% improvement in UPDRS motor "off" scores, 40% improvement in UPDRS ADL "off" scores and 23% improvement in dyskinesias. The UPDRS motor "on" scores improved by 1% and UPDRS ADL "on" scores improved by 30% with a 68% improvement in dyskinesias. Long-term results of GPi stimulation have been lacking. Ghika et al. *(51)* reported six PD patients with a mean age of 55 yr and disease duration of 16 yr with a minimum follow-up of 24 mo. The mean improvement in the UPDRS motor "off" scores and the ADL scores were more than 50%. The mean "off" time decreased from 40 to 10% and the dyskinesia scores were reduced by 30%. Although the improvements persisted beyond 2 yr after surgery, signs of decreased efficacy were seen after 12 mo. In a recently published multicenter trial, GPi DBS in 38 patients resulted in 38% improvement in motor performance and a marked reduction of involuntary movements *(51a)*.

2.6. Subthalamotomy

Hyperactivity of the STN is considered a hallmark of PD. The STN has many connections, including excitatory glutamatergic input directed at the GPi and substantia nigra. In experimental parkinsonism, modulation of STN activity has been shown to have therapeutic benefit *(52)*. In a pilot study, Alvarez et al. *(53)* reported their experience in 11 PD patients who underwent unilateral dorsal subthalamotomy. The mean age of their patients was 59.5 yr with disease duration of 11 yr. There was a significant improvement in the UPDRS ADL and motor scores in the "off" state at 12-mo follow-up. The effect was maintained in four patients up to 24 mo. Anti-parkinsonian medications were unchanged in all but one patient who stopped the medication. The dyskinesia scores did not change following surgery. The percentage of the waking day spent in "on" time was significantly improved. One patient had a large infarct several days postsurgery.

2.7. *Subthalamic Stimulation*

There are multiple reports of the antiparkinsonian effects of STN DBS *(54–61)*. These studies indicate that stimulation induces a 40–75% reduction in UPDRS "off" motor scores and all cardinal features of PD improve. UPDRS "on" motor scores are not significantly changed but there is a 40–80% reduction in dose of antiparkinsonian medication. Motor fluctuations and dyskinesias as well as ADL and patient quality of life scales have also shown significant improvement in multiple studies.

Long-term follow-up results for STN DBS are limited. Benabid et al. *(62)* have followed more than 50 patients for 1 yr who have maintained benefit. Thirty patients have been assessed at 2 yr, 16 patients at 3 yr, nine patients at 4 yr and 4 patients at 5 yr. They have observed adequate control of the cardinal features of PD and the reduced levodopa requirement has persisted. They have observed a tendency towards increased hypophonia and axial motor symptoms. Rodriquez et al. *(61)* reported initial results in 15 patients after 12 mo and in nine patients between 30 and 36 mo after surgery. They reported a 74% improvement in the UPDRS motor scores in the "off" state with a 55% reduction in the levodopa daily dose. Nine patients with long-term follow-up continued to have a 61% reduction in UPDRS motor scores and a 38% reduction in levodopa dosage. They reported two hemorrhages, and one infection that required the device to be explanted. Other device-related events that have been reported include scalp ulceration, hematoma in the stimulator pocket, replacement of the external extension and repositioning of the stimulator *(62)*. In the recently published multicenter trial comparing GPi and STN DBS *(51b)*, STN DBS in 96 patients resulted in 49% improvement in motor scores, a marked reduction of involuntary movements, and a significant reduction in dose of dopaminergic drugs.

2.8. *Transplantation*

Neural transplantation is a reasonable consideration for the treatment of PD. This is because the neuronal degeneration is site- and type-specific (dopaminergic), the target area is well-defined (striatum), postsynaptic receptors are relatively intact, and the neurons provide tonic stimulation of the receptors and appear to serve a modulatory function *(63)*. Although multiple sources of dopamine-producing cells like fetal nigral cells, sympathetic ganglia, carotid body glomus cells, PC-12 cells, and neuroblastoma cells have only been studied experimentally, human and porcine fetal nigral cells have been studied in humans. Although the initial study regarding the use of autologous adrenal medullary cells into the human putamen in PD patients reported significant clinical benefit *(64)*, other investigators using similar techniques failed to replicate these dramatic effects *(65)*. It is now generally accepted that the benefits of adrenal tissue implant do not justify the risks and the procedure has been abandoned.

In animal PD models, fetal nigral dopaminergic transplants have been shown to survive in the striatum, form synaptic connections, develop extensive striatal reinnervation, exhibit relatively normal electrical firing patterns, and improve motor function *(66–68)*. The results of fetal tissue implantation in PD patients have been inconsistent. This may be due to differences in transplant variables and the evaluations that are performed. Recently, Hauser et al. *(63)* reported six PD patients who underwent bilateral fetal nigral transplantation. Immunosuppresion was provided for 6 mo. Complications related to surgery were mild and transient. Mean total UPDRS scores improved by 32%, mean percentage of "on" time without dyskinesias improved from 22–60%. Mean putamenal fluorodopa on positron emission tomography (PET) scans improved significantly in comparison to baseline.

A recent double-blind study with a subgroup of patients receiving sham operations did not show a significant improvement in patients who had received fetal tissue *(69)*. To date, although over 250 PD patients have received fetal tissue implants this procedure remains investigational.

3. FUTURE

The future of the treatment of PD will consist of a better understanding of the cause and pathophysiology of the disorder. A cure or at least neuroprotective therapy may then be possible. Improved pharmacological therapy would lead to less long-term motor complications thus reducing the burden of the disease. Nonetheless, many patients now and probably in the future will be referred for surgery because of increased disability and reduction of quality of life.

Optimization of DBS is one clear goal for the future. It is unclear why some patients have a dramatic response to DBS while others do not. If this inconsistent response is simply due to poor electrode localization, then imaging and neurophysiologic methodologies need to be developed to provide more consistent and proper electrode placement. A more precise understanding of the mechanism of action of DBS would be helpful in plotting future ideas for improvement. Criteria for patient selection also need to be better defined. We need to know exactly which symptoms of PD will respond to surgery. For instance, are patients with poor postural stability, "on" period freezing, speech and gait problems ideal candidates for surgery? Furthermore, exclusion criteria for surgery need to be better developed. Unanswered questions include whether advanced patient age reduces the likelihood of a successful outcome or is a risk for surgical complications. Is there a certain level of cognitive dysfunction or type of cognitive decline, such as frontal lobe dysfunction, that should exclude a patient? What tests should be used to assess mentation? Generally, it would appear that better patient selection for surgery would result in a better outcome.

In the future, hopefully, research will better define the best anatomical site for surgery and precise means for localization of the target site. It is not currently known whether the GPi or STN is the preferred target or that certain symptoms might respond better to one anatomical localization or another. It is also possible that a yet undiscovered site will represent the optimal location for amelioration of PD symptoms.

The main risk of stereotactic surgery is intraoperative cerebral hemorrhage, which is estimated to occur in 3% of patients. Although the majority of these are asymptomatic and discovered by brain imaging, some patients are left with a persistent neurological deficit. If this risk could be eliminated then perhaps surgery could be preformed earlier in the course of the disease. This would be an obvious important advance in surgical treatment.

Another need for potential progress is device improvement. For instance, it may be possible to eliminate the need for an extension wire by the use of wireless technology. It is also expected that the IPG will be improved. In the future, one IPG will be used for control of bilateral DBS electrodes. It may also be possible to program the IPG by telephone rather than an office visit to reduce the need for frequent follow-up visits for reprogramming. Battery life needs to be extended to last longer than 5 yr. Also a system has been developed that will let patients easily know if the IPG is turned on or off. Many of these improvements are currently subjects of active investigation.

REFERENCES

1. Horsely, V. (1909) The Linacre Lecture on the function of the so-called motor area of the brain. *BMJ* **ii,** 125–132.
2. Horsely, V. (1890) Remarks on the surgery of the central nervous system. *BMJ* **ii,** 1286–1292.
3. Nazaroff, N. N. (1927) Uber Alkohol injectionen in die kortikale Hirnsubstanz bei Athetose. *Zentralbl. Chir.* **54,** 1478–1481.
4. Speelman, J. D. and Bosch, D. A. (1998) Resurgence of functional neurosurgery for Parkinson's disease: a historical perspective. *Mov. Disord.* **13,** 582–588.

5. Bucy, P. C. and Buchanan, D. N. (1932) Athetosis. *Brain* **55,** 479–492.
6. Bucy, P. C. and Case, T. J. (1939) Tremor. Physiologic mechanism and abolition by surgical means. *Arch. Neurol. Psychiatry* **41,** 721–746.
7. Putnam, T. J. (1940) Paralysis agitans and athetosis. Manifestations and methods of treatment. *Arch. Neurol. Psychiatry* **43,** 170–171.
8. Putnam, T. J. (1938) Results of treatment of athetosis by section of extrapyramidal tracts in the spinal cord. *Arch. Neurol. Psychiatry* **39,** 258–275.
9. Putnam, T. J. (1933) Treatment of athetosis and dystonia by section of the extrapyramidal motor tracts. *Arch. Neurol. Psychiatry* **29,** 504–521.
10. Meyers, R. (1951) Surgical experiments in the therapy of certain "extrapyramidal" diseases: a current evaluation. *Acta. Psychiatr. Neurol.* **67,** 1–42.
11. Meyers, R. (1968) The surgery of the hyperkinetic disorders. In: *Handbook of Clinical Neurology*, vol. 6 (Vinken, P. J. and Bruyn, G. W., eds.), North Holland Publishers, Amsterdam, pp. 844–878.
12. Dandy, W. E. (1930) Changes in our conceptions of localization of certain functions in the brain. *Am. J. Physiol.* **93,** 643–647.
13. Horsely, V. and Clarke, R. H. (1908) The structure and functions of the cerebellum examined by a new method. *Brain* **31,** 45–124.
14. Spiegel, E. A. and Wysic, H. T. (1952) *Stereoencephalotomy*. Part I. Methods and stereotaxic atlas of the human brain. Grune & Stratton, New York.
15. Spiegel, E. A. and Wysic, H. T. (1962) *Stereoencephalotomy*. Part II. Clinical and Physiological Applications. Grune & Stratton, New York.
16. Hassler, R. and Riechert, T. (1954) Indikationen und Lokalosations-methode der gezielten Hirnoperationen. *Nervearzt* **25,** 441–447.
17. Albe-Fessard, D., Arfel, G., and Guiot, G. (1963) Activities electriques caracteristoques de auelques structures cerebrales chez l'homme. *Ann. Chirurgie* **17,** 1185–1214.
18. Fukamachi, A., Ohye, C. H., and Narabayashi, H. (1973) Delineation of the thalamic nuclei with a microelectrode in stereotaxic surgery for parkinsonism and cerebral palsy. *J. Neurosurg.* **39,** 214–225.
19. Narabayashi, H. (1982) Surgical approach to tremor. In: *Movement Disorders* (Marsden, C. D. and Fahn, S., eds.), Butterworth Scientific, London, pp. 292–299.
20. Selby, G. (1967) Stereotactic surgery for the relief of Parkinson's disease. 2. An analysis of the results in a series of 303 patients (413 operations). *J. Neurol. Sci.* **5,** 343–375.
21. Kelly, P. J. and Gillingham, F. J. (1980) The long-term results of stereotaxic surgery and L-dopa therapy in patients with Parkinson's disease. A 10-year follow-up study. *J. Neurosurg.* **53,** 332–337.
22. Koller, W. C., Wilkinson, S., Pahwa, R., and Miyawaki, E. K. (1998) Surgical treatment options in Parkinson's disease. *Neurosurg. Clin. North Am.* **9,** 295–306.
23. Kelly, P. J., Ahlskog, J. E., Goerss, S. J., Daube, J. R., Duffy, J. R., and Kall, B. A. (1987) Computer-assisted stereotactic ventralis lateralis thalamotomy with microelectrode recording control in patients with Parkinson's disease. *Mayo Clin. Proc.* **62,** 655–664.
24. Linhares, M. N. and Tasker, R. R. (2000) Microelectrode-guided thalamotomy for Parkinson's disease. *Neurosurgery* **46,** 390–395; discussion 395–398.
25. Nagaseki, Y., Shibazaki, T., Hirai, T., Kawashima, Y., Hirato, M., Wada, H., et al. (1986) Long-term follow-up results of selective VIM-thalamotomy. *J. Neurosurg.* **65,** 296–302.
26. Jankovic, J., Hamilton, W. J., and Grossman, R. G. (1997) Thalamic surgery for movement disorders. *Adv. Neurol.* **74,** 221–233.
27. Diederich, N., Goetz, C. G., Stebbins, G. T., Klawans, H. L., Nittner, K., Koulosakis, A., et al. (1992) Blinded evaluation confirms long-term asymmetric effect of unilateral thalamotomy or subthalamotomy on tremor in Parkinson's disease. *Neurology* **42,** 1311–1314.
28. Selby, G. (1987) Stereotaxic surgery. In: *Handbook of Parkinson's Disease* (Koller, W. C., ed.), Marcel Dekker, New York, pp. 421–435.
29. Blond, S., Caparros-Lefebvre, D., Parker, F., Assaker, R., Petit, H., Guieu, J. D., et al. (1992) Control of tremor and involuntary movement disorders by chronic stereotactic stimulation of the ventral intermediate thalamic nucleus. *J. Neurosurg.* **77,** 62–68.
30. Speelman, J. D. and Bosch, D. A. (1995) [Continuous electric thalamus stimulation for the treatment of tremor resistant to pharmacotherapy]. *Ned. Tijdschr. Geneeskd.* **139,** 926–930.
31. Alesch, F., Pinter, M. M., Helscher, R. J., Fertl, L., Benabid, A. L., and Koos, W. T. (1995) Stimulation of the ventral intermediate thalamic nucleus in tremor dominated Parkinson's disease and essential tremor. *Acta. Neurochir.* **136,** 75–81.
32. Benabid, A. L., Pollak, P., Gao, D., Hoffmann, D., Limousin, P., Gay, E., et al. (1996) Chronic electrical stimulation of the ventralis intermedius nucleus of the thalamus as a treatment of movement disorders. *J. Neurosurg.* **84,** 203–214.
33. Ondo, W., Jankovic, J., Schwartz, K., Almaguer, M., and Simpson, R. K. (1998) Unilateral thalamic deep brain stimulation for refractory essential tremor and Parkinson's disease tremor. *Neurology* **51,** 1063–1069.
34. Limousin, P., Speelman, J. D., Gielen, F., and Janssens, M. (1999) Multicentre European study of thalamic stimulation in parkinsonian and essential tremor. *J. Neurol. Neurosurg. Psychiatry* **66,** 289–296.
35. Koller, W., Pahwa, R., Busenbark, K., Hubble, J., Wilkinson, S., Lang, A., et al. (1997) High-frequency unilateral thalamic stimulation in the treatment of essential and parkinsonian tremor. *Ann. Neurol.* **42,** 292–299.

36. Pollak, P., Benabid, A. L., Limousin, P., and Benazzouz, A. (1997) Chronic intracerebral stimulation in Parkinson's disease. *Adv. Neurol.* **74,** 213–220.
37. Benabid, A. L., LeBas, J. F., Hoffman, D., et al. (1994) Chronic high frequency thalamic stimulation in Parkinson's disease. In: *Therapy of Parkinson's Disease* (Koller, W. C. and Paulson, G. W., eds.), Marcel Dekker, New York, pp. 381–402.
38. Schuurman, P. R., Bosch, D. A., Bossuyt, P. M., Bonsel, G. J., van Someren, E. J., de Bie, R. M., et al. (2000) A comparison of continuous thalamic stimulation and thalamotomy for suppression of severe tremor. *N. Engl. J. Med.* **342,** 461–468.
39. Laitinen, L. V., Bergenheim, A. T., and Hariz, M. I. (1992) Leksell's posteroventral pallidotomy in the treatment of Parkinson's disease. *J. Neurosurg.* **76,** 53–61.
40. Favre, J., Burchiel, K. J., Taha, J. M., and Hammerstad, J. (2000) Outcome of unilateral and bilateral pallidotomy for Parkinson's disease: patient assessment. *Neurosurgery* **46,** 344–353; discussion 353–345.
41. Baron, M. S., Vitek, J. L., Bakay, R. A., Green, J., Kaneoke, Y., Hashimoto, T., et al. (1996) Treatment of advanced Parkinson's disease by posterior GPi pallidotomy: 1-year results of a pilot study. *Ann. Neurol.* **40,** 355–366.
42. Baron, M. S., Vitek, J. L., Bakay, R. A., Green, J., McDonald, W. M., Cole, S. A., et al. (2000) Treatment of advanced Parkinson's disease by unilateral posterior GPi pallidotomy: 4-year results of a pilot study. *Mov. Disord.* **15,** 230–237.
43. Fine, J., Duff, J., Chen, R., Chir, B., Hutchison, W., Lozano, A. M., et al. (2000) Long-term follow-up of unilateral pallidotomy in advanced Parkinson's disease. *N. Engl. J. Med.* **342,** 1708–1714.
44. Hariz, M. I. and Bergenheim, A. T. (2001) A 10-year follow-up review of patients who underwent Leksell's posteroventral pallidotomy for Parkinson disease. *J. Neurosurg.* **94,** 552–558.
45. Alkhani, A. and Lozano, A. M. (2001) Pallidotomy for parkinson disease: a review of contemporary literature. *J. Neurosurg.* **94,** 43–49.
46. Siegfried, J. and Lippitz, B. (1994) Bilateral chronic electrostimulation of ventroposterolateral pallidum: a new therapeutic approach for alleviating all parkinsonian symptoms. *Neurosurgery* **35,** 1126–1129; discussion 1129–1130.
47. Pahwa, R., Wilkinson, S., Smith, D., Lyons, K., Miyawaki, E., and Koller, W. C. (1997) High-frequency stimulation of the globus pallidus for the treatment of Parkinson's disease. *Neurology* **49,** 249–253.
47a. Volkmann, J., Sturm, V., Weiss, P., Kappler, J., Voges, J., Koulousakis, A., et al. (1998) Bilateral high-frequency stimulation of the internal globus pallidus in advanced parkinson's disease. *Ann. Neurol.* **44,** 953–961.
48. Gross, C., Rougier, A., Guehl, D., Boraud, T., Julien, J., and Bioulac, B. (1997) High-frequency stimulation of the globus pallidus internalis in Parkinson's disease: a study of seven cases. *J. Neurosurg.* **87,** 491–498.
49. Krack, P., Pollak, P., Limousin, P., Hoffmann, D., Xie, J., Benazzouz, A., et al. (1998) Subthalamic nucleus or internal pallidal stimulation in young onset Parkinson's disease. *Brain* **121,** 451–457.
50. Kumar, R., Lang, A. E., Rodriguez-Oroz, M. C., Lozano, A. M., Limousin, P., Pollak, P., et al. (2000) Deep brain stimulation of the globus pallidus pars interna in advanced Parkinson's disease. *Neurology* **55,** S34–S39.
51. Ghika, J., Villemure, J. G., Fankhauser, H., Favre, J., Assal, G., and Ghika-Schmid, F. (1998) Efficiency and safety of bilateral contemporaneous pallidal stimulation (deep brain stimulation) in levodopa-responsive patients with Parkinson's disease with severe motor fluctuations: a 2-year follow-up review. *J. Neurosurg.* **89,** 713–718.
51a. The Deep-Brain Stimulation for Parkinson's Disease Study Group. (2001) Deep-brain stimulation of the subthalamic nucleus or the pars interna of the globus pallidus in Parkinson's disease. *N. Engl. J. Med.* **345,** 956–963.
52. Bergman, H., Wichmann, T., and DeLong, M. R. (1990) Reversal of experimental parkinsonism by lesions of the subthalamic nucleus. *Science* **249,** 1436–1438.
53. Alvarez, L., Macias, R., Guridi, J., Lopez, G., Alvarez, E., Maragoto, C., et al. (2001) Dorsal subthalamotomy for Parkinson's disease. *Mov. Disord.* **16,** 72–78.
54. Limousin, P., Krack, P., Pollak, P., Benazzouz, A., Ardouin, C., Hoffmann, D., et al. (1998) Electrical stimulation of the subthalamic nucleus in advanced Parkinson's disease. *N. Engl. J. Med.* **339,** 1105–1111.
55. Kumar, R., Lozano, A. M., Kim, Y. J., Hutchison, W. D., Sime, E., Halket, E., et al. (1998) Double-blind evaluation of subthalamic nucleus deep brain stimulation in advanced Parkinson's disease. *Neurology* **51,** 850–855.
56. Moro, E., Scerrati, M., Romito, L. M., Roselli, R., Tonali, P., and Albanese, A. (1999) Chronic subthalamic nucleus stimulation reduces medication requirements in Parkinson's disease. *Neurology* **53,** 85–90.
57. Molinuevo, J. L., Valldeoriola, F., Tolosa, E., Rumia, J., Valls-Sole, J., Roldan, H., et al. (2000) Levodopa withdrawal after bilateral subthalamic nucleus stimulation in advanced Parkinson disease. *Arch. Neurol.* **57,** 983–988.
58. Burchiel, K. J., Anderson, V. C., Favre, J., and Hammerstad, J. P. (1999) Comparison of pallidal and subthalamic nucleus deep brain stimulation for advanced Parkinson's disease: results of a randomized, blinded pilot study. *Neurosurgery* **45,** 1375–1382; discussion 1382–1374.
59. Houeto, J. L., Damier, P., Bejjani, P. B., Staedler, C., Bonnet, A. M., Arnulf, I., et al. (2000) Subthalamic stimulation in Parkinson disease: a multidisciplinary approach. *Arch. Neurol.* **57,** 461–465.
60. Bejjani, B. P., Gervais, D., Arnulf, I., Papadopoulos, S., Demeret, S., Bonnet, A. M., et al. (2000) Axial parkinsonian symptoms can be improved: the role of levodopa and bilateral subthalamic stimulation. *J. Neurol. Neurosurg. Psychiatry* **68,** 595–600.
61. Rodriguez-Oroz, M. C., Gorospe, A., Guridi, J., Ramos, E., Linazasoro, G., Rodriguez-Palmero, M., et al. (2000) Bilateral deep brain stimulation of the subthalamic nucleus in Parkinson's disease. *Neurology* **55,** S45–S51.
62. Benabid, A. L., Krack, P. P., Benazzouz, A., Limousin, P., Koudsie, A., and Pollak, P. (2000) Deep brain stimulation of the subthalamic nucleus for Parkinson's disease: methodologic aspects and clinical criteria. *Neurology* **55,** S40–S44.
63. Hauser, R. A., Freeman, T. B., Snow, B. J., Nauert, M., Gauger, L., Kordower, J. H., et al. (1999) Long-term evaluation of bilateral fetal nigral transplantation in Parkinson disease. *Arch. Neurol.* **56,** 179–187.

64. Madrazo, I., Drucker-Colin, R., Diaz, V., Martinez-Mata, J., Torres, C., and Becerril, J. J. (1987) Open microsurgical autograft of adrenal medulla to the right caudate nucleus in two patients with intractable Parkinson's disease. *N. Engl. J. Med.* **316,** 831–834.
65. Goetz, C. G., Olanow, C. W., Koller, W. C., Penn, R. D., Cahill, D., Morantz, R., et al. (1989) Multicenter study of autologous adrenal medullary transplantation to the corpus striatum in patients with advanced Parkinson's disease [see comments]. *N. Engl. J. Med.* **320,** 337–341.
66. Sladek, J. R. Jr., Collier, T. J., Haber, S. N., Roth, R. H., and Redmond, D. E. Jr. (1986) Survival and growth of fetal catecholamine neurons transplanted into primate brain. *Brain Res. Bull.* **17,** 809–818.
67. Redmond, D. E. J., Sladek, J. R. J., Roth, R. H., Collier, T. J., Deutch, A. Y., and Haber, S. N. (1986) Fetal neuronal grafts in monkeys given methylphenytetrahydropyridine. *Lancet* **1,** 1125–1127.
68. Arbuthnott, G., Dunnett, S. D., and MacLeod, N. (1985) Electrophysiological properities of single units in dopamine-rich mesencephalic transplants in rat brain. *Neurosci. Lett.* **57,** 205–210.
69. Fischbach, G. D. and McKhann, G. M. (2001) Cell therapy for Parkinson's disease. *N. Engl. J. Med.* **344,** 763–765.

II Surgical Therapy for Parkinson's Disease and Tremor

4

Patient Selection for Movement Disorders Surgery

Rajeev Kumar and Anthony E. Lang

1. INTRODUCTION

Patient selection is one of the most important tasks necessary to ensure a successful outcome from movement disorders surgery. A multidisciplinary team with involvement of a neurologist, neurosurgeon, neuropsychologist, and often, a psychiatrist is usually necessary to comprehensively evaluate a patient's suitability for surgery. This chapter will focus predominantly on deep brain stimulation (DBS) and lesioning of the subthalamic nucleus (STN), globus pallidus internus (GPi), and thalamus for Parkinson's disease (PD), tremor, and dystonia. After discussion of considerations common to patient selection for all types of movement disorders surgery, specific disorders will be discussed, highlighting where appropriate how the differing effects of various surgical procedures impact patient selection. Unfortunately, for most of these surgical procedures, criteria that specifically predict surgical outcome, including efficacy and adverse effects, have not been well-established. Best clinical practice must therefore be informed by examination of the type of patients operated upon and the results of different case series.

2. GENERAL CONSIDERATIONS

A number of criteria are typically used by experienced surgical centers to select patients for surgery that are common to all movement disorders stereotactic surgery.

1. Patients must have significant disability in performance of activities of daily living or tasks necessary for employment, despite appropriate maximal drug therapy.
2. Patients should be in reasonable general health without specific contraindications to the neurosurgical procedure and have the physical and mental stamina to provide appropriate feedback while awake during a lengthy and demanding procedure. Usually these procedures are performed with the patients awake; however, in some severely debilitated hyperkinetic patients (e.g., generalized dystonia) or in younger children, general anesthesia may be used for much of the procedure. Patients who are medically ill or debilitated or who have unstable or severe cardiac, pulmonary, renal, or hepatic function, uncontrolled hypertension, or cancer are poor candidates for surgery. The need for chronic anticoagulation does not necessarily contraindicate surgery, but requires careful perioperative management with discontinuation of warfarin and implementation of heparin to minimize the time off anticoagulation and the risk of intracerebral hemorrhage *(1)*.
3. The patient's biological age, life expectancy, and expected duration of benefit should justify the risks of surgery. Some, but not all, groups restrict surgery to those with a biological age less than 70.
4. Patients and their families should have reasonable expectations of the outcome of surgery (e.g., patients with Parkinson's disease should not expect to be "cured" or have symptoms respond that generally do not benefit from the surgery).

From: Current Clinical Neurology:
Surgical Treatment of Parkinson's Disease and Other Movement Disorders
Edited by: D. Tarsy, J. L. Vitek, and A. M. Lozano © Humana Press Inc., Totowa, NJ

5. Patients should have a good understanding of the risks of surgery, including especially the risk of hemorrhage, which may result in serious neurologic disability or death.
6. There should be no uncontrolled psychiatric illness, especially anxiety or mood disorder, which may cause significant intraoperative patient decompensation that may compromise the quality of patient feedback necessary to obtain optimal results. PD patients with untreated depression undergoing STN DBS may be predisposed to severe worsening postoperatively and even suicide in the face of motorically successful surgery (unpublished observations) *(2)*.
7. Patients must not be demented or have significant cognitive impairment. Demented patients may be unable to provide appropriate intraoperative feedback. Such patients undergoing DBS may be difficult to program postoperatively because of lack of insight into their own motor status or inability to manage their own stimulation (i.e., learning to turn the stimulators on and off when appropriate). Surgery may also worsen cognition in patients with preexisting cognitive problems, especially patients with PD *(3–6)*.
8. Emotional support must be available from family or other caregivers to help the patient adjust postoperatively to his new role with increased physical capabilities and less physical dependence. Patients who have been dependent for many years may have psychological problems learning to cope with a more independent life *(7)*. Family members also need to be fully aware of the need to adapt to the changes experienced by the patients. Caregivers must be available able to aid patients requiring multiple and frequent physician visits for DBS programming, especially PD patients who may need to attend clinic visits during antiparkinson drug withdrawal when they will experience poor mobility.
9. Pre-operative MRI should not reveal severe cerebral atrophy or extensive white matter T_2 signal changes, which may increase the risk of intracerebral hemorrhage *(7,8)*.

3. ROLE OF THE SURGICAL TEAM IN PATIENT SELECTION

Individual evaluation of a prospective surgical candidate by each member of a multi-disciplinary team can aid in selecting appropriate patients for surgery. The neurologist must ensure that the underlying diagnosis is correct, that maximal medical therapy has been provided, and that the patient still has substantial disability. The neurosurgeon should evaluate the patient's general health, potential neurosurgical contraindications, and carefully review the risks of surgery with the patient and family. Neuropsychological evaluation and, if necessary, psychiatric evaluation are mandatory in all cases of surgery for PD and are often also useful in surgery for tremor and dystonia *(6)*. This should include a full clinical interview with the patient and important caregivers. Behavioral abnormalities, any propensity towards anxiety or panic attacks in stressful or potentially claustrophobic situations, and symptoms suggestive of early dementia should be explored. For anxious individuals, teaching systematic relaxation techniques that the patient can employ intraoperatively may be useful. A detailed neuropsychological assessment should follow. Although, a discussion of the specific psychometric instruments that may be used is beyond the scope of this chapter, recommendations for screening, clinical, and research evaluations have recently been published *(2)*. A variety of domains should be assessed including estimation of premorbid intellectual capacity, attention, language function, memory for verbal and nonverbal information, executive function, as well as behavior and mood state. This examination should allow determination of the patient's cognitive strengths and weaknesses, aid in diagnosis of a possible co-morbid early dementia, and detect untreated depression or other psychiatric symptoms. Cognitive abnormalities in keeping with the underlying diagnosis of PD should not lead one to advise against surgery, but significant abnormalities not normally seen in uncomplicated PD (such as markedly impaired naming and verbal fluency) should lead one to question the patient's suitability for surgery *(2–6)*. It is often useful to hold periodic meetings of the entire surgical team to discuss results of the evaluations and make a final decision regarding a patient's suitability for surgery as well as the surgical procedure which may be most appropriate.

4. DEEP BRAIN STIMULATION VS LESIONING

Thalamic lesioning and DBS are of approximately the same efficacy for tremor, whereas data in PD suggest that lesioning the STN or GPi also have similar beneficial effects as stimulation *(5,7,9–25)*. However, DBS has fewer adverse neurologic effects compared with lesioning because much less tissue is destroyed with electrode implantation alone *(9)*. Stimulation is also adjustable in order to maximize benefit and minimize adverse effects. Unlike lesions, the hardware for DBS is quite costly and may be associated with both immediate and delayed complications relating to hardware infection, breakage, and battery changes *(26–28)*. Many follow-up visits are often necessary to adjust stimulation settings (especially with STN DBS for PD) and a large effort by physicians and patients is required *(16)*. This may not be practical in patients who live in geographically isolated locations far from surgery centers. Many patients often express a preference for one or another treatment modality. As a result, the choice of stimulation or lesioning must be individualized depending on resources available at the surgical center and a variety of patient specific factors.

5. PARKINSON'S DISEASE

Surgery should be considered for PD in patients with severe medication-refractory motor fluctuations and levodopa-induced dyskinesias, disabling medication-refractory tremor, or marked medication intolerance making medical management unsatisfactory. (Caution should be exercised with the latter criteria with respect to hallucinations or other psychiatric symptoms occurring on low doses of dopaminergic drugs since this is often a forewarning of subsequent dementia.) Nondopaminergic problems and nonmotor symptoms should not be the major source of disability as these are not markedly improved with surgery, though one group has preliminarily reported an improvement in nonmotor symptoms of parkinsonism with bilateral STN DBS *(29)*. With expert medical management alone, most patients with PD have sufficient reduction in disability to function well for 10 or more years after diagnosis. In addition to altering the dose and frequency of levodopa therapy, a variety of different medication strategies may be helpful in obviating the need for surgery in patients with motor fluctuations and dyskinesias and should be considered before proceeding with surgery:

1. High-dose dopamine agonists (e.g., pergolide 6–12 mg/d) and low-dose levodopa.
2. Addition of catechol-O-methyltransferase inhibitor (i.e., entacapone or tolcapone) and reduction of levodopa.
3. Liquid levodopa/carbidopa taken orally hourly or continuously via duodenal infusion.
4. Where available, apomorphine by intermittent injection or continuous subcutaneous infusion.
5. Use of antidyskinetic agents such as amantadine; fluoxetine; clozaril; propranolol; buspirone (amantadine is the most reliably useful antidyskinetic agent and also improves off-period parkinsonism and motor fluctuations).

Not all patients are suitable for each of these strategies and indeed, many physicians and patients would opt to proceed directly to surgery without a trial of liquid levodopa/carbidopa or apomorphine. For patients with severe tremor, medication trials should generally include high doses of levodopa/carbidopa (at least 1500 mg/d), anticholinergic therapy, and clozapine.

Although surgery for PD is effective late in the disorder, the timing of surgery should be assessed with respect to when the advantages of surgery outweigh the risks of surgery and the risks of medical treatment. Patient quality of life based on personal, professional, and social factors is an important factor that the patient must use to judge the risk:benefit ratio of surgery. However, surgery should not be delayed until the patient loses his job because of physical disability or there is loss of independence and ability to effectively participate in family or society affairs. It has been speculated that STN DBS or lesioning may alter the course of PD by potentially reducing excitotoxic glutamatergic outflow from the STN to a number of targets, but especially to the substantia nigra pars compacta *(30)*. If this is the case, there would be significant justification for performing surgery at a much earlier stage of the disease. Although there is supportive data in animal models of PD, there is no convincing clinical data in humans that STN surgery is neuroprotective *(31)*. Indeed, STN DBS might actually increase glutamate release *(32)*. Therefore, at this time the possibility of neuroprotection should not influence one's decision regarding surgery.

Some groups have found that older patients (especially those greater than 70 years of age), tend to benefit less from pallidotomy, though this has not been confirmed by other surgical teams *(18,19)*. This may reflect the greater frequency of levodopa-resistant symptoms that are seen in the elderly.

Elderly patients are less tolerant of surgery and more succeptable to intraoperative or postoperative confusion, especially when undergoing bilateral STN DBS. Furthermore, persistent postoperative decline is also more common in elderly patients with STN DBS, especially if there is any pre-operative cognitive dysfunction *(3)*.

There is very little published experience with surgery for atypical parkinsonian syndromes. Patients with multiple system atrophy (MSA) may initially respond well to levodopa, but this response typically wanes within a few years. It is possible that such patients might have some short-term benefit from GPi or STN surgery. One case of nonlevodopa responsive MSA has been reported with failure to improve following STN DBS *(7,33)*. Nevertheless, it may be appropriate to consider surgery for levodopa-related dystonia or dyskinesias in MSA patients with a clearly preserved levodopa response. On the other hand, patients with PD due to Parkin mutations reportedly have had an excellent response to STN DBS, in keeping with their young age of onset, excellent levodopa response, prominent and early levodopa-induced dyskinesias, and pathology typically restricted to the substantia nigra *(7)*.

Previous surgery for PD does not contraindicate additional surgery if the patient is otherwise an appropriate surgical candidate. There are reports of successful bilateral STN DBS in patients with prior unilateral thalamotomy, unilateral or bilateral thalamic DBS, unilateral pallidotomy and unilateral or bilateral GPi DBS who benefited from initial surgery but subsequently developed additional disability despite aggressive medical therapy *(7,34–37)*.

Severity of patient disability should be assessed not only through routine clinical interview and examination, but also using formal clinical rating scales. The Unified Parkinson's Disease Rating Scale (UPDRS) allows one to gauge the severity of disability with respect to mental function, activities of daily living, motor signs, and complications of drug therapy *(38)*. Clinical response to levodopa is predictive of the response to STN DBS and pallidotomy on off-period signs of parkinsonism *(15,39–41)*. Similarly, lentiform nucleus hypermetabolism on FDG-PET scanning correlates with the response to pallidotomy and also correlates with levodopa response *(39)*. Therefore, the levodopa challenge test after overnight withdrawal of all antiparkinson medication, using a supramaximal dose of levodopa is an important part of the evaluation to determine the degree of benefit obtainable with surgery. This process also educates the patient and family regarding appropriate expectations from surgery. Most symptoms resistant to a supramaximal levodopa dose fail to respond to surgery, though one report suggests that bilateral STN DBS in combination with levodopa may slightly improve preoperative on-period axial disability *(42)*. However, persistent on-period tremor can often be improved more with surgery than with levodopa *(7,14,43)*. How severe the motor signs of parkinsonism must be in the off-period to justify surgery is a highly subjective determination. However, some groups have arbitrarily set a minimum cut-off of 30/108 on the UPDRS motor (though most patients with PD for 10 to 20 years have a score of 40–80) except for tremor-dominant patients who may have a lower total score *(7)*. Determining what degree of expected improvement justifies surgery is also difficult. Some groups believe that a suprathreshold dose of levodopa should improve parkinsonism by at least 50% before proceeding with surgery *(7)*. Nevertheless, it may be reasonable to judiciously consider surgery in carefully selected patients with significant persistent on-period disability who may only be modestly improved by surgery. On the other hand, operating on patients with very poor on-period postural stability and frequent falls pre-operatively may put such patients at even higher risk of falls due to improved bradykinesia and faster gait. Furthermore, such patients may fracture or displace their DBS hardware due to falls if they receive DBS (unpublished observations).

Severe dyskinesia and motor fluctuations do not predict a poorer response to either GPi or STN surgery both of which markedly reduce dyskinesias, though by different mechanisms *(12)*. As a result, patients with significant disability due to severe motor fluctuations are likely to benefit more with surgery than those without such motor complications. Pre-operatively, the severity of motor complications may be evaluated using part IV of the UPDRS, motor fluctuation diaries, the Lang-Fahn dyskinesia rating scale *(43)* and dyskinesia rating scales obtained during the levodopa challenge test.

Many groups also incorporate the use of PD-specific quality of life scales such as the PDQ-39 into their pre-operative assessment of disability *(45–48)*.

As mentioned above, significant cognitive abnormalities on detailed neuropsychological testing are a contraindication to surgery. Simple cognitive screening tools which can be used in the clinic may be helpful to screen out some patients before referring them for more detailed testing. The Grenoble group excludes patients with a Mini-Mental Status Exam score ≤24/30 or with a Mattis Dementia Rating Scale Score ≤130/144 *(7)*. Drug-induced hallucinations and psychosis markedly worsen intraoperatively resulting in confusion and agitation which may persist for several days postoperatively. Such patients should be excluded from surgery *(2,3)*. It is an open question as to whether patients with any prior history of drug-induced hallucinations should be excluded from surgery. If such patients pass detailed neuropsychological testing and can be managed temporarily pre-operatively on a reduced but suboptimal dose of antiparkinson medication without neuroleptic therapy, surgery can be successfully performed without significant postoperative cognitive decline (unpublished observations). However, as mentioned previously, pre-operative occurrence of hallucinations is a strong predictor for the subsequent development of dementia and the increased probability of severe cognitive decline developing in the future needs to be taken into account. On the other hand, in highly select cases surgery might be considered in patients with the combination of mild pre-operative cognitive abnormalities and severe motor disability, where the potential for cognitive worsening with surgery is outweighed by the possibility of improved motor disability *(49)*.

5.1. *Thalamic Surgery*

DBS and lesioning of the thalamus, GPi and STN have been widely performed for advanced PD. The clinical effects of lesioning vs. stimulation at any one of these sites seem similar based on the published data *(9–25)*. However, the clinical effects of operating at each of these sites differ. Thalamic surgery has limited effects and can markedly improve tremor, moderately improve rigidity, and may also improve levodopa-induced dyskinesias, depending on the exact site of stimulation or lesioning *(9–11,51–53)*. Thalamic surgery does not significantly improve bradykinesia or gait disorders, which are usually the greatest sources of disability. Reports of improvement in bradykinesia are probably artifactual due to reduction in tremor-related interference with tasks used to measure bradykinesia *(11)*. Quality of life may be improved with thalamic DBS, but activities of daily living as measured by the UPDRS are often unchanged *(9–11)*. Because bradykinesia and gait are not improved, several patients initially treated with thalamic DBS for tremor-dominant PD have subsequently undergone STN DBS for their other symptoms of parkinsonism that have become more pronounced over time *(7)*. Since the anti-tremor effects of STN DBS seem comparable to those of thalamic DBS *(43,54)*, thalamic surgery may no longer have a significant place in the surgical treatment of PD.

5.2. *Subthalamic Nucleus and Globus Pallidus Surgery*

STN and GPi surgery can improve all of the cardinal features of Parkinson's disease, including tremor, bradykinesia, and rigidity in addition to improving levodopa-induced dyskinesias *(12–25)*. Nonrandomized studies suggest that bilateral STN DBS may improve off-period parkinsonism to a slightly greater degree than bilateral GPi DBS *(12,15)*. STN DBS predominantly reduces dyskinesias because of reduction in concomitant drug therapy (since STN DBS actually lowers the threshold for levodopa-induced dyskinesias), while GPi DBS or lesioning directly suppresses dyskinesias. Patient selection criteria for surgery at either site are quite similar since it is unknown what preoperative factors may suggest that a patient would have a better response to one surgery than another (e.g., severe dyskinesias, prominent axial disability, etc.). The STN may be a preferable target in that it is small and easily seen on MRI, has low spatial variability between patients, and good correlation of response to intraoperative stimulation and postoperative benefit *(7)*. Unlike GPi surgery, bilateral STN DBS allows a marked reduction in antiparkinson medication *(12)*. Approximately 5–10% of patients can be optimally improved and remain off all anti-Parkinson medication 1–2 yr after surgery; 30% remain off all levodopa, but take dopamine agonists, while the majority of patients take low-dose levodopa *(7,55)*. Average antiparkinson drug reduction is approx 50% *(12–14)*. This is particularly favorable in patients unable to tolerate adequate doses of antiparkinson medication because of somnolence, nausea, and vomiting despite domperidone and other anti-emetics, or psychiatric adverse effects in the absence of cognitive impairment. Levodopa and dopamine agonists may actually worsen on-period freezing in some patients. Therefore, STN DBS may improve on-period freezing by allowing a reduction in levodopa dose. If it is discovered that levodopa is actually toxic to nigral neurons, then the levodopa-sparing effect of STN surgery may also be an advantage. Less medication reduces cost and is less inconvenient for patients, especially if the number of drug doses per day is reduced. Likely, because the STN is a smaller target, DBS parameters are generally lower compared to the GPi which will result in longer battery life and need for fewer battery changes *(15)*. However, in comparison to GPi, STN DBS requires more frequent follow-up visits with complex adjustments of stimulation parameters and antiparkinson medication. In addition, other postoperative management problems are more common including stimulation-induced dyskinesias, mood changes, hypophonia, stimulation-induced dysarthria, and sialorrhea *(16)*.

Cognitively, both bilateral GPi DBS and bilateral STN DBS are well-tolerated in younger patients, including lack of detrimental effects on executive function. Both interventions result in mild decline in lexical fluency. STN DBS may result in mild improvement in working memory and psychomotor speed, which is not seen with GPi DBS *(56–58)*. On the other hand, bilateral STN DBS may adversely affect frontal executive function in patients greater than 69 yr of age and patients with borderline cognitive status risk postoperative decompensation, including even the development of a PSP-like syndrome *(3)*. Mood changes have been more frequently reported with STN DBS, including depression and abulia, in part secondary to levodopa withdrawal *(50)*. Severe stimulation-induced depression has also been reported associated with inadvertent substantia nigra reticulata stimulation *(59)*. STN DBS also seems to be associated with an increased risk of postoperative suicide. Mood-congruent laughter accompanied by stimulation-induced dyskinesias has also been induced with highly effective STN stimulation, possibly due to current spread to the limbic portion of the STN *(60,61)*. Mania and hypersexuality occasionally may occur in patients treated with bilateral STN DBS *(62)*.

GPi surgery may be performed unilaterally or bilaterally. Bilateral surgery has more pronounced antiparkinson and anti-dyskinetic effects. Unilateral surgery may be considered most appropriate in patients with highly asymmetric parkinsonism and levodopa-induced dyskinesias or dystonia. Although no overall cognitive decline has been reported with GPi DBS, a subgroup of elderly patients using high doses of levodopa may be at risk *(2,63)*. Left hemisphere lesions on the other hand result in reduced verbal fluency and loss of verbal learning and memory capacity, while right hemisphere lesions cause diminished visual-spatial constructional and mnemonic processes. Unilateral pallidotomy may also cause clinically significant behavioral abnormalities in approximately 25% of patients, especially impulsivity, poor judgment, disinhibition, and loss of insight *(2,4)*. Bilateral pallidotomy is associated with a high incidence of bulbar dysfunction, including dysarthria, hypophonia, dysphagia, and drooling *(5,64)*. A severe dysexecutive syndrome has also been reported in isolated cases *(64,65)*. As a result, bilateral pallidotomy cannot be recommended and either bilateral GPi DBS or unilateral pallidotomy with contralateral GPi DBS is preferred.

There is limited data available on the effects of STN lesioning, but recent reports suggest that unilateral or bilateral lesioning tends to be relatively well-tolerated with motor effects similar to STN DBS *(23–25)*. As with GPi surgery, bilateral STN DBS results in greater improvement than unilateral STN DBS with not only marked bilateral improvement in parkinsonism, but greater improvement in parkinsonism on each side *(54)*. As a result, bilateral GPi or STN surgery is preferable in most patients with advanced PD. Unilateral STN surgery may also result in problems balancing the effects of drugs and stimulation, since the stimulated side requires less antiparkinson medication and may become dyskinetic without drug reduction, while drug reduction may result in under treatment of the unstimulated side (a similar situation applies to unilateral STN stimulation combined with contralateral GPi DBS). Although this has been our experience with unilateral STN DBS, other investigators report less difficulty achieving the appropriate balance (J. Vitek, personal communication). Nevertheless, we have found that unilateral STN DBS may be effectively applied in patients with highly asymmetric tremor-dominant parkinsonism, including patients with a prior thalamotomy or unilateral thalamic DBS.

Although progression of predominately nonlevodopa-responsive axial symptoms has been reported on long term follow up of STN DBS, most of the benefit has been maintained *(7,55)*. Ghika has reported decreased efficacy of bilateral GPi DBS after more than 12 mo of follow up, requiring additional anti-parkinson medication and partial loss of the anti-dyskinetic effect *(66)*. There is very little other data reported on the long-term effects of bilateral GPi DBS. However, several patients who experienced waning benefit following bilateral GPi DBS have subsequently undergone bilateral STN DBS with significant benefit *(34)*. Long-term follow-up of the effects of unilateral pallidotomy suggest that significant improvement in contralateral off-period parkinsonism and on-period dyskinesias is maintained for at least 5 yr *(21)*. Nevertheless, as with GPi DBS, many such patients have subsequently required either contralateral GPi DBS or bilateral STN DBS *(67)*.

6. TREMOR

Severe nonparkinsonian tremor is a common cause of severe disability, requiring DBS or lesioning of the motor thalamus—usually the ventralis intermedius (Vim) nucleus, ventralis oralis posterior (Vop) nucleus, and occasionally the zona incerta. In general, thalamic DBS is preferable to thalamotomy because of the increased rate of adverse effects with unilateral thalamotomy, including alteration in speech in approx 30% of patients and possibly a greater improvement in quality of life with Vim DBS *(9)*. Selecting appropriate patients for surgery follows the same general guidelines previously outlined in this chapter.

6.1. Essential Tremor

Essential tremor (ET) is the most common cause of tremor. Although the majority of those affected never seek treatment because there is only mild tremor-related disability, approximately 75% of patients have some disability related to social embarrassment or tremor-related interference with writing, use of utensils, drinking from a cup or vocal tremor interfering with communication *(68)*. Although ET is manifest predominantly as postural tremor, a high proportion also have significant kinetic or intention tremor. This subgroup has higher tremor-related disability and is more likely to require surgery. The majority of patients have hand tremor with coexistent head tremor in 40%, vocal tremor in approximately 20% and trunk or leg tremor in less than 20%. ET is very slowly progressive with increasing tremor amplitude and decreasing tremor frequency with advancing disease *(69)*.

Prior to consideration of surgery, patients should have significant tremor-related disability, despite optimal medical therapy. All patients should receive an adequate trial of first line anti-tremor drugs—propranolol (240–360 mg q/d), primidone (250–750 mg q/d), and possibly gabapentin (1800–3600 mg q/d)—alone and/or in combination *(70)*. Reduction in tremor amplitude with these medications may significantly improve disability in some patients. Oral medications are more helpful for limb tremor than vocal or head tremor, which are typically improved more with botulinum toxin injections *(70)*. Judicious use of small amounts of alcohol taken intermittently may also be appropriate to facilitate certain tasks (e.g. handwriting, feeding) in select individuals, since approximately 50% of patients will improve with alcohol administration. If patients fail first-line therapy, trials of additional medications are not mandatory and may result in unnecessary delay in surgery, since there is relatively little chance of marked improvement with second-line (clonazepam, alprazolam, and mirtazapine) and third-line (clonidine, acetazolamide, flunarizine, and theophyline) agents *(70)*. Pre-operative assessment of tremor severity may be undertaken using the tremor rating scale (TRS), spiral drawing and handwriting rating, tremor-related disability questionnaire, Purdue pegboard test, and quality of life scales like the SF-36 or sickness impact profile (SIP). Accelerometry usually does not provide additional useful information *(71)*.

Thalamotomy and thalamic DBS result in approximately equal improvement in tremor control *(9)*. Thalamic surgery almost uniformly markedly improves or abolishes distal postural tremor, though treatment of intention tremor and severe proximal arm tremor is less efficacious. Patients with marked intention tremor have only approximately 50–75% long-term benefit with thalamic DBS *(51)*. Patients with severe bilateral tremor are best treated with bilateral Vim DBS, since bilateral thalamotomy is associated with a high rate of bulbar and cognitive adverse effects. Patients who have previously undergone unilateral thalamotomy and who have developed significant tremor ipsilateral to the lesion should be treated with contralateral thalamic DBS *(51)*. Although patients with prominent head, vocal, and trunk tremor may note some improvement with unilateral DBS, a better response is seen in these axial signs with bilateral DBS *(72)*. In contrast to patients with severe bilateral Parkinson's disease in whom bilateral STN or GPi DBS is most often performed simultaneously, bilateral thalamic surgery is frequently staged.

6.2. Cerebellar Tremor

Cerebellar tremor is most commonly problematic in patients with multiple sclerosis (MS), post-traumatic tremor, midbrain stroke, spinocerebellar ataxia, or the cerebellar subtype of multiple system atrophy. Disabling tremor is seen in approximately 5–10% of MS clinic patients *(73)*. Cerebellar tremor is characterized by unilateral or bilateral intention tremor (though postural tremor may also be present) that is less than 5 Hz *(69,73)*. Head and trunk titubation are common and may be the most disabling form of axial tremor. Although there is little data available regarding the natural history of these cerebellar tremors, in general they do not usually improve over time. Medical therapy with anticholinergic drugs, carbamazepine, clonazepam, L-5 hydroxytryptophan, and buspirone is rarely successful *(73,74)*. Occasional patients may improve mildly with high-dose propranolol. Superimposed ataxia often makes it difficult to sort out what component of the disability is due to ataxia and what is due to tremor. Deuschl has suggested simple inspection to assess this, examining the regularity of the movements when patients make typical movements that activate tremor *(69)*. For example, during examination of a patient attempting to drink from a cup, the examiner must decide if the disability is primarily due to rhythmic or arrhythmic movements. Physiologic assessment may help to predict those most likely to benefit from surgery. Upper extremity postural tremor frequency analysis using accelerometry was predictive in one series of Vim DBS. Patients with tremor >3Hz experienced tremor ablation, but those with tremor <3Hz did not improve with surgery *(74)*. Frequency analysis during a wrist-tracking task may also be predictive of response of action tremor to thalamotomy with 80% tremor reduction in those patients with just one frequency peak in the spectra and only 30% tremor reduction in those with multiple frequency peaks *(75)*.

MS patients also have multiple other nervous system lesions, causing other neurologic deficits. The effect of these deficits on the potential for improvement following surgery must also be considered. Patients with marked sensory impairment in the target limb, excessive arm weakness (less than grade 4/5), or marked truncal weakness resulting in a bed-bound state should not be offered surgery because significant functional improvement would not be achieved even if tremor were eliminated *(74)*. Alusi et al. *(74)* have suggested that a more comprehensive evaluation may be helpful in selecting MS patients for surgery. Besides the tremor-rating scales and motor testing suggested for ET, assessments of disability caused by ataxia and other MS lesions may be helpful including the extended disability status scale (EDSS), ataxia rating scales, speech and swallowing evaluation, and Barthel index *(74)*.

Previous reports of the effects of thalamotomy suggest that approximately 30% of MS patients are significantly improved *(76,77)*. There have been several recent studies of Vim DBS for MS-associated cerebellar tremor. Most have noted significant reduction in tremor although overall disability was only mildly improved, probably because of the presence of other neurologic deficits *(9,78,79)*. Additional important issues include the increased risk of adverse effects from surgery given the presence of multiple coexisting brain lesions and a possible negative effect on disease progression including postoperative exacerbation of MS due to breach of the blood/brain barrier (BBB) *(74)*.

6.3. *Holmes Tremor*

Holmes tremor is characterized by a combination of parkinsonian rest tremor and cerebellar intention tremor with a frequency of <4.5 Hz. This symptomatic tremor is due to a lesion in the cerebellar outflow pathway, typically in the midbrain, which also involves the substantia nigra or nigrostriatal tract *(69)*. Onset is commonly delayed after head trauma or midbrain stroke. Medical therapy with levodopa, dopamine agonists, and anticholinergics may be effective in some patients, though levodopa responders may develop dyskinesias. Surgery is appropriate for patients with significant disability due to medication-refractory tremor although significant weakness in the target limb is a relative contraindication. Pallidotomy, thalamotomy, and thalamic DBS have reportedly been helpful *(76,80,81)* but the best surgical target has not been established.

6.4. *Primary Writing Tremor*

This represents a task-specific tremor or a variant of dystonia in which tremor is only present during writing or predominantly during writing and not present with other fine motor tasks. Tremor may be either task-specific or position-specific. Some patients may partially respond to botulinum toxin injections and rarely patients may improve with anticholinergic drugs or propranolol *(82)*. We have also seen considerable improvement with the use of a simple writing device. Where optimal handwriting is necessary for work, this form of tremor may threaten employment. Both thalamic DBS and thalamotomy *(83)* have reportedly been successful.

7. DYSTONIA

Dystonia is a highly heterogeneous disorder with both primary (genetically-defined and idiopathic) and secondary etiologies, variable distribution (generalized, hemidystonia, segmental, and focal), and variable age at onset. There are no controlled studies of surgery for dystonia and the optimal target (GPi, thalamus, or other) has not been determined. There are no predictive clinical tests comparable to the levodopa response in PD. As a result, conclusions about appropriate patient selection for various surgeries for dystonia must be tempered in light of significant gaps in the current state of knowledge. Furthermore, there have been no contemporary systematic studies of the cognitive effects of surgery for dystonia. As with PD, surgery for dystonia should be restricted to those patients with significant functional disability despite maximal medical therapy. Unfortunately, with the exception of botulinum toxin injections for focal dystonias, medical therapy for dystonia has poor efficacy. Nevertheless, oral medications are sometimes helpful and therapy should be tailored to the individual with consideration given to trials of anticholinergic drugs, oral baclofen, benzodiazepines, dopamine depleters (e.g., tetrabenazine), and dopamine receptor blockers alone or in combination. The role of intrathecal baclofen in the management of dystonia is uncertain. This should probably be considered before other CNS surgery, especially in patients with symptomatic dystonia with associated spasticity (e.g., cerebral palsy) *(84,85)*. Patients who require surgery typically have generalized dystonia, hemidystonia, segmental dystonia involving at least one limb, or severe cervical dystonia with botulinum toxin resistance. The severity of motor disability in these patients may be quantified using rating scales predominantly developed for patients with widespread dystonia such as the Burke-Fahn-Marsden scale and the Unified Dystonia Rating Scale or for cervical dystonia such as the Toronto Western Spasmodic Torticollis Rating Scale.

7.1. Thalamotomy

Based largely on series published by Tasker, Andrew, and Cooper in which a high proportion of operated patients had generalized dystonia, thalamotomy is thought to be most effective for dystonia affecting distal limbs and least effective for axial dystonia *(86–88)*. The placement of thalamic lesions was variable in these reports but generally involved the Vim and/or Vop with lesions frequently expanded to the centromedian nucleus or other adjacent regions of the thalamus. Improvement was commonly progressive for up to 6 mo postoperatively. However, some patients demonstrated only transient improvement followed by deterioration. Patients with idiopathic, nonprogressive, familial disease seemed to respond better than patients without a family history of dystonia. Andrew found that patients with symptomatic hemidystonia fared better than patients with primary dystonia *(87)*. As in PD, bilateral thalamotomy was associated with a high incidence of dysarthria and dysphagia *(86–88)*. Thalamotomy has also been reported to be helpful in tardive dystonia and has been successfully used for occasional cases of writer's cramp *(89,90)*.

7.2. Pallidotomy

The initial rationale for pallidotomy in dystonia was the improvement in levodopa off-period dystonia following pallidotomy for PD. Close to 100 cases of pallidotomy for dystonia have been reported in the past five years since several groups first reported striking benefits *(91–97)*. Similar to PD, the sensorimotor portion of the GPi has been used as the target in dystonia. However, the best place to lesion the pallidum in dystonia is unknown. Although axial signs may initially be improved with unilateral pallidotomy, this benefit tends to be lost relatively quickly if the contralateral side is not lesioned *(91,93,97)*. Most reported patients underwent bilateral lesioning and the high incidence of bulbar weakness and dysphonia that occurred following bilateral pallidotomy in PD has not been observed. Delayed onset improvement occurs commonly with a distal to proximal order of progressive improvement. Younger patients have generally improved more than older patients, though the duration of follow-up has been relatively short. Indeed, some patients with an initial excellent response to pallidotomy now seem to be gradually worsening with a few patients subsequently undergoing GPi DBS (unpublished observations). Thus the duration of benefit from pallidotomy is unknown. The greatest and most uniform improvements have been seen in patients with primary dystonia (especially those who are DYT-1 positive), though improvements have been reported in Hallervorden-Spatz syndrome, tardive dystonia, post-anoxic dystonia, and exercise-induced dystonia *(91–99)*. In keeping with these observations, Yoshor et al. performed a retrospective single center comparison of the effects of pallidotomy and thalamotomy and found significantly greater benefit with pallidotomy than with thalamotomy in patients with primary dystonia, but little difference between the two procedures in patients with secondary dystonia *(100)*.

7.3. Thalamic DBS

Only a handful of cases of dystonia treated with thalamic DBS have been reported. Sellal et al. noted improvement with DBS of the VPL nucleus of the thalamus in a patients with symptomatic hemidystonia who pre-operatively noted reduction in dystonic posturing with superficial sensory stimulation *(101)*. The Grenoble group has performed Vim DBS on ten patients with a variety of forms of dystonia with mild to moderate improvement in about half. Some of these patients have gone on to subsequently receive GPi stimulation with greater benefit *(102)*. A patient with severe tardive dystonia undergoing simultaneous implantation bilateral into GPi and Vim obtained benefit only with GPi DBS and no additional improvement with concurrent Vim stimulation *(103)*. Higher stimulation pulse widths and voltages have usually been required compared to PD, which necessitates more frequent battery changes.

7.4. GPi DBS

Several small case series have reported dramatic benefits in both children and adults *(91,102,104–109)*. Secondary orthopedic abnormalities were also slowly improved in some patients. As with pallidotomy, the greatest improvements were seen in children with DYT-1 generalized dystonia with lesser improvements in adults and patients with non-DYT-1 primary dystonia *(102,104)*. Follow-up for 1–4 yr in children with DYT-1 dystonia suggests sustained improvement allowing for reduction or discontinuation of anti-dystonia medications *(104)*. Both axial and limb dystonia is improved with bilateral GPi DBS. In general, patients with primary dystonia have had less variable outcomes than patients with secondary dystonia, and in agreement with this impression, the presence of an abnormal MRI scan seems to reduce the likelihood of an optimal response *(102,108)*. Bilateral GPi DBS has also been beneficial in two small series of patients with cervical dystonia resulting in significant improvements in both neck pain and posturing *(106,107)*.

On initiation of stimulation, progressive improvement is typically seen over hours to weeks with gradual return of dystonia over minutes to hours on discontinuation of stimulation. Several groups have found that high stimulation settings are necessary to achieve benefit in some patients, resulting in short battery life and the need for frequent battery replacements. Although this surgical approach seems to be the most promising, further investigations are necessary to explore the effects of surgery on aditional targets such as STN since GPi surgery is clearly not effective in all patients, especially those with secondary dystonia.

8. CONCLUSION

Patient selection for movement disorders surgery requires a multidisciplinary approach taking into account the patient's neurologic condition, prior medial therapy, co-morbid illnesses, and psychiatric and cognitive status. Thereafter, the appropriate surgical procedure for each patient can be selected. This is a rapidly evolving field and it is likely that the boundaries of who may potentially benefit from surgery will continue to expand. Bearing this in mind, it is the job of each surgical team to exercise judgment and discretion in selecting patients who have an appropriate risk: benefit ratio for surgery. It is a difficult task to find an appropriate balance between conservatism in patient selection and attempting to make this form of treatment available to all who might benefit.

ACKNOWLEDGMENTS

Supported in part by the Colorado Neurological Institute and the National Parkinson Foundation.

REFERENCES

1. Heit, J. A. (2001) Perioperative management of the chronically anticoagulated patient. *J. Thromb. Thrombolysis* **12,** 81–87.
2. Saint-Cyr, J. A. and Trepanier L. L. (2000) Neuropsychologic assessment of patients for movement disorder surgery. *Mov. Disord.* **15,** 771–783.
3. Saint-Cyr, J. A., Trepanier, L. L., Kumar, R., Lozano, A. M., and Lang, A. E. (2000) Neuropsychological consequences of chronic bilateral stimulation of the subthalamic nucleus in Parkinson's disease. *Brain* **123,** 2091–2108.
4. Trepanier, L. L., Saint-Cyr, J. A., Lozano, A. M., and Lang, A. E. (1998) Neuropsychological consequences of posteroventral pallidotomy for the treatment of Parkinson's disease. *Neurology* **51,** 207–215.
5. Scott, R., Gregory, R., Hines, N., Carroll, C., Hyman, N., Papanasstasiou, V., et al. (1998) Neuropsychological, neurological and functional outcome following pallidotomy for Parkinson's disease. A consecutive series of eight simultaneous bilateral and twelve unilateral procedures, *Brain* **121,** 659–675.
6. Saint-Cyr, J. A. and Trepanier, L. L. (2000) Neuropsychological considerations in movement disorder surgery. *Prog. Neurol. Surg.* **15,** 266–271.
7. Pollak, P. (2000) Deep Brain Stimulation. Annual Course of the American Academy of Neurology, Innovative surgical treatment of movement disorders 3AC.0006. San Diego.
8. Tan, E.-K. and Jankovic, J. (2000) Movement disorder surgery: patient selection and evaluation of surgical results. *Prog. Neurol. Surg.* **15,** 78–90.

9. Schuurman, P. R., Bosch, D. A., Bossuyt, P. M., Bonsel, G. J., van Someren, E. J., de Bie, R. M., et al. (2000) A comparison of continuous thalamic stimulation and thalamotomy for suppression of severe tremor. *N. Engl. J. Med.* **342,** 461–468.
10. Koller, W., Pahwa, R., Busenbark, K., et al. (1997) High frequency unilateral thalamic stimulation in the treatment of essential and parkinsonaim tremor. *Ann. Neurol.* **42,** 292–299.
11. Limousin, P., Speelman, J. D., Gielen, F., Janssens, M. and study collaborators. (1999) Multicentre European study of thalamic stimulation in parkinsonsian and essential tremor. J. *Neurol. Neurosurg. Psychiatry* **66,** 289–296.
12. DBS Study Group. (2001) Deep-brain stimulation of the subthalamic nucleus or the pars interna of the globus pallidus in Parkinson's disease. *N. Engl. J. Med.* **345,** 956–963.
13. Limousin, P., Krack, P., Pollak, P., Benazzouz, A., Ardouin, C., Hoffmann, D., and Benabid, A. L. (1998) Electrical stimulation of the subthalamic nucleus in advanced Parkinson's disease. *N. Engl. J. Med.* **339,** 1105 –1111.
14. Kumar, R., Lozano, A. M., Kim, Y. J., Hutchison, W. D., Sime, E., Halket, E., and Lang, A. E. (1998) Double-blind evaluation of subthalamic nucleus deep brain stimulation in advanced Parkinson's disease. *Neurology* **51,** 850–855.
15. Krack, P., Pollak, P., Limousin, P., Hoffmann, D., Xie, J., Benazzouz, A., and Benabid, A. L. (1998) Subthalamic nucleus or internal pallidal stimulation in young onset Parkinson's disease. *Brain* **121,** 451–457.
16. Volkmann, J., Allert, N., Voges, J., Weiss, P. H., Freund, H. J., and Sturm, V. (2001) Safety and efficacy of pallidal or subthalamic nucleus stimulation in advanced PD. *Neurology* **56,** 548–551.
17. Kumar, R., Lang, A. E., Rodriguez, M. C., Lozano, A. M., Limousin, P., Pollak, P., et al. (2000) Deep brain stimulation of the globus pallidus pars interna in advanced Parkinson's disease. *Neurology* **55(Suppl. 6),** S34–S39.
18. Lang, A. E., Lozano, A. M., Montgomery, E., Duff, J., Tasker, R., and Hutchinson, W. (1997) Posteroventral medial pallidotomy in advanced Parkinson's disease. *N. Engl. J. Med.* **337,** 1036–1042.
19. Uitti, R. J., Wharen, R. E. J., Turk, M. F., Lucas, J. A., Finton, M. J., Graff-Radford, N. R., et al. (1997) Unilateral pallidotomy for Parkinson's disease: comparison of outcome in younger versus elderly patients, *Neurology* **49,** 1072–1077.
20. Baron, M., Vitek, J., Bakay, R., Green, J., Kaneoke, Y., Hashimoto, T., et al. (1996) T reatment of advanced Parkinsons disease by posterior GPi pallidotomy: 1-year results of a pilot study. *Ann. Neurol.* **40,** 355–366.
21. Fine, J., Duff, J., Chen, R., Hutchison, W., Lozano, A. M., and Lang, A. E. (2000) Long-term follow-up of unilateral pallidotomy in advanced Parkinson's disease. *N. Engl. J. Med.* **342,** 1708–1714.
22. Samii, A., Turnbull, I. M., Kishore, A., Schulzer, M., Mak, E., Yardley, S., and Calne, D. B. (1999) Reassessment of unilateral pallidotomy in Parkinson's disease. A 2-year follow-up study. *Brain* **122,** 417–425.
23. Gill, S. S. and Heywood, P. (1997) Bilateral dorsolateral subthalamotomy for advanced Parkinson's disease. *Lancet* **350,** 1224.
24. Alvarez, L., Macias, R., Guridi, J., Lopez, G., Alvarez, E., Maragoto, C., et al. (2001) Dorsal subthalamotomy for Parkinson's disease. *Mov. Disord.* **16,** 72–78.
25. Barlas, O., Hanagasi, H. A., Imer, M., Sahin, H. A., Sencer, S., and Emre, M. (2001) Do unilateral ablative lesions of the subthalamic nucleu in parkinsonian patients lead to hemiballism? *Mov. Disord.* **16,** 306–310.
26. Schwalb, J. M., Riina, H. A., Skolnick, B., Jaggi, J. L., Simuni, T., and Baltuch, G. H. (2001) Revision of deep brain stimulator for tremor. Technical note. *J. Neurosurg.* **94,** 1010–1012.
27. Koller, W. C., Lyons, K. E., Wilkinson, S. B., Troster, A. I., and Pahwa, R. (2001) Long-term safety and efficacy of unilateral deep brain stimulation of the thalamus in essential tremor. *Mov. Disord.* **16,** 464–468.
28. Lyons, K. E., Koller, W. C., Wilkinson, S. B., and Pahwa, R. (2001) Surgical and device-related complications with deep brain stimulation. *Neurology* **56(Suppl. 3),** A147.
29. Witjas, T., Kaphan, E., Azulay, J. P., Regis, J., Cherif, A. A., and Peragut, J. C. (2001) Effects of subthalamic nucleus (STN) deep brain stimulation (DBS) on non-motor fluctuations (NMF) on Parkinson's disease. *Neurology* **56(Suppl. 3),** A274.
30. Rodriguez, M. C., Obeso, J. A., and Olanow, C. W. (1998) Subthalamic nucleus-mediated excitotoxicity in Parkinson's disease: a target for neuroprotection. *Ann. Neurol.* **44(Suppl. 1),** S175–S188.
31. Piallat, B., Benazzouz, A., and Benabid, A. L. (1996) Subthalamic nucleus lesion in rats prevents dopaminergic nigral neuron degeneration after striatal 6-OHDA injection: behavioural and immunohistochemical studies. *Eur. J. Neurosci.* **8,** 1408–1414.
32. Meissner, W., Reum, T., Paul, G., Harnack, D., Sohr, R., Morgenstern, R., and Kupsch, A. (2001) Striatal dopaminergic metabolism is increased by deep brain stimulation of the subthalamic nucleus in 6-hydroxydopamine lesioned rats. *Neurosci. Lett.* **303,** 165–168.
33. Krack, P., Dowsey, P. L., Benabid, A. L., Acarin, N., Benazzouz, A., Kunig, G., et al. (2000) Ineffective subthalamic nucleus stimulation in levodopa-resistant postischemic parkinsonism. *Neurology* **54,** 2182–2184.
34. Houeto, J. L., Bejjani, P. B., Damier, P., Staedler, C., Bonnet, A. M., Pidoux, B., et al. (2000) Failure of long-term pallidal stimulation corrected by subthalamic stimulation in PD. *Neurology* **55,** 728–730.
35. Merello, M. (1999) Subthalamic stimulation contralateral to a previous pallidotomy: an erroneous indication? *Mov. Disord.* **14(5),** 890.
36. Moro, E., Esselink, R. A., Van Blercom, N., Caputo, E., Pollak, P., Limousin, P., and Hariz, M. I. (2000) Bilateral subthalamic nucleus stimulation in a parkinsonian patient with previous unilateral pallidotomy and thalamotomy. *Mov. Disord.* **15,** 753–755.

37. Foncke, E., van der Linden, C., Vandewalle, V., Colle, H., and Caemaert, J. (2001) Chronic bilateral stimulation of the subthalamic nucleus (STN) in 15 patients with advanced Parkinson's disease previously treated with unilateral internal globus pallidus (GPi) stimulation. *Neurology* **56(Suppl. 3),** A272.
38. Fahn, S. and Elton, R. L., and UPDRS Development Committee. (1987) Unified parkinson's disease rating scale. In: *Recent Developments in Parkinson's Disease* (Fahn, S., et al., eds.), Macmillan, New York, pp. 153–163.
39. Kazumata, K., Antonini, A., Dhawan, V., Moeller, J. R., Alterman, R. L., Kelly, P., et al. (1997) Preoperative indicators of clinical outcome following stereotaxic pallidotomy. *Neurology* **49,** 1083–1090.
40. Bonnet, A. M., Welter, M.-L., Houeto, J.-L., Mesnage, V., Pidoux, B., Dormont, D., et al. (2001) Subthalamic stimulation in Parkinson's disease: perioperative predictive factors. *Neurology* **56(Suppl. 3),** A277.
41. Welter, M.-L., Houeto, J.-L., du Montcel, S. T., Mesnage, V., Bonnet, A. M., Pidoux, B., et al. (2001) Preoperative clinical factors preict the effects of subthalamic stimulation in Parkinson's disease (PD). *Neurology* **56(Suppl. 3),** A146.
42. Bejjani, B. P., Gervais, D., Arnulf, I., Papadopoulos, S., Demeret, S., Bonnet, A. M., et al. (2000) Axial parkinsonian symptoms can be improved: the role of levodopa and bilateral subthalamic stimulation. *J. Neurol. Neurosurg. Psychiatry* **68,** 595–600.
43. Krack, P., Benazzouz, A., Pollak, P., Limousin, P., Piallat, B., Hoffmann, D., et al. (1998) Treatment of tremor in Parkinson's disease by subthalamic nucleus stimulation. *Mov. Disord.* **13,** 907–914.
44. Parkinson Study Group. (2001) Evaluation of dyskinesias in a pilot, randomized, placebo-controlled trial of remacemide in advanced Parkinson disease. *Arch. Neurol.* **58,** 1660–1668.
45. Schrag, A., Jahanshahi, M., and Quinn, N. (2000) What contributes to quality of life in patients with Parkinson's disease? *J. Neurol. Neurosurg. P*sychiatry **69,** 308–312.
46. Troster, A. I., Fields, J. A., Lyons, K. E., Straits-Troster, K. A., Wilkinson, S. B., Pahwa, R., and Koller, W. C. (2001) Predictors and correlates of quality of life improvements after subthalamic nucleus deep brain stimulation in Parkinson's disease. *Neurology* **56(Suppl. 3),** A277.
47. Lagrange, E., Moro, E., Ardouin, C., van Blercom, N., and Pollak, P. P. (2001) Quality-of-life benefit induced by bilateral subthalamic nucleus stimulation in Parkinson's disease. *Neurology* **56(Suppl. 3),** A275.
48. Drapier, S., Lallement, F., Rivier, I., Lajat, Y., and Verin, M. (2001) Bilateral subthalamic or pallidal stimulation for Parkinson's disease: impact on quality of life. *Neurology* **56(Suppl. 3),** A275-A276.
49. Wheelock, V. J., King, D. S., Levine, D. K., Duke, C. M., Yu, J. T., Na-Lee, C. K., et al. (2001) Efficacy of pallidotomy and thalamotomy in cognitively impaired Parkinson disease patients. *Neurology* **56(Suppl. 3),** A277-A278.
50. Funkiewiez, A., Caputo, A., Ardouin, C., Krack, P., Fraix, V., Benabid, A. L., and Pollak, P. (2001) Behavioral and mood changes associated with bilateral stimulation of the subthalamic nucleus: a consecutive series of 98 parkinsonian patients. *Neurology* **56(Suppl. 3),** A274.
51. Benabid, A. L., Pollak, P., Gao, D. M., Hoffmann, D., Limousin, P., Gay, E., et al. (1996)Chronic electrical stimulation of the ventralis intermedius nucleus of the thalamus as a treatment of movement disorders. *J. Neurosurg.* **84,** 203–214.
52. Caparros-Lefebvre, D., Blond, S., Feltin, M. P., Pollak, P., and Benabid, A. L. (1999) Improvement of levodopa induced dyskinesias by thalamic deep brain stimulation is related to slight variation in electrode placement: possible involvement of the centre median and parafascicularis complex. *J. Neurol. Neurosurg. Psychiatry* **67,** 308–314.
53. Narabayashi, H., Yokoshi, F., and Nakajima, Y. (1984) Levodopa-induced dyskinesia and thalamotomy. *J. Neurol. Neurosurg. Psychiatry* **47,** 831–839.
54. Kumar, R., Sime, E., Halket, E., Lozano, A. M., and Lang, A. E. (1999) Comparative effects of unilateral and bilateral subthalamic nucleus deep brain stimulation. *Neurology* **53,** 561–566.
55. Rodriguez-Oroz, M. C., Zamarbide, I. D., Guridi, J., and Obeso, J. A. (2001) Deep brain stimulation of the subthalamic nucleus and globus pallidus pars interna in Parkinson's disease: 4-year follow-up. *Neurology* **56(Suppl. 3),** A273.
56. Ardouin, C., Pillon, B., Peiffer, E., Bejjani, P., Limousin, P., Damier, P., et al. (1999) Bilateral subthalamic or pallidal stimulation for Parkinson's disease affects neither memory nor executive functions: a consecutive series of 62 patients. *Ann. Neurol.* **46,** 217–223.
57. Jahanshahi, M., Ardouin, C. M., Brown, R. G., Rothwell, J. C., Obeso, J., Albanese, A., et al. (2000) The impact of deep brain stimulation on executive function in Parkinson's disease. *Brain* **123,** 1142–1154.
58. Pillon, B., Ardouin, C., Damier, P., Krack, P., Houeto, J. L., Klinger, H., et al. (2000) Neuropsychological changes between "off" and "on" STN or GPi stimulation in Parkinson's disease. *Neurology* **55,** 411–418.
59. Bejjani, B. P., Damier, P., Arnulf, I., Thivard, L., Bonnet, A. M., Dormont, D., et al. (1999) Transient acute depression induced by high-frequency deep-brain stimulation. *N. Engl. J. Med.* **340,** 1476–1480.
60. Kumar, R., Krack, P., and Pollak, P. (1999) Transient acute depression-induced by high-frequency deep-brain stimulation [letter]. *N. Engl. J. Med.* **341,** 1003–1004.
61. Krack, P., Kumar, R., Ardouin, C., Limousin-Dowsey, P., McVicker, J. H., Benabid, A.-L., and Pollak, P. (2001) Mirthful laughter induced by subthalamic nucleus stimulation. *Mov. Disord.* **16,** 867–875.
62. Ghika, J., Vingerhoets, F., Albanese, A., and Villemure, J. G. (1999) Bipolar swings in mood in patient with bilateral subthalamic nucleus deep brain stimulation (DBS) free of antiparkinson medication [abstract]. *Parkinsonism Rel. Disord.* **5(Suppl. 1),** 104.
63. Vingerhoets, G., van der Linden, C., Lannoo, E., Vandewalle, V., Caemaert, J., Wolters, M., and Van den Abbeele, D. (1999) Cognitive outcome after unilateral pallidal stimulation in Parkinson's disease. *J. Neurol. Neurosurg. Psychiatry* **66,** 297–304.

64. Merello, M., Starkstein, S., Nouzeilles, M. I., Kuzis, G., and Leiguarda, R. (2001) Bilateral pallidotomy for treatment of Parkinson's disease induced corticobulbar syndrome and psychic akinesia avoidable by globus pallidus lesion combined with contralateral stimulation. *J. Neurol. Neurosurg. Psychiatry* **7,** 611–614.
65. Ghika, J., Ghika-Schmid, F., Fankhauser, H., Assal, G., Vingerhoets, F., Albanese, A., et al. (1999) Bilateral contemporaneous posteroventral pallidotomy for the treatment of Parkinson's disease: neuropsychological and neurological side effects. Report of four cases and review of the literature. *J. Neurosurg.* **91,** 313–321.
66. Ghika, J., Villemure, J. G., Fankhauser, H., Favre, J., Assal, G., and Ghika-Schmid, F. (1998) Efficiency and safety of bilateral contemporaneous pallidal stimulation (deep brain stimulation) in levodopa-responsive patients with Parkinson's disease with severe motor fluctuations: a 2-year follow-up review. *J. Neurosurg.* **89,** 713–718.
67. Galvez-Jimenez, N., Lozano, A., Tasker, R., Duff, J., Hutchison, W., and Lang, A. E. (1998) Pallidal stimulation in Parkinson's disease patients with a prior unilateral pallidotomy. *Can. J. Neurol. Sci.* **25,** 300–305.
68. Louis, E. D., Barnes, L., Albert, S. M., Cote, L., Schneier, F. R., Pullman, S. L., and Yu, Q. (2001) Correlates of functional disability in essential tremor. *Mov. Disord.* **16,** 914–920.
69. Deuschl, G., Raethjen, J., Lindemann, M., and Krack, P. (2001) The pathophysiology of tremor. *Muscle Nerve* **24,** 716–735.
70. Louis, E. D. (2001) Clinical practice. Essential tremor. *N. Engl. J. Med.* **345,** 887–891.
71. Alusi, S. H. and Bain, P. G. (2001) Tremor clinical measurement of impairment, disability, and handicap. In: *Clinical Trials in Neurology* (Guiloff, R. J., ed.), Springer, London, pp. 339–346.
72. Taha, J. M., Janszen, M. A., and Favre, J. (1999) Thalamic deep brain stimulation for the treatment of head, voice, and bilateral limb tremor. *J. Neurosurg.* **91,** 68–72.
73. Alusi, S. H., Worthington, J., Glickman, S., and Bain, P. G. (2001) A study of tremor in multiple sclerosis. *Brain* **124,** 720–730.
74. Alusi, S. H., Aziz, T. Z., Glickman, S., Jahanshahi, M., Stein, J. F., and Bain, P. G. (2001) Stereotactic lesional surgery for the treatment of tremor in multiple sclerosis: a prospective case-controlled study. *Brain* **124,** 1576–1589.
75. Liu, X., Aziz, T. Z., Miall, R. C., Rowe, J., Alusi, S. H., Bain, P. G., and Stein, J. F. (2000) Frequency analysis of involuntary movements during wrist tracking: a way to identify ms patients with tremor who benefit from thalamotomy. *Stereotact. Funct. Neurosurg.* **74,** 53–62.
76. Goldman, M. S. and Kelly, P. J. (1992) Symptomatic and functional outcome of stereotactic ventralis lateralis thalamotomy for intention tremor. *J. Neurosurg.* **77,** 223–229.
77. Speelman, J. D. and Van Manen, J. (1984) Stereotactic thalamotomy for the relief of intention tremor of multiple sclerosis. *J. Neurol. Neurosurg. Psychiatry* **47,** 596–599.
78. Montgomery, E. B. Jr., Baker, K. B., Kinkel, R. P., and Barnett, G. (1999) Chronic thalamic stimulation for the tremor of multiple sclerosis. *Neurology* **53,** 625–628.
79. Geny, C., Nguyen, J. P., Pollin, B., Feve, A., Ricolfi, F., Cesaro, P., and Degos, J. D. (1996) Improvement of severe postural cerebellar tremor in multiple sclerosis by chronic thalamic stimulation. *Mov. Disord.* **11,** 489–494.
80. Miyagi, Y., Shima, F., Ishido, K., Moriguchi, M., and Kamikaseda, K. (1999) Posteroventral pallidotomy for midbrain tremor after a pontine hemorrhage. Case report. *J. Neurosurg.* **91,** 885–888.
81. Krauss, J. K. and Mundinger, F. (1996) Thalamic stimulation for severe action tremor after lesion of the superior cerebellar peduncle. *J. Neurol. Neurosurg. Psychiatry* **61,** 234.
82. Bain, P. G., Findley, L. J., Britton, T. C., Rothwell, J. C., Gresty, M. A., Thompson, P. D., and Marsden, C. D. (1995) Primary writing tremor. *Brain* **118,** 1461–1472.
83. Ohye, C., Miyazaki, M., Hirai, T., Shibazaki, T., Nakajima, H., and Nagaseki, Y. (1982) Primary writing tremor treated by stereotactic selective thalamotomy. *J. Neurol. Neurosurg. Psychiatry* **45,** 988–997.
84. Ford, B., Greene, P., Louis, E. D., Petzinger, G., Bressman, S. B., Goodman, R., et al. (1996) Use of intrathecal baclofen in the treatment of patients with dystonia. *Arch. Neurol.* **53,** 1241–1246.
85. Albright, A. L., Barry, M. J., Painter, M. J., and Shultz, B. (1998) Infusion of intrathecal baclofen for generalized dystonia in cerebral palsy. *J. Neurosurg.* **88,** 73–76.
86. Tasker, R. R., Doorly, T., and Yamashiro, K. (1988) Thalamotomy in generalized dystonia. *Adv. Neurol.* **50,** 615–631.
87. Andrew, J., Fowler, C. J., and Harrison, J. G. (1983) Stereotaxic thalamotomy in 55 cases of dystonia. *Brain* **106,** 981–1000.
88. Cooper, I. S. (1976) 20-year follow-up of the neurosurgical treatment of dystonia musculoram deformans. *Adv. Neurol.* **14,** 423–452.
89. Hillier, C. E., Wiles, C. M., and Simpson, B. A. (1999) Thalamotomy for severe antipsychotic induced tardive dyskinesia and dystonia. *J. Neurol. Neurosurg. Psychiatry* **66,** 250–251.
90. Goto, S., Tsuiki, H., Soyama, N., Okamura, A., Yamada, K., Yoshikawa, M., et al. (1997) Stereotactic selective Vo-complex thalamotomy in a patient with dystonic writer's cramp. *Neurology* **49,** 1173–1174.
91. Vitek, J. L., Evatt, M., Zhang, J.-Y., et al. (1999) Pallidotomy and deep brain stimulation as a treatment for dystonia. *Neurology* **52(Suppl. 2),** A294.
92. Vitek, J. L., Chockkan, V., Zhang, J. Y., Kaneoke, Y., Evatt, M., DeLong, M. R., et al. (1999) Neuronal activity in the basal ganglia in patients with generalized dystonia and hemiballismus. *Ann. Neurol.* **46(1),** 22–35.
93. Vitek, J. L. and Lenz, F. A. (1998) Pallidal surgery: a new option for surgical treatment of dystonia. In: *Pallidal Surgery for the Treatment of Parkinson's Disease and Movement Disorders* (Krauss, J. K., Grossman, R. G., and Jankovic, J., eds.), Lippincott-Raven, Philadelphia, PA, pp. 267–274.

94. Justesen, C. R., Penn, R. D., Kroin, J. S., and Egel, R. T. (1999) Stereotactic pallidotomy in a child with Hallervorden-Spatz disease. *J. Neurosurg.* **90,** 551–554.
95. Lozano, A. M., Kumar, R., Gross, R. E., et al. (1997) Globus pallidus internus pallidotomy for generalized dystonia. *Mov. Disord.* **12(6),** 865–870.
96. Lin, J.-J., Lin, G.-Y., Shih, G., Lin, S.-Z., Chang, D.-C., and Lee, C.-C. (1999) Benefit of bilateral pallidotomy in the treatment of generalized dystonia. *J. Neurosurg.* **90,** 974–976.
97. Ondo, W. G., Desaloms, J. M., Jankovic, J., and Grossman, R. G. (1998) Pallidotomy for generalized dystonia. *Mov. Disord.* **13(4),** 693–698.
98. Weetman, J., Anderson, I. M., Gregory, R. P., and Gill, S. S. (1997) Bilateral posteroventral pallidotomy for severe antipsychotic induced tardive dyskinesia and dystonia. *J. Neurol. Neurosurg. Psychiatry* **63,** 554–556.
99. Bhatia, K. P., Marsden, C. D., and Thomas, D. G. (1998) Posteroventral pallidotomy can ameliorate attacks of paroxysmal dystonia induced by exercise. *J. Neurol. Neurosurg. Psychiatry* **65,** 604–605.
100. Yoshor, D., Hamilton, W. J., Ondo, W., Jankovic, J., and Grossman, R. G. (2001) Comparison of thalamotomy and pallidotomy for the treatment of dystonia. *Neurosurgery* **48,** 818–824.
101. Sellal, F., Hirsch, E., Barth, P., Blond, S., and Marescaux, C. (1993) A case of symptomatic hemidystonia improved by ventroposterolateral thalamic electrostimulation. *Mov. Disord.* **8(4),** 515–518.
102. Vercueil, L., Pollak, P., Fraix, V., Caputo, E., Moro, E., Benazzouz, A., et al. (2001) Deep brain stimulation in the treatment of severe dystonia. *J. Neurol.* **248,** 695–700.
103. Trottenberg, T., Paul, G., Meissner, W., Maier-Hauff, K., Taschner, C., and Kupsch, A. (2001) Pallidal and thalamic neurostimulation in severe tardive dystonia. *J. Neurol. Neurosurg. Psychiatry* **70,** 557–559.
104. Coubes, P., Roubertie, A., Vayssiere, N., Hemm, S., and Echenne, B. (2000) Treatment of DYT1-generalised dystonia by stimulation of the internal globus pallidus. *Lancet* **355,** 2220–2221.
105. Kumar, R., Dagher, A., Hutchison, W. D., Lang, A. E., and Lozano, A. M. (1999) Globus pallidus deep brain stimulation for generalized dystonia: clinical and PET investigation. *Neurology* **53,** 871–874.
106. Krauss, J. K., Pohle, T., Weber, S., Ozdoba, C., and Burgunder, J. M. (1999) Bilateral stimulation of globus pallidus internus for treatment of cervical dystonia. *Lancet* **354,** 837–838.
107. Parkin, S., Aziz, T., Gregory, R., and Bain, P. (2001) Bilateral internal globus pallidus stimulation for the treatment of spasmodic torticollis. *Mov. Disord.* **16,** 489–493.
108. Roubertie, A., Cif, L., Vayssiere, N., et al. (2000) Symptomatic generalized dystonia: neurosurgical treatment by continuous bilateral stimulation of the internal globus pallidus in eight patients. *Mov. Disord.* **15(Suppl. 3),** 156.
109. Loher, T. J., Hasdemir, M. G., Burgunder, J.-M., and Krauss, J. K. (2000) Long-term follow-up study of chronic globus pallidus internus stimulation for post-traumatic hemidystonia. Case Report. *J. Neurosurg.* **92,** 457-460, **101,** 77–87.

5

Methods of Patient Assessment in Surgical Therapy for Movement Disorders

Esther Cubo and Christopher G. Goetz

1. INTRODUCTION

In the biological and social sciences, rating scales are commonly employed for the purposes of measurement. The ability to measure specific movement disorder features over time allows for comparability of outcomes, helps interpretation of results, and minimizes errors of measurement due to standardization.

Measurement is the assignment of numerals to symptoms, behaviors, or clinical signs according to previously agreed-upon rules. Scales are the means used in clinical medicine for assigning numbers to observable qualities *(1)*. The scales used in clinical medicine can be classified as nominal, ordinal, interval, or ratio scales. In nominal or categoric scales, the basic relationship described is equality or difference and therefore signs are present or absent. In an ordinal scale, an attribute is classified according to its rank order. However, the steps in the scale are not necessarily presumed to be equal. The basic relationship described in an ordinal scale is greater or less. Most of the rating scales used in neurology are ordinal, for example the well-known disability status of Kurtzke *(2)*. Interval scales, like ordinal scales, order behaviors, but all steps in the scale are presumed to be equal so that the difference between 30 and 35 is the same as the difference between 60 and 65. The basic relationships described in an interval scale are equality or difference of intervals. True interval scales are rare in neurology. Ratio scales have equal intervals, but, in addition, they have a true (nonarbitrary) zero, for example, the Kelvin temperature scale is a ratio scale because it is based on absolute zero *(1)*.

The ability of scales to produce consistent results and to therefore be useful instruments to monitor patients and conduct research depends on their psychometric properties. Reliability is the extent to which a measure yields the same results on repeated trials. This is the proportion of variation in any given measurement that is the result of true variation and not error. Reliability can be classified as intra-rater and inter-rater reliability. The former refers to the reproducibility of a single examinater's rating on separate occasions (test-retest); the latter to the reproducibility of ratings when multiple examiners independently examine the same patient. Dimensionality refers to the ability of a rating instrument to measure several subdomains of a particular construct. Dimensionality and internal consistency of a scale are important in forming composite measures of subscale scores. Internal consistency is the extent to which the items making up a composite score are measuring the same latent factor. Finally, validity is the extent to which an instrument measures what it is truly designed to assess *(1)*.

To be widely adopted, a scale must be easy to apply and to analyze statistically. Historical precedence has shown that complicated scales are quickly abandoned by clinicians. No single scale is perfect, and a balance must be effected between practicality and detail. Scales designed to obtain a general

From: Contemporary Clinical Neurology:
Surgical Treatment of Parkinson's Disease and Other Movement Disorders
Edited by: D. Tarsy, J. L. Vitek, and A. M. Lozano © Humana Press Inc., Totowa, NJ

overview may be criticized as being unfocused, whereas those that are designed to address a particular problem may be criticized as being too limited and of little clinical pertinence. Historically, surgical treatments of Parkinson's disease (PD) and other movement disorders have not been rigorously evaluated with standardized testing. More recently, several scales, originally developed for use in clinical pharmacologic trials, have been used to assess surgical treatments. Although surgical and pharmacological trials have often been evaluated with similar scales, special adaptations of traditional scales have been created to focus on issues pertinent to operative interventions. This chapter will present and discuss these scales in detail. They will not be reproduced here but references for all of them have been provided.

2. PARKINSON'S DISEASE

Clinical evaluation of PD remains a complex objective. The disease itself presents with multiple symptoms and signs, the presence and intensity of which differ from one patient to another, and in advanced disease from moment to moment. The evaluation of PD has been modified over time. Initially, the main objective was to assess the severity of disease manifestations in relation to pathological changes (clinical-anatomical method). Over the last 30 years, the aim has focused on the evaluation of drug therapy. From the mid-1970s forward, methods for evaluating the effects of chronic treatment (dyskinesias, on-off phenomena, neuropsychological effects) have been incorporated as well *(3,4)*. At the same time, better knowledge of PD has allowed investigators to supplement rating scales to assess other PD features such as dementia, psychosis, pain, and sleep disturbances *(5,6)*.

Two methods are used to evaluate parkinsonian patients: subjective evaluation, using patient derived scales to assess symptoms of functional disability and objective evaluation, using investigator-based assessments to measure performance on simple or sophisticated tests. A combination of both methods is frequently used and has been recommended *(5)*.

For both types of assessment quantitative measure scales have been developed. These can be complex or simple. Complex methods are time-consuming, and require stereotypic test conditions and often expensive or sophisticated equipment *(7)*. The results obtained by means of such complex tests may be authentic measures, but they have not gained general acceptance because of their limitations in time and space. These complicated tests are not useful in evaluating the large number of patients involved in most current clinical trials.

Simpler and more rapidly applied quantitative methods are usually ordinal measures of primary domains of disability and they are occasionally supplemented by timed tests that provide data for interval scales *(8)*. Several scales currently used in PD assessment are discussed below, each with its advantages and disadvantages highlighted.

2.1. Standard Scales

2.1.1. Hoehn and Yahr Staging Scale

The Hoehn and Yahr staging scale *(9)* was developed prior to the introduction of levodopa, to measure disease progression and provide a general sense about severity of disease. It ranges from 0 to 5. The scale focuses on the bilaterality of involvement and impairment of postural reflexes.

2.1.1.1. Advantages

This is a brief scale that is easy to administer. Psychometric properties include high inter-rater reliability *(10)* and good convergent validity with other PD rating scales *(10–12)*. It focuses on motor disability, progression of postural reflex impairment, and independence in walking.

2.1.1.2. Disadvantages

The scale provides little specific information about the presence or absence of tremor, rigidity, or bradykinesia. The change from one stage to another cannot be considered linear, so parametric statistics cannot be applied. Because it only has 5 points, significant clinical improvement or deterioration may not be detected by this scale. Increments of 0.5 have recently been suggested to overcome this problem *(13)*.

2.1.2. *Schwab and England Activities of Daily Living Scale*

This is a rapidly administered questionnaire *(12)* that may be used to measure the patient's perception of functional independence. It is not specific for PD. The scale includes general questions about ability to perform activities of daily living with scores registered as percentages of normal: 100% (completely normal), 90% (completely independent, able to do all chores with some degree of slowness), and so forth, until 0%, (completely bedridden, and vegetative functions are not functioning).

2.1.2.1. Advantages

This scale is easy to apply. Convergent validity between this scale and other PD rating scales, including the UPDRS, is high *(14)*. As a continuous scale, data can be analyzed parametrically.

2.1.2.2. Disadvantages

Reliability has not been assessed. In addition, patients may find it difficult to determine whether they perform chores twice as slowly or four times as slowly as normal, since normality is not defined. In addition, patients are not questioned regarding their ability to perform a specific set of chores, and they may have trouble assigning a number to their function because their abilities may vary from task to task.

2.1.3. *Unified Parkinson's Disease Rating Scale*

The Unified Parkinson's Disease Rating Scale (UPDRS) *(15)* was developed to provide clinical investigators with a detailed assessment of specific areas of disability as well as a global measure of PD function for use in practice and research. The UPDRS has four primary sections to assess clinical problems associated with PD: Part I: Behavior (cognition, mood, psychosis, and motivation scores); Part II: Activities of daily living; Part III: Motor examination (patients may be assessed either while "on" or while "off"); Part IV: Additional complications of disease or therapy (dystonia, dyskinesia, and motor fluctuation estimates). In clinical trials, the Hoehn and Yahr staging *(9)*; and Schwab and England Activities of daily living scale *(12)* are often attached to the UPDRS.

Part III is based on a neurological examination, and requires observation of the patient sitting quietly at rest, carrying out movements, standing, walking and in response to challenged postural reflexes. Parts I, II, and IV are assessed by patient interview.

2.1.3.1. Advantages

The UPDRS has rapidly become the most widely used assessment device for studies involving patients with PD *(16)*. It has been the major outcome variable in multicenter studies of new interventions, including the evaluation of new surgical and medical treatments *(17,18)*. Several studies have examined the inter-rater reliability when both raters were neurologists *(14,19)*, reporting moderate to excellent agreement between raters. In an attempt to improve the consistency and reliability of data collected by researchers dealing with parkinsonian rating scales, a teaching video tape with the motor section of the UPDRS has been published *(20)*. The factor structure of the motor subscale of the UPDRS during "on" and "off" states *(21,22)* reveals that there are high degrees of internal consistency and that the same factors hold for "on" and "off" states. Its construct validity as assessed by examining the relationship among the UPDRS motor subscales and Hoehn and Yahr stage is also high *(14,23)*. The UPDRS has been used extensively in surgical reports and is a component of the CAPIT *(24)* and CAPSIT *(25)* scales for surgery (*see* below).

2.1.3.2. Disadvantages

The UPDRS has low inter-rater reliability for some items and redundancy of others. The UPDRS is also deficient in multiple areas, especially those assessing complications not verified by a trained observer. It is also not possible to establish a DSM-IV diagnosis of dementia or depression based on

Part I. Whereas Part III can be performed rapidly as part of general neurological practice, the entire scale is too time-consuming to be used regularly outside of a research setting.

2.1.4. *Short Parkinson's Evaluation Scale*

The Short Parkinson's Evaluation Scale (SPES) is a brief scale derived from the UPDRS *(26)*, but based on a zero-to-three point assessment and limited to fewer items. Items from the UPDRS considered difficult to evaluate, redundant, or of minor clinical significance were omitted. In developing a 0–3 scale to measure larger increments of disability, the scale designers hoped to improve inter-rater reliability.

2.1.4.1. ADVANTAGES

This scale is easier to apply and quicker to complete than the UPDRS. Psychometric properties have been fully studied, showing good inter-rater reliability and a high degree of internal consistency *(23)*.

2.1.4.2. DISADVANTAGES

This scale has not been extensively used in clinical and research settings, outside of those reported by the scale designers. The collapse to a 4-point scale limits detection of small changes that still may be potentially of clinical significance.

2.1.5. *Summary*

The UPDRS *(15)*, especially the UPDRS motor subscale, is a reliable and valid assessment of global PD severity as well as distinct multiple areas of physical disability. It is widely used and well known. It is also used as the major outcome measure of new interventions including the evaluation of new surgical and medical treatments. To date, the correlation of Part III with the remaining subject derived portions of the scale has not been fully elicited and therefore the subscales may be measuring complementary but different aspects of the disease. Though not widely adopted, the SPES *(26)* has the potential to become more useful for assessments of PD function especially in a practice setting.

The Hoehn and Yahr scale *(9)* is useful as a global measure of Parkinson's disease function regarding clinical treatment outcomes especially as they relate to bilateral clinical impairment and balance. Because it is known even outside the world of movement disorders, it is especially important when communicating to general neurologists and medical audiences.

The Schwab and England Activities of Daily Living Scale *(12)* is a useful complement to the activities of daily living portion of the UPDRS for assessing global function, and assigning a number to the assessment of independence in patients with chronic diseases.

2.2. *Specialized Scales*

2.2.1. *Tremor*

Tremors are usually classified according to their phenomenology and their anatomical distribution. Phenomenologically, they are classified by the action that is associated with maximal intensity, such as resting, postural, kinetic, action (postural and kinetic), and intention or end point tremor *(27)*. Anatomically, they are classified by the body part affected. Tremor at rest is almost always a sign of parkinsonism, whereas postural tremor is most commonly a sign of essential tremor (ET). The latter condition will usually be even more pronounced with action and often with intention. Predominant intention tremor typically occurs with lesions of the cerebellar outflow pathway, and when severe, usually spreads to become a postural tremor as well.

Studies evaluating drug trials and stereotactic surgery of PD and ET, have used a number of methods to estimate tremor severity which can be divided into four categories *(28)*: 1) Electronic-physiologic indices of tremor magnitude (e.g., accelerometric and electromyographic data, or gyroscopic techniques); 2) Impairment as measured by clinical rating scales; 3) Objective functional performance test measurements (e.g., nine-hole pegboard test or the amount of water spilled from a cup); and 4) Subjective measures that assess tremor severity as perceived by the patient, and the impact on the patient's quality of life. Clinical assessment by blinded observers who rate global severity from randomized videotape sequences *(29)* may be reasonable, but do not allow for quantification of small changes or qualification of different aspects of tremor *(30)*. Considerations in designing or using a scale for tremor include whether tremor magnitude is scored separately for different parts of the body as well as for different tremor components, e.g., rest, postural, or kinetic tremor. Accelerometer recording has been popular with some research investigators *(31)*, but this method ordinarily requires a laboratory setting and specialized instrumentation, which is not feasible for most neurologists. Furthermore, it cannot be used in isolation because it may overestimate the benefit of therapy in patients with ET. As an example, one study showed 50% reduction in acceleration but this did not translate to a similar alleviation of disability of handicap as determined by other measures *(32)*.

Although the UPDRS Part III assesses parkinsonian resting tremor and postural tremor, other scales have been developed to assess tremor in more detail. These scales can be applied to PD and other tremor conditions.

2.2.1.1. The Clinical Tremor Rating Scale

The Clinical Tremor Rating Scale (CTRS) *(30)* is divided into three parts (A, B, and C), each yielding a subtotal score that can be combined for a total score or can be used for independent analysis. In addition to the task-specific quantitative scores, a global assessment (by the patient and by the examiner) is also obtained at each visit.

Part A (nine items) quantifies tremor at rest, with posture, and with action and intention maneuvers for nine body parts. Severity of tremor in each of the nine body parts is rated by amplitude. Whether the tremor is intermittent or always present is not a factor in the severity score. Action and intention tremor are given a single score. Part B (five items) relates to action tremors of the upper extremities, particularly writing and pouring liquids. Severity is determined by watching the patient carry out the aforementioned activities. Part C (7 items) assesses functional disability, evaluating the severity of tremor with speaking, eating, bringing liquids to the mouth, hygienic care, dressing, and working, including domestic tasks. These scores, with the exception of speaking, are provided by patients, who are asked to evaluate their ability to carry out these tasks. Voice tremor is assessed by the examiner. In addition, the global assessment of overall severity by the examiner and the patient, is a subjective scale that calculates the percent of impairment in carrying out activities of daily living and the cosmetic effect of tremor.

2.2.1.1.1. Advantages. This scale allows the clinical quantification of tremor severity in all its forms. No special tools are required other than a pencil, paper, and two cups to hold water. This rating scale can be used to assess tremors of different etiologies. Because this scale is used with standard sets of conditions and definitions for tremor severity, it facilitates intra-rater and inter-rater consistency *(30)*.

2.2.1.1.2. Disadvantages. This rating scale has not yet been statistically evaluated for validity and reliability. In addition, emphasis is placed on a prescribed set of activities and many tremor patients have task-specific tremors which may not be evaluated because of the rigid protocol *(28)*.

2.2.1.2. The Unified Tremor Rating Scale

The Unified Tremor Rating Scale (UTRE) was developed by the Tremor Investigation and Research Group (TIRG) *(33)* and is used to assess the functional severity of different types of tremor. This detailed assessment scale is divided into five major sections. The first section consists of 10 activities of daily living (ADL) questions inquiring about functional disability. These are all scored from 0 (not affected) to 4 (completely unable to perform the task). The second section rates amplitude-based observations of tremor at rest, posture, and kinesis around all major limb joints, as well as trunk, face, head, voice, tongue, and arm tremor in the "wing beating" position (a total of 62 data points rated from 0–4 in 0.5 point increments). The third section evaluates bilateral water-pouring tests, which are scored from 0 (normal) to 4 (tremor with greater than 50% spillage). The fourth section includes spirographs that are drawn "normally" with the hand resting on the paper (0–4 score in 0.5 point increments). The fifth section includes triaxial accelerometry over the third metacarpal joint in each hand. Fifty-second epochs in both arms are measured in the outstretched position and in the wing beating position. A total of the four trials (200 total seconds) is used for statistical analysis.

2.2.1.2.1. Advantages. In this scale, subjective and objective assessments are included. This rating scale can also be used to assess tremors of different etiologies including ET, postural tremor associated with PD, or action and end-point tremors associated with other conditions such as multiple sclerosis (MS). Because it has few gradations (0–4 scale), it is more easily scored than those with more increments. In addition, scoring tremor in spirals or handwriting has been found to be particularly useful for patients with tremor *(34)*.

2.2.1.2.2. Disadvantages. The psychometric properties of this scale have not well-established. In this type of scale, a single point difference represents a marked change so that small but potentially important changes cannot be detected. Although the inclusion of accelerometry may increase the validity of the scale it adds sophisticated instrumentations that is not always available in a practice setting.

2.2.1.3. Washington Heights-Inwood Tremor Rating Scale

In this scale *(35,36)* the patient is first tested with the arms held in front of the body with wrists pronated and then in the "wing beating" position. The tremor is rated from 0 (normal) to 3 (large amplitude tremor). Tremor is also rated 0–3 while pouring water between two cups (10 repetitions using cups filled to the three-quarters mark), drinking water from a cup (cup filled to the three-quarter mark and raised 10 times from lap level to the mouth); using a spoon to drink water (10 repetitions, hand raised form lap level to mouth), performing finger-to-nose movements (10 repetitions), and drawing Archimedes spirals.

2.2.1.3.1. Advantages. This scale allows the rater to evaluate postural and kinetic tremor separately, to evaluate kinetic tremor during multiple explicitly defined maneuvers, to rate both extremities separately, and to rate severity of tremor based on amplitude, presence of oscillations, and constancy of tremor. Psychometric studies have shown high inter-rater and intra-rater reliability, and validity *(36)*.

2.2.1.3.2. Disadvantages. Because the ratings range from 0–3, subtle differences in tremor severity may not be picked up. In addition, specific tremor components such as resting tremor and anatomical distribution are not included. The impact of the tremor on patient's ADLs is also not included. This scale is not designed for the predominant resting tremor of PD and therefore, if used in PD research, must be accompanied by another assessment tool for PD rest tremor.

2.2.1.4. Bain, Findley Rating Scale

This is a questionnaire *(34)* where 25 activities about ADLs (cutting food with a knife and fork, using a spoon, pouring milk, tying up the shoelaces, etc.), are scored using a four-point rating scale (1 = able to do the activity without difficulty; 4 = cannot do the activity by yourself).

2.2.1.4.1. Advantages. This is a very brief scale and easy to complete. It has successfully fulfilled criteria for inter-rater and intra-rater reliability and validity *(34)*.

2.2.1.4.2. Disadvantages. The information is obtained by patient's impression with no objective data collection. In addition, the description of severity can be interpreted differently by various users. The scale is based on patient's perceptions, without validation by the examiner and has prominent limitations. Anatomical and tremor components are not included.

2.2.1.5. Summary

Measuring tremor is a surprisingly difficult task because tremor behaves in a complex way with natural fluctuations in amplitude and frequency *(37)*. In routine clinical practice, scoring a patient's tremor using a rating scale that divides tremor phenomenologically and anatomically allows good clinical characterization. In therapeutic trials, evaluation should be multidimensional and include subjective clinical measures, a functional performance test, a disability measurement, and a physiologic technique. According to these criteria, the CTRS and UTRS *(30,33)* are the most complete scales.

2.2.2. *Dyskinesias*

Although clinical manifestations of dyskinesias are visible or audible, there is considerable difficulty in objectively quantifying them. One factor contributing to this difficulty is the significant variety of movements that can affect an individual at any given time. To assess severity, one must consider multiple variables like frequency, phenomenology, intensity, body distribution, and interference with activities important to normal function. Second, symptoms vary with activity and dyskinesias observed at rest may give an unreliable idea of dyskinesia disability in a life setting. Ideally, a scale that evaluates dyskinesia should provide five types of information. It should define the phenomenology of the movements, their anatomical distribution, the impact of maximal movements on activities of daily living, should be brief enough to provide multiple assessments, and should meet psychometric criteria.

2.2.2.1. Abnormal Involuntary Movement Scale

The abnormal involuntary movement scale (AIMS) *(38)* was originally developed for the evaluation of tardive dyskinesia but has also been applied to Huntington's disease (HD) and levodopa dyskinesias in PD *(39,40)*. The scale includes specific instructions to standardize the evaluation and requires the examiner to observe the patient sitting quietly at rest and also while the patient carries out selected motor tasks. Seven body areas are rated: muscles of facial expression, lips and perioral area, jaw, tongue, upper and lower extremities, and trunk. A five-point scheme, ranging from 0 = normal to 4 = severe, is used to assess each body part. There are also three global ratings to complete: overall severity, incapacitation for the patient, and the patient's awareness of the dyskinesias. Finally, two interview questions for the patient concentrate on dental hygiene and the wearing of dentures.

2.2.2.1.1. Advantages. This scale has been used for many years in psychiatry so that its psychometric properties have been fully studied. It provides an anatomic view of involuntary movements and a total numeric score for the entire body. It is easy and quick to apply, so repetitive scores can be obtained approximately every 15 min without fatiguing the patient.

2.2.2.1.2. Disadvantages. The AIMS does not provide any information concerning the type of movement disorder observed and consequently all existing movements are merged during the rating. Furthermore, the tasks required in the protocol are not all activities of daily living so that a full assessment of the impact of movements on the subject's life is difficult to determine. Because it was originally developed for rating tardive dyskinesia, the scale places a preferential emphasis on orolingual movements. Finally the severity ratings of "minimal, mild, moderate, and severe" have no descriptive anchors.

2.2.2.2. Unified Parkinson's Disease Rating Scale (UPDRS Part IV)

As part of the larger UPDRS *(15)*, Part IV has four historical questions that cover the presence of dyskinesias over the previous week. These questions assess duration of the waking day in which the patient is affected by dyskinesia, a rating of the patient's perception of disability from dyskinesia, degree of pain resulting from dyskinesias, and a yes/no question on early morning dystonia. The information obtained is based on patient interview and responses are recorded without input from the examiner or objective evaluation.

2.2.2.2.1. Advantages. Because the UPDRS is so widely used in clinical research and practice, the section on dyskinesias is routinely completed by many physicians. It is simple and takes less than three minutes to complete.

2.2.2.2.2. Disadvantages. The scale is based on patient perceptions unvalidated by the examiner and has significant limitations. Patient accuracy concerning presence of dyskinesias especially when they are mild is notoriously poor *(41)*. No anatomic information is gathered and the scale cannot be used to monitor dyskinesia though a drug cycle because the scale specifically covers the past week. No specific ADLs are included in the scale because it covers historical information that would include the patient's entire repertoire of behaviors over the monitored time. The question on pain is difficult to interpret and lacks specificity because most painful spasms are dystonic, although severe choreic neck dyskinesias can also cause radicular paresthesias that are painful. It has not been tested psychometrically.

2.2.2.3. Obeso Dyskinesia Rating Scale

This scale combines the patient's historical assessment of function along with the examiner's ratings of dyskinesia *(42)*. Disability is assessed using two categories of information, intensity and duration. These scores are handled arithmetically to provide a single score based on the mean of the two subscores. The intensity score combines two clinical features, patient awareness of the movements and the observed intensity of the movement. The duration score, similar to the UPDRS Part IV question on duration, divides the waking day onto segments.

2.2.2.3.1. Advantages. This is a speedy assessment and has been adapted officially in the Core Assessment Protocol for Intracerebral Transplantation (CAPIT) *(24)* (see below). It is therefore widely used in research efforts dealing with neurotransplantation.

2.2.2.3.2. Disadvantages. As a scale that combines patient perceptions with observer derived information, all possible combinations of responses are not listed on the scale, and the same movement is rated differently depending on whether the patient recognizes its presence or not. This fusion of objective information and patient perception, especially in the context of dementia or drug-induced confusion that may be present in PD is limiting. The scale does not gather anatomic or phenomenologic information and cannot be used for multiple assessments during a drug cycle.

2.2.2.4. Rush-Dyskinesia Scale-Modified from Obeso Scale

To address the limitations of the above scale Goetz et al. *(43)* modified the Obeso dyskinesias scale to create an objective rating scale for dyskinesia assessment during activities of daily living. They chose three activities to evaluate: walking, putting on a coat and buttoning it, and drinking from a cup. The scale calls for rating the most severe dyskinesias seen during any of three tasks and ranges from 0 (no dyskinesia) to 4 (violent dyskinesia). The rating is based completely on objective observation with no patient interview and the score is tied directly to the successful performance of ADLs. In addition to the intensity rating, the most pronounced type of dyskinesia associated with disability is identified (e.g., chorea, dystonia, myoclonus).

2.2.2.4.1. Advantages. The scale is easy to use and quick to complete. This objectively based scale focuses on ADLs with tasks selected specifically for evaluating dyskinesia involving small, large, and axial muscles. The original article included a videotape with demonstrated cases covering the range of scores, severities, and types of dyskinesias so that researchers using the scale can test their own interrater reliability in order to enhance standardized use. Phenomenology is detected for all dyskinesias as well as the most disabling and the intensity score is directly linked to activities that a patient must perform in daily life. The short-assessment permits repeated examinations during a drug-cycle or over several hours in studies of motor fluctuations. The scale's psychometric properties have been examined and both physicians and study coordinators used the scale with high inter- and intra-rater reliability.

2.2.2.4.2. Disadvantages. The scale does not isolate anatomic distribution of dyskinesias. The protocol limits activities to three tasks, and, conceptually, individual patients may have more dyskinesias during tasks other than the ones chosen. The tasks do not include speaking, an activity that often activates dyskinesias.

2.2.2.5. Summary

For objective evaluation of dyskinesias the combined use of the AIMS *(38)* and Rush scales *(43)* provide anatomical information, severity, and motor impairment information. For historical information, the UPDRS, Part IV *(15)* complements the aforementioned scales and assesses patient perceptions of dyskinesias outside of the hospital or office setting. The Obeso scale *(42)* attempts to collapse all elements into a single assessment but this reductionism may lead to important ambiguities. Of the available dyskinesias scales, the Rush-Dyskinesia Scale-Modified from Obeso *(43)* is one which succeeds better than the rest although useful modifications may still be envisioned.

2.2.3. *Quality of Life Scales*

Quality of life refers to the perception and evaluation by the patient of the impact that the disease and its consequences have produced on their daily life *(44)*. The diversity of symptoms associated with PD and its management affect an individual's usual or expected physical, social, and mental well being, referred to here as health-related quality of life (HQL). The goal of therapeutic interventions is to manage the symptoms of PD, thereby mitigating their effect on HQL. Twelve areas of HQL have been identified as particularly relevant to PD: Physical function, mental health/emotional well being, self-image, social function, health-related distress, cognitive function, communication, sleep and rest, eating, role function, energy/fatigue, and sexual function *(44)*.

The most important disease-specific HQL are the Parkinson's disease Questionnaire-39 *(45)*, the Parkinson's disease Quality-of-life Questionnaire *(46)*, and the Medical Outcome Study 36-Item Short Form Health Survey *(47)*.

2.2.3.1. Parkinson's Disease Questionnaire-39

The PD questionnaire (PDQ-39) *(45)* consists of 39 items that are aggregated into scales: mobility, activities of daily living, emotional well being, stigma, social support, cognition, communication, and bodily discomfort. The scales address all 12 HQL areas, except for self-image and sexual function. This scale is relatively brief and has been designed and validated to be self-completed by patients. Patients respond to each question on a 5-point scale: Never = 0, occasionally = 1, sometimes = 2, often = 3, and always = 4. The PDQ-39 was developed in the United Kingdom and has been validated and translated into 12 languages.

2.2.3.1.1. Advantages. PDQ-39 is a specific quality of life scale for PD. The PDQ-39 has high internal consistency, reliability, and validity as assessed by correlation on PDQ-39 and SF-36 scale scores, Hoehn and Yahr stages, and the Columbia Rating Scale *(48)*. In addition, PDQ-39 appears to be sensitive to changes in health status over time, and has been used in clinical trials of pharmaceutical interventions in several countries *(49)*. Further, the PDQ-39 has been validated in clinic-based as well as community-based samples.

2.2.3.1.2. Disadvantages. If used for new therapeutics trials, unanticipated effects may be not captured because it does not measure all elements within each HQL area. For instance, the PDQ-39 asks specifically about 7 of the 11 emotions identified in the mental health/emotional well being area. In mental health/function well being, the PDQ-39 does not address paranoia, panic disorders, sense of loss or frustration, sexual dysfunction, and self-image.

2.2.3.2. Parkinson's Disease Quality of Life Questionnaire

The PD quality of life questionnaire (PDQL) consists of 37 questions aggregated into four scales: parkinsonian symptoms, systemic symptoms, emotional functioning, and social functioning *(46)*. The PDQL was developed in the Netherlands and was translated and adapted for the United Kingdom using appropriate cross-cultural adaptation methods *(46)*. Patients respond to each question on a 5-point scale: all of the time, most of the time, some of the time, a little of the time, and never. Although designed as a self-completed survey, it can be interviewer-administered to patients requiring assistance. Scoring is described in the PDQL publication *(46)* and is based on computing the mean item score within each of the four scales and overall, with lower scores representing poorer HQL.

2.2.3.2.1. Advantages. PDQL scale scores have demonstrated good internal consistency, reliability, and significant associations with general HQL scores and patient-reported ADLs. Administration time has not been formally evaluated but based on its length we believe that patients can complete the PDQL in less than 30 min.

2.2.3.2.2. Disadvantages. Psychometric properties and responsiveness to changes in the disease are less well-developed than in PDQ-39. The PDQL addresses 10 of the 12 HQL areas, with eating and role function representing the missing areas. Permission for use must be granted from the developers. Scoring, administration, and interpretation guidelines are not available. Like the PDQ-39 scale, if used for monitoring new therapies, the PDQL may not capture unanticipated effects.

2.2.3.3. Medical Outcomes Study 36-Item Short Health Survey

The 36-Item Short Form Health Survey (SF-36) is a new generic health status measure developed from the Medical Outcomes Study in the United States *(47,50)*. The SF-36 measures eight HQL items including physical functioning and bodily pain (10 items, and 2 items, respectively), social functioning and role limitations-physical (4 items and 2 items, respectively), general health (5 items), energy (4 items), mental health (5 items), role limitations-emotional (3 items), and one dimension assessing change in health status over the last year. This survey has been constructed for self-administration by persons 14 years of age and older and for administration by a trained interviewer in person or by telephone. In the Core Assessment Program for Surgical Interventional Therapies in Parkinson's disease (CAPSIT-PD) *(25)*, which is the revised version of the CAPIT protocol, the combination of the generic SF-36 and a disease-specific HQL has been recommended for the assessment of patients undergoing neurosurgical interventions for PD.

2.2.3.3.1. Advantages. The popularity of SF-36 appears to be largely driven by its brevity and comprehensiveness. It has high levels of reliability and validity in neurologically disabled patients including PD *(50–52)*, and appears to be very sensitive to disease severity when correlated with Hoehn and Yahr staging scale *(53)*.

2.2.3.3.2. Disadvantages. This scale was not specifically developed for PD. This generic measure is broad in scope and has been developed for the widest possible range of health problems. Furthermore, it has not been specifically developed to measure change over time. Thus, a theoretical disadvantage with this scale is that it may lack sensitivity and responsiveness to change when administered to patients with PD. In addition, SF-36 does not take into consideration special features of PD such as disabilities in cognition, communication, activities of daily living, and self-perceived social stigma. Other HQL concepts such as sexual functioning, sleep disorders, and health distress are also not included.

2.2.3.4. Summary

PDQ-39 *(45)* is a specific quality of life scale for PD that can present a health profile, providing a wide picture of the wide range of issues that affect quality of life in patients with PD. Because it has been validated and translated into other languages, it improves the standardization of measures among different international clinical trials in PD. The PDQL *(46)* covers several areas with less depth than the PDQ-39. The SF-36 *(47)* is not specific for PD but has been validated, translated in several languages, and has been used in many drug trials. It is usually used as a complement to a PD-specific scale.

2.2.4. Surgical Scales

Because in 1989 there was a growing development of transplantation programs for PD and each program had a small number of subjects, research leaders involved in intracerebral transplantation proposed common methods for patient diagnosis and evaluation. This led to the formation of a working committee and to the publication of the Core Assessment Program for Intracerebral Transplantation (CAPIT) *(24)*, providing the minimal requirements for a common patient evaluation protocol. Because pallidotomy and deep brain stimulation emerged as additional treatment modalities, the European Union Biomed 2 program developed a new Core Assessment Program for Surgical Interventional Therapies in PD (CAPSIT-PD) *(25)*.

2.2.4.1. Core Assessment Program for Intracerbral Transplantations

CAPIT *(24)* was formed to develop a series of recommendations for a common diagnostic and methodologic core evaluation that could be used by all groups, including clinical diagnostic criteria for PD, levodopa responsiveness, definition of "off" and "on" periods, clinical rating scales, pharmacological testing, issues relating to fetal age, and imaging techniques. This discussion focuses only on the rating scale recommendations.

CAPIT includes: the UPDRS *(14)*, Hoehn and Yahr staging *(9)*, and the Obeso Dyskinesia Scale Score *(42)*. All of these have already been discussed. The main advantage of CAPIT is the definition of clinical state: "practically defined off state." Added to these measures are self reporting diaries, timed testing, and a levodopa challenge with hourly ratings using the UPDRS, that permits "area under the curve" analysis. All these tests should be done in patients in both the best "on" and practically defined "off" states. If possible, the patients should be videotaped during test sessions.

Self-reporting

The patients should record their condition on an hourly basis each day, for at least 1 wk prior to each visit, using simple symbols to record one of five conditions. The five conditions are as follows: complete on = A; on with dyskinesias = D; partial on = P; complete off = F; sleep = S. No specific training or validation of these diaries was obtained in the CAPIT protocol.

Timed Testing

The following four timed tests were recommended as part of the core evaluation. All four should be performed in both the best "on" and practically defined "off" conditions:

- Pronation-Supination Test

This timed test of motor performance records the time in seconds required for the patient to perform 20 successive cycles of alternating tapping movements of the palm and dorsum of the hand on the knee while seated with both feet flat on the floor. Two data sets consisting of 20 cycles (trials) each should be recorded for each hand and the better set recorded as the result for each hand.

- Hand/Arm Movement Between Two Points

This timed test performance records the time in seconds required for the patient to tap the index finger of the right or left hand between 2 points on a table surface placed 30 cm apart horizontally. The test should be performed independently for each hand, and for consistency, each test should begin with the left target. Two data sets of 20 successive taps should be performed with each hand, and the better set for each hand saved as the final result.

- Finger Dexterity

The time required for tapping the thumb with the forefinger and then with each finger in rapid succession for 10 times should be measured in seconds with each hand independently. Two data sets should be recorded with each hand, and the better set for each hand used as the final result.

- Stand-walk-sit-test

This timed performance test of postural and gait control records the time in seconds required to stand up from a chair, walk seven meters, turn, walk back to the chair, and sit down. This test should be performed twice and the faster time should be recorded as the final result.

2.2.4.1.1. Advantages. This conglomerate rating tool provides a group consensus, minimal standard requirement for a common surgical protocol. It became a model for surgical evaluation and has been incorporated in several surgical publications. Although the CAPIT was initially designed to be applied only for intracerebral transplantation it has been extended to other surgical treatment modalities such as thalamotomy, pallidotomy, and deep brain stimulation (DBS).

2.2.4.1.2. Disadvantages. The CAPIT is time consuming and requires neurological expertise, sometimes not readily available to surgical teams without movement disorder specialty support. It also lacks evaluations of cognitive function and quality of life measures.

2.2.4.2. Core Assessment Program for Surgical Interventional Therapies in Parkinson's Disease

CAPSIT-PD *(25)* was designed to achieve two main goals: to propose a new assessment program for all kinds of surgical interventional therapies in PD, and to organize a registry of operated patients regardless of which surgical technique was used. The CAPSIT-PD was developed as a series of recommendations for a common diagnostic and methodologic core evaluation that could be used by all groups including clinical diagnostic criteria for PD, levodopa responsiveness, definition of "off "and "on" periods, cognitive and behavioral criteria, clinical rating scales, pharmacological testing, medication adjustment, and imaging criteria. This discussion focuses on the clinical rating scales.

CAPSIT-PD includes: the UPDRS *(15)*, Hoehn and Yahr staging *(9)*, and quality of life assessment using the SF-36 *(47)* all of which have been previously discussed. Self reporting, timed testing, and dyskinesia rating scales were partially modified from prior scales

- Self-reporting

Before the patient completes self-reporting, an educational program for accurate completion of the diary was recommended by this committee. It was also recommended that the patient perform the self-reporting as regularly as possible for one week per month during the three preoperative months and then for 12 or, if possible, 24 mo after surgery. It was also recommended to score additional optional items during each week of self-reporting including number of falls, number of freezing episodes, and the number of "off" episodes with dystonia.

- Timed Tests

In the previous CAPIT program *(24)*, some of the timed tests such as the finger dexterity and pronation-supination tests were criticized because of the limitation of the data interpretation due to variability in difficulty of performing these tests. The repetitive hand-arm movement between two points was regarded by most committee members as the simplest and most reproducible test. In conclusion, the hand-arm movements between two points and the stand-walk-sit test were retained. These tests should be performed during the drug challenge and in the "defined-off" and "defined-on" conditions.

- Dyskinesia Rating Scale

In this program, it was recommended that the Obeso scale *(42)* and AIMS *(38)* be used, suggesting that items from these scales could be combined and that a separate dystonia rating scale should be added in addition to the ratings performed by the patient using a self-reporting diary. These combined rating scales have been been found to have significant reliability *(54)*. Ratings are performed at least once in conjunction with the patient in defined "off" and "on" conditions. For quantification, the patient is sitting in a chair and observed at rest. The patient is then asked to perform the tests in the UPDRS motor scale. The predominant types of abnormal movements are recorded.

- Cognitive and Behavioral Assessment

The goal of the CAPSIT-PD evaluation was to add neuropsychological inclusion/exclusion criteria as well as a test battery for pre- and postoperative assessments. Behavioral alterations represent well-known side effects in bilateral pallidal and striatal lesions. Furthermore, cognitive alterations including memory and executive functions deficits have been reported *(55,56)*. PD patients' executive functions, short-term and working memory, episodic memory, and especially recall and procedural memory are clearly more impaired than instrumental functions and seem to be the core deficit in nondemented PD *(57–59)*.

Pre- and postoperative cognitive evaluations must incorporate tests sensitive to frontal lobe function to detect possible alterations produced by surgical manipulations and should be selected according to the following considerations: 1) The tests need to be especially sensitive for executive tasks including working memory, episodic memory tasks, and procedural memory tasks. 2) Retest effect should be minimal or parallel forms must be available. 3) The tests must be sufficiently sensitive to assess preoperative patient status and to detect positive or negative changes induced by the surgical procedure. 4) Completion of the test battery should not require more than 90 min.

To minimize psychiatric abnormalities that could interfere with neurological assessment patients with major behavioral disorders or severe psychiatric illness are excluded from surgical consideration. It is recommended also to have a psychiatric evaluation including the Minnesota Multiphasic Inventory *(60)* and the Montgomery and Asberg depression rating scale *(61)* to exclude patients with a high risk for psychiatric complications after surgery.

2.2.4.2.1. Advantages. The main advantage of this program are the inclusion of new evaluations such as cognitive assessment and quality of life. Compared to the previous CAPIT program, the CAPSIT-PD has tried to simplify motor evaluation and avoid sophisticated assessment procedures requiring testing in highly specialized centers.

2.2.4.2.2. Disadvantages. Because it has been recently proposed as a new surgical evaluation program in PD, it has not been formally used in clinical or research surgical trials in PD and applicability in practice is still lacking. Because of the incorporation of new evaluations such as cognitive assessment and quality of life scales, it is time-consuming and requires the addition of neuropsychologists to the movement disorder team.

2.2.4.3. SUMMARY

The CAPIT protocol *(24)*, originally designed for intracerebral transplantation, has been extensively used since its development for surgical and pharmacological trials. Because of the development of new neurosurgical procedures in PD and a growing appreciation of quality of life and neuropsychological outcomes the CAPSIT-PD *(25)* provides an enhancement. The CAPSIT-PD has not been extensively applied as yet but its comprehensive nature and standardized "package" offer international teams a common ground for multicenter collaborative efforts.

3. DYSTONIA

The symptomatic treatment of dystonia has markedly improved over the last two decades, particularly as a result of botulinum toxin and advances in surgical treatments. The assessment of various therapeutic interventions in dystonia is problematic for the following reasons *(62)*: 1) Dystonia and its effects on function are difficult to quantitate and therefore most trials utilize rating scales that have not been properly evaluated or validated. 2) Dystonia is a syndrome with different etiologies, anatomic distributions, and heterogeneous clinical manifestations producing a large and varied array of disabilities. 3) Some patients have transient spontaneous remissions. Three primary rating scales for dystonia have been developed: the Burke-Fahn-Marsden Evaluation Scale for Dystonia (BFM) *(63)*, the Toronto Western Spasmodic Torticollis Rating Scale (TWSTRS) *(64)*, and the Unified Dystonia Rating Scale (UDRS) *(65)*.

3.1. The Burke-Fahn-Marsden Evaluation Scale

This scale has two sections *(63)*: a Movement Scale based on examination of the patient and a Disability Scale based on the patient's view of his/her disability in ADLs. The Movement Scale score is the sum of individual scores for each nine body regions. The individual score for each region is the product of two factors, the provoking factor and the severity factor, each rated from 0 (lowest) to 4 (highest). The provoking factor quantifies dystonia in a given body region by rating the circumstances in which dystonia appears while the severity factor quantifies the severity of dystonia in a region regardless of the circumstances in which dystonia appears. After each region is rated for the provoking and severity factor, the two are multiplied to give a product of that region. For the eyes, mouth, and neck the product is further multiplied by 0.5 to down weight the score for those regions since their involvement seems to add less to overall disability. The Disability Scale score is the sum of individual ratings based on guidelines for seven activities of daily living.

3.1.1. Advantages

This scale allows the clinician to rate dystonic movements while taking many different aspects of dystonia—including anatomical distribution and total disability—into account. Its psychometric properties have been studied and it performs well *(63)*.

3.1.2. Disadvantages

This scale was designed to primarily assess generalized torsion dystonia, so that its assessment of individual body regions in focal forms of dystonia is limited. In addition, many forms of secondary dystonia occur in the context of other neurological disabilities and it is ambiguous whether the score should reflect neurological impairment from dystonia alone or from all neurological abnormalities. For example, a child with dystonia due to cerebral palsy may also have limb ataxia, weakness, and spasticity that cause inability to grasp or stand. Consequently, a rating of all neurological deficits with the scale could give high scores even when there is little pure dystonia *(63)*. In addition, this scale may be insensitive to changes in focal dystonia, where multiple dimensions of function need to be assessed. Finally the weighting system and multiplication paradigm are complicated.

3.2. The Toronto Western Spasmodic Torticollis Rating Scale

The Toronto Western Spasmodic Torticollis Rating Scale (TWSTRS) is a specific and composite scale for cervical dystonia *(64)* with subscales for severity, disability, and pain. This scale includes a videotape protocol so that all patients are viewed in a standardized fashion. The motor subscale for severity is rated from 0 = normal to 5 = greatest severity (some items have only 3 subscores), and is subdivided into six different parts, which assess: A) Maximal excursion of the torticollis (rotation, laterocollis, anterocollis/retrocollis, lateral shift, and sagital shift). B) Duration factor, which provides an overall score of maximal head deviation (weighted × 2). C) Effect of sensory tricks. D) Shoulder elevation/anterior displacement. E) Range of motion (without the aid of sensory tricks). F) Time up to 60 s that the patient is able to maintain the head within the 10º of the neutral position without the use of sensory tricks. The disability subscale is a seven-item subjective patient assessment of ADLs. The pain subscale is a three-item subjective assessment of pain severity, duration, and disability.

3.2.1. Advantages

This scale allows the examiner to evaluate torticollis in a focussed and detailed manner, taking into account multiple different aspects of clinical importance including maximal excursion, different postures (e.g., rotation, tilt, shift), duration of involuntary movements, and effect of sensory tricks. It has showed high inter-rater reliability and validity *(64,66)*. It is well-known, has been applied in several treatment trials, and is easily and quickly completed. A teaching videotape has been developed for the scoring of the motor symptoms, which both provides a tool for uniform application to cervical dystonia and promotes collaborative research among diverse examiners *(67)*.

3.2.2. Disadvantages

This scale can only be used for cervical dystonia and is not useful for other forms of focal dystonia. The instructions for the range of motion component do not clearly define the midline and full range for each of the three axes of movements. In addition, assessment of dystonic tremor is not included with this instrument.

3.3. The Unified Dystonia Rating Scale

The Unified Dystonia Rating Scale (UDRS) was developed by the Dystonia Study Group to provide a standard instrument for the assessment of all forms of dystonia *(65)*. The UDRS is an extension of the BFM and was designed to allow a more detailed assessment. Like several other scales used in movement disorder studies, items are rated from 0 (lowest) to 4 (highest), which includes ratings for 14 body regions including eyes and upper face; lower face, tongue, larynx and jaw; neck; shoulder and proximal arm; distal arm and hand; pelvis, upper and distal leg, foot, and trunk, with a maximal score of 56. Each body part has a severity and duration score. The latter is comprised of two components: duration of dystonia at rest or with action for the specific time that body area is examined and the overall preponderance of maximal or submaximal dystonia during the time dystonia is present.

The UDRS also has standard sets of conditions and definitions for the evaluation of dystonia and its anatomical distribution, which allows for a standard assessment.

3.3.1. *Advantages*

The UDRS permits the physician to assess focal or generalized dystonia in a practice and research setting. It focuses on the basic character of dystonia as an action exacerbated movement disorder. The UDRS demonstrates high inter-rater reliability and shows concurrent validity with the BFM in emphasizing dystonia at rest and during action *(65)*.

3.3.2. *Disadvantages*

The UDRS gives a general overview of dystonia, but some details such as presence of tremor, the impact of sensory tricks, or the effect of individualized positions are lacking. In addition, a subjective scale of impairment of daily living activities by the patient is not present. The scale takes several minutes to complete and may be excellent for a primary outcome measure but less useful for regular clinical follow-up.

3.4. *Summary*

For assessment of cervical dystonia the TWSTRS remains the most useful and widely used scale. The UDRS *(65)* can also be used in this setting but is more oriented towards evaluating multiple body regions. It avoids the weighting scheme and multiplication elements of the earlier BFM scale *(63)*. None of these scales capture details that would be applicable to unusual forms of dystonia like paroxysmal dystonia. With regard to surgical interventions where deep brain stimulation is studied, each scale can be administered with the stimulator "on" or "off" with two scores reported as outcome measures.

4. FUTURE PERSPECTIVES

The evaluation of surgical outcomes for the treatment of movement disorders relies on accurate rating measures that capture the full breadth of impairment. Because surgical intervention protocols usually require a multicenter approach to provide adequate numbers of patients to evaluate safety and efficacy, scales that can reliably be used by many investigators in different centers are particularly important. This chapter has focused on a discussion of scales of motor impairment. However, movement disorders and surgical interventions can be associated with a large array of nonmotor deficits, such as cognitive and behavioral changes. A comprehensive evaluation of new therapies also should include standardized assessments of these functions. Each of the clinical scales discussed has limitations and many suggestions have been offered to amend or adapt them. However, the adaptation or reworking of a scale carries the implicit disadvantage that patients evaluated with earlier versions can no longer be followed longitudinally for meaningful interpretation of chronic effects, and contemporary and future studies cannot be compared with previous studies utilizing earlier versions of the scales. For this reason, movement disorders researchers have favored the development of "unified" scales composed of essential elements of existing scales, rather than the alteration of well-established scales. With the advent of new technologies and more sophisticated rating tools, these advances can be easily added to existing clinical scales without modifying the core clinical evaluation. This additive strategy typified by the CAPIT and CAPSIT-PD provides a standardized framework for clinical evaluation with sufficient flexibility to be adapted to future advances and tailored to the evaluation of a variety of surgical procedures.

REFERENCES

1. LaRocca, N. G. (1989) Statistical and Methodologic considerations in Scale Construction. In: *Quantification of Neurologic Deficit* (Munsat, T. L., ed.), Butterworth, Boston, MA, pp. 49–67.
2. Kurtze, J. (1983) Rating neurological impairment in multiple sclerosis: an Expanded Disability Status Scale (EDSS). *Neurology* **33,** 1444–1452.

3. Fahn, S. (1974) "On-off" phenomenon with levodopa therapy in parkinsonism. *Neurology* **24,** 431–441.
4. Larsen, T. A., Calne, S., and Calne, D. B. (1984) Assessment of Parkinson's disease. *Clin. Neuropharmacol.* **7,** 165–169.
5. Martinez-Martin, P., Carrasco de la Pena, J. L., Ramo, C., et al. (1986) Estudio previo sobre fiabilidad de escalas en enfermedad de Parkinson. Abstracts of the International Symposium on Movement Disorders, Barcelona, Spain.
6. Lakke, J. P. W. F., Barbeau, A., Duvoisin, R. C., et al. (1981) Classification of extrapyramidal disorders. *J. Neurol. Sci.* **51,** 311–327.
7. Potvin, A. R. and Tourtellotte, W. W. (1975) The neurological examination: advancements in its quantification. *Arch. Phys. Med. Rehabil.* **56,** 425–437.
8. Montgomery, G. K., Reynolds, N. C., and Warren, R. M. (1985) Qualitative assessment of Parkinson's disease: study of reliability and data reduction with an abbreviated Columbia scale. *Clin. Neuropharmacol.* **8,** 83–92.
9. Hoehn, M. M. and Yahr, M. D. (1967) Parkinsonism: onset, progression, and mortality. *Neurology* **17,** 427–442.
10. Ginanneschi, A., Degl'Innocenti, F., Maurello, M. T., et al. (1991) Evaluation of Parkinson's disease: a new approach to disability. *Neuroepidemiology* **10,** 282–287.
11. Duvoisin, R. C. (1971) The evaluation of extrapyramidal disease. In: *Monoamines, noyaux gris centraux et syndrome de Parkinson* (De Ajuriaguerra, J. and Gauthier, G., eds.), Georg, Geneve, pp. 313–325.
12. Schwab, J. F. and England, A. C. (1969) Projection technique for evaluating surgery in Parkinson's disease. In: *Third Symposium on Parkinson's Disease* (Billingham, F. H. and Donaldson, M. C., eds.), Livingstone, Edinburgh, pp. 152–157.
13. Jankovic, J., McDermott, M., Carter, R. N., et al. (1990) Variable expression of Parkinson's disease: a base-line analysis of the DATATOP cohort. *Neurology* **40,** 1529–1534.
14. Martinez-Martin, P., Gil-Nagel, A., Morlan Gracia, L., et al. (1994) The Cooperative Multicentric Group. Unified Parkinson's Disease Rating Scale characteristics and structure. *Mov. Disord.* **9(1),** 76–83.
15. Fahn, S., Elton, R. L., and the UPDRS Development Committee. (1987) Unified Parkinson's disease rating scale. In: *Recent Developments in Parkinson's Disease,* vol. 2 (Fahn, S., Marsden, C. D., Calne, D., and Goldstein, M., eds.), Macmillan Healthcare Information, Florham Park, NJ, pp. 153–163.
16. Martinez-Martin, P. and Bermejo-Parja, F. (1988) Rating scales in Parkinson's disease. In: *Parkinson's Disease and Movement Disorders* (Jankovic, J. and Tolosa, E., eds.), Urban & Schwarzenberg, Baltimore, MD, pp. 235–242.
17. Parkinson Study Group. (1989) Effect of deprenyl on the progression disability in early Parkinson's disease. *N. Engl. J. Med.* **321,** 1364–1371.
18. Goetz, C. G., Stebbins, G. T., Klawans, H. L., et al. (1990) United Parkinson Foundation neurotransplantation registry: multicenter US and Canadian database: presurgical and 12 month follow-up. Neural transplantation: from molecular basis to clinical application. In: *Progress in Brain Research,* vol. 82 (Dunnett, S. B. and Richards, S. J., eds.), Elsevier, Amsterdam, pp. 611–618.
19. Richards, M., Marder, K., Cote, L., et al. (1994) Interrrater reliability of the Unified Parkinson's Disease Rating Scale Motor Examination. *Mov. Disord.* **9(1),** 89–91.
20. Goetz, C. G., Stebbins, G. T., Chmura, T. A., et al. (1995) Teaching tape for the motor section of the Unified Parkinson's Disease Rating Scale. *Mov. Disord.* **10,** 263–266.
21. Stebbins, G. T. and Goetz, C. G. (1998) Factor structure of the Unified Parkinson's Disease Rating Scale Motor Examination Section. *Mov. Disord.* **13,** 633–636.
22. Stebbins, G. T., Goetz, C. G., Lang, A. E., and Cubo, E. (1999) Factor analysis of the Unified Parkinson's Disease Rating Scale during the off-state. *Mov. Disord.* **14,** 585–589.
23. Van Hilten, J. J., van der Zwan, A. D., Zwinderman, A. H., et al. (1994) Rating impairment and disability in Parkinson's disease: evaluation of the Unified Parkinson's disease rating scale. *Mov. Disord.* **9,** 84–88.
24. Langston, J. W., Widner, H., Goetz, C. G., et al. (1991) Core Assessment Program for Intracerebral Transplantations (CAPIT). In: *Intracerebral Transplantation in Movement Disorders* (Lindvall, O., Bjorklund, A., Widner, H., eds.), Elsevier, Amsterdam, The Netherlands, pp. 227–241.
25. Defer, G. L., Widner, H., Marie, R. M., et al. (1999) Core assessment program for surgical interventional therapies in Parkinson's disease. *Mov. Disord.* **14,** 572–584.
26. Rabey Martin, J., Bass, H., Bonucelli, U., et al. (1997) Evaluation of the short Parkinson's evaluation scale: a new friendly scale for the evaluation of Parkinson's disease in clinical drug trials. *Clin. Neuropharmacol.* **20,** 322–337.
27. Guy, W. ECDEU Assessment Manual for Psychopharmacology.US Government Printing Office, Washington, DC, 1976.
28. Bain, P. G. (2000) Tremor assessment and quality of life measurements. *Neurology* **54(Suppl. 4),** S26–S29.
29. Duquette, P., Pleines, J., and du Souich, P. (1985) Isoniazid for tremor in multiple sclerosis: a controlled trial. *Neurology* **35,** 1772–1775.
30. Fahn, S., Tolosa, E., and Martin, C. (1988) Clinical rating scale for tremor. In: *Parkinson's Disease and Movement Disorders* (Jankovic, J. and Tolosa, E., eds.), Urban, and Schwarzenberg, Baltimore, MD, pp. 225–234.
31. Koller, W. C. (1984) Propranolol therapy for essential tremor of the head. *Neurology* **34,** 1077–1079.
32. Bain, P. G. (1997) The effectiveness of treatments for essential tremor. *Neurologist* **3,** 305–321.
33. Koller, W., Pahwa, R., and Busenbark, K. (1997) High frequency unilateral thalamic stimulation in the treatment of essential and parkinsonian tremor. *Ann. Neurol.* **42,** 292–299.
34. Bain, P. G., Findley, L. J., Atchison, P., et al. (1993) Assessing tremor severity. *J. Neurol. Neurosurg. Psychiatry* **56,** 868–873.
35. Louis, E. D. (1997) Movement Disorders. In: *On Call Neurology* (Marshall, R. and Mayer, S., eds.), W.B. Saunders Co., Philadelphia, PA, pp. 325–334.

36. Louis, E. D., Ford, B., and Bismuth, B. (1998) Reliability between two observers using a protocol for assessing essential tremor. *Mov. Disord.* **13,** 287–293.
37. Cleeves, L. and Findley, L. J. (1987) Variability in amplitude of untreated essential tremor. *J. Neurol. Neurosurg. Psychiatry* **50,** 704–708.
38. Gardos, G., Cole, J. O., and Rapkin, R. M. (1984) Anticholinergic challenge and neuroleptic withdrawal. *Arch. Gen. Psychiatry* **41,** 1030–1035.
39. Mouradian, M. M., Heuser, I. J. E., Baronti, F., et al. (1989) Pathogenesis of dyskinesias in Parkinson's disease. *Ann. Neurol.* **25,** 523–526.
40. Bonifati, V., Fabrizio, E., Cipriani, R., Vanacore, N., and Meco, G. (1994) Buspirone in L-dopa-induced dyskinesias. *Clin. Neuropharmacol.* **17,** 73–82.
41. Goetz, C. G., Stebbins, G. T., Blassucci, L. M., et al. (1997) Efficacy of a patient-training videotape on motor fluctuations for on-off diaries in Parkinson's disease. *Mov. Disord.* **12,** 1039–1041.
42. Obeso, J. A., Grandas, F., Vaamonde, J., et al. (1989) Motor complications associated with chronic L-dopa therapy in Parkinson's disease. *Neurology* **39(Suppl. 2),** 11–19.
43. Goetz, C. G., Stebbins, G. T., Shale, H. M., et al. (1994) Utility of an objective dyskinesias rating scale for Parkinson's disease inter-and intrarater reliability assessment. *Mov. Disord.* **9,** 390–394.
44. Damiano, A. M., Snyder, C., Strausser, B., et al. (1999) A review of health-related quality-of-life concepts and measures for Parkinson's disease. *Quality of Life Res.* **8,** 235–243.
45. Peto, V., Jenkinson, C., Fitzpatrick, R., and Greenhall, R. (1995) The development and validation of a short measure of functioning and well being for individuals with Parkinson's disease. *Quality of Life Res.* **4,** 241–248.
46. De Boer, A. G. E. M., Wojker, W., Speelman, J. D., et al. (1996) Quality of life in patients with Parkinson's disease: development of a questionnaire. *J. Neurol. Neurosurg. Psychiatry* **61,** 70–74.
47. Stewart, A. L., Hays, R. D., and Ware, J. E. (1988) The MOS Short-Form General Health Survey, Reliability and validity in a patient population. *Med. Care* **26,** 724–735.
48. Fitzpatrick, R., Peto, V., Jenkinson, C., et al. (1997) Health-related quality of life in Parkinson's disease: a study of out-patient clinic attenders. *Mov. Disord.* **12,** 916–922.
49. Fitzptrick, R., Jenkinson, C., Peto, V., et al. (1997) Desirable properties for instruments assessing quality of life: evidence form the PDQ-39. *J. Neurol. Neurosurg. Psychiatry* **62,** 104.
50. Ware, J. E., Brook, R. H., Williams, K. N., et al. (1980) *Conceptualization and Measurements of Health for Adults in Health Insurance Study, vol. 1: Model of Health and Methodology*. Rand Corp, Santa Monica, CA, pp. 216–242.
51. Ware, J. E., Snow, K. K., Kosinski, M., et al. (1993) *Health Survey: Manual and Interpretation Guide*. New England Medical Centre Health Institute, Boston, MA.
52. Lyons, R. A., Lo, S. V., and Littlepage, B. N. (1994) Comparative health status of patients with 11 common illnesses in Wales. *J. Epidemiol. Community Health* **48,** 388–390.
53. Hobson, J. P. and Menra, R. J. (1997) Is the SF-36 health survey questionnaire suitable as a self-report measure of the health status of older adults with Parkinson's disease? *Quality of Life Res.* **6,** 213–216.
54. Hagell, P. and Widner, H. (1999) Clinical rating of dyskinesias in Parkinson's disease. Utility and reliability of a new rating scale. *Mov. Disord.* **14,** 448–455.
55. Laplane, D., Levasseur, M., Pillon, B., et al. (1989) Obsessive-compulsive and other behavioral changes with bilateral basal ganglia lesions. A neuropsychological magnetic resonance imaging and positron tomography study. *Brain* **112,** 699–785.
56. Cummings, J. L. (1993) Frontal-subcortical circuits and human behavior. *Arch. Neurol.* **50,** 873–880.
57. Twedy, J. R., Langer, K. G., and McDowell, F. H. (1982) The effect of semantic relations on the memory deficit associated with Parkinson's disease. *J. Clin. Neuropsychol.* **4,** 235–247.
58. Saint-Cyr, J. A., Taylor, A. E., and Lang, A. E. (1988) Procedural learning and neostriatal dysfunction in man. *Brain* **111,** 941–959.
59. Pillon, B., Dubois, B., Ploska, A., et al. (1991) Neuropsychological specificity of dementia in Alzheimer's, Huntington's, Parkinson's diseases and progressive supranuclear palsy. *Neurology* **41,** 634–6543.
60. Hathaway, S. R. and McKinley, J. C. (1991) Manual for administration and scoring MMPI 2. University of Minnesota Press, Minneapolis, MN.
61. Montgomery, S. A. and Asberg, M. A. (1975) A new depression scale designed to be sensitive to change. *Br. J. Psychiatry* **134,** 382–389.
62. Jankovic, J. and Fahn, S. (1998) Dystonic disorders. In: *Parkinson's Disease and Movement Disorders*, 3rd ed. (Jankovic, J. and Tolosa, E., eds.), Williams and Wilkins, Baltimore, MD, pp. 513–551.
63. Burke, R. E., Fahn, S., Marsden, C. D., et al. (1985) Validity and reliability of a rating scale for the primary torsion dystonias. *Neurology* **35,** 73–77.
64. Consky, E. S. and Lang, A. E. (1994) Clinical assessments of patients with cervical dystonia. In: *Therapy with Botulinum Toxin* (Jankovic, J. and Hallett, M., eds.), Marcel Dekker, New York, pp. 211–237.
65. Comella, C. L., Leurgans, S., Chmura, T., et al. (1999) The Unified Dystonia Rating Scale: initial concurrent validity testing with other dystonia scales. *Neurology* **52(Suppl. 2),** A292.
66. Consky, E. S., Basinski, A., Belle, L., et al. (1990) The Toronto Western Spasmodic Torticollis Rating Scale (TWSTRS): assessment of validity and inter-rater reliability. **40(Suppl. 1),** 445.
67. Comella, C. L., Stebbins, G. T., Goetz, C. G., et al. (1997) Teaching tape for the motor section of the Toronto Western Spasmodic Torticollis Scale. *Mov. Disord.* **4,** 570–575.

6
Target Localization in Movement Disorders Surgery

Michael G. Kaplitt, William D. Hutchison, and Andres M. Lozano

1. INTRODUCTION

The success of a stereotactic neurosurgical procedure is influenced by a number of factors. Proper patient selection is important in order to avoid treating patients unlikely to benefit from the procedure. Careful preoperative evaluation should identify factors that may result in avoidable complications or a difficult postoperative course. When surgery is deemed appropriate, the choice of anatomic target and method of treatment (lesion vs deep brain stimulation [DBS]) are the next major determinants of outcome.

Following these evaluations, effective target localization is necessary to maximize therapeutic efficacy while minimizing unwanted adverse effects. The accuracy of target localization can be influenced by a variety of factors, including the choice and placement of stereotactic frames, imaging modality and method of image-based targeting, and use of electrophysiological methodologies. No study has definitively proven that any single approach influences outcome, and methods of target localization therefore continue to vary widely among practitioners. Nonetheless, numerous studies have evaluated each of these factors and have provided data that can serve to guide surgeons in choosing effective methods for target localization. This chapter will review the use of different imaging modalities for initial target identification, factors that may influence the accuracy of each modality, the use of intraoperative electrophysiological methods for target refinement including the use of microelectrode recording and macrostimulation, and methods and indications for lesioning and DBS.

2. IMAGING

Until recently, ventriculography was considered the gold standard imaging technique for functional neurosurgery, because it has been used and refined over several decades *(1–3)*. Among the possible imaging modalities, this approach is perhaps least subject to distortions secondary to computer reconstruction of images. Obviously, visualization of only the ventricular system prohibits direct visual targeting of intraparenchymal structures and imaging accuracy is dependent on the experience of the surgeon. Ventriculography is also an invasive procedure, and significant morbidity has been associated with gaining ventricular access and infusion of air or contrast medium into the ventricular system *(4)*. With the advent of modern noninvasive imaging, localization by computerized tomography (CT) and magnetic resonance imaging (MRI) have become increasingly popular. Several studies have now confirmed equivalent accuracy of CT and MRI compared with ventriculographic methods of target localization *(2–4)*. These results together with the ease, familiarity, and low-morbidity of noninvasive imaging have reduced the need for ventriculography and eliminated its use in most centers.

From: Contemporary Clinical Neurology:
Surgical Treatment of Parkinson's Disease and Other Movement Disorders
Edited by: D. Tarsy, J. L. Vitek, and A. M. Lozano © Humana Press Inc., Totowa, NJ

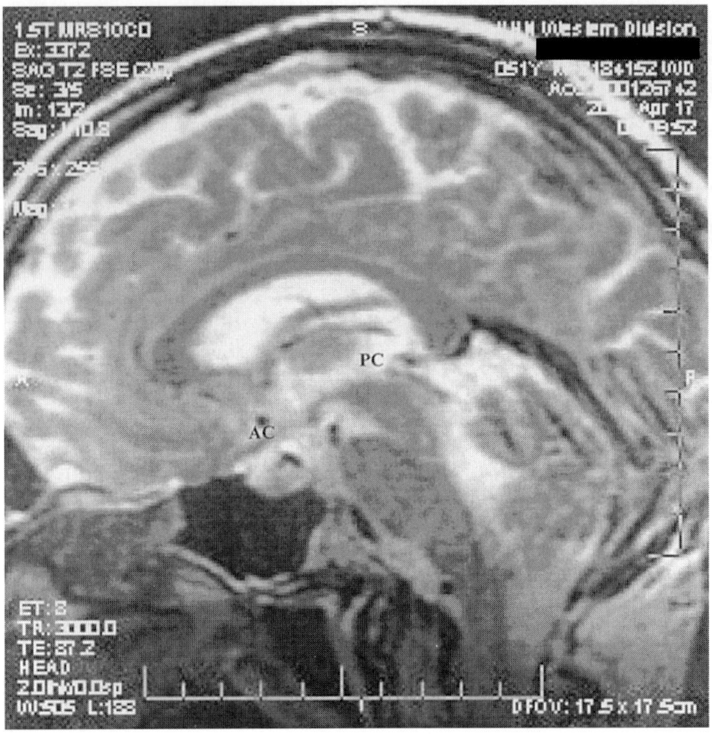

Fig. 1. Mid-sagittal T2-weighted MRI section demonstrating the location of the anterior commissure (AC) and posterior commissure (PC). Note that PC lies dorsal to the tectal plate, while AC lies inferior to the anterior fornices.

In addition to reducing morbidity, the development of modern imaging techniques has created new methods of target localization. Ventriculography resulted in identification of periventricular structures, in particular the anterior commissure (AC) and posterior commissure (PC). Deep brain structures could then be indirectly targeted using fixed distances from these coordinates and the resulting intercommissural line *(5)*. CT and MRI permit highly accurate localization of these same structures, thereby facilitating indirect targeting in a more standardized fashion that is also associated with lower morbidity *(4,6)* (Figs. 1 and 2). The anatomic resolution of CT is limited, however, and images can only be obtained in the axial plane (although even poorer resolution 3D reconstructions are now available). Another method of indirect targeting uses an atlas-based method *(7,8)* (Fig. 3). Since the atlas is adjusted to the intercommissural distance of a specific patient, it is also subject to errors in imaging AC and PC. Although the Schaltenbrand-Wahren atlas *(7)* is clearly the most popular among functional neurosurgeons, it has been suggested that other atlases may improve the accuracy of this technique since they may more closely correlate with functional activity *(9)*.

Direct visual localization of deep brain targets only became a reality with the widespread use of high field strength MRI (Fig. 4). MRI has sufficient resolution for visual targeting as well as flexibility with respect to plane of image and image modality, which can be adjusted to highlight specific locations *(2,3, 10,11)*. However, this does not guarantee that a visually identified target is functionally significant. This issue will be further discussed later. A recent study also demonstrated that indirect targeting of the subthalamic nucleus (STN) using standard distances from the midcommissural point appeared to correlate more closely with the final target than was the case with direct visual targeting *(9)*. This was surprising, given the widely held view that the STN on a T2 or "spoiled grass" coronal image is readily visible. This suggests either that imaging errors may produce a visually "obvious" target that is not anatomically accurate and/or that functionally significant regions do not necessarily correlate with anatomic appearance.

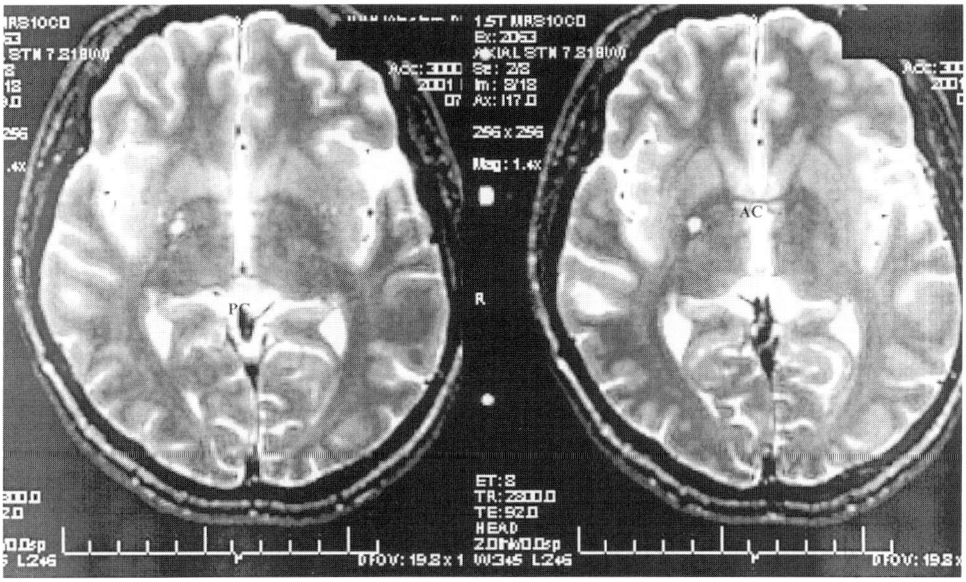

Fig. 2. T2-weighted axial sections used to identify the coordinates of the posterior commissure (PC) and anterior commissure (AC) for all indirect targeting methods.

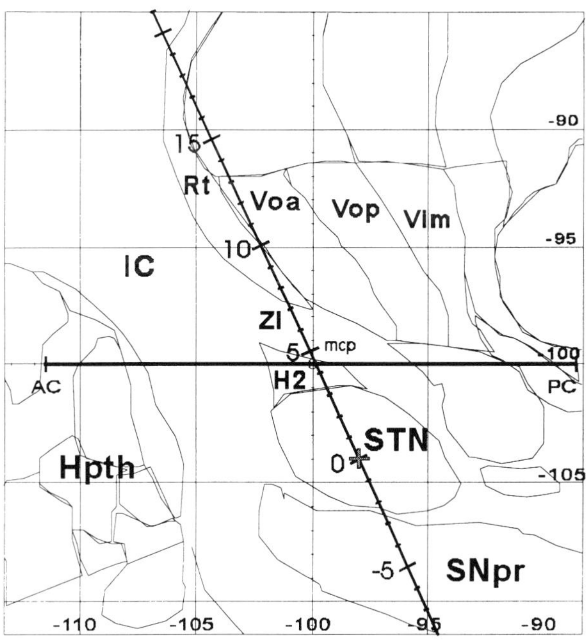

Fig. 3. A typical trajectory for microelectrode recording of the subthalamic nucleus (STN) mapped onto an a parasagittal atlas image (12.5 mm from midline) adjusted to conform to the intercommissural distance of the individual patient. The numbers represent the stereotactic coordinates for the Leksell frame in the Y direction (horizontal axis) and Z direction (vertical axis). Note the relationship of the STN to the midcommisural point (MCP), substantia nigra pars reticulata (SNpr), the zona incerta/fields of forel (ZI,H2), and the internal capsule (IC). Rt = reticular thalamus, Voa/Vop = ventralis oralis anterior/posterior, Vim = ventral intermediate nucleus.

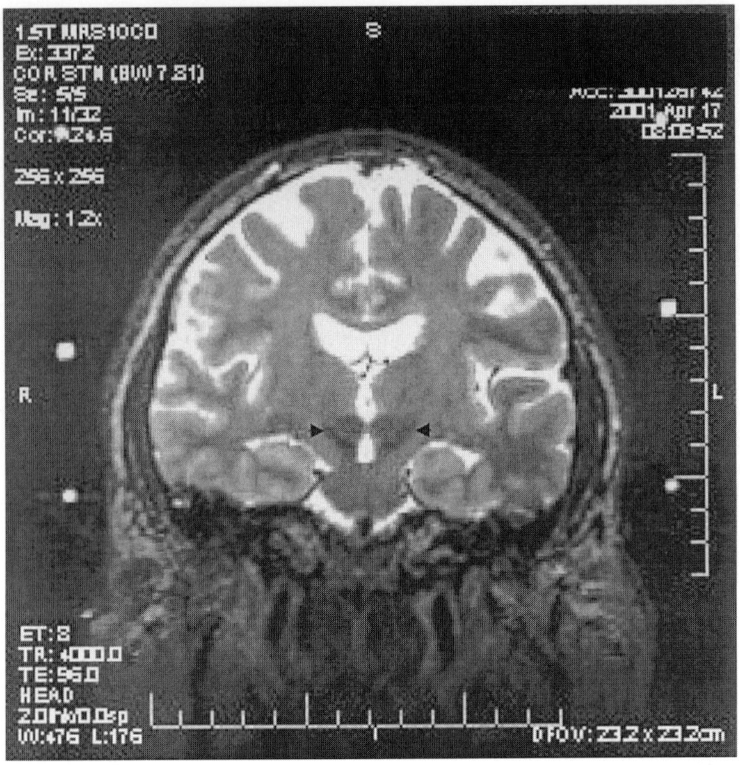

Fig. 4. T2-weighted coronal image for direct targeting of the subthalamic nuclei bilaterally (arrowheads). Notice that the substantia nigra lies ventromedial to the STN, the red nucleus lies dorsomedial, and the internal capsule runs lateral to the STN as it projects inferiorly toward the cerebral peduncle.

There is a continuing debate concerning the relative accuracy of CT and MRI for target localization in functional neurosurgery. MRI is subject to error due to spatial distortion from magnetic field heterogeneity and influences of the frame on image acquisition *(11,12)*. Recently, for example, we have noted that significant distortion can occur when MRI images are acquired with a low-band width protocol, which is optimal for visualizing the STN. Regular testing of MRI protocols with phantom targets as well as diligent attention to preoperative studies are necessary for early recognition of image heterogeneities. Often, such distortions can be minimized by altering various acquisition parameters in a stepwise fashion, but this can be at the expense of optimal resolution of other brain structures.

CT scanning is based on X-ray technology, and therefore is not subject to as many sources of error as MRI. Slice thickness and spacing between slices however, can introduce errors with both techniques *(13)*. MRI has been repeatedly validated as a technique with acceptable accuracy, however comparison of MRI and CT has revealed small but significant differences in target coordinates *(11)*. Some studies have revealed minor differences between ventriculography and MRI, which do not appear sufficiently substantial to overcome the benefits of MRI *(2,3)*. Since these three modalities have not been compared directly and have not been correlated clearly with outcome, it is difficult to determine whether differences between MRI and CT are functionally significant. Some have suggested that computer fusion technology can use CT to improve the accuracy of MRI while retaining the advantages of better resolution *(14,15)*. These are widely available, and practitioners of radiosurgery have been routinely using these techniques for several years, with some reports suggesting improved accuracy. In most functional neurosurgery centers, neurophysiological confirmation of the lesion or DBS target obviates the importance of minor errors related to a given imaging modality. If direct or indirect image-based targeting alone were proven to be satisfactory for functional neurosurgical procedures, then wider application of imaging technologies to improve accuracy may have greater significance.

3. MICROELECTRODE RECORDING VS MACROSTIMULATION

Physiological assessment of the activity of deep brain nuclei is an attractive method of localizing functionally significant targets in stereotactic neurosurgery. These methods generally involve microelectrode recording and macrostimulation. Microelectrode recording permits single-unit recording of neuronal firing. Numerous primate and human studies have identified characteristic firing patterns for various deep brain structures. In addition, the absence of neuronal activity can help identify boundaries between gray and white matter. High-frequency stimulation may produce symptomatic improvement, suggesting proper localization of the stimulating electrode. Adverse effects resulting from intraoperative stimulation in the awake patient can also indicate unacceptable proximity to vital structures, resulting in alteration of the final target. The application and relative merits of these two methods of physiological refinement will be discussed below.

3.1. Microelectrode Recording Equipment and Surgical Technique

Microelectrode recording in the human brain began in the early 1960s *(16)*. The earliest reports utilized electrodes which only recorded field potentials. However, higher impedance microelectrodes were soon employed that were capable of recording single-unit activity. Improvements in equipment used to amplify and filter signals while limiting noise have resulted in sufficient technical reproducibility to permit widespread use of microelectrode recording in modern clinical practice. The arguments put forth and data supporting or disputing the value of microelectrode recording will be discussed below; here we will focus on technical methods and analysis of microelectrode recording data.

3.1.1. Recording Equipment

A number of commercial sources provide complete systems for the recording, amplification, and filtering of single units with microelectrodes. While some systems provide for only a single channel of data, others are capable of recording several channels simultaneously, which, although technically more demanding, may prove useful if one electrode produces suboptimal recordings. The microelectrodes employed at our institution are tungsten with tip sizes of 15–25 um, plated with gold and platinum before use to reduce impedance at the tip (from 1.2 MOhm to about 0.2–0.4 MOhm) providing a better signal-to-noise ratio. The electrodes are mounted on 25-cm stainless-steel extender tubes insulated with a kapton sleeve suitable for use with a stereotactic guide tube. The neuronal signals are amplified with a gain of 5000–10,000 and filtered to allow bandpass of the frequency of interest for single unit discrimination (highpass filter setting of 250–5500 Hz and lowpass filter setting of about 10–20 kHz). The signals are sent to an audio monitor, oscilloscopes (or computer monitor in oscilloscope mode), a spike discriminator to determine firing rates, and a digital data recorder for further offline analysis. Many currently available systems have online spike discriminators with either a single level crossing that registers the number of spikes that pass a given voltage level per second, or more sophisticated "template" algorithms that sample the shape of the waveforms in a signal and then set up templates to match with the spikes in the record. The former is probably easier to use in practice because there can be significant noise in operating room recordings that interferes with template matching. Usually a relatively short period of time is spent at each level to identify the cell types and firing frequency in order to move to the next site without sufficient time to set up template matching. Our system of data storage uses an 8-channel video data recorder (Instrutech, NY) that allows storage of about 2 h of neuronal recordings along with simultaneous EMG, accelerometry, and other signals of interest.

3.1.2. Surgical Methods

After the frame has been applied and CT or MRI has been performed, an image-based target is chosen by one or more of the direct or indirect methods described earlier. At the Toronto Western Hospital, we use an atlas-based method adjusted to the intercommissural line to target Vim or GPi, and a direct visual target from a coronal T2 MRI to target STN. A guide tube is then inserted to a depth approx 10–15 mm superior to the optimal imaging-based target, and the trajectory is drawn on a scaled map to record electrophysiological data. The microelectrode assembly attached to a microdrive is then inserted into the guide tube under sterile conditions. The microdrive is used to move the microelectrode toward the target, stopping at multiple points in which new physiological data is obtained or questions are to be asked. We also utilize a dual microelectrode assembly with independent microdrivers to allow recording of two neurons at the same level or to permit simultaneous microstimulation and recording *(17)*. Based on data from the initial tract, one or more additional tracts are used to create an electrophyiological map from which the final target is generated. If bilateral procedures are performed, the initial contralateral tract uses this final target from the first side. This routinely reduces the number of tracts and time needed to complete the procedure on the contralateral side.

3.2. Physiological Targeting of the Internal Globus Pallidus

The initial target, whether by one of the indirect or direct imaging methods, is usually near Laitinen's original target of 20 mm lateral to midline, 3–6 mm below the intercommisural line and 2–3 mm anterior to the midcommissural point*(5)*. The major structures to be identified are the sensorimotor GPi, optic tract, and internal capsule *(8,18,19)*. Mapping the optic tract and internal capsule are important in addition to identifying GPi cells, since significant morbidity or reduced efficacy are encountered with lesions or DBS that are too close to these structures. When starting 10–15 mm superior to the target, recording usually begins within the external pallidum (GPe). Primate studies have identified two types of GPe cells with low frequency discharge *(20)*. Bursting cells (LFD-B) discharge at a rate of 5–10 Hz, with short bursts of 300–500 Hz. These cells are infrequent in primate GPe but are believed to characteristically identify this area. Slow-frequency cells with pauses (SFD-P) are far more common, but may be less pathognomonic. These cells discharge at a rate of 20–60 Hz, irregularly interrupted by pauses of 150–300 ms. We often observe similar cells in human patients *(8,19,21)*, however no study has yet made a definitive correlation of primate findings with human GPe physiology. GPe cells in the sensorimotor portion of the structure may respond to active or passive movement.

The GPe and GPi are separated by a white matter lamina, which is often identified by a significant decrease in overall signal as the GPe is exited. At the borders of GPe and GPi cells have been identified in primates and humans, which may be found while transiting this quieter white matter region. These "border" cells have a more regular firing pattern than GPe cells with a frequency of 30–40 Hz, but the amplitude is often smaller than GPe and GPi cells *(8,19,21)*. Border cells are less likely to respond to limb movement compared with their pallidal counterparts.

Entrance into the GPi is often first characterized by an overall increase in background noise *(8,19)*. As with the GPe, two types of cells can be encountered. The typical GPi cell has a larger amplitude than GPe cells with a frequency of 60–100 Hz. These cells also have a more regular firing pattern, compared with the irregular patterns encountered in GPe, and when recording in the sensorimotor territory of GPi they may respond to active and passive movements. A second cell type may be present in some patients with tremor. These show a firing pattern, which is synchronous with the patient's contralateral limb tremor.They are called "tremor cells" and are similar to those seen in the thalamus, although less frequently encountered than thalamic tremor cells *(8,22)*.

Mapping of vital structures near the pallidum is another rationale for microelectrode recording. The optic tract lies beneath the globus pallidus and the internal capsule is posteromedial to GPi. Identification of these structures helps to avoid complications secondary to encroachment of the lesion or lead and provides additional information for localization of the optimal final target. In both cases, entry into white matter tracts can be identified by the electrical silence that occurs when the microelectrode enters the tract. Axonal electrical activity is occasionally found and is characterized by narrow spikes. Two methods can be used to identify these structures. Stimulation of the optic tract (with either a microelectrode or a macroelectrode) usually causes light or color sensations or scotomata in the contralateral visual field. The proximity to the optic tract can be determined based upon stimulation threshold. We find that thresholds of 1 uA to 20 uA suggest that the electrode is in the optic tract while higher thresholds (up to 100 uA) indicate that the tip is near but not in the tract. Similarly, stimulation of the internal capsule may result in tetanic contractions or paresthesias of the contralateral limbs, again with lower thresholds suggesting closer proximity of the electrode to the capsule. Microelectrode recording of optic tract potentials in response to flashing or strobe lights can also confirm the location of the optic tract, but comparable recordings are not available for the internal capsule *(19,23)*. Occasionally, there is a discordance between stimulation of the optic tract and microelectrode recordings of strobe light responses. One study has suggested a greater discordance between microstimulation and visual evoked potentials when compared with macrostimulation alone, and in this study one-third of patients with negative responses to macrostimulation had positive visual responses *(23)*. Localizing microelectrode recordings in the absence of positive stimulation effects suggests that reliance on microstimulation or macrostimulation for mapping without microelectrode recording may not adequately reflect the physiological activity of the brain regions under study.

3.3. *Physiological Targeting of the Subthalamic Nucleus*

Trajectories to target the STN begin 2–3 cm from midline at the coronal suture and usually pass, in order of occurrence, anterior thalamic nuclei, the zona incerta, and the Fields of Forel prior to encountering the STN *(24)*. Below the STN is the substantia nigra, which in parkinsonian patients is almost exclusively the pars reticulata (SNpr). Identification of these structures defines the major boundaries of the STN (Fig. 3). Recording is usually initiated 10–15 mm above the STN as defined by direct visual targeting from a T2-weighted or "spoiled grass" coronal MRI (Fig. 4). We will occasionally modify this target based on the adjusted atlas map, although a recent study has suggested that indirect targeting using standard distances from the midcommissural point may be more accurate than both of these methods *(9)*. The ideal trajectory will begin with recording of thalamic cells in the reticular nucleus, ventralis oralis anterior (Voa), or ventralis oralis posterior (Vop) nuclei. These nuclei are populated by cells with similar firing patterns, and two cell types are encountered. "Bursting" cells have a mean firing rate of 15Hz with fairly regular, characteristic bursts. Nonbursting cells have a slightly higher frequency, with a mean of 30Hz *(24,25)*. Bursting cells tend to be more frequently identified in the reticular thalamus. If the initial recordings are quiet for several millimeters, it suggests that the electrode is traversing the white matter of the internal capsule anterolateral to the thalamus. Unlike pallidal procedures, we do not attempt to intentionally identify the internal capsule, but we begin a more posterior or medial tract if there is difficulty identifying clear neuronal activity in proximal portions of the initial tract.

As the thalamus is exited, a significant decrease in overall electrical activity is observed as the electrode tip passes through the white matter of the Fields of Forel *(24)*. The thalamic and lenticular fasciculi are separated by the zona incerta, which is a small gray matter strip in which a few cells may be recorded. Zona incerta cells may occasionally have properties similar to STN neurons, including responses to movement, so that clear mapping of the STN and the SNr is necessary to avoid inadvertently choosing the zona incerta as a target *(24)*. Because the zona incerta is bounded by white matter tracts, any confusion regarding cellular electrical activity should be resolved when electrical silence is again encountered prior to entering the subthalamic nucleus.

Entry into the STN is accompanied by an obvious increase in background noise, as described for other areas in which the electrode leaves white matter and enters a pathologically hyperactive nucleus.

Characteristic STN cells have a frequency of 25–45 Hz with high-amplitude spikes and an irregular firing pattern *(24)*. As with other deep nuclei, tremor cells may be encountered in patients with tremor in the contralateral limb. The likelihood of encountering tremor cells appears to correlate with the severity of the clinical tremor. STN neurons in the sensorimotor portion of the structure may respond to active and passive movement. The widest portion of STN is approximately 6 mm, but the tapered shape of this nucleus may result in STN cells spanning only 3 mm if the tract does not traverse the center of the nucleus. The density of these cells should be high in the true STN in which numerous cells are readily encountered. This is another feature that distinguishes STN from the zona incerta, which contains only sparse neurons. Arrest or reduction of tremor can be seen with stimulation of STN, but this is not a reliable finding and few centers rely on this for target localization.

The lower edge of the STN is bordered by the SNr. SNr neurons have a characteristic firing pattern, which is more regular than STN cells and has a higher discharge frequency (60–90 Hz), although some lower frequency cells can be encountered *(24)*. This pattern is similar to cells encountered in the GPi, which is physiologically related to the SNr *(8)*. The primary value of stimulation in this setting is to identify the proximity of the tract or target to the medial lemniscus posterior to STN. Paresthesias resulting from low threshold stimulation suggest unacceptably close proximity to the medial lemniscus and usually require a more anterior placement. Although we usually identify this structure, if all other regions are clearly identified and an appropriate length of STN is mapped, the lead may be placed without identification of the medial lemniscus. The internal capsule is found anterior and lateral to the STN. Stimulation-induced motor contractions or patient reports of "pulling" sensations (suggesting motor rather than sensory stimulation) can also help identify targets, which are too close to this structure. Finally, the fibers of the third cranial nerve are medial to the STN, and stimulation in medial portions of the STN too close to the oculomotor nerve can result in stimulation-induced ocular movements.

3.4. Physiological Targeting of Motor Thalamus for Tremor

Stereotactic lesioning or stimulation of the motor thalamus has been widely performed for many years. The surgical target is the ventral intermediate nucleus (Vim), which is the cerebellar receiving area. Anterior to this are the two pallidal receiving areas, ventral oralis anterior (Voa) and ventral oralis posterior (Vop). Posterior to Vim is the lemniscal receiving area, the ventrocaudal nucleus (Vc), which is the major thalamic sensory relay nucleus. The internal capsule lies lateral to Vim. The initial trajectory targets a site slightly anterior to the posterior commissure, which often passes through the posterior border of Vim or through Vc. The lower border of Vim is usually targeted, particularly with DBS, so that all four contacts of the DBS electrode span a large portion of the motor thalamus. As a result, initiating recordings 10–15 mm above the target usually identifies cells of either Vc or motor thalamus, depending on the anterior-posterior position of the tract. If recording is started at higher positions, very slow discharge cells (0.1–10 Hz) may be encountered representing the caudate nucleus, or a quiet area with few slow bursting cells may be found slightly deeper in the dorsal thalamus. These activities do not respond to movement.

Upon entry into motor thalamus, cells responsive to movement and/or tremor cells will be encountered. Tremor cells discharge in a pattern synchronous with the patients contralateral limb tremor, as described for GPi and STN. These cells are more frequently encountered in the thalamus, however, possibly owing in part to the fact that most patients undergoing thalamic surgery have significant tremor as their main disability. It has been suggested that substantial therapeutic benefit can be derived from lesion or lead placement within a few millimeters of a concentrated cluster of tremor cells *(26)*. Kinesthetic cells (which respond to involuntary movements) or voluntary cells can be mapped, as can more quiet ventral regions which suggest one is exiting from ventral thalamus into white matter. Posterior to motor thalamus, cells can be found which respond to deep muscle pressure or to light tactile stimuli thereby defining Vc.

Both macrostimulation and microstimulation can help define the borders of motor thalamus and confirm the functional significance of the final surgical target. Stimulation of areas posterior to the optimal target produces paresthesias and a low threshold for sensory changes indicates the location of the electrode within Vc. Contralateral muscle contractions at low threshold stimulation indicate that the electrode is unacceptably close to the internal capsule and a more medial target should be explored. Induction of tremor arrest without adverse side effects following stimulation further confirms the location of Vim and raises confidence in the clinical significance of the chosen target.

3.5. Is Microelectrode Recording Necessary for Target Localization?

Any discussion of the value of microelectrode recording (MER) should begin with the recognition that no study to date has compared the outcomes of any functional neurosurgical procedure performed with or without MER refinement in a prospective, double-blind fashion. The debate regarding the relative value of microelectrode recording is unlikely to be definitively settled without such a multicenter trial. In the absence of such a study, the theoretical rationale for MER and currently available data largely support the value of this technique in obtaining optimal targets. Microelectrode recording provides physiological data regarding gray matter/white matter boundaries, and characteristic patterns of neuronal firing have been identified for individual deep nuclei. This collective data provides an individualized physiological map for each patient. As discussed earlier, errors from the stereotactic frame and imaging modality can be reduced but not entirely eliminated. Therefore, even if it were accepted that errors from visual targeting or atlas/coordinate based targeting were relatively small, these may be magnified by other sources of error that cannot be eliminated.

Most current literature supports the use of some form of microelectrode refinement in targeting deep brain structures for movement disorder surgery. One study has shown that combination of all image-based modalities can significantly reduce error, but there is still some variation from the MER-defined target *(9)*. Numerous other studies have reported that MER changed the final target in most or all cases, regardless of choice of deep brain target and regardless of whether lesioning or stimulation was employed *(9,27–32)*. In one pallidotomy study, for example, 98% of cases had targeting changes, with 12% of cases resulting in a change of 4 mm or more from the original, image-based target *(28)*. It has also been suggested that some recording results within a nucleus can influence outcome. A retrospective study of 15 patients revealed that lesions placed within 2 mm of a cluster of "tremor" cells resulted in resolution of tremor in all patients *(26)*. Although identification of vital structures bordering target nuclei can often be performed with stimulation, variable results using this method may make negative responses unreliable. For example, we have on several occasions obtained negative results from microstimulation within the optic tract while recordings from visual evoked responses at the same site were positive. This is supported by recent data, which appear to demonstrate that microelectrode mapping of visual evoked potentials more accurately and reliably defines the borders of GPi and the optic tract as compared with microstimulation or macrostimulation *(23)*. Thus, MER appears to provide a patient-specific physiological map that may not only be more anatomically accurate than image-based targeting, but that also may be more functionally relevant for final target determination and provide better definition of vital structures to be avoided.

The paucity of objective data proving the value of MER continues to fuel the debate regarding the practical necessity of this technique for target localization. Few practitioners argue against the utility of MER for research. However, MER is time-consuming and therefore contributes to some patient discomfort. There is also a theoretical but uncertain increased risk of brain hemorrhage following use of multiple recording tracts. Because no study has yet been undertaken to definitively prove that MER improves surgical outcomes, questions remain regarding the need for MER in clinical practice. It has been suggested that direct visual targeting or atlas/coordinate-based methods may provide satisfactory results alone if imaging errors can be minimized. For example, one study used computed tomography/magnetic resonance imaging (CT/MRI) fusion to minimize distortion errors from MRI while retaining better resolution than CT alone to permit target refinement based on individual anatomic variations *(33)*. Their thalamotomy results (65% improvement in tremor) were less impressive than other published studies in which MER was used, but their pallidotomy results were comparable to other reports.

Additionally, 6% of their pallidotomy patients developed hemiparesis, suggesting that absence of MER may result in reduced safety as well as reduced efficacy. Techniques for image-based targeting of STN with macrostimulation have also been reported, although no outcome data was provided *(34)*. Perhaps the most provocative data is contained in the study by Zonenshayn et al. *(9)*, which supports the use of MER data. Their best target from image and coordinate-based mapping, however, varied from the physiology-defined target by an average of only 1.3 mm *(9)*. Further studies are necessary to determine whether this degree of variability is functionally significant.

3.6. *Lesioning vs Deep Brain Stimulation*

The ultimate goal of most functional neurosurgical procedures is to alter the activity of selected deep brain nuclei in order to achieve symptomatic improvement of neurological symptoms. There are currently two major methods for achieving this outcome. Ablative lesioning has been used for many years to treat essential tremor, Parkinson's disease, and dystonia *(35–38)*. Thalamotomy and pallidotomy have been the most widely performed ablative procedures. However, some centers are performing subthalamotomy as well. Lesions are generally performed using a radiofrequency lesion generator and lesioning electrode. Macrostimulation can first be performed through this electrode to determine whether the probe is too close to vital structures to safely perform the lesion. Lesions are then made by first heating to a moderate temperature (usually 50–60°C) for 60–90 s. If this is well-tolerated, the temperature is increased to 80–90°C for variable times until the lesion is complete *(39)*.

Chronic DBS has been introduced more recently as an alternative method for blocking or altering activity of deep brain nuclei. As indicated earlier, intraoperative macrostimulation has long been used as a localizing method prior to performing lesions. The advent of permanently implantable, flexible electrodes and subcutaneous pulse-generators has led to a rapid increase in application of chronic DBS for thalamic, pallidal, and subthalamic blockade *(40–42)*. Target localization using microelectrode recording and/or macrostimulation is performed similarly for either lesioning or DBS. After the target is identified, a DBS electrode containing four electrode contacts at its tip is inserted in the target. Fluoroscopic guidance is used after placement to insure that the electrode does not move during subsequent manipulation and fixation. Pulse generators are then inserted subcutaneously into the anterior chest wall and connected by an extension to the DBS electrode in the head. This second stage involves subcutaneous tunneling, necessitating the use of general anesthesia.

Several criteria may be used to decide whether lesioning or DBS is the appropriate treatment for a given patient. The major advantages of DBS is that it is reversible and adjustable. If DBS causes adverse effects, the stimulus intensity or pulse width can be reduced and various electrode contact combinations can be tested to optimize results, whereas adverse effects following lesions are more likely to be long-lasting or permanent. Furthermore, if symptoms return over time, DBS parameters can often be adjusted to regain control of symptoms. This may explain why some groups have observed better long-term results with DBS and fewer complications from bilateral DBS compared with bilateral lesioning *(43,44)*. DBS is costly however and, in the case of GPi or STN DBS, often requires numerous programming sessions over several weeks or months to optimize parameters. If cost is a concern or if patients live in areas remote from a physician with DBS programming capability, lesioning may be a preferable option. Lesioning can also be performed entirely under local anesthesia, whereas DBS requires general anesthesia to tunnel and internalize the stimulating hardware, which may be a consideration for some patients. Finally, patients who develop hardware-related adverse effects such as lead fracture or scalp infections may be candidates for lesioning.

4. SUMMARY

A variety of effective methods for target localization in stereotactic and functional neurosurgery have been reported. Although there is no clear consensus regarding the best technique to use at each stage of a given stereotactic procedure, scrupulous attention to detail at each step should optimize outcome. Any modern frame system can be used successfully. However, careful frame placement and properly centering the frame and patient within the scanner can minimize error. Both MRI and CT are reliable imaging modalities. While CT is less subject to distortion, MRI is more appropriate for visual targeting. Direct or indirect targeting methods are all subject to some variability, and the optimal technique for a given deep brain region continues to be the subject of debate. Even when all possible sources of imaging error are eliminated, there remains discordance between image-based targets and MER refined targets in most studies. The functional significance of this difference is unclear, and several practitioners remain unconvinced of the value of MER outside of research. Current literature, however, appears to favor the use of MER as outcomes in studies using MER refinement appear to be more favorable and consistent. Because stereotactic procedures are designed to correct pathological activity, we believe it is likely that the bias among neurosurgeons will continue to favor the use of MER to physiologically define the target and surrounding structures. It is hoped that advances in technology will further minimize error and promote increasing consensus regarding optimal methods for targeting localization.

ACKNOWLEDGMENTS

The support of the Parkinson's Foundation of Canada (W.D.H. and A.M.L.) is gratefully acknowledged. M.G.K. is a recipient of a fellowship and A.M.L is a Clinician Scientist of the Canadian Institute for Health Research.

REFERENCES

1. Hariz, M. I. and Bergenheim, A. T. (1990) A comparitive study on ventriculographic and computerized tomography-guided determination of brain targets in functional stereotaxis. *J. Neurosurg.* **73,** 565–571.
2. Mandybur, G., et al. (1995) Comparison of MRI and ventriculographic target acquisition for posteroventral pallidotomy. *Stereotact. Funct. Neurosurg.* **65(1–4),** 54–59.
3. Schuurman, P. R., et al. (1999) A prospective comparison between three-dimensional magnetic resonance imaging and ventriculography for target-coordinate determination in frame-based functional stereotactic neurosurgery. *J. Neurosurg.* **91(6),** 911–914.
4. Alterman, R. L., et al. (1995) Stereotactic ventrolateral thalamotomy: is ventriculography necessary? *Neurosurgery* **37(4),** 717–721.
5. Laitinen, L. V., Bergenheim, A. T., and Hariz, M. I. (1992) Leksell's posteroventral pallidotomy in the treatment of Parkinson's disease. *J. Neurosurg.* **76,** 53–61.
6. Tasker, R. R., Dostrovsky, J. O., and Dolan, E. J. (1991) Computerized tomography (CT) is just as accurate as ventriculography for functional stereotactic thalamotomy. *Stereotact. Funct. Neurosurg.* **57,** 157–166.
7. Schaltenbrand, G. and Wahren, W. (1977) *Atlas for Stereotaxy of the Human Brain*. Thieme, Stuttgart.
8. Lozano, A., et al. (1996) Methods for microelectrode-guided posteroventral pallidotomy [see comments]. *J. Neurosurg.* **84(2),** 194–202.
9. Zonenshayn, M., et al. (2000) Comparison of anatomic and neurophysiological methods for subthalamic nucleus targeting. *Neurosurgery* **47(2),** 282–292.
10. Reich, C. A., et al. (2000) A high-resolution fast spin-echo inversion-recovery sequence for preoperative localization of the internal globus pallidus. *AJNR Am. J. Neuroradiol.* **21(5),** 928–931.
11. Holtzheimer, P. E. III, Roberts, D. W., and Darcey, T. M. (1999) Magnetic resonance imaging versus computed tomography for target localization in functional stereotactic neurosurgery. *Neurosurgery* **45(2),** 290–297; discussion 297–298.
12. Burchiel, K. J., et al. (1996) MRI distortion and stereotactic neurosurgery using the Cosman-Roberts-Wells and Leksell frames. *Stereotact. Funct. Neurosurg.* **66(1–3),** 123–136.
13. Maciunas, R., Galoway, R., and Latimer, J. (1994) The application accuracy of stereotactic frames. *Neurosurgery* **35,** 682–695.
14. Cohen, D. S., Lustgarten, J. H., and Miller, E. (1995) Effects of coregistration of MR to CT images on MR stereotactic accuracy. *J. Neurosurg.* **82,** 772–779.
15. Alexander, E. A., et al. (1995) Magnetic resonance image-directed stereotactic neurosurgery: use of image fusion with computerized tomography to enhance spatial accuracy. *J. Neurosurg.* **83,** 271–276.
16. Gildenberg, P. L. (2000) History of movement disorder surgery. In: *Movement Disorder Surgery* (Lozano, A. M., ed.), Karger, Basel, pp. 1–20.
17. Dostrovsky, J. O., et al. (2000) Microstimulation induced inhibition of neuronal firing in human globus pallidus. *J. Neurophysiol.* **84(1),** 570–574.

18. Lozano, A. M., et al. (1997) Microelectrode recording-guided posteroventral pallidotomy in patients with Parkinson's disease. *Adv. Neurol.* **74,** 167–174.
19. Lozano, A. M., et al. (1998) Microelectrode recordings define the ventral posteromedial pallidotomy target. *Stereotact. Funct. Neurosurg.* **71(4),** 153–163.
20. DeLong, M. R. (1971) Activity of pallidal neurons during movement. *J. Neurophysiol.* **34,** 414–427.
21. Hutchinson, W. D., et al. (1994) Differential neuronal activity in segments of globus pallidus in Parkinson's disease. *Neuroreport* **5,** 1533–1537.
22. Hutchison, W. D., et al. (1997) Identification and characterization of neurons with tremor-frequency activity in human globus pallidus. *Exp. Brain Res.* **113(3),** 557–563.
23. Yokoyama, T., et al. (1999) Visual evoked potentials during posteroventral pallidotomy for Parkinson's disease. *Neurosurgery* **44(4),** 815–822; discussion 822–824.
24. Hutchison, W. D., et al. (1998) Neurophysiological identification of the subthalamic nucleus in surgery for Parkinson's disease. *Ann. Neurol.* **44(4),** 622–628.
25. Raeva, S. N., Lukashev, A., and Lashin, A. (1991) Unit activity in human thalamic reticular nucleus. I. Spontaneous activity. *Electroenceph. Clin. Neurophysiol.* **79,** 133–140.
26. Lenz, F. A., et al. (1995) Statistical prediction of the optimal site for thalamotomy in parkinsonian tremor. *Mov. Disord.* **10(3),** 318–328.
27. Guridi, J., et al. (1999) Stereotactic targeting of the globus pallidus internus in Parkinson's disease: imaging versus electrophysiological mapping [see comments]. *Neurosurgery* **45(2),** 278–287; discussion 287–289.
28. Alterman, R. L., et al. (1999) Microelectrode recording during posteroventral pallidotomy: impact on target selection and complications. *Neurosurgery* **44(2),** 315–321.
29. Forster, A., et al. (1999) Audit of neurophysiological recording during movement disorder surgery. *Stereotact. Funct. Neurosurg.* **72,** 154–156.
30. Kirschman, D. L., et al. (2000) Pallidotomy microelectrode targeting: neurophysiology-based target refinement. *Neurosurgery* **46(3),** 613–622; discussion 622–624.
31. Tsao, K., et al. (1998) Pallidotomy lesion locations: significance of microelectrode refinement. *Neurosurgery* **43(3),** 506–512; discussion 512–513.
32. Bejjani, B. P., et al. (2000) Bilateral subthalamic stimulation for Parkinson's disease by using three-dimensional stereotactic magnetic resonance imaging and electrophysiological guidance. *J. Neurosurg.* **92(4),** 615–625.
33. Giller, C. A., et al. (1998) Stereotactic pallidotomy and thalamotomy using individual variations of anatomic landmarks for localization. *Neurosurgery* **42(1),** 56–62; discussion 62–65.
34. Yoon, M. S. and Munz, M. (1999) Placement of deep brain stimulators into the subthalamic nucleus. *Stereotact. Funct. Neurosurg.* **72(2–4),** 145–149.
35. Lozano, A. M., et al. (1997) Globus pallidus internus pallidotomy for generalized dystonia. *Mov. Disord.* **12(6),** 865–870.
36. Lozano, A. M., et al. (1995) Effect of GPi pallidotomy on motor function in Parkinson's disease. *Lancet* **346(8987),** 1383–1387.
37. Guridi, J. and Lozano, A. M. (1997) A brief history of pallidotomy. *Neurosurgery* **41(5),** 1169–1180.
38. Shahzadi, S., Tasker, R. R., and Lozano, A. (1995) Thalamotomy for essential and cerebellar tremor. *Stereotact. Funct. Neurosurg.* **65(1–4),** 11–17.
39. Linhares, M. N. and Tasker, R. R. (2000) Thalamotomy with microelectrode recording. In: *Movement Disorder Surgery* (Lozano, A. M., ed.), Karger, Basel, pp. 156–171.
40. Starr, P. A., Vitek, J. L., and Bakay, R. A. (1998) Deep brain stimulation for movement disorders. *Neurosurg. Clin. North Am.* **9(2),** 381–402.
41. Kumar, R., et al. (1998) Double-blind evaluation of subthalamic nucleus deep brain stimulation in advanced Parkinson's disease. *Neurology* **51(3),** 850–855.
42. Kumar, K., Kelly, M., and Toth, C. (1999) Deep brain stimulation of the ventral intermediate nucleus of the thalamus for control of tremors in Parkinson's disease and essential tremor. *Stereotact. Funct. Neurosurg.* **72(1),** 47–61.
43. Tasker, R. R., et al. (1997) Deep brain stimulation and thalamotomy for tremor compared. *Acta Neurochir. Suppl. (Wien.)* **68,** 49–53.
44. Kumar, R., et al. (1998) Pallidotomy and deep brain stimulation of the pallidum and subthalamic nucleus in advanced Parkinson's disease. *Mov. Disord.* **13(Suppl. 1),** 73–82.

7
Thalamotomy for Tremor

Sherwin E. Hua, Ira M. Garonzik, Jung-Il Lee, and Frederick A. Lenz

1. INTRODUCTION

Since the 1960s, stereotactic surgery for tremor has targeted the ventral nuclear group of thalamus. According to Hassler's classification *(1)*, the nuclei in the ventral nuclear group, from anterior to posterior, are a pallidal relay nucleus (ventral oral, Vo), a cerebellar relay nucleus (ventral intermediate, Vim), and the principal somatosensory nucleus (ventral caudal, Vc) *(2,3)*. On the basis of surgical experience, Hassler proposed that the anterior portion of Vo, the nucleus ventralis oralis anterior (Voa), was a better target for rigidity, whereas the posterior portion, the nucleus ventral oral posterior (Vop), was better for the relief of tremor. With the aid of microelectrode recordings, an area posterior to Vop was later found to have rhythmic bursting activity close to the frequency of tremor *(4)*. Many subsequent studies have demonstrated that the nucleus in this location, Vim, is the target of choice for treatment of tremor of all types.

2. STEREOTACTIC SURGICAL TECHNIQUE

Many techniques can be used to carry out functional stereotactic procedures within the standard of care. The goal of thalamotomy is to lesion a population of cells within Vim that is involved in the mechanism of tremor. Combined radiologic and physiologic landmarks provide the most accurate localization of the target. At our institution, we have localized the anterior commissure (AC), posterior commissure (PC), and the border between the internal capsule and thalamus radiologically with CT and MRI scans. We refine the radiologic estimate of location by microelectrode physiologic localization *(5)* and then carry out radiofrequency lesioning. Alternative approaches are to localize radiologically by ventriculography or CT/MR fusion techniques, to localize physiologically by semi-microelectrode recording or macrostimulation or both, and to lesion by radiosurgery. The relative efficacy and safety of these different techniques have not been examined systematically.

2.1. *Radiologic Localization*

Radiologic targeting usually uses MRI or CT to determine the location of the AC and PC by ventriculography. AC and PC predict the locations of the different thalamic nuclei in stereotactic space. At our institution the transparent templates of the sagittal sections of the Schaltenbrand and Bailey atlas *(6)* overlay graph paper marked with the positions of the anterior and posterior commissures in stereotactic space. In this way the nuclear locations predicted radiographically in that patient are displayed in the coordinates of the Leksell frame. The laterality of the target is determined from a fast inversion recovery MR sequence. This sequence is used to determine the position of the capsule and the medial

From: Contemporary Clinical Neurology: Surgical Treatment of Parkinson's Disease and Other Movement Disorders
Edited by: D. Tarsy, J. L. Vitek, and A. M. Lozano © Humana Press Inc., Totowa, NJ

dorsal nucleus (MD) as a large dorsal periventricular thalamic high intensity signal (Lenz, Eckell, Bryant, unpublished observations). Because the MD forms the medial boundary of Vim and Vop, the center of Vim is midway between the lateral border of MD and the medial border of the capsule *(6)*. This central plane is matched to the closest sagittal section of the atlas. The first microelectrode trajectories target Vc in this plane; physiologic observations are recorded on the graph paper. Alternative approaches to targeting Vim from the AC-PC line include the geometric construction for approximating nuclear location as described by Guiot *(7,8)*.

Determination of the radiologic position of the AC-PC line is usually accomplished by CT and MRI scanning. MRI scanning is slightly less accurate than CT scanning due to systematic errors (2 mm mean and 4 mm maximum) such as inhomogenieties in the magnetic field *(9,10)*. Attempts to decrease errors in MRI scans due to these artifacts include software modifications and overlapping (fusion) of the MRI database with the CT database, which is not prone to these types of artifacts *(11)*. Targeting in thalamotomy can then be accomplished by computer programs that overlay radiologic images and atlas maps. These programs display atlas maps transformed either to match the AC-PC line in isolation *(12)* or to match the AC-PC line and other structures, such as the margins of the third ventricle or the internal capsule *(13,14)*.

2.2. *Physiologic Localization*

Radiologic targeting can be further refined by identifying the different thalamic nuclei, including Vim, Vop, and Vc, on the basis of their electrophysiologic properties. These properties are defined in terms of spontaneous activity, neuronal response to passive and active movements, and sensory responses to natural or electrical stimulation. Physiologic localization has been carried out by stimulation with a macroelectrode (impedance < 1000 Ohms), or by stimulation and recording with a semi-microelectrode (impedance < 100 kOhms) or a microelectrode (impedance > 500 kOhms).

2.2.1. Microelectrode Localization

Microelectrodes for physiologic monitoring and recording are designed to isolate single action potentials *(15,16)*. In addition, the electrode must be durable to withstand microstimulation, which degrades the insulation. Typically these characteristics are achieved by constructing electrodes from a platinum-iridium alloy or from tungsten, producing a tapered tip, and insulating with glass *(15,17, 18)*. The electrode impedance is usually greater than 500 kOhms *(15,16,19)*. Passing current through the electrode during microstimulation will degrade insulation and lower impedance, which makes it harder to isolate single units.

The assembled electrode is attached to a hydraulic microdrive and mounted on the stereotaxic frame. The signal from the microelectrode is amplified and filtered. Multiple neuronal discharges of various sizes may be seen on an oscilloscope and heard by use of an audio monitor. In addition to recording, microstimulation of subcortical structures through the microelectrode may be employed in physiologic localization. Current may be delivered through the same electrode that is used for recording by disconnecting it from the preamplifier and connecting it to the output of a current-isolation stimulator. The current used in stimulation determines the amount of local current spread. Stimulation in Vc will evoke somatic sensations *(20)*, while stimulation in Vim may alter the ongoing tremor *(21)* or dystonia *(22)*.

Cells responding to sensory stimulation in small, well defined, receptive fields are found in Vc *(23)*. Anterior to Vc, in Vim and Vop a large percentage of neuronal activity demonstrates statistical changes in rate of firing related to active movement (voluntary cells) (*see* Fig. 1) *(24,25)*. Some neurons respond during both active movement and somatosensory stimulation (combined cells) *(24,26)*. Combined cells fire in response to passive movements of a joint and during active movements of the same joint. The sensory cells are found in Vc and thus are located posterior to the cells with responses during active movement.

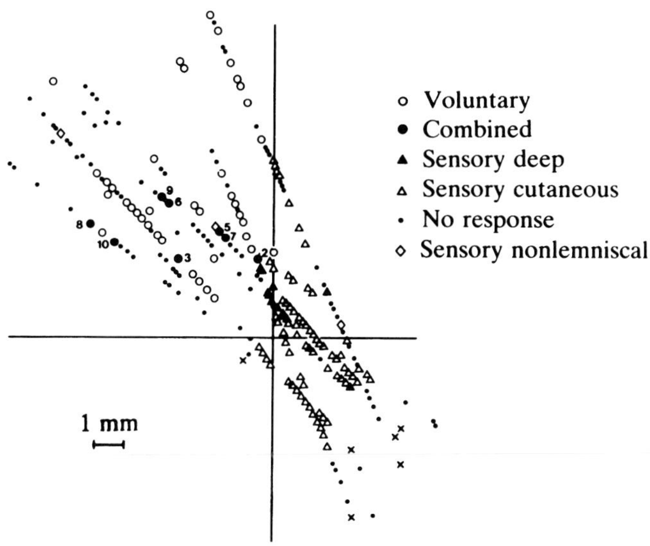

Fig. 1. Relative locations of cells identified by functional category from microelectrode studies during thalamotomy for tremor. The results have been pooled from planes in several patients where the majority of cells had activity related to hand and wrist movements. The horizontal line represents the AC-PC line. The vertical line represents the anterior-posterior position of the most anterior cell responding to sensory stimulation. Therefore the principal sensory nucleus Vc is to the right of the vertical and the cerebellar relay Vim is to the left. Numbers apply to combined cells. Each x marks the site where the last somatic action potential was recorded along that trajectory. Adapted with permission from ref. *(24)*.

Cells in Vc, Vim, and Vop often exhibit activity at about the frequency of tremor. Correlations between thalamic neuronal activity and tremor have been suggested previously by visual or auditory inspection *(16,27–29)*. Quantitative analysis techniques have allowed clearer demonstration of correlation between thalamic neuronal firing and EMG activity during tremor *(30–32)*, as shown in Fig. 2.

2.2.2. Localization with Macrostimulation and/or Semi-microelectrode

Semi-microelectode recordings are carried out using microelectrodes with impedances of less than 100 kOhms. The semi-microelectrode signal is often amplified against a concentric ring electrode that is located on a radius of 0.4 mm around the microelectrode *(8,33,34)*. Bipolar stimulation has been used through a concentric ring electrode alone or in combination with recording through a semi-microelectrode or with recording of scalp EEG *(35,36)*.

Macrostimulation through a low impedance electrode (impedance often less than 1000 Kohms) can reliably identify the capsule by stimulation-evoked tetanic contraction of skeletal muscle at low threshold *(35)*. Stimulation of intralaminar nuclei, medial to Vc or Vim may evoke the recruiting response—long latency, high voltage, negative waves—occurring over much of cortex at the frequency of stimulation (usually less than 10 Hz) *(2,37)*. The target area in Vim can be identified by stimulation-evoked increase or decrease in the amplitude of tremor *(38)*. Although macrostimulation in Vc evokes paresthesiae, similar sensations can be evoked by stimulation in Vim *(38)*. Therefore, recording of responses to tactile stimulation localizes Vc more accurately *(35)*.

Semi-microelectrode recordings *(8,13,34)* reveal patterns of neuronal activity parallel to those of microelectrode recordings. Vc can be identified by a high level of neural activity and by responses to tactile stimulation. Vim, and perhaps Vop, can be identified by the presence of responses to stimulation

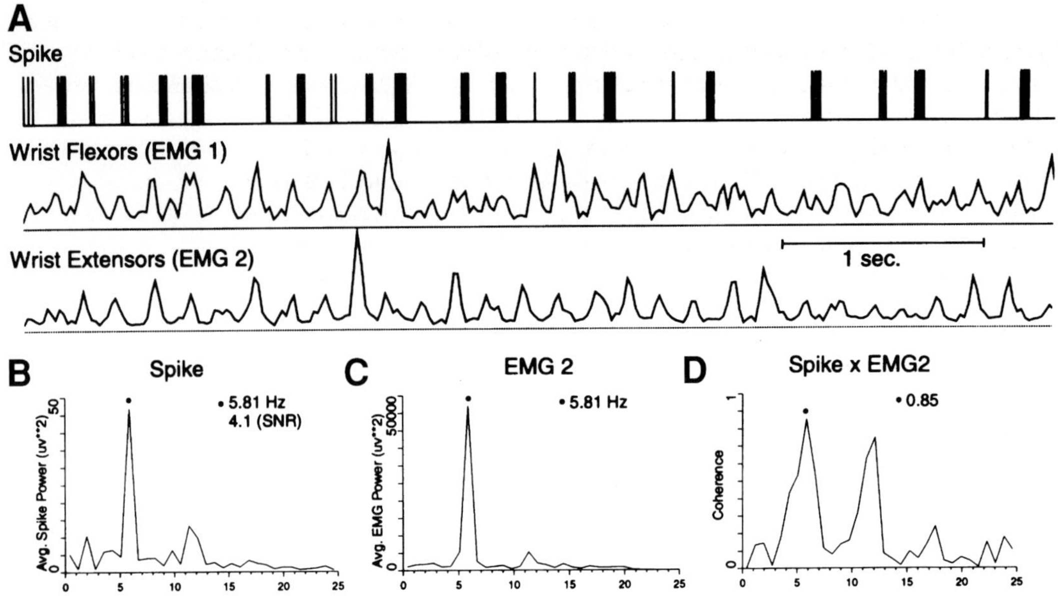

Fig. 2. Simultaneous recording of thalamic single neuron activity and peripheral EMG during tremor in a patient with essential tremor. (**A**) digitized spike train (upper trace) and EMG channels (lower two traces). (**B**) Autopower spectrum of the spike train illustrated in (A). (**C**) Autopower spectrum for EMG 2. (**D**) Coherence spectrum of the spike x EMG2 function *(31)*. The autopower spectrum measures power or the intensity of the signal as a function of frequency. The coherence is a statistical function used to estimate the probability that two signals are correlated at a given frequency. As computed by this method, a coherence ≥0.42 indicates significant probability ($p < 0.05$) of a linear relationship between the two signals. This figure adapted with permission from ref. *(31)*.

of deep structures (e.g., squeezing tendons) or movement of joints *(27)*. Phasic tremor frequency activity can also be recorded in the Vim and, to a lesser extent, in Vop *(39,40)*. Vim may also be identified by median or tibial nerve evoked potentials, which invert as the electrode traverses from Vim into Vc *(8,41)*. It has been reported that Vop may also be identified by spindles, an EEG pattern characterized by a 7–10/s rhythm that waxes and wanes over many seconds *(8)*. Semi-microelectrode recordings are simpler and less time-consuming than microelectrode recordings but they do not provide the spatial resolution of single cell recordings.

2.3. Stereotactic Lesioning

2.3.1. Stereotactic Lesioning Technique: Radiofrequency

In our technique, coordinates are taken from both radiographic studies and physiologic observations to predict the best target to lesion those neurons involved in tremor. A recent study suggests that the optimal target for treating parkinsonian tremor is the site where cells with activity related to tremor are located *(42)*, i.e., 2 mm anterior to Vc and 3 mm above the AC-PC line. Other approaches have been applied to define the optimal site for thalamotomy: 1) anterior to the site at which evoked potentials can be recorded in response to cutaneous stimulation of the fingers *(13,43,44)*; 2) in the region where electrical stimulation produces effects on tremor and anterior to the region where electrical stimulation evokes sensations *(38)*; 3) in the region where cells respond to somatosensory stimulation of muscle, joint, and tendon *(45)*.

One or two lesions are then made at the target defined by the above algorithms. Lesions are made by the technique of radiofrequency coagulation by use of an electrode with a 1.1 mm outer diameter and a 3 mm exposed tip and a thermister at the tip of the electrode (TM electrode, Radionics Inc., Burlington, MA). Temperature is held constant at 60°C over a 1-min interval. The temperature is increased in 5–10°C steps during subsequent 1-min intervals to a level of approx 80°C. Because temperature is increased in steps of about 10°, the time to make the lesion is 4 min. Neurologic examination stressing lemniscal sensory function, pyramidal function, cerebellar function, and speech should be carried out before, during, and after each stage of lesion-making. The coagulum of such each separate lesion made by this technique is approximated by a cylinder with a diameter of 3 mm and a length of 5 mm *(42,46,47)*.

2.3.2. Stereotactic Lesioning Technique: Radiosurgery

The use of MR imaging to provide radiologic localization has led to the development of stereotactic radiosurgical thalamotomy using the gamma knife. Lesions with a volume of approx 250 mm^3 are created *(48,49)*. The lesion placement is estimated from the usual location of Vim in relation to the anterior and posterior commissures and the internal capsule, without physiological confirmation *(48, 49)*. A good to excellent result was reported in 78% ($n = 34$) and 88% ($n = 27$) of cases *(48,49)*. Complications were reported in neither of these series. The conclusion of these reports *(48,49)* as well as a recent review *(50)* is that radiosurgical thalamotomy may have a role in the treatment of tremor in patients with significant medical contraindications for microelectrode-guided thalamotomy.

3. TREMOR OF PARKINSON'S DISEASE

Parkinsons's disease affects approximately 1% of the population over 65 yr *(51)*. The three cardinal signs of Parkinson's disease are resting tremor, cogwheel rigidity, and bradykinesia. Parkinsonian tremor often does not respond to medication *(52,53)*, so that some of these patients may be candidates for thalamic surgical procedures *(54)*.

3.1. Mechanism of Tremor in Parkinson's Disease

Two mechanisms have been proposed as the basis for the tremor of Parkinson's disease *(55,56)*. The central oscillator hypothesis proposes that tremor is caused by pacemaker cells located in the basal ganglia or thalamus. Alternatively, the peripheral hypothesis suggests that parkinsonian tremor results from peripheral feedback loops that have become unstable and oscillate.

3.1.1. The Central Oscillator Hypothesis

The thalamus could be the site of a central oscillator that drives tremor. Thalamic neurons function in either the transfer mode or the oscillatory mode *(57)*. The oscillatory mode occurs during drowsiness and slow wave sleep and is associated with neuronal hyperpolarization leading to a firing pattern characterized by repetitive bursting, with a stereotyped intraburst pattern of activity. The central oscillator hypothesis for parkinsonian tremor predicts that overactivity in the internal segment of the globus pallidus (GPi) would cause a relative hyperpolarization of cells in Vop, a pallidal relay nucleus. Thus the repetitive bursting activity during hyperpolarization suggests that thalamic cells could be the central oscillator *(58,59)*. In recordings from Vim and Vop of parkinsonian patients undergoing thalamotomy. the stereotyped intraburst pattern of firing was found in only 1 of 118 cells *(60)*. This cell had tremor-related activity *(30)* but was located in Vim, not in Vop as predicted by the model.

Alternatively, thalamic tremor-related bursting could arise from transmission of bursting activity from GPi to cells in Vop which are in the transfer mode. The transfer mode occurs during waking and is a characterized by a relatively constant firing rate (i.e., cells are slightly depolarized). This suggests that Gpi drives thalamic tremor related activity and is the central pattern generator. This hypothesis would suggest that activity correlated with tremor, should be maximal in the pallidal relay nucleus of thalamus. However, the incidence of tremor-related activity was less in Vop (21%) than in Vim (25%) *(26)*. Furthermore, GPi activity at tremor frequency is rarely correlated with tremor in Parkinson's disease *(61,62)* or in monkey models of parkinsonism *(63)*. Therefore the activity of cells in thalamus and pallidum is not consistent with a pallidal generator for parkinsonian tremor.

3.1.2. The Peripheral Feedback Hypothesis

The other major hypothesis of the generation of parkinsonian tremor involves abnormal sensory feedback to the central nervous system (CNS). According to this hypothesis, stretch reflex arcs traverse motor cortex in much the same way that tendon tap reflexes traverse the spinal cord *(64–66)*. The increased gain of these reflexes may cause tremor in Parkinson's disease similar to the way that increased tendon tap reflexes cause clonus in spasticity *(65–67)*. This hypothesis has been studied by comparing the activity of thalamic relay cells with sensory inputs to that of relay cells without sensory inputs *(24,26)*. Tremor-related activity of sensory cells in the sensory relay nucleus Vc lags behind parkinsonian tremor *(26)* because of the conduction delay from the peripheral sensory afferents to the thalamus. Combined cells are those cells activated in response to passive movement and in advance of active movement, and so can be distinguished from sensory cells *(24)*. Combined cell activity is correlated with and phase-advanced on tremor, which suggests that activity of these cells may be involved in the generation of parkinsonian tremor by a feedback mechanism *(26)*. Systems analysis demonstrates a feedback mechanism in the transfer function relating thalamic activity to tremor for greater than 90% of cells in the Vim and Vop *(68)*. Thus, peripheral feedback loops appear to play an important role in the mechanism of tremor. This feedback may be involved in an unstable reflex loop or may modulate the activity of a central oscillator.

3.2. Indications for Thalamotomy in Parkinson's Disease

Medical therapy is the mainstay of treatment for parkinsonian tremor with levodopa-carbidopa and anticholinergics as the most effective agents *(53)*. After an adequate trial of medical therapy, parkinsonian patients with significant tremor and minimal other parkinsonian symptoms may be candidates for unilateral thalamotomy. Such patients should satisfy the following criteria *(69,70)*: 1) Parkinson's disease (idiopathic, juvenile, and postencephalitic) *(71)* with disabling unilateral or asymmetric tremor or drug-induced dyskinesias; 2) poor response to or intolerance for optimal medical management. Contraindications include Parkinson's plus syndromes (multiple system atrophy, striatonigral degeneration, Shy Drager syndrome, etc.), significant dementia, and significant medical illness. Bilateral procedures are now relatively contraindicated because of the high incidence of dysarthria and other voice disturbances following the second lesion *(70)*. Therefore deep brain stimulation (DBS) may be a viable option for treatment of tremor on the second side. Deep brain stimulation in Vim (Vim-DBS) involves implantation of a stimulator to block both neuronal activity and tremor during stimulation. Side effects complicating Vim-DBS, like voice disturbance, may be reversible by altering stimulation.

3.3. Results of Thalamotomy for Tremor in Parkinson's Disease

Recent series with long-term followup report complete abolition in 86% *(69)* to 82% of cases *(72)*. All patients had severe, asymmetrical, medically intractable parkinsonian tremor. Thalamotomies were guided by CT localization and microelectrode recording. In one large series, complete abolition of contralateral tremor was seen in 94% of cases (34/36 patients) at the time of discharge *(69)*. At 3 mo, 31/36 patients had no tremor, while at 3 yr, 13/16 patients remained tremor-free *(69)*. Eighty-four percent of patients reported that they would undergo the procedure again *(69)*.

In addition to the reduction of tremor symptoms, several studies have shown that patients require less or no levodopa after thalamotomy *(69,72)*. This decreased requirement for levodopa helps to reduce the amount of drug-related side effects (e.g., dyskinesias). Independent of this reduction of levodopa, thalamotomy has been shown to reduce levodopa-induced dyskinesias *(69)*. Narabayashi et al. *(74)* reported that although levodopa dyskinesias are ameliorated by Vim thalamotomy, the optimal site for a lesion to relieve dyskinesias may be Vop, just anterior to Vim. The reduction of dopa-related dyskinesia by thalamotomy allows some patients to tolerate higher doses of levodopa for treatment of other parkinsonian symptoms such as bradykinesia and rigidity *(53)*.

3.4. *Summary*

Thalamotomy is a safe and effective procedure for the treatment of asymmetric, severe, and medically intractable parkinsonian tremor *(69,75,76)*. Recent experience has confirmed the early observation that thalamotomy is not effective for treatment of bradykinesia, micrographia, or difficulty with gait or speech in Parkinson's disease *(54)*. Rigidity may be improved in some cases. Computerized imaging should be used for radiologic localization and microelectrode recording should be used for physiologic localization *(70)*.

Patients with the tremor-predominant Parkinson's disease often go on to develop other symptoms which to not respond to thalamic procedures. Thus neurosurgeons are reluctant to make a lesion which may make future interventions ineffective. Such interventions might include stimulation in Vim (Vim DBS), GPi (GPi DBS), or subthalamus (STN DBS) *(77–79)*. These latter two procedures may be considered later in the course of the disease for symptoms that develop after tremor. For these reasons, Vim stimulation may now be preferable to thalamotomy for treatment of parkinsonian tremor *(21,70)*. In turn, Gpi-DBS and STN-DBS can be effective against many symptoms of Parkinson's disease in addition to tremor *(77,78)*, so that these procedures may replace thalamic procedures for the treatment of Parkinson's tremor.

4. ESSENTIAL TREMOR

Essential tremor is a bilateral, largely symmetrical, postural and/or action tremor that occurs in the absence of any condition or drug known to cause enhanced physiologic tremor, in the absence of cerebellar signs and symptoms, and in the absence of other conditions causing tremor, such as Parkinson's disease *(80,81)*. It preferentially affects both upper extremities and the head while the lower extremities are affected to a lesser extent.

4.1. *Mechanism of Essential Tremor*

A familial form of the essential tremor exists that is transmitted in an autosomal dominant pattern with high penetrance *(80,82)*. The etiology of this condition is poorly understood however, despite investigations into the neurophysiologic mechanisms. Animals treated with β-carboline drugs such as harmaline develop a tremor similar to essential tremor *(83,84)*. Harmaline tremor has been shown to originate in the inferior olive and to be expressed through the cerebellobulbospinal pathways.

In essential tremor, PET scans have shown that the cerebellum, contralateral red nucleus, thalamus, and sensorimotor cortex display overactivity *(85)*. Thalamic single neuron activity recorded during thalamotomy has been compared with forearm EMG activity (Fig. 2). These studies indicate that thalamic cells have tremor frequency firing patterns that are linearly related to forearm EMG signals during essential tremor (tremor-related activity). One-third of cells with tremor-related activity responded to sensory stimulation. Surgical lesions in the thalamus abolish essential tremor *(69,86,87)*. Therefore it seems likely that thalamic mechanisms are involved in essential tremor, perhaps by transmission of cerebellar tremor-related activity to the periphery via the cortex *(31)*.

4.2. *Indications for Thalamotomy in Essential Tremor*

Surgery is an option for patients with disabling essential tremor who are unresponsive to or intolerant of optimal medical management and who do not have significant medical illness *(69,86,87)*.

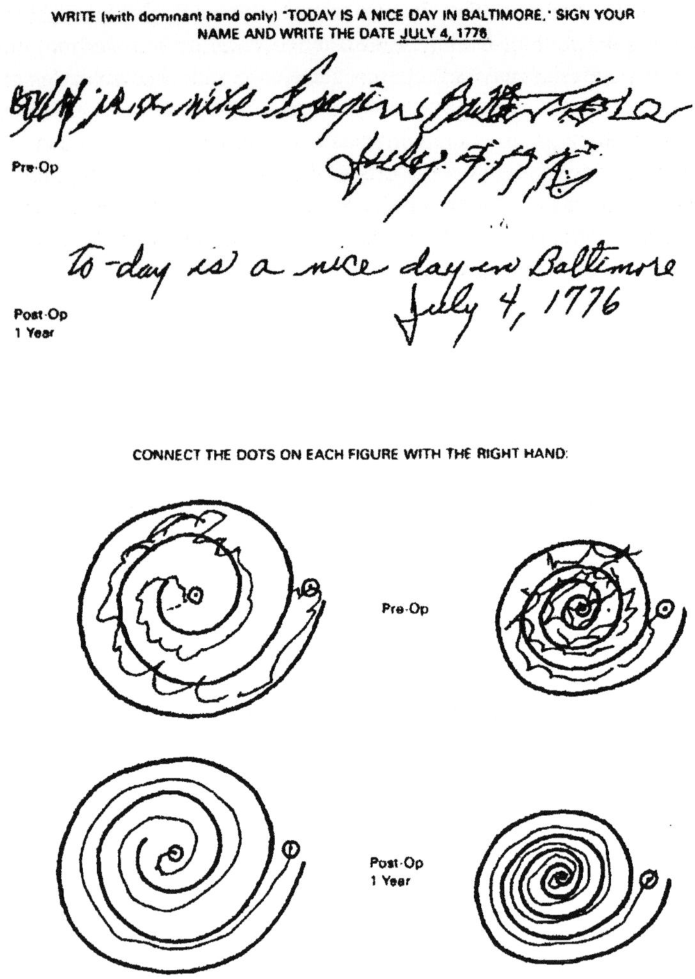

Fig. 3. Example of the handwriting/drawing component of the standard rating scale of tremor in a patient with essential tremor. The preoperative sample is shown above in each case, and the 1 yr postoperative sample is shown below. Reproduced with permission from ref. *(86)*.

4.3. Results

Dramatic reductions in essential tremor can be achieved with thalamotomy, as illustrated in Fig. 3. The results of several clinical series of thalamotomies for essential tremor have been published. Although these studies have been conducted by different operative techniques, each has demonstrated that the majority of patients undergoing the procedure have a significant reduction in tremor. In these studies complete or slight residual tremor was reported in between 68–83% of cases, whereas moderate reductions in tremor were reported in the remainder *(69,87–89)*. Most patients were able to discontinue their pharmacological therapy and many were able to return to work *(88)*. In one series voice tremor was abolished or significantly improved in 71% of patients *(87)*.

4.4. Summary

Essential tremor is the ideal indication for thalamotomy since, unlike Parkinson's disease, other symptoms do not develop with time. Since the benefit is long-lasting, no further procedures are required for this monosymptomatic condition. The alternative to thalamotomy for essential tremor is Vim DBS. Thalamotomy produces good, long-lasting control for essential tremor without the need for maintenance of the device, battery changes, and the like. Unlike the radiofrequency lesion of thalamotomy, which is permanent, DBS can be adapted to treat the patient's symptoms and decrease the side effects *(21,91)*. By reducing, modifying, or stopping stimulation, some side effects can be reduced or eliminated. This is particularly advantageous for bilateral procedures where the incidence of dysarthria approaches 30–60% of patients after bilateral thalamotomy *(69,86,87)*. The decision to carry out thalamotomy or Vim-DBS is based on the patients bias to accept the somewhat higher risk (thalamotomy) or the lifelong maintenance of an implanted device (Vim DBS) *(79)*.

5. CEREBELLAR TREMOR

Cerebellar tremor is characterized by tremor with intention, that is, tremor which increases in amplitude as the target is approached during visually guided movements. Specifically, cerebellar tremor is defined as a unilateral or bilateral intention tremor with frequency usually below 5 Hz. Postural tremor may be present, but not rest tremor *(80)*. Cerebellar tremor may occur from multiple etiologies encompassing the range of inherited, traumatic, inflammatory, neoplastic, and vascular disorders that can affect the cerebellum or cerebellar outflow pathways.

5.1. Mechanism of Cerebellar Tremor

Tremor may be related to interruption of cerebellar feedforward control of motor cortex that is responsible for the antagonist muscle activity that brakes movement *(93)*. In the absence of cerebellar feedforward control of antagonists, sensory (feedback) control may take precedence so that cortical activity related to antagonists lags behind rather than leads movement. Thus cerebellar tremor is the result of a delay in the control signal to antagonist muscles during movement *(94,95)*. This pathologic delay should be reflected in thalamic activity since cerebellar efferents project to motor cortex *(96,97)* via the thalamus *(98)*.

Thalamic recordings in patients with cerebellar tremor provide support for this model. Neurons in Vim of patients with cerebellar tremor *(99)* have significantly lower firing rates than in Vim of patients operated for the treatment of pain (controls). The degree of correlation between the thalamic and EMG activities during tremor was not significantly different between neurons in Vim and Vop. Cellular activity lagged behind EMG activity more often in Vim than in Vop. The phase lag in Vim of cerebellar tremor patients is in contrast to studies of normal monkeys carrying out active wrist oscillations in which thalamic activity is correlated with and leads wrist oscillations *(100)*. This suggests that cerebellar feedback to motor cortex is delayed by cerebellar lesions, leading to tremor during movement.

5.2. Indications for Thalamotomy for Cerebellar Tremor

As with the other types of tremor, surgery is an option for patients with disabling cerebellar tremor who are unresponsive to or intolerant of optimal medical management and who do not have significant medical contraindications to surgery. Medical management of this condition is less effective than for the other types of tremor *(101)*.

5.3. Results of Thalamotomy for Cerebellar Tremor

Recent studies demonstrate complete abolition or significant reduction in 44–82% of patients with intention tremors of different etiologies *(87,102,103)*. A recent case control study of surgical treatment of intention tremor in multiple sclerosis found significant improvements in tremor-related disability, contralateral upper extremity postural and kinetic tremors, and head tremor *(111)*. No significant difference was found in measures of general disability, activities of daily living, and speech or swallowing between surgical cases and controls. Patients with a prior thalamotomy had complicated postoperative courses and epilepsy recurred postoperatively in two patients. Thus surgery was recommended in patients whose primary disability was from tremor and in whom there was no history of a prior thalamotomy or of epilepsy *(111)*.

5.4. *Summary*

Comparisons of the results of thalamotomy for parkinsonian or essential tremor with that for cerebellar tremor make it clear that thalamotomy is less effective for cerebellar tremor than for other tremors. Patients with cerebellar tremor are more disabled, however, because their tremor occurs with action and thus interferes directly with voluntary movement. In addition, many patients with cerebellar tremor suffer other motor or sensory deficits in the affected limb due to the underlying cause of the tremor. A good result in these patients, although less common than with other tremors, is particularly satisfying for everyone involved. Thalamic DBS is not approved in the United States for these patients and experience is limited. However, it can be of some benefit *(21,104)*. Thus thalamotomy is still the ablative procedure of choice for treatment of disabling, medically intractable cerebellar tremor.

6. COMPLICATIONS

Complications from Vim thalamotomy fall into two categories: those that result from neural injury related to lesion making and those considered to be general risks of stereotactic surgery. Both types of complications are not directly related to the indication for thalamotomy. Therefore, we will discuss complications of thalamotomy for parkinsonian, essential, and cerebellar tremor together.

Complications from stereotactic surgery can arise from infection *(105)*, intracranial hemorrhage *(106)*, or epilepsy *(111)*. Infection of pin sites and meningitis has been reported in about 1% of stereotactic surgeries *(105)*. Hemorrhages comprise a significant percentage of operative mortalities in stereotactic surgery with rates reported from 1–6% *(106)*. Hemorrhages may occur at the lesion site or at cortical sites, resulting in intracerebral or subdural hematomas. In four recent large series of thalamotomies ($n = 242$ patients), no hemorrhages were reported *(69,72,88,89)*. In the same series mortality after thalamotomy was limited to a single death from a pulmonary embolus. Two deaths were reported in recent small series of patients ($n = 53$) operated on for treatment of cerebellar tremor *(87,102,103,107)*.

Functional deficits account for the majority of postoperative complications in thalamotomy. Functional deficits can be explained by lesion-induced disruption of the cerebello-thalamo-cortical pathway or damage to thalamic nuclei and nearby structures. Large or incorrectly placed lesions may be responsible for deficits. Lesions made posterior to Vim in ventralis posterior (Vc) may cause sensory deficits. A laterally placed lesion may injure internal capsule fibers, leading to weakness. Inferiorly placed lesions may cause hemiballismus by damage to the subthalamic nucleus. Additionally, left sided or dominant hemispheric thalamic lesions may be associated with postoperative dysarthria and verbal memory impairment *(108)*.

In a series of 60 patients with essential, parkinsonian, or cerebellar tremor functional deficits in the immediate postoperative period were reported in 58% of patients *(69)*. These transient deficits included weakness (34%), dysarthria (29%), ataxia (8%), dystonia (5%), and sensory deficits (3%). Transient deficits may have occurred from edema surrounding the acute lesion site *(109)*. Functional deficits persisted in 23% but were generally mild and did not increase disability *(69)*. In a series of 105 patients with essential tremor, Mundinger and coworkers reported that 9 patients had persistent side effects *(89)*. Five patients had contralateral weakness; 1 had a verbal dysarthria, and 3 showed signs of cerebellar dysfunction. Nagaseki et al. reported that among 43 patients undergoing Vim thalamotomy for essential or parkinsonian tremor *(88)* there was 1 case each of meningitis and limb weakness. Thus the rate of permanent functionally significant postoperative deficits is low.

7. THALAMOTOMY VS THALAMIC DEEP BRAIN STIMULATION

The primary alternative to Vim thalamotomy for tremor has been stimulation through deep brain stimulating electrodes implanted in Vim (Vim DBS). Although thalamotomy produces good tremor control for this condition, it was postulated that using stimulation rather than thermal coagulation would reduce the frequency of long-lasting neurologic side effects from these procedures. Unlike the radiofrequency lesion of thalamotomy, which is permanent, Vim DBS can be adapted to tailor the stimulation patterns to match the patient's symptoms *(21,91)*. By reducing, modifying, or stopping stimulation, unpleasant or disabling side effects can be reduced or eliminated. These effects are particularly advantageous for bilateral procedures.

Schuurman et al. *(110)* carried out a prospective, randomized study of Vim-DBS versus thalamotomy for both Parkinson's disease and essential tremor. Vim-DBS had a better outcome based on a validated disability scale and the number of patients with complete or almost complete relief of tremor. There were significantly more side effects from thalamotomy than from Vim-DBS, although the only postoperative death was due to an intracranial hemmorhage that occurred in a patient in the Vim DBS group. Equipment-related complications occurred in 30% of patients in the Vim DBS group and often required revision of the device. Finally, DBS assumes the cost and inconvenience of periodic readjustment of the stimulator and changing the battery at 3–5-yr intervals. DBS carries the obvious advantage of being reversible and adjustable, which makes bilateral procedures safer and more practical. Therefore, the patient's input is a critical factor in balancing the higher complication rate of thalamotomy vs the cost and inconvenience of lifelong maintenance of the DBS device.

ACKNOWLEDGMENT

Some of the studies reported here were funded by the NIH (RO1 NS38493 and NS40059).

REFERENCES

1. Hassler, R. (1982) Architectonic organization of the thalamic nuclei. In: *Stereotaxy of the Human Brain* (Schaltenbrand, G. and Walker, A. E., eds.), Thieme, Stuttgart, pp. 140–180.
2. Jones, E. G. (1985) *The Thalamus.* Plenum, New York.
3. Hirai, T. and Jones, E. G. (1989) A new parcellation of the human thalamus on the basis of histochemical staining. *Brain Res. Rev.* **14,** 1–34.
4. Guiot, G., Hardy, J., and Albe-Fessard, D. G. (1962) Delimitation precis des structures sous-corticales et identification de noyaux thalamiques chez l'homme par l'electrophyiologie stereotactic. *Neurochirurgia* **5,** 1–18.
5. Mandir, A. S., Rowland, L. H., Dougherty, P. M., and Lenz, F. A. (1997) Microelectrode recording and stimulation techniques during stereotactic procedures in the thalamus and pallidum. *Adv. Neurol.* **74,** 159–168.
6. Schaltenbrand, G. and Bailey, P. (1959) *Introduction to Stereotaxis With an Atlas of the Human Brain.* Thieme, Stuttgart.
7. Guiot, G. and Derome, P. (1969) The principle of stereotaxic thalamotomy. In: *Correlative Neurosurgery* (Kahn, E. A., Crosby, E. C., Schneider, R. C., and Taren, J., eds.), Charles C. Thomas, Springfield, IL, pp. 376–401.
8. Burchiel, K. J. (1995) Thalamotomy for movement disorders. In: *Neurosurgery Clinics of North America* (Gildenberg, P. L., ed.), W.B. Saunders Company, Philadelphia, PA, pp. 55–71.
9. Kondziolka, D., Dempsey, P. K., Lunsford, L. D., Kestle, J. R. W., Dolan, E. J., Kanal, E., and Tasker, R. R. (1992) A comparison between magnetic resonance imaging and computed tomography for stereotactic coordinate determination. *Neurosurgery* **30,** 402–407.
10. Holtzheimer, P. E. I., Roberts, D. W., and Darcey, T. M. (1999) Magnetic resonance imaging versus computed tomography for target localization in functional stereotactic neurosurgery. *Neurosurgery* **45,** 290–298.
11. Alexander, E., Kooy, H. M., van Herk, M., Schwartz, M., Barnes, P. D., Tarbell, N., et al. (1995) Magnetic resonance image-directed stereotactic neurosurgery: use of image fusion with computerized tomography to enhance spatial accuracy. *J. Neurosurg.* **83,** 271–276.
12. Dostrovsky, J. O. (1998) The use of inexpensive personal computers for map generation and data analysis. In: *Textbook of Stereotactic and Functional Neurosurgery* (Gildenberg, P. L. and Tasker, R. R., eds.), McGraw-Hill, New York, pp. 2031–2036.
13. Kelly, P. J., Ahlskog, J. E., Goerss, S. J., Daube, J. R., Duffy, J. R., and Kall, B. A. (1987) Computer-assisted stereotactic ventralis lateralis thalamotomy with microelectrode recording control in patients with Parkinson's disease. *Mayo Clinic Proc.* **62,** 655–664.

14. Cooper, I. S., Bergmann, L. L., and Caracalos, A. (1963) Anatomic verification of the lesion which abolishes parkinsonian tremor and rigidity. *Neurology* **13,** 779–787.
15. Lenz, F. A., Dostrovsky, J. O., Kwan, H. C., Tasker, R. R., Yamashiro, K., and Murphy, J. T. (1988) Methods for microstimulation and recording of single neurons and evoked potentials in the human central nervous system. *J. Neurosurg.* **68,** 630–634.
16. Jasper, H. H. and Bertrand, G. (1966) Thalamic units involved in somatic sensation and voluntary and involuntary movements in man. In: *The Thalamus* (Purpura, D. P. and Yahr, M. D., eds.), Columbia University Press, New York, pp. 365–390.
17. Umbach, W. and Ehrhardt, K. J. (1965) Micro-electrode recording in the basal ganglia during stereotaxic operations. *Confinia Neurolog.* **26,** 315–317.
18. Ohye, C. (1982) Depth microelectrode studies. In: *Stereotaxy of the human brain. Anatomical, physiological and clinical applications* (Schaltenbrand, G. and Walker, A. E., eds.), Thieme, Stuttgart, pp. 372–389.
19. Vitek, J. L., Bakay, R. A. E., Hashimoto, T., Baron, M. S., Kaneoke, Y., Turner, R., and DeLong, M. R. (1998) Microelectrode-guided pallidotomy: technical approach and application for treatment of medically intractable Parkinson's disease. *J. Neurosurg.* **88,** 1027–1043.
20. Lenz, F. A., Seike, M., Lin, Y. C., Baker, F. H., Richardson, R. T., and Gracely, R. H. (1993) Thermal and pain sensations evoked by microstimulation in the area of the human ventrocaudal nucleus (Vc). *J. Neurophysiol.* **70,** 200–212.
21. Benabid, A. L., Pollak, P., Gao, D., Hoffmann, D., Limousin, P., Gay, E., et al. (1996) Chronic electrical stimulation of the ventralis intermedius nucleus of the thalamus as a treatment of movement disorders. *J. Neurosurg.* **84,** 203–214.
22. Lenz, F. A., Seike, M. S., Jaeger, C. J., Reich, S. G., Lin, Y. C., DeLong, M. R., and Vitek, J. L. (1999) Thalamic single neuron activity in patients with dystonia: dystonia-related activity and somatic sensory reorganization. *J. Neurophysiol.* **82,** 2372–2392.
23. Lenz, F. A., Dostrovsky, J. O., Tasker, R. R., Yamashiro, K., Kwan, H. C., and Murphy, J. T. (1988) Single-unit analysis of the human ventral thalamic nuclear group: somatosensory responses. *J. Neurophysiol.* **59,** 299–316.
24. Lenz, F. A., Kwan, H., Dostrovsky, J. O., Tasker, R. R., Murphy, J. T., and Lenz, Y. E. (1990) Single unit analysis of the human ventral thalamic nuclear group: activity correlated with movement. *Brain* **113,** 1795–1821.
25. Crowell, R. M., Perret, E., and Siegfried, J. (1968) "Movement units" and "tremor phasic units" in the human thalamus. *Brain Res.* **11,** 481–488.
26. Lenz, F. A., Kwan, H. C., Martin, R. L., Tasker, R. R., Dostrovsky, J. O., and Lenz, Y. E. (1994) Single neuron analysis of the human ventral thalamic nuclear group: tremor-related activity in functionally identified cells. *Brain* **117,** 531–543.
27. Raeva, S. N. (1972) Unit activity of some deep nuclear structures of the human brain during voluntary movements. In: *Neurophysiology Studied in Man* (Somjen, G. ed.), Excerpta Med, Amsterdam, pp. 64–78.
28. Bertrand, C., Martinez, S. N., Hardy, J., et al. (1973) Stereotactic surgery for parkinsonism: microelectrode recording, stimulation, and oriented sections with a leucotome. In: *Progress in Neurological Surgery* (Krayenbuhl, H., Maspes, P. E., and Sweet, W. H., eds.), Karger, Basel, pp. 79–112.
29. Hongell, A., Wallin, G., and Hagbarth, K. E. (1973) Unit activity connected with movement initiation and arousal situations recorded from the ventrolateral nucleus of the human thalamus. *Acta Neurol. Scand.* **49,** 681–698.
30. Lenz, F. A., Tasker, R. R., Kwan, H. C., Schnider, S., Kwong, R., Murayama, Y., et al. (1988) Single unit analysis of the human ventral thalamic nuclear group: correlation of thalamic "tremor cells" with the 3-6 Hz component of parkinsonian tremor. *J. Neurosci.* **8,** 754–764.
31. Hua, S. E., Lenz, F. A., Zirh, T. A., Reich, S. G., and Dougherty, P. M. (1998) Thalamic activity correlated with essential tremor. *J. Neurol. Neurosurg. Psychiatry.* **64,** 273–276.
32. Lenz, F. A., Tasker, R. R., Kwan, H. C., Schnider, S., Kwong, R., and Murphy, J. T. (1985) Cross-correlation analysis of thalamic neurons and EMG activity in parkinsonian tremor. *Appl. Neurophysiol.* **48,** 305–308.
33. Taren, J., Guiot, G., Derome, P., and Trigo, J. C. (1968) Hazards of stereotactic thalamectomy. *J. Neurosurg.* **29,** 173–182.
34. Ohye, C. (1998) Neural noise recording in functional neurosurgery. In: *Textbook of Stereotactic and Functional Neurosurgery* (Gildenberg, P. L. and Tasker, R. R., eds.), McGraw-Hill, New York, pp. 941–948.
35. Ojemann, G. A. and Ward, A. A. Jr. (1982) Abnormal movement disorders. In: *Neurological Surgery* (Youmans, J. R., ed.), W.B. Saunders Company, Philadelphia, PA, pp. 3821–3857.
36. Laitinen, L. V. and Hariz, M. I. (1996) Movement disorders. In: *Neurological Surgery* (Youmans, J. R., ed.), W.B. Saunders Company, Philadelphia, PA, pp. 3575–3609.
37. Fisher, R. S., Uematsu, S., Krauss, G. L., Cysyk, B. J., McPherson, R., Lesser, R. P., et al. (1992) Placebo-controlled pilot study of centromedian thalamic stimulation in treatment of intractable seizures. *Epilepsia* **33,** 841–851.
38. Tasker, R. R., Organ, L. W., and Hawrylyshyn, P. (1982) *The Thalamus and Midbrain in Man: a Physiologic Atlas Using Electrical Stimulation.* Charles C. Thomas, Springfield, IL, pp. 1–503.
39. Fukamachi, A., Ohye, C., and Narabayashi, H. (1973) Delineation of the thalamic nuclei with a microelectrode in stereotaxic surgery for parkinsonism and cerebral palsy. *J. Neurosurg.* **39,** 214–225.
40. Lucking, C. H., Struppler, A., Erbel, F., et al. (1972) Stereotactic recording from human subthalamic structures. In: *Neurophysiology Studied in Man* (Somjen, G. G., ed.), Excerpta Med., Amsterdam, pp. 95–99.
41. Albe-Fessard, D. (1998) Evoked potential recording in functional neurosurgery part I: use of thalamic evoked potentials to improve the stereotactic localization of electrodes in the human brain. In: *Textbook of Stereotactic and Functional Neurosurgery* (Gildenberg, P. L. and Tasker, R. R., eds.), McGraw-Hill, New York, pp. 911–924.

42. Lenz, F. A., Normand, S. L., Kwan, H. C., Andrews, D., Rowland, L. H., Jones, M. W., et al. (1995) Statistical prediction of the optimal lesion site for thalamotomy in parkinsonian tremor. *Mov. Disord.* **10,** 318–328.
43. Kelly, P. J., Derome, P., and Guiot, G. (1976) Thalamic spatial variability and the surgical results of lesions placed with neurophysiologic control. *Surg. Neurol.* **9,** 307–315.
44. Guiot, G., Derome, P., Arfel, G., et al. (1973) Electrophysiological recordings in stereotaxic thalamotomy for parkinsonism. In: *Progress in Neurological Surgery* (Krayenbuehl, H., Maspes, P. E., and Sweet, W. H., eds.), Karger, Basel, pp. 189–221.
45. Ohye, C. H. and Narabayashi, H. (1979) Physiological study of presumed ventralis intermedius neurons in the human thalamus. *J. Neurosurg.* **50,** 290–297.
46. Tasker, R. R., Yamashiro, K., Lenz, F. A., et al. (1988) Thalamotomy in Parkinson's disease: microelectrode techniques. In: *Modern Stereotactic Surgery* (Lundsford, D., ed.), Academic Press, Norwell, MA, pp. 297–313.
47. Cosman, E. R. and Cosman, B. J. (1985) Methods of making nervous system lesions. In: *Neurosurgery* (Wilkins, R. H. and Rengachary, S. S., eds.), McGraw-Hill, New York, pp. 2490–2499.
48. Duma, C. M., Jacques, D. B., Kopyov, O. V., Mark, R. J., Copcutt, B., and Farokhi, H. K. (1998) Gamma knife radiosurgery for thalamotomy in parkinsonian tremor: a five year experience. *J. Neurosurg.* **88,** 1044–1049.
49. Young, R. F., Shumway-Cook, A., Vermeulen, S. S., Grimm, P., Blasko, J., Posewitz, A., et al. (1998) Gamma knife radiosurgery as a lesioning technique in movement disorder surgery. *J. Neurosurg.* **89,** 183–193.
50. Kondziolka, D. and Lunsford, L. D. (1998) Functional radiosurgery using the gamma knife: current and future applications. In: *Textbook of Stereotactic and Functional Neurosurgery* (Gildenberg, P. L. and Tasker, R. R., eds.), McGraw-Hill, New York, pp. 871–880.
51. Adams, R. D., Victor, M., and Ropper, A. H. (1996) *Principles of Neurology.* McGraw-Hill, New York.
52. Paulson, H. L. and Stern, M. B. (1997) Clinical manifestations of Parkinson's disease. In: *Movement Disorders: Neurologic Principles and Practice* (Watts, R. L. and Koller, W. C., eds.), McGraw Hill, New York, pp. 183–199.
53. Poewe, W. and Granata, R. (1997) Pharmacologic treatment of Parkinson's disease. In: *Movement Disorders: Neurologic Principles and Practice* (Watts, R. L. and Koller, W. C., eds.), McGraw-Hill, New York, pp. 201–220.
54. Tasker, R. R., Siqueira, J., Hawrylyshyn, P. A., and Organ, L. W. (1983) What happened to VIM thalamotomy for Parkinson's disease? *Appl. Neurophysiol.* **46,** 68–83.
55. Marsden, C. D. (1984) Origins of normal and pathological tremor. In: *Movement Disorders: Tremor* (Findley, L. J. and Capildeo, R., eds.), Macmillan Press Ltd., London, pp. 37–85.
56. Stein, R. B. and Lee, R. G. (1981) Tremor and clonus. In: *Handbook of Physiology. Section I: Nervous System. Volume II: Motor Control Part II* (Brooks, V. B., ed.), American Physiological Society, Bethesda, MD, pp. 325–343.
57. Steriade, M. and Deschenes, M. (1984) The thalamus as a neuronal oscillator. *Brain Res. Rev.* **8,** 1–63.
58. Alexander, G. E., DeLong, M. R., and Strick, P. L. (1986) Parallel organization of functionally segregated circuits linking basal ganglia and cortex. *Ann. Rev. Neurosci.* **9,** 357–381.
59. Pare, D., Curro Dossi, R., and Steriade, M. (1990) Neuronal basis of the parkinsonian resting tremor: a hypothesis and its implications for treatment. *Neuroscience* **35,** 217–226.
60. Zirh, A. T., Lenz, F. A., Reich, S. G., and Dougherty, P. M. (1997) Patterns of bursting occurring in thalamic cells during parkinsonian tremor. *Neuroscience* **83,** 107–121.
61. Lemstra, A. W., Verhagen Metman, L., Lee, J.-I., Dougherty, P. M., and Lenz, F. A. (1999) Tremor-frequency (3-6Hz) activity in the sensorimotor arm representation of the internal segement of the globus pallidus in patients with Parkinson's disease. *Neurosci. Lett.* **267,** 129–132.
62. Hutchinson, W. D., Benko, R., Dostrovsky, J. O., Lang, A. E., and Lozano, A. M. (1998) Coherent relation of rest tremor to pallidal tremor cells in Parkinson's disease patients. *Mov. Disord.* **13(Suppl. 2),** 204.
63. Raz, A., Fiengold, A., Vaadia, E., Abeles, M., and Bergman, H. (1998) Neuronal oscillations in the globus pallidus of tremulous MPTP-treated monkeys: are they synchronized? *Mov. Disord.* **13(Suppl. 2),** 184.
64. Lenz, F. A., Tatton, W. G., and Tasker, R. R. (1983) Electromyographic response to displacement of different forelimb joints in the squirrel monkey. *J. Neurosci.* **3,** 783–794.
65. Lenz, F. A., Tatton, W. G., and Tasker, R. R. (1983) The effect of cortical lesions on the electromyographic response to joint displacement in the squirrel monkey forelimb. *J. Neurosci.* **3,** 795–805.
66. Desmedt, J. E. (1978) *Progress in Clinical Neurophysiology. Cerebral Motor Control in Man: Long Loop Mechanisms.* Karger, Basel.
67. Lenz, F. A., Tasker, R. R., Tatton, W. G., and Halliday, W. (1987) Long-latency reflex activity in squirrel monkeys with occlusion of the middle cerebral artery. *EEG Clin. Neurophysiol.* **67,** 238–246.
68. Schnider, S. M., Kwong, R. H., Lenz, F. A., and Kwan, H. C. (1989) Detection of feedback in the central nervous system using system identification techniques. *Biolog. Cybernet.* **60,** 203–212.
69. Jankovic, J., Cardoso, F., Grossman, R. G., and Hamilton, W. J. (1995) Outcome after stereotactic thalamotomy for parkinsonian, essential and other types of tremor. *Neurosurgery* **37,** 680–687.
70. Hallett, M., Litvan, I., and Members of the Task Force on Surgery for Parkinson's Disease of AAN Therapeutics and Technology Assessment Commitee (1999) Evaluation of surgery for Parkinson's disease. *Neurology* **15,** 1910–1921.
71. Tasker, R. R. (1998) Ablative therapy for movement disorders. does thalamotomy alter the course of Parkinson's disease. *Neurosurg. Clin. North Am.* **9,** 375–380.
72. Fox, M. W., Ahlskog, E. J., and Kelly, P. J. (1991) Stereotactic ventrolateralis thalamotomy for medically refactory tremor in post-levodopa era Parkinson's disease patients. *J. Neurosurg.* **75,** 723–730.
73. Lenz, F. A., Dougherty, P. M., and Reich, S. G. (1996) The effectiveness of thalamotomy for treatment of tremor and dystonia. *Mov. Disord.* **11(Suppl. 1),** 18.

8
Pallidotomy for Parkinson's Disease

Diane K. Sierens and Roy A. E. Bakay

1. INTRODUCTION

Pallidotomy is a longstanding surgical procedure that was rediscovered in the 1990s and, with the development of modern imaging and electrophysiological techniques, has become an effective treatment for Parkinson's disease (PD). Pallidotomy was performed in the 1950s by Fenelon, Guiot, Cooper, Spiegel, Wycis, Talairach, Riechert, Narabayashi, and Leksell *(1)* in attempts to palliate the symptoms of PD. At that time, the focus was primarily on tremor, which is often the least disabling but most noticeable symptom of PD. The work of Hassler, Riechert, and Mundinger popularized the ventral lateral region of the thalamus and led to abandonment of the pallidum as the surgical target of choice for tremor alleviation for PD *(2)*. With the introduction of L-dopa therapy in the 1960s *(3)*, surgical approaches for the treatment of PD were performed infrequently. Despite advances in medical treatment, however, patients often developed severe disabling medication-induced dyskinesias and motor fluctuations. The reintroduction of Leksell's posteroventral pallidotomy by Laitinen in 1992 *(4)* generated a new interest in this procedure among neurologists and neurosurgeons. Not only were the primary motor symptoms improved but medication-induced dyskinesias were also reduced. Patients in the modern era of surgery for PD differ from the pre-L-dopa era in several ways. First, contemporary patients are generally very advanced in the course of their disease. Second, today's patients are all on antiparkinsonian medications and frequently suffer from drug-induced side effects in the form of motor fluctuations and drug-induced dyskinesia. Third, there are no longer large numbers of postencephalitic parkinsonian patients. Finally, many forms of parkinsonism other than idiopathic PD have been identified. Today, the standard to which new surgical therapies are compared is the posteroventral pallidotomy.

2. PALLIDOTOMY RATIONALE

Basal ganglia pathophysiology and circuitry are discussed elsewhere in this volume. The primary symptoms of PD are related to dysfunction of the sensorimotor circuit. The posterior ventral internal segment of the globus pallidus (GPi) is the final relay in the pallidal-thalamocortical sensorimotor loop. Loss of dopamine producing cells in the substantia nigra pars compacta leads to altered rates and patterns of neuronal activity in the GPi that may induce changes in rate and pattern of thalamic cells that are considered responsible for the development of parkinsonian motor signs *(5)*. Most effects of pallidotomy are acute. However, physiologic normalization of thalamic neuronal activity after pallidotomy may require time to occur. This may explain the delay in tremor alleviation following pallidotomy *(6)*. Although mean discharge rates are increased in GPi in PD, recent hypotheses have emphasized the change

From: Contemporary Clinical Neurology:
Surgical Treatment of Parkinson's Disease and Other Movement Disorders
Edited by: D. Tarsy, J. L. Vitek, and A. M. Lozano © Humana Press Inc., Totowa, NJ

in pattern of neuronal activity in addition to the change in mean discharge rate as a key factor underlying the development of parkinsonian motor signs and dyskinesia.

2.1. Operative Indications

Posteroventral pallidotomy is a symptomatic treatment for idiopathic PD. Since the benefits of pallidotomy are predominantly unilateral, surgery is typically directed toward the patient's worst side first. The highest ranking indication for pallidotomy is L-dopa dyskinesia *(7)*. On-off fluctuations, off-period dystonia, rigidity, tremor, and bradykinesia are also good indications. Freezing, gait disturbance, and voice problems are considered marginal indications and are less likely to be benefited by pallidotomy.

2.2. Inclusion Criteria

1. Patients with idiopathic PD who have disabling motor symptoms despite maximal medical therapy.
2. A clear response to L-dopa should be documented by a movement disorders specialist.
3. Hoehn and Yahr Stage III or greater.
4. No evidence for other causes of parkinsonism.
5. Normal cognitive and psychiatric function.

2.3. Exclusion Criteria

1. Atypical parkinsonism or parkinson-plus syndromes.
2. Dementia.
3. Medical conditions or bleeding disorders which make the risk for surgery unacceptable.

Two weeks prior to surgery, all antiplatelet agents should be discontinued. Preoperative cognitive evaluation should be performed on all surgical candidates. As a general rule, patients with more than a mild impairment in cognitive function should be excluded. Patients should be examined in both the "on" and "off" states. Marked motor fluctuation is a good predictor of response. The United Parkinson's Disease Rating Scale (UPDRS), the Hoehn and Yahr Staging Scale (H&Y), and the Schwab and England Activities of Daily Living Scale (ADL) are most frequently used for documenting and quantifying severity of PD *(8)*. The neurologist should also rank dyskinesia and dystonia, and perform timed tests for motor evaluation. The Core Assessment Program for Surgical Interventional Therapies in Parkinson's Disease (CAPSIT-PD) gives detailed guidelines for the evaluation of PD patients *(9)*.

3. SURGICAL APPROACH

The treatment of movement disorders, including pallidotomy, has evolved into a multidisciplinary team approach involving neurosurgeons trained in functional neurosurgery, neurologists specialized in movement disorders, and neurophysiologists with extensive understanding of basal ganglia physiology and electrophysiological techniques. Holding antiparkinson medications the morning of surgery is recommended to achieve a "practical off" state for intraoperative neurological testing. Image-guided stereotactic localization, microelectrode mapping, and macrostimulation are commonly used in conjunction to localize the sensorimotor portion of GPi and surrounding structures before making the radiofrequency lesion.

4. IDEAL STEREOTACTIC TARGET

The Cosman-Roberts-Wells (CRW) or Leksell series G are the two most commonly used stereotactic head frames in North America *(7)*. With any system, magnetic resonance imaging (MRI) should be acquired in planes that are orthogonal to the frame axis. Aligning the anterior posterior frame axis parallel to the orbitomeatal line keeps all images parallel to the anterior commissure-posterior commissure (AC-PC) line *(10)*. The optimal target within the globus pallidus has been a subject of debate *(11–16)*. In the pre-L-dopa era, the anterior dorsal GPi was targeted at lateral 15–17 mm to the AC-PC

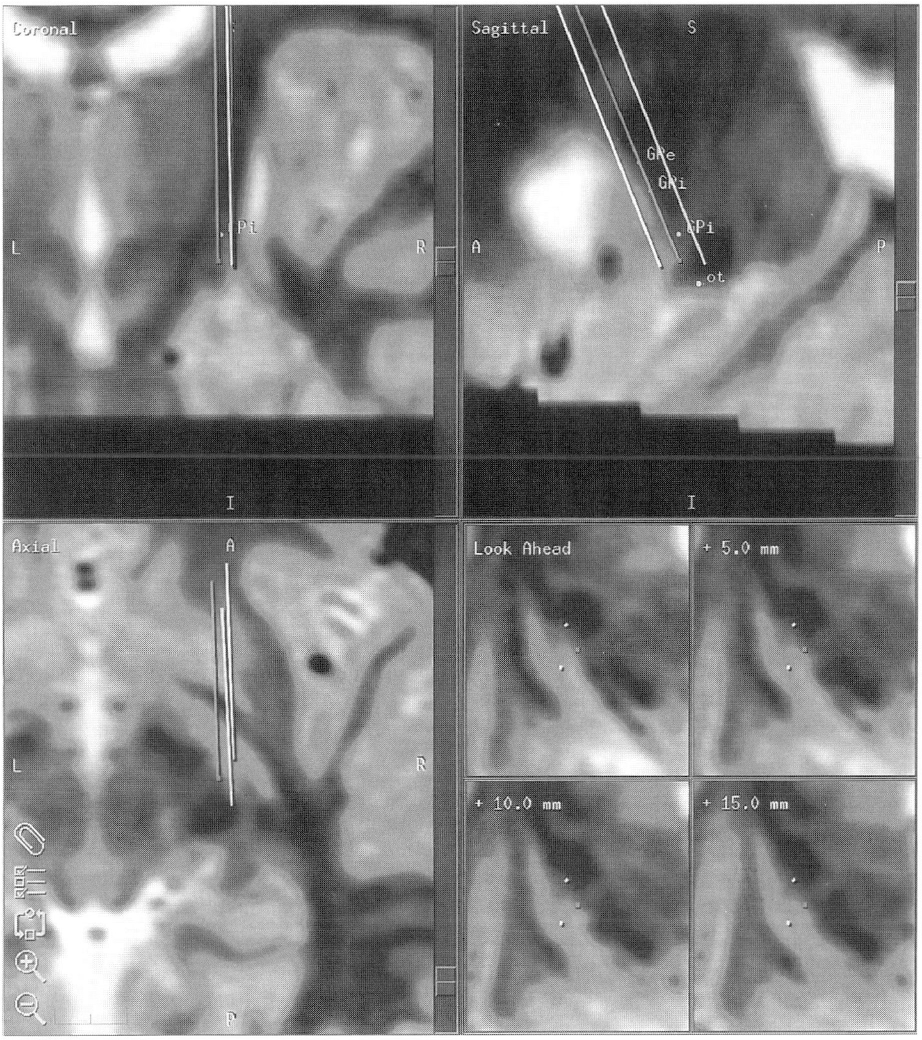

Fig. 1. This is an example of Stealth Station® image-guided three dimensional reconstructions demonstrating three parallel trajectories through the GPi down to the optic tract. Sagittal, coronal, and axial images are displayed along with look ahead views in the lower right hand quadrant.

line, and 0–5 mm posterior to the anterior commissure. This target produced inconsistent benefit predominately in rigidity and is not the location of the sensorimotor area of the GPi. The target most commonly used today is in posteroventral GPi, 2–6 mm ventral to the AC-PC line, 20–22 mm lateral to AC-PC line, and 0–4 mm anterior to the midpoint of the AC-PC line *(13)*. Since anatomic variation between individuals significantly affects the accuracy of targeting, an axial and coronal MRI are obtained with 2 mm slice thickness and 0 interslice interval, using an inversion recovery sequence (TE = 40, TI = 200, TR = 3000) to directly visualize the border of the GPi *(17)*. Three dimensional surgical planning software such as the Medtronic StealthStation®, Treatment Guidance System FrameLink™, and Stereotactic Linking System or SurgiPlan® from Elekta Instruments AB, are recommended as a parallel planning reference. This allows for simultaneous visualization of each trajectory on multiple planes in a probe's eye fashion (Fig. 1).

Table 1
Drugs and Pallidotomy

Drugs to be avoided in patients for Pallidotomy			
Buchadin	Haldol	Phenergan	Taracton
Compazine	Ketamine	Prolixin	Thorazine
Demerol	Loxitane	Reglan	Tigan
Droperidol	Moban	Resperpine	Torecon
Emete-con	Morphine	Serentil	Versed
Etomidate	Navane	Stelazine	Vontrol
Drugs to be used in smaller than usual doses if necessary			
Fentanyl	Propofol	Sufentanil	Zofran

5. SURGICAL PREPARATIONS

Minimal medication should be used as cooperation of the awake patient is essential (Table 1). Intravenous sedation (propofol) along with local anesthetic can be used for opening and closing. Blood pressure should be controlled to a mean of <90 mmHg. The patient's face must be visible. The entry point is positioned at 90° to the AC-PC line so that instruments enter the brain in a true parasagittal plane. Image guidance systems can be very helpful to correct for any asymmetry of the head in the frame by assuring the target is in proper alignment to the AC-PC line. The anterioposterior axis entrance is 45–60 degrees with respect to the AC-PC line. A craniectomy burr hole is used to allow multiple parallel passes of the microelectrode. Fibrin glue is used to prevent leakage of cerebrospinal fluid (CSF).

6. LOCALIZATION TECHNIQUES

The sensorimotor area resides in the most posterior and lateral region of the GPi. The sensorimotor territory is bounded by the ambiens cistern and the optic tract ventrally and the internal capsule at the medial wall (Fig. 2). Corticospinal fibers to the mouth, face, and upper extremity are located in an anterior to posterior position. These landmarks greatly facilitate target localization. Microelectrode recording allows exact identification of the targeted nucleus and its boundaries as well as the optic tract and corticospinal tract. Specific firing patterns of cells within the caudate, external segment of the globus pallidus (GPe), GPi, and optic tract allow for physiological mapping of the region *(18,19)*. A silent zone is encountered as the microelectrode passes through laminae between GPe and GPi. High-frequency irregular discharges are characteristic of neurons in the GPi *(18)*. The optic tract is confirmed by fluctuations in neuronal activity when a bright light is flashed into the eyes of the patient in the darkened operating room. Visual evoked potentials can also be recorded. The optic tract, separated from the GPi by an arachnoid plane, can be variable in its location. If the initial track is well-placed, only two additional tracks are needed to define the posterior and lateral border of GPi. The posterior margin of GPi and location of the corticospinal tract can be confirmed by repositioning of the microelectrode posteriorly, the distance of which is based on the length of the trajectory through GPi. The lateral boundary of GPi is then confirmed by moving lateral to the initial tracts, the distance again is determined based on the information gained in the initial microelectrode passes. The Shaltenbrand and Bailey Human Brain Atlas *(20)* in the parasagittal plane is used to map the best fit. The somatotopy of the GPi demonstrates predominance of neurons responding to joint movement in the leg with more medial tracks and in the arm with more lateral tracks *(21)*.

6.1. Ablation

After the sensorimotor area of the GPi is clearly identified and the internal capsule and optic tract are safeguarded by microelectrode recording, the electrode is replaced by the lesion probe used for

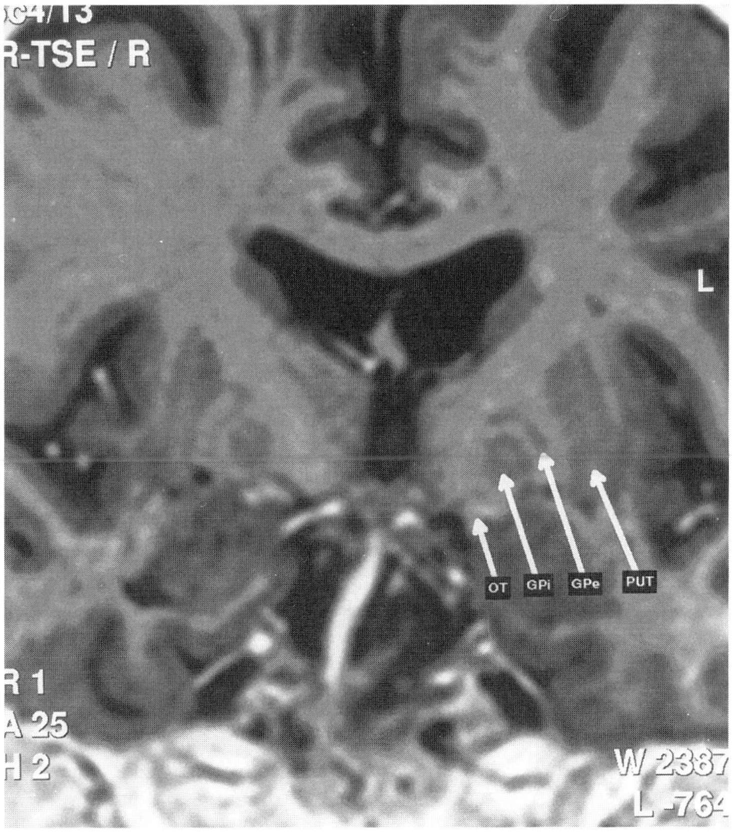

Fig. 2. A coronal MRI anterior to the mamillary bodies demonstrates the anatomy of the GPi bounded by the optic tract (OT) ventrally, the internal capsule medially, and the external segment of the globus pallidus (GPe) and putamen (PUT) laterally.

macrostimulation and producing lesions. Macrostimulation can also serve as a guide to avoid injury to the optic tract and internal capsule. Some centers rely solely on macrostimulation to define the target physiologically and do not perform microelectrode recording *(22–28)*. However, many neurosurgeons agree that it is preferable to obtain more information on which to base an ablative lesion. Two year results comparing lesions using microelectrode recording *(29)* and macrostimulation alone *(23)* suggest that benefits may be more sustained with lesions based on microelectrode mapping. However, there is no current data to allow a firm conclusion concerning this issue. Using the Radionics RFG 3B Lesion generator, a geometric target is lesioned at multiple depths with parallel trajectories to create a lesion matching the sensorimotor GPi. By gradually increasing the temperature from 60° to 70–90°C for 60 s, lesions are created while the patient is continuously monitored for development of a visual field cut, limb weakness, or speech difficultly. A second lesion is placed superiorly to lengthen the lesion column. Multiple lesion tracts (Fig. 3) may be used at lower temperatures to shape the lesion to the posterior third of the GPi (ie. a triangular shape) *(30)*.

7. OUTCOME

After a decade of performing posteroventral pallidotomy throughout the world, the results have provoked a contentious debate among neurosurgeons and neurologists. Although patients are all diagnosed with the same disease, because of its complexity, a great deal of variability is unavoidable. Different methodologies involving patient selection, assessment, medical therapy, surgical technique, and outcome

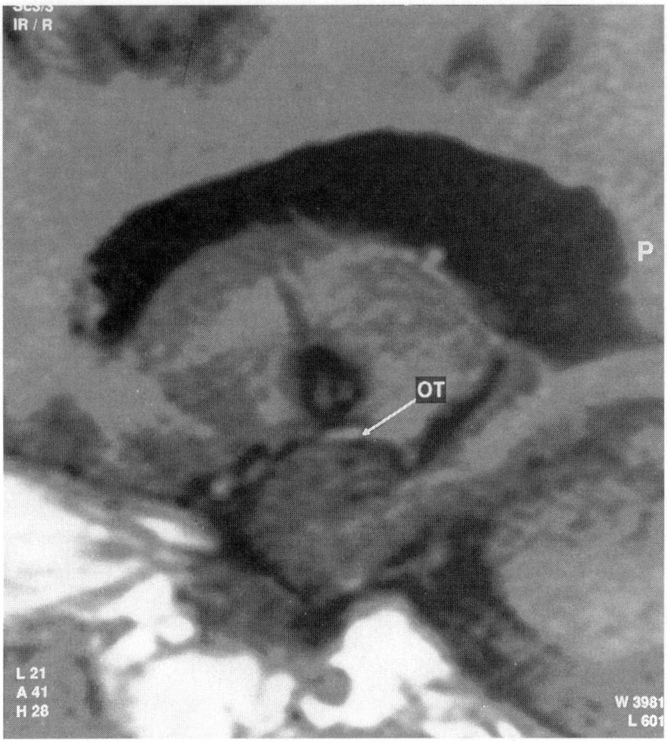

Fig. 3. A sagittal MRI demonstrates two lesions of the posterior aspect of the Gpi avoiding the internal capsule posteriorly and the optic tract inferiorly. The two central necroses and a third lesion medial to the anterior lesion will result in a single overlapping lesion in a triangular fashion to mirror the shape of the posterior sensorimotor area of the Gpi.

criteria make side-by-side comparisons of clinical outcomes difficult at best and cannot lead to any rational conclusion. Most of the measures used such as the United Parkinson's Disease Rating Scale (UPDRS), motor and activities of daily living (ADL) scales, and Hoehn & Yahr (H & Y) Scale are evaluations that depend on patient cooperation and examiner experience. Some studies try to provide more objective evaluations by blinding raters or by recording videos before and after pallidotomy *(31,32)*. The majority of studies have included no controls and are not randomized or blinded. Two randomized clinical trials have compared the outcome of pallidotomy versus best medical management for PD *(31,32a)*. Another study attempted to compare the outcome of pallidotomy with effects of GPi deep brain stimulation (DBS) in a prospective randomized comparison *(33)*. The results from 22 different centers published between 1992 and 2001 are summarized in Table 2. It is difficult to draw solid conclusions by making comparisons among centers when each vary their target, localization technique, ablation protocol, and neurological assessment.

7.1. Dyskinesias

Contralateral drug-induced dyskinesias respond very well to pallidotomy. Nearly every study has documented improvement in L-dopa dyskinesias from 61–82% *(22–24,26–29,31,34–45)*. Ipsilateral relief of dyskinesias can also occur but to a lesser degree than contralateral effects. The longevity of pallidotomy for relief of dyskinesias is interesting. In a 10-year follow up, patients with posteroventral pallidotomy remained free of this symptom on the contralateral side despite increases in dopaminergic medications *(44)*. The NIH randomized clinical trial observed continued of benefits at two years *(31)*.

7.2. Tremor

Most patients with PD have tremor. Hence the title of the classic 1817 monograph by Dr. James Parkinson, "Essay on the Shaking Palsy." Before L-dopa was introduced in 1967, tremor was the chief indication for surgical intervention. Today, tremor alone is not an indication for pallidotomy. Tremor improves by 33–90% at 6 mo following pallidotomy. Findings by Lang et al. *(46)* suggested these effects were immediate and were maintained for more than two years. The wide variability in tremor response to surgery may be due to lesion location and/or patient selection *(15)*.

7.3. Rigidity

Rigidity is defined as a velocity-independent increase in passive tone in a limb, an important clinical sign that correlates with subjective limb stiffness in PD. The reported benefit of pallidotomy on rigidity is variable. Several studies suggest no difference in rigidity *(22,36,39,43–45,47)*. Other studies report improvement in contralateral rigidity from 25–55% *(23,24,26,28,29,31,34,37,38,40–42)*. The NIH randomized clinical trial reports 55% improvement in rigidity in the "off" state at 6 mo, which remains significantly improved at 2 yr *(31)*. Rigidity is one cause of limb pain which some patients experience. A significant reduction in overall pain scores at 6 wk and 1 yr has been reported following pallidotomy *(48)*.

7.4. Bradykinesia

Of the three cardinal features of Parkinson's disease, bradykinesia or slowness of movement is usually the most disabling symptom. Akinesia is impairment in voluntary willed movement. Patients often describe this symptom as an inability to get their muscles to obey the commands of their mind. Bradykinesia and akinesia are usually the key features of parkinsonian "off" states. Unfortunately, the effect of pallidotomy on bradykinesia has been variable among studies performed, with some reporting no significant change *(22,36,43–45,47)* and others reporting significant improvement. A randomized clinical trial reports 27 and 39% improvement in contralateral bradykinesia in the "on" and "off" states, respectively *(31)*.

7.5. Gait Difficulty

The so-called festinating gait disorder is often responsive to L-dopa therapy. However, only modest improvement in gait has been documented following pallidotomy. However, few studies have evaluated gait in detail. Improvement of gait from 7–30% is reported in these studies *(23,26,31,37,41)*. In the NIH randomized trial, gait improved significantly at 6 mo but not at 2 yr. A 10-year follow-up study of 13 patients originally operated by Laitinen *(4)* showed that five required additional stereotactic surgery and that, as a group, they suffered progressive motor and cognitive decline during the mean follow-up period of 10.5 yr *(44)*. Importantly, axial symptoms affecting gait, balance, and speech did not appear to be benefited in these patients but L-dopa dyskinesias did remain suppressed on the side contralateral to pallidotomy.

8. ACTIVITIES OF DAILY LIVING

The UPDRS ADL scale depends at least in part on the quality and quantity of "on" time, reflecting the patient's overall level of functional independence. ADL scores improved between 24–33% following pallidotomy in some studies *(26,28,29,37,45)* but showed no significant change at 6 mo to 1 yr in others *(24,40,43,47)*. Vitek et al., in their randomized trial, stated there is no improvement in ADL scores in the "on" state and 23% improvement in the "off" state *(31)*. One review at 2 yr appears to show 30% improvement in ADL scores *(49)*.

Table 2
Summary of Results of Pallidotomies for the Treatment of Parkinson's Disease

Source and year	No. patients	Age range	Target	Localization	Ablation	Neurological Assessment Scores	Follow-up	Outcomes: Dyskinesia	Tremor	Rigidity	Brady-kinesia Akinesia	Gait	ADL	Permanent Complications
Laitinen *(4)* (1992)	38 (4 bilat)	30–80 (60.3)	PVP GPi	MRI Macro	RF 72–80°C 60–90 s	Neuro exam: writing drawing gait	2–71 mo 28 mo	?	81% of patients with relief	92% of patients with relief	92% of patients with relief	?	?	14% visual field deficit
Dogali *(35)* (1995)	18 (7 med therapy)	42–79 (59.8)	GPi	MRI Micro	RF 80°C 60 s	UPDRS CAPIT on/off	12 mo	+	+	+	+	?	?	1-sexually disinhibited 1-MCA stroke 7 mo after surgery
Sutton *(36)* (1995)	5 (4 bilat)	60–75 (67)	PVP GPi (medial)	MRI + CT Macro	RF 72–80°C 60 s	UPDRS H&Y ADL	2 mo	+	–	–	–	?	?	2-visual field deficit 1-worsened speed
Iacono *(34)* (1995)	126 (68 bilat)	31–80 (62)	PVP GPi	MRI Semi-Micro	RF 65–80°C 30–60 s	UPDRS H&Y	6 mo–3 yr (11.4 mo)	+	60–90% reduction in tremor	+	+	?	?	Permanent 3.2% 3-hemianopsia 1-hemiparesis 1-abscess 3-subcortical hematoma
Friedman *(47)* (1996)	4	61–74	Right Gpi	MRI Gamma Knife	Gamma knife 180 Gy	UPDRS	12 mo	Only 1 patient responded	–	–	–	?	–	1-psychosis
Baron *(37)* (1996)	15	38–71 (55.6)	Gpi sensori-motor	MRI Micro	RF 60–80°C 60 s	CAPIT UPDRS 30% improvement ADL	12 mo	+	+	+	+	+	24% +	2-asymptomatic hemorrhage 1-quadrantanopsia
Kopyov *(38)* (1997)	29	?	PVP (medial)	MRI Micro	RF 80–85°C 85 s	CAPIT UPDRS blinded video	3 mo	+	89% of patients with relief	+	+	?	+	0
Kishore *(23)* (1997)	24	34–74	GPi (medial)	CT Macro	RF 80°C 60 s	CAPIT blinded video	12 mo	76% +	79% +	55% +	43% +	+	+	1-facial paresis
Johansson *(22)* (1997)	22	43–78 (63.8)	PVP	CT or MRI Macro	RF 75–83°C 30–60 s	UPDRS video H&Y ADL	12 mo	++	Mod +	–	–	?	?	?

Lang *(29)* (1997)	40	44–72 (58.8)	PVP (medial)	MRI Micro	RF 90°C 60 s	CAPIT UPDRS ADL	27 pt 12 mo 11 pt 24 mo	82% ++	53% improvement at 12 mo only	51% +	36% +	-	30% +	1-intracerebral hemorrhage
Uitti *(39)* (1997)	20	49–78 (65.5)	GPi	MRI Micro	RF 70°C 60 s	CAPIT UPDRS 22% improvement	3 mo	++	?	?	?	?	+	0
Masterman *(26)* (1998)	36	34–82 (65.3)	GPi	MRI Micro	RF 75–80°C 60 s	UPDRS 22% improvement	6 mo	61% +	43% +	28% +	19% +	30% +	30% +	0
Shannon *(40)* (1998)	26	(59.3)	GPi	MRI Micro	RF 75°C 60 s	CAPIT UPDRS 15% improvement	6 mo	+	+	+	+	–	–	1-death 3-intracerebral hemorrhage
Scott *(27)* (1998)	12 (8 bilat)	44–70	PVP	MRI and CT Macro	RF 75°C 60–90 s	UPDRS	3 mo	+	–	+	?	?	?	1-death (GI bleed) 2 deaths: 1-intracerebral hemorrhage
Samuel *(41)* (1998)	26	(55.9)	GPi	CT Micro	RF 70–72°C 60–80 s	CAPIT UPDRS 27% improvement	12 mo	67% +	33% +	25% +	24% +	7% +		1-hemorrhage infarct 2-hemorrhage 1-neglect; dysarthria
Merello *(42)* (1999)	10	56.1	PVP	MRI Micro Ventriculo-gram angiogram	RF 75°C 60 s	CAPIT UPDRS	12 mo	++	+	+	+	?	?	?
Kondziolka *(24)* (1999)	58 (7 bilat)	40–79 (67)	PVP	MRI Macro	RF 70–80°C 60–70 s	UPDRS 22% improvement	6–24 mo	++	+	+	+	–	–	0
Lai *(28)* (2000)	89	40–76 (62)	GPi	MRI Micro	RF 75°C 60 s	UPDRS 35.5% improvement	12–18 mo	65% +	70% +	50% +	?	?	33% +	1-hematoma hemiparesis resolved after 6 mo
Favre *(43)* (2000)	39 (22 uni) (17 bilat)	33–84 (65)	GPi	MRI Micro	RF 84°C 60 s	Patient questionnaires only	7 mo	++	–	–	–	–	–	?
Hariz *(44)* (2001)	13 (2 bilat)	43–72 (58.5)	PVP	CT Macro	RF	Neuro exam	10 yr	+	+/–	–	–	–		2-scotoma 2-repeat PVP
Van Horn *(45)* (2001)	32	48–76	PVP	MRI Micro	RF 80°C 60 s	CAPIT UPDRS 32% improvement	12 mo	++	–	–	–	–	27% +	?
Vitek *(31)* (2001)	36	?	PVP	MRI Micro	RF	*Randomized UPDRS 32% improvement v/s medical therapy only 5% worsening	6–24 mo	75% ++	70% +	55% +	39% +	+	23% +	1 seizure 1 transient speech problem

Table 3
Major Complications of Pallidotomy Correlates with Experience

Series of patients	Percentage complications
0–60	6.7%
61–120	3.3%
121–180	1.7%
181–240	1.7%
241–300	0%
301–360	3.3%
>361	0%

9. TECHNICAL REVIEW

Despite the variability of reported results in many uncontrolled studies, two randomized controlled trials *(31,31a)* and one case control study *(42)* of unilateral pallidotomy, each of which compared surgery to best medical therapy, demonstrated improvement in the cardinal symptoms of PD as well as drug-induced dyskinesias. In addition to patient selection, details of the surgical procedure also have a profound influence on clinical benefit. Thirteen groups listed in Table 2 routinely used microelectrode recording (micro) for pallidotomy while seven used macrostimulation (macro) alone. The remaining two studies used either a semi-microelectrode or gamma knife. Upon assessment of the different outcomes reported, lesions placed only a few millimeters from each other may have vastly different short-and long-term effects on parkinsonian symptoms *(30)*. Most of these publications are initial reports representing a center's learning curve for performance of pallidotomy. There also appears to be a learning curve for complications (Table 3) as well as for optimizing outcome.

10. COMPLICATIONS

Because the globus pallidus rests just dorsal to the optic tract and lateral to the internal capsule, misdirected lesions can impinge on visual or motor pathways. Patients can develop hemiparesis or hemianopsia either transiently or permanently. Complications are likely related to individual surgical experience. As already mentioned, current reported complication rates may reflect the fact that most reports have been from centers still on a learning curve (Table 3). Among 735 patients reported in 22 different series there were four deaths. Alkani and Lozano *(50)* reviewed contemporary articles on pallidotomy. In 85 articles, 1959 patients with PD underwent pallidotomy at 40 centers in 12 countries. There were 1735 unilateral (88.6%) and 224 bilateral (11.4%) procedures. Overall mortality rate was 0.4% and the rate of persistent adverse effects was estimated at 14%. Major adverse events, including intracerebral hemmorhage, contralateral weakness, and visual field defects occurred in 5.3% of patients reported.

On a historical note, Leksell's pallidotomies from 1958–1962 reported a mortality rate of 0.8% *(51)*, which compares favorably with today's results. Intracerebral, pallidal, or subcortical hemorrhages were reported in eight patients (1.0%). The incidence of asymptomatic hemorrhage may be skewed because not all centers routinely obtain postoperative imaging. Asymptomatic hemorrhage was documented in only two patients. The remaining permanent deficits included six additional patients with hemianopsia, quadrantanopsia, or scotoma (0.8%), excluding those originally reported by Laitinen *(4)*. The incidence of visual field deficits after pallidotomy is highly variable and dependent on whether formal visual field testing is routinely performed. Laitinen *(4)* reported a 14% incidence of visual field deficits before moving his target more laterally in the pallidum. Three cases of permanent hemiparesis (0.4%) were documented with one patient suffering a middle cerebral artery stroke 7 mo after surgery. There was one abscess and two reoperations for a second lesion. Other uncommon complications include psychosis, sexual disinhibition, dysarthria, hypophonia, dysphagia, hypersalivation, blepharospasm, impaired memory, depression, seizure, and urinary symptoms (50). In a study of 18 patients, preliminary findings by Kubu et al. *(52)* found that patients who underwent a left-sided pallidotomy had a clinically significant decline in the Controlled Oral Word Association (COWA) test, a measure of phonemic word fluency. This decline was only evident in patients with late-onset PD. Lang et al. *(53)* found mild cognitive impairment in several patients and suggested that its incidence may depend on lesion location *(16)*. The NIH randomized trial *(31)* found no significant cognitive changes regardless of lesion side.

11. BILATERAL PALLIDOTOMY

Bilateral pallidotomy is more effective than unilateral pallidotomy but is much less frequently performed. In a survey reviewing the current practice of pallidotomy in a limited sample of 28 centers in North America, all centers performed unilateral pallidotomies and 15 centers performed staged bilateral procedures with only four centers performing simultaneous bilateral procedures *(7)*. Controversy exists when comparing the benefits and side effects of unilateral versus bilateral procedures. Very few authors believe that bilateral pallidotomy carries no increased risk of speech or swallowing difficulties *(4,34)*. A recent report compares 22 patients undergoing unilateral and 17 patients undergoing bilateral simultaneous pallidotomy *(43)*. In this study, bilateral pallidotomy carried a 53% risk of speech deterioration. This compares to only 37% of patients who experienced speech deterioration with a unilateral procedure *(43)*. There was no significant difference between the two groups in swallowing or drooling. Another study confirms that bilateral simultaneous pallidotomy may also be associated with emotional, behavioral and cognitive deficits as well as abulia and disabling corticobulbar dysfunction *(54)*. By contrast, however, retrospective analysis of 14 patients who underwent contralateral pallidotomy because of recurrent motor symptoms 5–15 mo after initially successful unilateral pallidotomy showed improved motor function with relatively little morbidity *(55)*. Bulbar symptoms were few although mild hypophonia occurred in five patients. Gait and postural instability were not improved. Similar to previous studies, dyskinesias were virtually abolished in all patients.

12. WHAT TO AVOID?

PD is a progressive disease with a clinically progressive course, which is unaltered by medical or surgical therapy. The best we can do is to palliate symptoms as the disease continues to progress. We must be honest regarding which symptoms we are trying to alleviate with our chosen surgical therapy. Patient selection is a key factor. Surgical therapy should be avoided in patients with a poor response to L-dopa, unusually rapid progression of motor symptoms, or dementia. Bilateral ablative therapy should be avoided, especially since new nonablative and restorative therapies are on the horizon. Additionally, it has been shown *(47,56)* that gamma knife surgery is usually not suitable for routine pallidotomy, although it has apparently been used successfully in very selected patients *(57)*.

13. WHO TO INCLUDE?

Patients who are severely disabled by asymmetrical L-dopa dyskinesias appear to be the best candidates for pallidotomy. With the exception of tremor, symptoms responsive to L-dopa therapy appear to show the greatest improvement. A multidisciplinary team approach providing close collaboration between experienced neurologists, neurosurgeons and neurophysiologists is critical in selecting the most appropriate patients for the procedure and maximizing a successful outcome. Choosing increased technological sophistication (microelectrode and macroelectrode electrophysiological mapping) allows more precise lesion targeting, further decreasing the incidence of complications and making pallidotomy even safer and more effective.

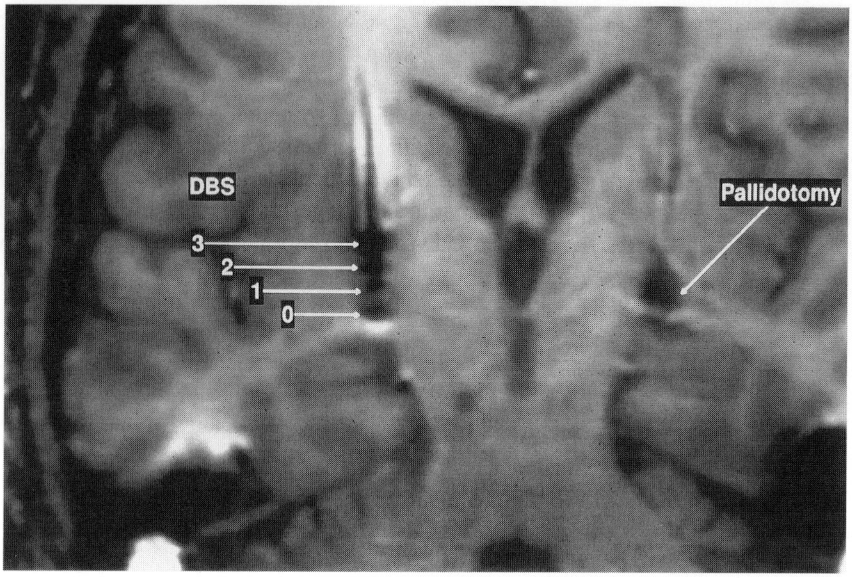

Fig. 4. A coronal MRI of an old left pallidotomy and a newly placed right DBS. A large number of unilateral pallidotomies are now being combined with DBS on the contralateral side. The DBS has the advantage of adjustability and seems to avoid many of the complications seen with bilateral pallidotomy.

14. CONCLUSIONS

It is difficult to assess the results of a surgical procedure that is nonuniformly performed and evaluated on a diverse group of patients whose disease varies in degree of severity and rate of progression *(58)*. Unilateral posteroventral pallidotomy is a safe and effective palliative surgery for drug-induced dyskinesias. Much progress has been made understanding the nature of PD since James Parkinson's "Essay on the Shaking Palsy" in 1817, especially in the past four decades. Much remains to be discovered about this disease and even more about better forms of treatment. Thalamic DBS has proven just as effective and safer than thalamotomy *(59)*; the same is probably true for pallidal DBS compared with pallidotomy (Fig. 4); and subthalamic DBS is now emerging as a favored surgical treatment in increasing numbers of patients. Whatever its relationship to DBS, pallidotomy will remain a good option for the treatment of PD.

REFERENCES

1. Guridi, J. and Lozano, A. M. (1997) A brief history of pallidotomy. *Neurosurgery* **41(5),** 1169–1180; discussion 1180–1183.
2. Payne, B. R., Bakay, R. A. E., and Vitek, J. L. (2001) Pallidotomy for treatment of Parkinson's Disease. In: *Surgery for Parkinson's Disease and Movement Disorders* (Krauss, J. K., Jankovic, J., and Grossman, R. G., eds.), Lippincott, Williams, and Wilkins, Philadelphia, PA, pp. 161–169.
3. Cotzias, G. C., Van Woert, M. H., and Schiffer, L. M. (1967) Aromatic amino acids and modification of parkinsonism. *N. Engl. J. Med.* **276(7),** 374–379.
4. Laitinen, L. V., Bergenheim, A. T., and Hariz, M. I. (1992) Leksell's posteroventral pallidotomy in the treatment of Parkinson's disease. *J. Neurosurg.* **76(1),** 53–61.
5. Pare, D., Curro'Dossi, R., and Steriade, M. (1990) Neuronal basis of the parkinsonian resting tremor: a hypothesis and its implications for treatment. *Neuroscience* **35(2),** 217–226.
6. Giroux, M. L. and Vitek, J. L. (1998) Pallidotomy: a treatment for Parkinsonian tremor? In: *Pallidal Surgery for the Treatment of Parkinson's Disease and Movement Disorders* (Krauss, J. K., Grossman, R. G., and Jankovic, J., eds.), Lippincott-Raven, Philadelphia, PA, pp. 291–296.

7. Favre, J., Taha, J. M., Nguyen, T. T., et al. (1996) Pallidotomy: a survey of current practice in North America. *Neurosurgery* **39(4),** 883–890; discussion 890–892.
8. Langston, J. W., Widner, H., Goetz, C. G., et al. (1992) Core assessment program for intracerebral transplantations (CAPIT). *Mov. Disord.* **7(1),** 2–13.
9. Defer, G. L., Widner, H., Marie, R. M., et al. (1999) Core assessment program for surgical interventional therapies in Parkinson's disease (CAPSIT-PD). *Mov. Disord.* **14(4),** 572–584.
10. Starr, P. A., Vitek, J., and Bakay, R. A. E. Surgery for movement disorders. In: *Operative Neurosurgery* (Kaye, A. H. and Black, P. M., eds.), Churchill Livingston, London, in press.
11. Krauss, J. K. and Grossman, R. G. (1998) Optimal target of pallidotomy: a controversy. In: *Pallidal Surgery for the Treatment of Parkinson's Disease and Movement Disorders* (Krauss, J. K., Grossman, R. G., and Jankovic, J., eds.), Lippincott-Raven, Philadelphia, PA, pp. 291–296.
12. Laitinen, L. V. (1998) Optimal target of pallidotomy: a controversy. In: *Pallidal Surgery for the Treatment of Parkinson's Disease and Movement Disorders* (Krauss, J. K., Grossman, R. G., and Jankovic, J., eds.), Lippincott-Raven, Philadelphia, PA, pp. 285–289.
13. Bakay, R. A. E. and Starr, P. A. (1998) Optimal target of pallidotomy: a controversy. In: *Pallidal Surgery for the Treatment of Parkinson's Disease and Movement Disorders* (Krauss, J. K., Grossman, R. G., and Jankovic, J., eds.), Lippincott-Raven, Philadelphia, PA, pp. 275–283.
14. Hariz, M. I. and Hirabayashi, H. (1997) Is there a relationship between size and site of the stereotactic lesion and symptomatic results of pallidotomy and thalamotomy? *Stereotact. Funct. Neurosurg.* **69(1–4 Pt 2),** 28–45.
15. Gross, R. E., Lombardi, W. J., Lang, A. E., et al. (1999) Relationship of lesion location to clinical outcome following microelectrode-guided pallidotomy for Parkinson's disease. *Brain* **122(Pt 3),** 405–416.
16. Lombardi, W. J., Gross, R. E., Trepanier, L. L., et al. (2000) Relationship of lesion location to cognitive outcome following microelectrode-guided pallidotomy for Parkinson's disease: support for the existence of cognitive circuits in the human pallidum. *Brain* **123(Pt 4),** 746–758.
17. Reich, C., Hudgins, P., Sheppard, S., Starr, P., and Bakay, R. A. E. (1997) A high-resolution fast spin-echo inversion-recovery sequence for pre-operative localization of the internal globus pallidus. Presented at American Society of Neuroradiology, Toronto, Canada.
18. Vitek, J. L., Bakay, R. A., Hashimoto, T., et al. (1998) Microelectrode-guided pallidotomy: technical approach and its application in medically intractable Parkinson's disease. *J. Neurosurg.* **88(6),** 1027–1043.
19. Lozano, A., Hutchison, W., Kiss, Z., et al. (1996) Methods for microelectrode-guided posteroventral pallidotomy. *J. Neurosurg.* **84(2),** 194–202.
20. Shaltenbrand, G. B. P. (1959) *Introduction to Stereotaxis with an Atlas of the Human Brain.* Thieme, Stuttgart.
21. Starr, P. A., Vitek, J., DeLong, M., Mewes, K., and Bakay, R. A. E. (1999) Pallidotomy: theory and technique. *Techn. Neurosurg.* **5(1),** 31–45.
22. Johansson, F., Malm, J., Nordh, E., et al. (1997) Usefulness of pallidotomy in advanced Parkinson's disease. *J. Neurol. Neurosurg. Psychiatry* **62(2),** 125–132.
23. Kishore, A., Turnbull, I. M., Snow, B. J., et al. (1997) Efficacy, stability and predictors of outcome of pallidotomy for Parkinson's disease. Six-month follow-up with additional 1-year observations. *Brain* **120(Pt 5),** 729–737.
24. Kondziolka, D., Bonaroti, E., Baser, S., et al. (1999) Outcomes after stereotactically guided pallidotomy for advanced Parkinson's disease. *J. Neurosurg.* **90(2),** 197–202.
25. Samii, A., Turnbull, I. M., Kishore, A., et al. (1999) Reassessment of unilateral pallidotomy in Parkinson's disease. A 2-year follow-up study. *Brain* **122(Pt 3),** 417–425.
26. Masterman, D., DeSalles, A., Baloh, R. W., et al. (1998) Motor, cognitive, and behavioral performance following unilateral ventroposterior pallidotomy for Parkinson disease. *Arch. Neurol.* **55(9),** 1201–1208.
27. Scott, R., Gregory, R., Hines, N., et al. (1998) Neuropsychological, neurological and functional outcome following pallidotomy for Parkinson's disease. A consecutive series of eight simultaneous bilateral and twelve unilateral procedures. *Brain* **121(Pt 4),** 659–675.
28. Lai, E. C., Jankovic, J., Krauss, J. K., et al. (2000) Long-term efficacy of posteroventral pallidotomy in the treatment of Parkinson's disease. *Neurology* **55(8),** 1218–1222.
29. Lang, A. E., Lozano, A. M., Montgomery, E., et al. (1997) Posteroventral medial pallidotomy in advanced Parkinson's disease. *N. Engl. J. Med.* **337(15),** 1036–1042.
30. Vitek, J. L., Bakay, R. A., and DeLong, M. R. (1997) Microelectrode-guided pallidotomy for medically intractable Parkinson's disease. *Adv. Neurol.* **74,** 183–198.
31. Vitek, J. L., Bakay, R., Freeman, A., Evatt, M. L., Green, J., McDonald, W., Haber, M., et al. (1998) Randomized clinical trial of pallidotomy versus medical therapy for Parkinson's disease. *Ann. Neurol.* In press.
32. Ondo, W. G., Jankovic, J., Lai, E. C., et al. (1998) Assessment of motor function after stereotactic pallidotomy. *Neurology* **50(1),** 266–270.
32a. de Bie, R. M., de Haan, R. J., Nijssen, P. C., et al. (1999) Unilateral pallidotomy in Parkinson's disease: a randomised, single-blind, multicentre trial. *Lancet* **354(9191),** 1665–1669.
33. Merello, M., Nouzeilles, M. I., Kuzis, G., et al. (1999) Unilateral radiofrequency lesion versus electrostimulation of posteroventral pallidum: a prospective randomized comparison. *Mov. Disord.* **14(1),** 50–56.
34. Iacono, R. P., Shima, F, Lonser, R. R., et al. (1995) The results, indications, and physiology of posteroventral pallidotomy for patients with Parkinson's disease. *Neurosurgery* **36(6),** 1118–1125; discussion 1125–1127.
35. Dogali, M., Fazzini, E., Kolodny, E., et al. (1995) Stereotactic ventral pallidotomy for Parkinson's disease. *Neurology* **45(4),** 753–761.

36. Sutton, J. P., Couldwell, W., Lew, M. F., et al. (1995) Ventroposterior medial pallidotomy in patients with advanced Parkinson's disease. *Neurosurgery* **36(6),** 1112–1116; discussion 1116–1117.
37. Baron, M. S., Vitek, J. L., Bakay, R. A., et al. (1996) Treatment of advanced Parkinson's disease by posterior GPi pallidotomy: 1-year results of a pilot study. *Ann. Neurol.* **40(3),** 355–366.
38. Kopyov, O., Jacques, D., Duma, C., et al. (1997) Microelectrode-guided posteroventral medial radiofrequency pallidotomy for Parkinson's disease. *J. Neurosurg.* **87(1),** 52–59.
39. Uitti, R. J., Wharen, R. E. Jr., Turk, M. F., et al. (1997) Unilateral pallidotomy for Parkinson's disease: comparison of outcome in younger versus elderly patients. *Neurology* **49(4),** 1072–1077.
40. Shannon, K. M., Penn, R. D., Kroin, J. S., et al. (1998) Stereotactic pallidotomy for the treatment of Parkinson's disease. Efficacy and adverse effects at 6 months in 26 patients. *Neurology* **50(2),** 434–438.
41. Samuel, M., Caputo, E., Brooks, D. J., et al. (1998) A study of medial pallidotomy for Parkinson's disease: clinical outcome, MRI location and complications. *Brain* **121,** 59–75.
42. Merello, M., Nouzeilles, M. I., Cammarota, A., et al. (1999) Comparison of 1-year follow-up evaluations of patients with indication for pallidotomy who did not undergo surgery versus patients with Parkinson's disease who did undergo pallidotomy: a case control study. *Neurosurgery* **44(3),** 461–467; discussion 467–468.
43. Favre, J., Burchiel, K. J., Taha, J. M., et al. (2000) Outcome of unilateral and bilateral pallidotomy for Parkinson's disease: patient assessment. *Neurosurgery* **46(2),** 344–353.
44. Hariz, M. I. and Bergenheim, A. T. (2001) A 10-year follow-up review of patients who underwent Leksell's posteroventral pallidotomy for Parkinson disease. *J. Neurosurg.* **94(4),** 552–558.
45. Van Horn, G., Hassenbusch, S. J., Zouridakis, G., et al. (2001) Pallidotomy: a comparison of responders and nonresponders. *Neurosurgery* **48(2),** 263–271; discussion 271–273.
46. Lozano, A. M., Lang, A. E., and Hutchison, W. D. (1998) Pallidotomy for tremor. *Mov. Disord.* **13(Suppl. 3),** 107–110.
47. Friedman, J. H., Epstein, M., Sanes, J. N., et al. (1996) Gamma knife pallidotomy in advanced Parkinson's disease. *Ann. Neurol.* **39(4),** 535–538.
48. Honey, C. R., Stoessl, A. J., Tsui, J. K., et al. (1999) Unilateral pallidotomy for reduction of parkinsonian pain. *J. Neurosurg.* **91(2),** 198–201.
49. Lang, A. E., Duff, J., Saint-Cyr, J. A., et al. (1999) Posteroventral medial pallidotomy in Parkinson's disease. *J. Neurol.* **246(Suppl. 2),** II28–II41.
50. Alkhani, A. and Lozano, A. M. (2001) Pallidotomy for parkinson disease: a review of contemporary literature. *J. Neurosurg.* **94(1),** 43–49.
51. Laitinen, L. V. (2000) Leksell's unpublished pallidotomies of 1958–1962. *Stereotact. Funct. Neurosurg.* **74(1),** 1–10.
52. Kubu, C. S., Grace, G. M., and Parrent, A. G. (2000) Cognitive outcome following pallidotomy: the influence of side of surgery and age of patient at disease onset. *J. Neurosurg.* **92(3),** 384–389.
53. Lang, A., Lozano, A., Tasker, R., Duff, J., Tasker, R., Duff, J., et al. (1997) Neuropsychological and behavioral changes and weight gain after medial pallidotomy (letter). *Ann. Neurol.* **41(6),** 834–836.
54. Ghika, J., Ghika-Schmid, F., Fankhauser, H., et al. (1999) Bilateral contemporaneous posteroventral pallidotomy for the treatment of Parkinson's disease: neuropsychological and neurological side effects. Report of four cases and review of the literature. *J. Neurosurg.* **91(2),** 313–321.
55. Counihan, T. J., Shinobu, L. A., Eskandar, E. N., Cosgrove, G. R., and Penney, J. B. (2001) Outcomes following staged bilateral pallidotomy in advanced parkinson's disease. *Neurology* **56,** 799–802.
56. Okun, M. S., Stover, N. P., Subramanian, T., et al. (2001) Complications of gamma knife surgery for Parkinson disease. *Arch. Neurol.* **58,** 1995–2002.
57. Young, R. F., Shumway-Cook, A., Vermeulen, S. S., Grimm, P., Blasko, J., Posewitz, A., et al. (1998) Gamma knife radio surgery as a lesioning technique in movement disorder surgery. *J. Neurosurg.* **89(2),** 183–193.
58. Kelly, P. J. (1995) Pallidotomy in Parkinson's disease. *Neurosurgery* **36(6),** 1154–1157.
59. Schuurman, P. R., Bosch, D., Bossuyt, P. M. M., et al. (2000) A comparison of continuous thalamic stimulation and thalamotomy for suppression of severe tremor. *N. Engl. J. Med.* **342,** 461–468.

9

Bilateral Pallidotomy for Parkinson's Disease

Costs and Benefits

Simon Parkin, Carole Joint, Richard Scott, and Tipu Z. Aziz

1. INTRODUCTION

Pallidotomy for alleviation of the symptoms of Parkinson's disease (PD) is one of the oldest stereotactic procedures in functional neurosurgery. Early series described by Cooper *(1)*, Speigel and Wycis *(2)*, and Reichert *(3)* in the 1950s found rigidity was alleviated in 80% and tremor in about 45% of their patients with no effect on bradykinesia, although such an effect was claimed by Krayenbuhl in his series *(4)*. With the more predictable suppression of tremor via a thalamic lesion, pallidotomy eventually fell out of favor. Later, with the advent of L-dopa therapy for PD in 1969 *(5)*, all surgical options for these movement disorders declined in popularity. This process was accelerated by Hoehn and Yahr's longitudinal study in 1969 *(6)*, in which they found that although up to 80% of patients may lose tremor and rigidity after a thalamotomy, because of persisting akinesia only 17% were functionally better.

However, long-term experience with dopaminergic therapy for parkinsonism muted the early optimism that medical therapy alone would manage the disease. It was found that after five years of L-dopa therapy over 60% of patients developed side effects of medication, including dyskinesia, dystonia, and on-off effects, that were often as disabling as the untreated condition *(7)*. Medical strategies to alleviate these problems have been developed (reduction and splitting of L-dopa doses, dopamine agonists, COMT inhibitors, amantadine, continuous apomorphine infusion) with varying degrees of success.

Lack of basic understanding of the neural mechanisms underlying PD meant that surgical developments could not advance. All this was changed with the report by Davis et al. *(8)* of a young individual who developed parkinsonism after intravenous administration of 1-methyl-4-phenyl-1,2,3,6-tetrahydropyridine (MPTP). Further cases were reported by Langston *(9)*. Forno *(10)* confirmed that the neuropathology was indistinguishable from idiopathic PD. In 1983 Burns *(11)* reported that MPTP could induce parkinsonism in the experimental primate. This led rapidly to detailed studies into the neural mechanisms of the disease. Early electrophysiological studies *(12–14)* and the 2-DG metabolic studies of Crossman *(15)* were able to create a heuristic model of parkinsonism that, despite many reservations, has stood the test of time.

In this model, loss of nigrostriatal dopamine leads to unrestricted overactivity of the subthalamic nucleus (STN), which in turn drives the medial pallidum to excessively inhibit the motor thalamus and upper brainstem. Within the broad strokes of this simplified model, it appeared that lesioning the subthalamic nucleus might alleviate parkinsonism. Bergmann et al. *(16)* found that excitotoxic lesions

From: Contemporary Clinical Neurology:
Surgical Treatment of Parkinson's Disease and Other Movement Disorders
Edited by: D. Tarsy, J. L. Vitek, and A. M. Lozano © Humana Press Inc., Totowa, NJ

of the STN did alleviate the cardinal signs of parkinsonism in the MPTP exposed primate and Crossman's group *(17)* showed that standard radiofrequency lesions had the same effect. Benazzouz et al. showed that high-frequency stimulation of STN was also effective *(18)*. These observations led to a tidal wave of optimism in the future of surgical alleviation of parkinsonism.

In spite of these experimental findings, for several reasons there was a delay in development of STN surgery for PD. The primary concern was risk of inducing intractable hemichorea or hemiballismus in place of parkinsonism. Vascular events involving the subthalamic area were well-known to cause hemiballismus and a case report of subthalamic haemorrhage in a parkinsonian patient described hemichorea with subsequent alleviation of the condition *(19)*. Secondly, in Crossman's primate series *(20)* two of six primates who underwent subthalamotomy suffered intracerebral haemorrhages, indicating that the surgical risks might be high. Finally there was concurrent evidence, both clinically and from primate studies, that the medial pallidum might be an alternative target. GABA infusion into the medial pallidum of parkinsonian primates was found to alleviate parkinsonian symptoms *(21)*. More important, were the clinical observations by Laitinen *(22)* who resurrected the findings of Svenillson *(23)* that posteroventral pallidotomy could alleviate the cardinal signs of parkinsonism.

The globus pallidus was a surgical target with a long history and one that surgeons felt comfortable with. As a consequence there was a plethora of publications on the effects of pallidotomy in PD. In some small series results were disappointing *(24)* while others with larger numbers provided little useful detail *(25)*. Nevertheless, well-documented publications on unilateral pallidotomy *(26–37)* did appear to demonstrate that such procedures reduce the total United Parkinson's Disease Rating Scale (UPDRS) by up to 30% with significant improvement in contralateral tremor, rigidity, bradykinesia, and dyskinesia. It was tempting to double the benefit by lesioning the globus pallidus on both sides. However, although anecdotal reports showed significant benefits, bilateral pallidotomy has not become a widely adopted procedure. This has largely been based on fear of producing hyphonia and/or severe cognitive side effects though there has been relatively little documentation of this in the literature. It is also the case that bilateral lesions do not double the UPDRS changes. Based on our own series, unilateral pallidotomy can be expected to reduce total UPDRS by 30% and a bilateral procedure by 40%. The balance of risk vs gain has been thought too unfavorable for it to have a future role in functional surgery.

As pallidotomy began to fall from grace, the pioneering work of Benabid *(38)* resurrected the subthalamic nucleus as a surgical target. His group has used their extensive experience in deep brain stimulation (DBS) to modulate STN activity with impressive results which historically had not been achieved with pallidal surgery *(39)*. Nevertheless, DBS is an expensive procedure that will likely remain beyond the resources of most of the world's parkinsonian population. By contrast, we believe that ablative surgery will continue to have a place but prior to offering it one must be fully aware of its effects. With this in mind, we have studied a large cohort of our own patients who have undergone bilateral pallidotomy (BPVP).

In 1993, two developments led the Oxford group to consider the use of magnetic resonance imaging (MRI) and computed tomography (CT) fusion techniques in functional surgery. The work of Alexander *(40,41)* describing methodology for volumetrically fusing MRI scans to CT scans in acquisition of targets for radiosurgery in order to eliminate MRI field distortions led to the ImageFusion™ program. This, in combination with a stereotactic planning system, StereoPlan® (both prototypes developed by Radionics) allowed for direct and accurate targeting of the medial pallidum. As a result, anatomical localisation combined with careful intra-operative examination of the patient allowed for accurate lesion placement. Furthermore, in collaboration with Radionics, the Schaltenbrand and Wahren *(42)* functional atlas was incorporated in the software with the ability to alter the proportions in a manner to make it applicable to the patient's individual anatomy. We describe our technique using ImageFusion™ and StereoPlan® in performing BPVP without microelectrode guidance.

We aimed from the beginning to answer several questions: Is BPVP effective for alleviation of Parkinson's disease, and who benefits most? Does the neurological improvement correlate with improved

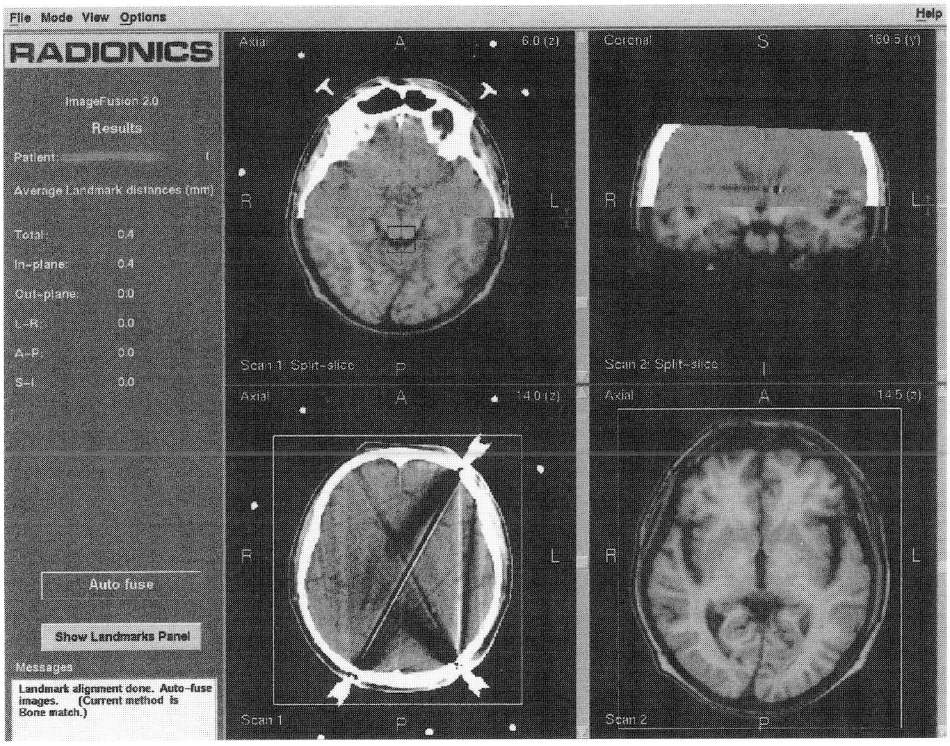

Fig. 1. An illustration of volumetrically fusing the MRI scan to the steeotactic CT scan after alignment using anatomical landmarks.

quality of life? Are there any cognitive trade-offs? What is the overall complication rate? The surgeon was to remain independent of the assessments. Functional surgery is a multidisciplinary speciality *(43)* and our group was comprised of a neurosurgeon, neurologist, neuropsychologist, neuroanaesthetist, neurophysiologist, and a specialist nurse.

2. SURGICAL TECHNIQUE

First, a pre-operative T-1 weighted MRI scan using a 3-D Turbo-FLASH sequence (TE7 ms, TR15 ms) and a Siemens 1.5T Magnetom Vision Scanner is acquired. Immediately before the operation and under general anaesthesia, the Cosman-Roberts-Wells (CRW™) head ring is fixed to the patient's head low enough to acquire a CT scan of the entire skull. We prefer to use general anaesthesia during this stage for patient comfort and to avoid patient movement. Stereotactic CT of the entire skull is acquired using 3mm contiguous slices. Next the MRI and stereotactic CT are transferred to the StereoPlan workstation. Using the ImageFusion software, the MRI is aligned to the stereotactic CT with at least three anatomic landmarks (Fig. 1). We use the lenses of both eyes and the pineal gland. Once alignment is complete the ImageFusion software volumetrically correlates the MRI image set to the stereotactic CT, independently scaling X, Y, Z, and all rotational axes. Upon completion of the correlation of the MRI to the stereotactic CT, the StereoPlan software is employed to pre-operatively plan a surgical trajectory for electrode placement. The spatially corrected and volumetrically correlated MRI is used for anatomic localization of the GPi that is clearly seen on the Turbo-FLASH MRI images (Fig. 2). Further anatomic verification is performed with the AtlasPlan module of StereoPlan. The Schaltenbrand and Wahren Atlas (used in the software with permission from Thieme) is co-registered with patient

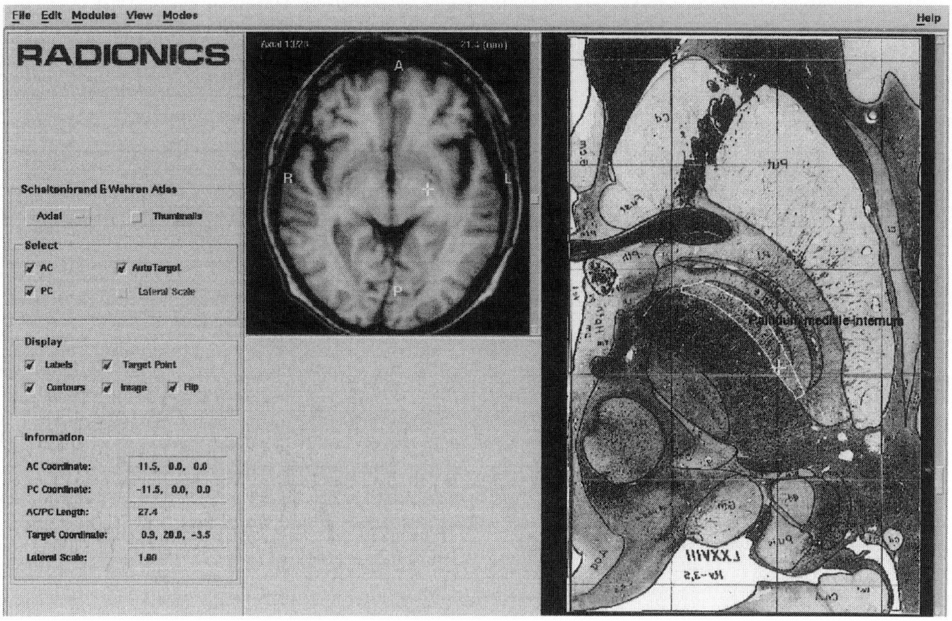

Fig. 2. Use of the Steroplan module to localize the posterior half of the medial pallidum.

anatomy by the anterior commissure (AC) and posterior commisure (PC) points as well as a known lateral landmark (we compare the putaminopallidal boundary of the patient's scan to that in the atlas). The AtlasPlan module then shows the placement of the target on the Schaltenbrand and Wahren Atlas images. The planned trajectory can be evaluated with the StereoPlan software once the arc angles are set to enter from an entry point 1.0 cm anterior to the coronal suture and 5.0–6.0 cm lateral to the mid-line with the CRW arc system in place.

While planning the procedure the patient is awakened after insertion of an arterial line to monitor blood pressure (BP). The patient's BP is maintained at 20 mm hg below their normal systolic BP using intravenous hydralazine, labetalol, or sublingual nifedipine. We do not routinely shave the patient's head but clean it on the operating table with aqueous and alcoholic chlorhexidine and then shave a small area at the point of entry. A dermal skin punch is used to incise the skin and a 4 mm twist drill made along the planned trajectory. The dura is then punctured with a biopsy cannula. This prevents any significant spinal fluid leakage that would cause brain shift. For posteroventral pallidotomy (PVP), an entry point 1.0 cm anterior to the coronal suture and 5.0–6.0 cm lateral to the mid-line is chosen. This approach avoids passing through the internal capsule and allows for lesions to be placed from medial to lateral in a single pass of the electrode.

Having determined the co-ordinates using ImageFusion and StereoPlan, the electrode (2 mm exposed tip, 1.8 mm diameter) is passed to the target. We choose the initial target to be in the medial globus pallidus, just beyond the border between external globus pallidus (Gpe) and internal globus pallidus (Gpi). All lesions are placed ventromedially (Fig. 3). This avoids encroaching into the lateral globus pallidus, which may have untoward effects *(44)*. However, despite the large numbers of published cases, there is still no generally agreed on precise pallidal target that one should aim for to obtain reliably good results. However, neurophysiologic studies in animals have demonstrated that neurons in posterior GPi are involved in movement, whereas studies in humans have reported that the optimal benefit in parkinsonian motor signs occurs following lesions in the posterior "sensorimotor" portion of GPi *(44a,44b,44c)*.

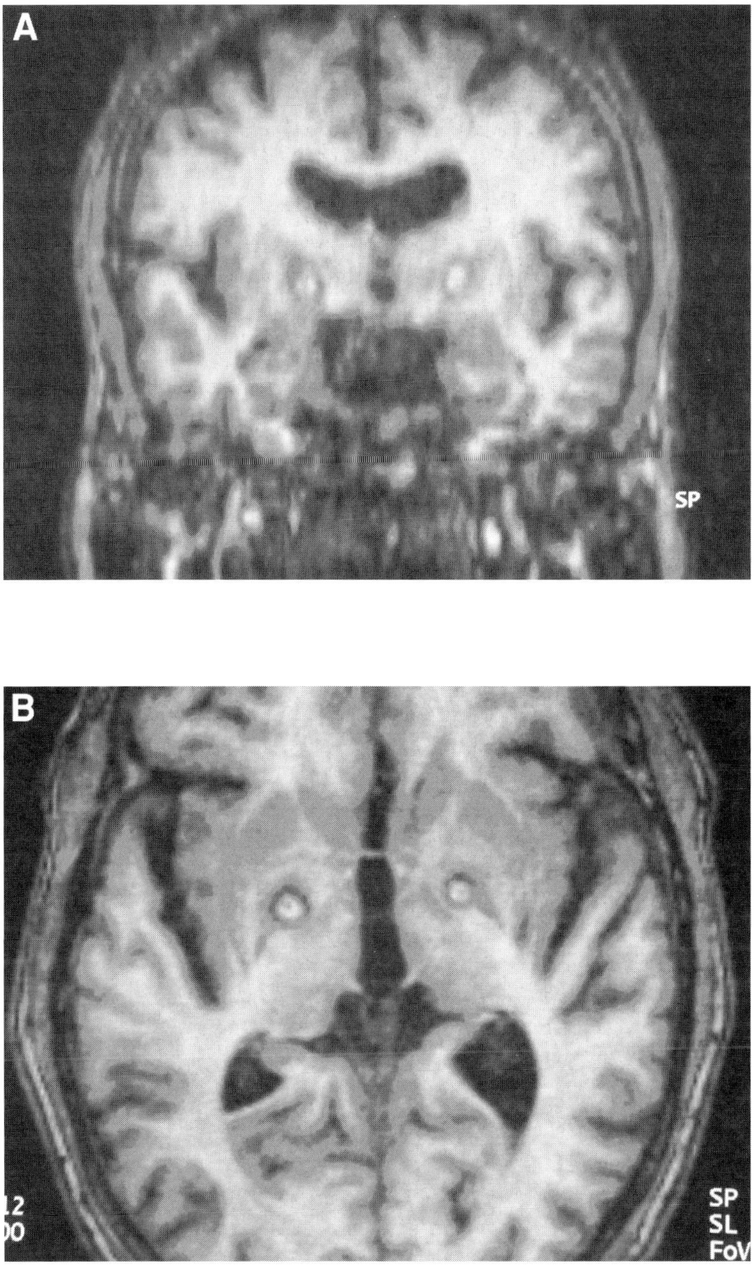

Fig. 3. Axial (**A**) and coronal (**B**) views immediately following bilateral pallidotomies.

Thus, we feel that in the anterior-posterior direction, the posterior half of the Gpi should be the target region. In the coronal plane the lesions are localized in Gpi without a great deal of encroachment into the ansa lenticularis.

Impedance in the pallidum using this electrode is 500–700 ohms. Stimulation at 100Hz is begun 2.0 mm above the calculated target while the attending neurologist examines the patient. The electrode is advanced in 1.0 mm steps while repeated testing is carried out. The optimal site is that point at which rigidity, bradykinesia and tremor, if present, are alleviated at 0.5–1.0V at 100Hz. Very occasionally patients may show exacerbation rather than alleviation of symptoms. We feel that it is important to examine the patient during the first pass of the electrode as impedance is measured since the stunning effect of passing the electrode to the anticipated end target may render subsequent neurological examination unhelpful due to injury to pallidal neurons. This phenomenon may also be why some groups do not find macrostimulation and clinical examination to be helpful.

The electrode is then advanced until the impedance begins to rise to about 800–1100 ohms. This indicates that the bottom of the medial pallidum has been reached and no further advancement is made. If capsular motor responses are not obtained at less than 2.0V and 2Hz and there are no visual phosphenes on stimulation at 3.5–4.0V it is safe to begin lesioning. We have observed that tongue "bobbing" (rhythmic contraction produced by macrostimulation at 2Hz and 2.0V) also indicates correct placement. A temporary "lesion" is generated using 45°C for 60 s. If no adverse effects are observed the first permanent lesion is placed (75°C for 30 s). Two further lesions are than made at 2.0 and 4.0 mm above the target (75°C for 60 s, 90 s if unilateral). It is not unusual to observe what we call "release dyskinesias" on completing the lesions. These tend to predict a good clinical outcome and vary in duration from a few minutes to a few days. The lesions thus obtained are 100–150 mm^3 in volume. With bilateral PVP we aim to make the lesions asymmetrical with a smaller lesion (~100 mm^3) in the non-dominant hemisphere and the larger lesion (~150 mm^3) on the dominant side.

3. OXFORD MOVEMENT DISORDER GROUP PATIENT SERIES

Patients with PD were selected from those referred to movement disorder clinics staffed by a neurologist and neurosurgeon in each centre. All patients satisfied United Kingdom PD Society brain bank diagnostic criteria for idiopathic PD *(45)*. Most had intractable drug-induced dyskinesia and had exhausted all available medical options. Any general medical, surgical, or neuropsychological contraindications were identified including, for example, significant dysarthria, dysphagia, excessive salivation/drooling, gait freezing 'on' medication, dementia, or major psychiatric disorder. Patients had to be L-dopa responsive and show that, if only for a brief period during the day, there were windows of quality time. On average, approximately one in three patients seen in the movement disorders clinic were considered appropriate for PVP.

The demographic features of our series are shown in Table 1. Outcome was assessed in 53 patients from the Radcliffe Infirmary (Oxford), Charing Cross Hospital (London), and The Princess Alexandra Hospital (Brisbane). Sequential BPVP was reserved for patients in whom unilateral PVP resulted in inadequate symptomatic relief ($n = 6$). Simultaneous BPVP ($n = 47$) was performed in cases where there were essentially bilateral symmetrical symptoms. All patients underwent identical neurological assessments at each of the three participating centres. Changes in medication were avoided until after the first postoperative assessment.

4. NEUROLOGICAL ASSESSMENTS

Neurological assessments were performed independent of the surgeon. The assessment protocol comprised the UPDRS, Hoehn and Yahr staging, and Schwab and England scores. Confrontational visual fields were plotted using a Humphrey field analyser. Initial outcome assessments were performed at 3–6 mo as it was not feasible to assess all patients at a strictly defined time-point postoperatively. Further assessments were made at about 12 mo postoperatively and have continued annually.

5. STATISTICAL ANALYSIS

Individual items from the UPDRS are described with median values and the interquartile range. Significance was tested with the Wilcoxon Signed Rank Sum test using paired, two-tailed exact tests. For subscores and medications, mean values with 95% confidence intervals are reported and tested

Table 1
Demographics of Patients Undergoing Bilateral Pallidotomy

Follow-up group	3 mo (values are means with 95% CI)	12 mo (values are means with minimum and maximum range)[a]
Total included in analysis	53	17
Simultaneous/staged procedure	47/6	15/2
Age at surgery (yr)	64 (61.2–66.6)	65 (45–78)
Length of PD history at surgery (yr)	14.9 (13.2–16.5)	16.3 (5–35)
Follow up time (mo)	3.4 (3.2–3.7)	12 (9–15)
Modified Hoehn & Yahr staging (median with interquartile range)	4 (3–5) OFF	4 (2.5–5) OFF
	3 (2.5–3.875) ON	3 (2–4) ON
Total UPDRS	94 (87–101) OFF	87 (51–134) OFF
	54 (49–50) ON	44.6 (21–66) ON
L-dopa (mg)	1017 (881–1152)	891 (0–2000)
Dopa-agonist (equivalent L-dopa dose) (mg)	89 (56–123)	47 (0–250)
L-dopa equivalent unit (LEU) total (mg)[b]	1107 (971–1244)	938 (0–2000)

[a]Used because the small number of values in this group are non-normally distributed.
[b]Calculated on basis of L-dopa adjusted for COMT inhibitors and theoretical equivalency of dopamine agonists.

with Student's two-tailed *t*-test for paired values. To minimize the chance of false positive results (in view of the large number of analyses performed) we accepted a p value of <0.001 as evidence for significant change. However, since effect size and confidence intervals should also be taken into account, we have also reported p values of less than 0.05. It should be borne in mind that equally large positive and negative changes within a group of scores will not affect the overall distribution and will therefore appear nonsignificant. The limited range (0–4) of scores for items in the UPDRS may create a "floor" effect and, to a lesser extent, a "ceiling" effect on changes. This is particularly problematic as most 0 scores mean "normal," which is realistically unlikely to be achieved and therefore sets the "floor" for an individual item at a score of 1.

The results have been described in charts as percentage reductions in postoperative scores compared to the preoperative baseline. This has the advantage of allowing easy comparison of different groups and outcome measures. However, it also tends to emphasize changes to lower scores (e.g., 10 reducing to 3 = 70%, but 4 reducing to 1 = 75%).

5.1. Results from 3- and 12-mo Follow Up

5.1.1. Off Period Scores (Fig. 4)

All scores improved significantly at 3 mo. Motor scores (UPDRS, Part III) were reduced by 31% with a greater effect on tremor and rigidity than bradykinesia and gait. In the group followed to 12 mo similar results were observed but only improvements in activities of daily living (ADL) (UPDRS, Part II) and gait remained significant at the later assessment. All other scores were improved from baseline but failed to reach statistical significance ($0.05 < p > 0.001$).

5.1.2. On Period Scores

Motor scores (UPDRS, Part III), ADL scores (UPDRS, Part II), and gait were significantly improved at 3 mo. Improvements in bradykinesia, tremor and rigidity were borderline significant. At 12 mo these improvements had diminished and were no longer significant.

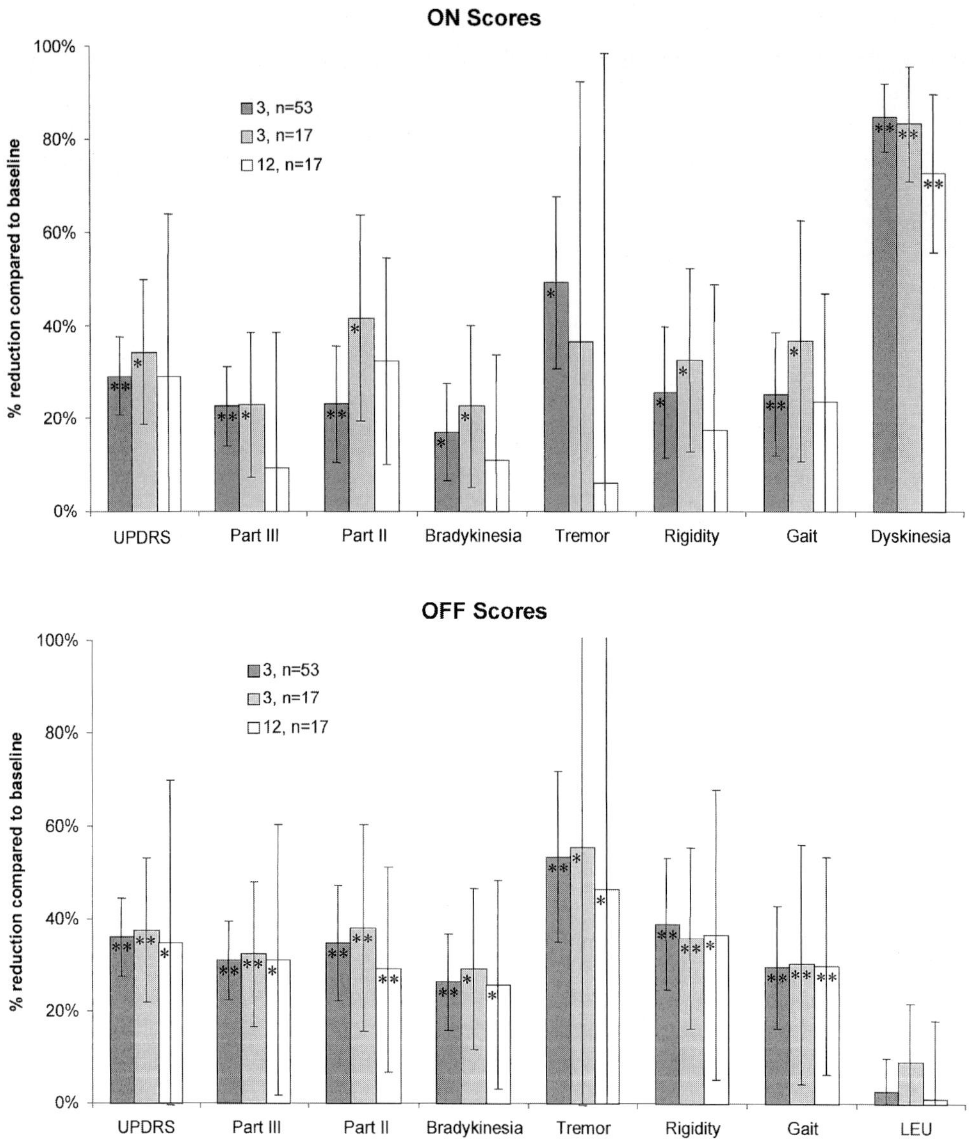

Fig. 4. Reduction in UPDRS scores in medication ON and OFF state compared to baseline at 3 mo ($n = 53$ and $n = 17$) and 12 mo ($n = 17$). The same group of 17 patients was studied at 3 and 12 months. Lines indicate 95% confidence intervals. $*p < 0.05$, $**p < 0.001$. LEU is L-dopa equivalent units (100 mg L-dopa; 133 mg sustained release L-dopa; 1 mg pergolide; 10 mg bromocriptine, 1 mg pramipexole, 1 mg cabergoline, 6 mg ropinirole, 1 mg lisuride, 20 mg apomorphine were assumed to be equivalent.

5.1.3. Dyskinesia

Overall dyskinesia score was significantly reduced by 85% at 3 mo. This declined to 73% in the group followed to12 mo.

5.1.4. Medications

There were no significant postoperative changes in medications and medication doses.

5.1.5. Other Relevant Changes

At 3-mo follow up ($n = 53$) early morning dystonia, unpredictable off periods, and sudden off periods were abolished in 63, 78, and 88% of patients, respectively. However, between 3 and 12 mo there was a return of early morning dystonia in 30% of patients. Time spent in the off state was improved significantly in 33% of patients. This was maintained at 12 mo but failed to reach statistical significance.

5.2. Long-Term Outcome

Although we attempted to continue annual assessment of patients, several patients declined to return and a few underwent further procedures at this centre. Those ($n = 10$) who were assessed at 24 mo or longer are presented in Fig. 5. The longest follow-up assessments averaged 35 mo, with a range of 24–48 mo. In this subgroup, improvements in UPDRS scores at 3 mo generally matched or exceeded those reported for the larger group of 53 patients. At this point most of the on medication improvements had deteriorated almost to baseline state. Rigidity and dyskinesia continued to be reduced but only the dyskinesia score approached statistical significance. Improvements while off medication deteriorated less at the longest follow-up evaluation. All scores except for bradykinesia approached statistical significance. Changes in medication dosage did not achieve statistical significance.

5.2.1. Operative Complications

No major complications such as haemorrhage, stroke, infection, or visual-field deficit were encountered in any of the patients undergoing bilateral pallidotomy, including those patients excluded from statistical analysis.

5.2.2. Adverse Effects

Given the irreversible nature of ablative surgery, adverse events are of particular importance. We looked for items of the UPDRS that had worsened at the 3–6 mo postoperative assessment. Only speech while on medication, as reported by the patient, significantly worsened ($p = 0.04$). However, using the five-point scale, it is possible that scores that were low preoperatively, such as while on medication, are more likely to worsen due to a “floor” effect. However, based on our clinical experience, we feel that some of these changes may be clinically relevant.

Speech or salivation was worsened in 26–30% of patients, both on and off medication, by an average of 1.2 points. Our impression is that speech may become more hypophonic and dysarthric after surgery. Of greater concern is that 23% of patients reported a worsening of gait freezing on medication, by an average of almost two points. This was recognized quite early in the series as it often occurred in patients who had never suffered on-period gait freezing before surgery. Up to 25% of patients reported deterioration in one or more measures of bradykinesia while on medication including handwriting. Again, these changes averaged only one point. Three patients developed difficulty opening their eyes postoperatively due to eyelid opening apraxia.

6. NEUROPSYCHOLOGICAL AND FUNCTIONAL ASSESSMENTS

Neuropsychological testing, psychiatric screening, and questionnaire measures of psychological symptomatology, functional disability, and quality of life, were obtained routinely on all patients presenting for pallidotomy to the Oxford Movement Disorder Group. To date, 88 patients have been reviewed in a consecutive series of 34 bilateral and 54 unilateral procedures. Patients were assessed at preoperative baseline, and at 3–6 mo postoperatively. The first eight patients to be tested following simultaneous bilateral pallidotomy were reexamined at 3 mo and have been reported in detail elsewhere *(46)*. This was extended to 6 mo for the latter part of the series. All assessments were carried out with patients in their optimal state while on medication.

The analysis of changes in the group mean scores on psychometric test measures following bilateral pallidotomy has revealed surprisingly selective changes given the concerns that have been expressed

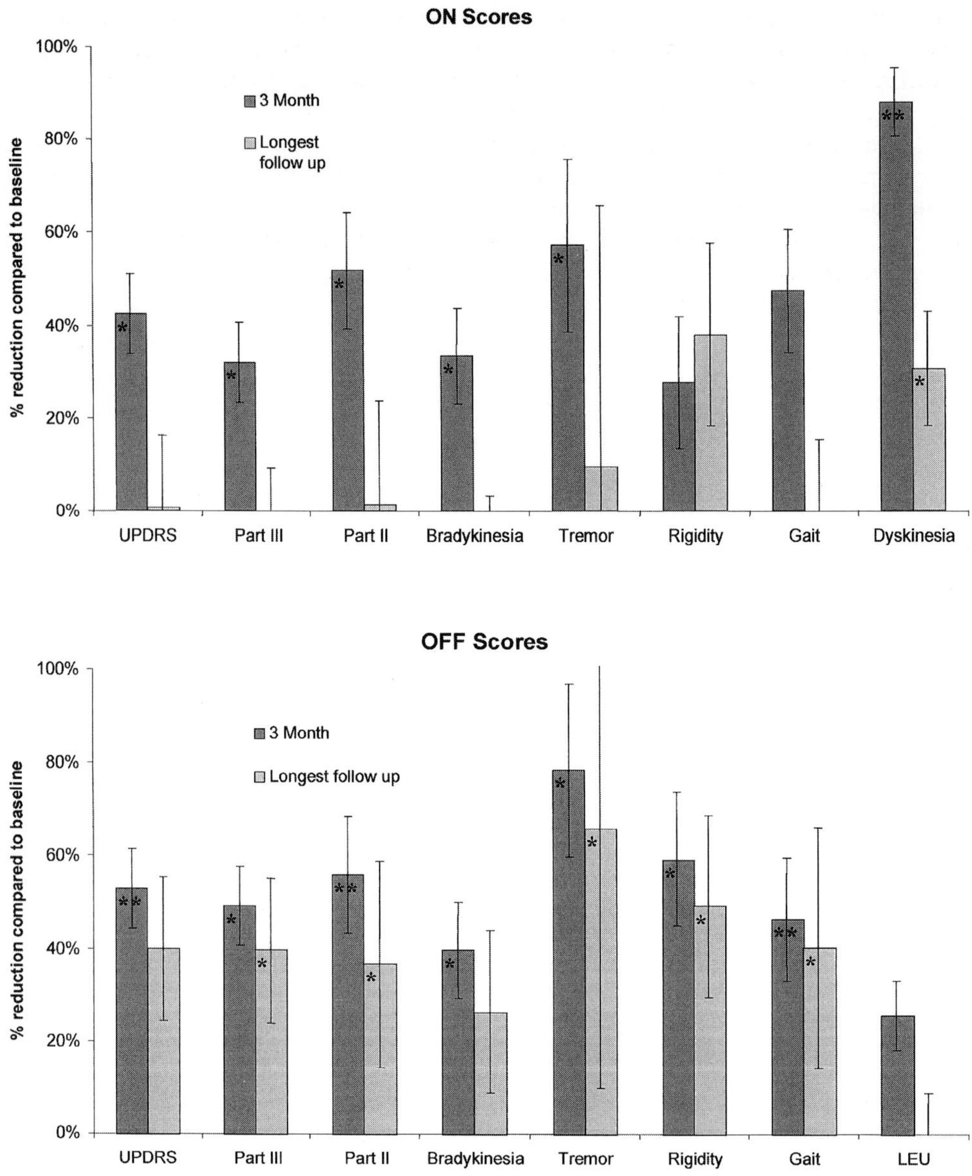

Fig. 5. Reduction in UPDRS scores in medication ON and OFF states at 3 mo and longest follow-up (mean 35 mo, $n = 10$) compared to baseline. $*p < 0.05$, $**p < 0.001$.

in the literature about cognitive risks associated with this procedure. In our series there has been only one case of global cognitive deterioration *(46)*. However, there was a clear pattern of deterioration in performance on tests of both categorical and phonemic verbal fluency. This deterioration was more marked for phonemic fluency (25%) than categorical verbal fluency (15%). Early data on tests of speech articulation rate *(46)* suggested postoperative deterioration, but the data from the complete series suggest no such change and on the same test, we have observed improvements following unilateral procedures. This finding is in contrast to the relatively high rate of subjective reports of a worsening in motor speech function following bilateral pallidotomy. However, a number of subjective symptoms are not infrequently concerned with hypophonia and/or increased hypersalivation and drooling. In our larger series, we have also identified a 10% deterioration in performance on the Boston naming test. There have been no changes in spatial functions despite the fact that right unilateral pallidotomy was associated with a 20% deterioration in performance on the Judgement Of Line Orientation test. Although effects of bilateral pallidotomy might be expected to reflect combined sequelae of left and right unilateral pallidotomy, in this series simultaneous bilateral pallidotomy has been performed with a smaller nondominant lesion. Surgical technique may therefore explain this apparent discrepancy.

A significant group deterioration in performance on the digit span subtest has also been observed together with a trend towards deterioration in performance on a constellation of other tests of attention-executive function such as tests of word list learning, the Stroop test, and drawing of a complex geometrical figure. We have conducted other more detailed studies of attention-executive function in a smaller series of 12 patients undergoing bilateral pallidotomy and confirmed the finding of a consistent postoperative failure in ability to perform extra-dimensional attentional set-shifting.

There were no psychiatric symptoms following bilateral pallidotomy. Questionnaire measures of psychological symptomatology showed no significant change in symptoms of depression but some evidence for reduction in pre-operative anxiety. Although no quantitative measures were applied, approx 16–20% of patients reported postoperative changes in personality consistent with a "dys-executive" syndrome, including flattening of affect or poor impulse control. A similar rate of change in these categories has been reported in patients undergoing unilateral pallidotomy *(47)*.

Disease-specific and generic quality of life questionnaire measures including the SF-36, the Parkinson's Disease Questionaire-39, the Hospital Anxiety and Depression Scale, and the Functional Limitations Profile (FLP) (UK version of the Sickness Impact Profile) have shown significant improvements in group mean scores following bilateral pallidotomy. Unilateral pallidotomy has been associated with similar improvements, but these have been confined to the mobility and ADL sub-scales of the PDQ-39 and the social and physical subscales of the SF-36. We have found no significant improvement on any of the FLP subscales following unilateral pallidotomy. Bilateral pallidotomy has been associated with significant improvements in communication, cognition, bodily discomfort, stigma, and emotion as measured by the PDQ-39. Similarly, both physical and psychosocial subscales of the FLP improve significantly.

In order to investigate the validity and meaning of patient-rated questionnaire findings, a caregiver-rated version of the FLP was also given to a subsample of 16 patients undergoing bilateral pallidotomy. There was no significant difference between patient and caregiver ratings pre-operatively, However, postoperatively a significant discrepancy emerged between patient and caregiver ratings of improvements in psycho-social function, with patients rating 30% improvement and carers rating only 15% improvement despite general agreement on the level of physical disability and percentage of postoperative improvement. Because of deterioration in attention and executive functions following this procedure, the differences that emerge between caregiver and patient ratings on postoperative quality of life measures may be explained by abnormalities in patient insight. Long-term follow-up of functional disability indices over 5 yr suggest that following immediate postoperative gains of approx 30%, patients group mean scores return to baseline levels of functional disability at 3.5–4 yr, postoperatively.

7. DISCUSSION

7.1. Extent and Longevity of Benefit

Bilateral pallidotomy alleviates the motor side effects associated with long-term medical therapy and alleviates most symptoms of parkinsonism. The principal benefit following pallidotomy is reduced L-dopa dyskinesia. The procedure is reliable and has a low risk for major complications. Many PD patients experience good results from medical therapy for years until the appearance of dyskinesia, dystonia, and motor fluctuations. All of these can be significantly improved by pallidotomy thereby allowing patients to continue to enjoy the benefit of medical therapy. During "off" periods the most disabling symptoms of rigidity, tremor, gait impairment, and bradykinesia are alleviated by pallidotomy.

These benefits are maintained for at least 1 yr and our long-term data suggests this can continue relative to baseline for 2–4 yr in individual cases and with respect to certain symptoms.

Using our surgical technique, a bilateral procedure can be performed within 1 h, which is easily tolerated by most patients and may reduce operative complications such as deep venous thrombosis and infection. The simplicity and reliability of using macrostimulation and clinical assessment allows the technique to be applied in centres where time or cost considerations are a limiting factor. Repeat operation is rarely required and no further intervention other than optimisation of medical therapy is needed. This contrasts with DBS procedures that require many hours of postoperative adjustment and replacement of the pulse generator every 3–5 yr.

7.2. *Costs and Limitations*

Based on the UPDRS, some symptoms of parkinsonism deteriorate in up to 30% of patients after surgery. Those most commonly reported are worsening of speech and increased salivation both while on and off medication. Others that deteriorate less commonly but that are of significant concern are gait freezing, handwriting, and bradykinesia. These are predominantly worsened in the "on" state lending support to what is sometimes reported by patients, a "blunting" of benefit from medication. In some cases this leads patients to increase the dose or frequency of medication in an effort to achieve the therapeutic effect experienced before surgery. It has also been our experience that some patients, despite obvious improvements in their "on" and "off" state after surgery, complain of less apparent benefit from medication. Possible explanations for this include an actual change in the subjective benefit produced by medication, a slowing of the switch from "off" to "on" state, and a narrowing of the difference between symptoms in the "off" and "on" state. Despite improvements in off medication symptoms and motor fluctuations, most of our patients did not report significantly less "off" time after surgery and the need for frequent medication doses remained unchanged.

The improvement in dyskinesia declines over time. Although we have observed that any return of limb dyskinesia tends to be mild and nondisabling, there was a marked increase in reported dyskinesia in the long-term follow-up group. Review of these cases suggests that many had axial (orofacial, neck, trunk) dyskinesia before surgery, which does not appear to show long-term improvement following pallidotomy. Since observing this, we have considered axial dyskinesia to be a contraindication for pallidotomy, although it may still develop after otherwise successful surgery in suitable candidates.

The improvements in UPDRS scores appear to be maximal within the first 6 mo after surgery with a gradual decline thereafter. The small number of longer-term follow-up assessments limits our conclusions but it seems clear that within 12 mo, improvements while on medication are lost and patients may gradually return to their preoperative level within 3 yr. Although functional gains are proportionally greater for bilateral than unilateral pallidotomy, benefits appear to return to baseline levels over a similar period of time.

Other than the high risk for decline in word finding ability and our more recent findings of a selective "dysexecutive" deficit, our analysis of group central nervous system (CNS) effects and subjective reports suggests that bilateral pallidotomy can be a relatively benign procedure from a cognitive viewpoint. However, these findings may be misleading, because inspection of individual pre- and postoperative neuropsychological testing suggests considerable individual variation, which is masked by group mean scores. Individual patients have shown improvement as well as decline in scores in several cognitive domains. A possible cause of improvement may be attentional gains following relief of distracting motor symptoms. Although patients and caregivers have been satisfied with functional and quality of life outcomes following BPVP, our findings suggest that this procedure should only be employed while using extremely careful patient selection together with explicit and detailed consenting. The clinical significance of the cognitive deficits we have identified in patients with advanced PD who undergo pallidotomy remains uncertain. Special caution may need to be exercised with respect to bilateral pallidotomy in children with generalized dystonia *(48)* as there may be delayed functional sequelae if lesions are acquired at or before the completed emergence of executive skills in the middle years of childhood *(49)*.

8. CONCLUSIONS

Bilateral pallidotomy has definite advantages over unilateral pallidotomy for reduction of symptoms and side effects of medication. Moreover, benefits may not be apparent from UPDRS scores alone as we have found that questionnaire measures of functional disability reported by patients and caregivers may be more sensitive to these gains. Nevertheless, it must be questioned whether the additional benefits from the bilateral procedure outweigh the increased risks. Adverse effects are approximately double those of unilateral pallidotomy for deterioration in speech, salivation, and "on" period gait freezing. In most cases the need for a bilateral procedure is due to bilaterally disabling dyskinesia but in our experience the procedure is more effective for limb than axial dyskinesia.

The initial benefits of pallidotomy are experienced both while on and off medication. However this benefit appears to decline gradually over time. Patients continue to require medical therapy, which exposes them to the risk of future adverse effects. Patients likely to need further surgical intervention after bilateral pallidotomy may not experience the same benefit as surgically naïve candidates and it is likely that the risk of adverse effects will be higher. In our limited experience of performing subthalamic surgery in these situations the results have been poor.

Since the development of pallidal and STN DBS there have been increasing numbers of publications with favorable results *(39,50–53)*. As a nonlesional procedure it may minimize permanent side effects and may therefore be performed bilaterally. Stimulation parameters can be adjusted postoperatively to achieve maximal effect. Bilateral pallidal and STN DBS have produced results that appear to surpass those of unilateral or bilateral pallidotomy. However, there have been no direct comparisons of lesioning and DBS surgery and, as the experience with DBS grows, it seems unlikely that a decisive randomized trial will be carried out. An argument has been made to abandon lesioning surgery altogether in view of these developments. However it has not yet been established that DBS has greater long-term benefit than lesioning surgery. At present DBS procedures are lengthy and, similar to some opinions concerning lesioning surgery, are believed by many to require microelectrode recording to properly position the DBS electrode. The more prolonged procedure required by microelectrode recording may be poorly tolerated by some patients and, because of multiple electrode insertions, may possibly increase the risk of haemorrhage although this point has not been established in prospective trials *(54)*. The cost of the equipment and necessary replacement of some components may be prohibitive for many healthcare delivery systems and out of reach for the majority of undeveloped countries. The need for repeated postoperative adjustment and assessment places strain on both the patient and clinical resources and may not be practical in situations where the patient cannot easily travel. Finally, the implantation and adjustment of DBS probably requires a greater degree of technical skill and experience than lesioning surgery, which is also likely to delay availability to larger numbers of suitable patients.

As DBS becomes more commonplace, it is likely that the cost implications will remain a factor in its provision. Whether these costs can be offset by reduced drug usage or a net reduction in dependency on the healthcare delivery system remains to be seen. What is certain is that the aging Western population will provide an increasing number of candidates for surgery and that, as the safety of these procedures improves, the proportion of those considered suitable will also increase.

We believe that bilateral pallidotomy can be performed reliably and reasonably safely with significant benefits for symptoms of L-dopa dyskinesia, motor fluctuations, tremor, rigidity, gait disturbance, and bradykinesia. The benefits of surgery diminish over time but some persist for at least 3–4 yr. Bilateral pallidotomy may therefore continue to be a useful surgical procedure in carefully selected patients. Inevitably, the decision on which surgical procedure to offer individual patients will continue to be influenced by financial constraints, geography, and individual preference.

REFERENCES

1. Cooper, I. S. (1954) Intracerebral injection of procaine into the globus pallidus in hyperkinetic disorders. *Science* **119,** 417–418.
2. Spiegel, E. A. and Wycis, H. T. (1954) Ansotomy in paralysis agitans. *Arch. Neurol. Psychiatry* **71,** 598–614.
3. Reichert, T. (1962b) Long term follow up of results of stereotaxic treatment of extrapyramidal disorders. *Confinia Neurol.* **22,** 356–363.
4. Krayenbuhl, H. O., Wyss, O., et al. (1961) Bilateral thalamotomy and pallidotomy as treatment for bilateral parkinsonism. *J. Neurosurg.* **16,** 429–444.
5. Cotzias, G., Papavasiliou, P., et al. (1969) Long term effects of DOPA on parkinsonism: a proposal. In: *Third Symposium on Parkinson's Disease.* Livingstone, Edinburgh.
6. Hoehn, M. M. and Yahr, M. D. (1969) Evaluation of the long term results of surgical therapy. In: *Third Symposium on Parkinson's Disease* Livingstone, Edinburgh, UK, pp. 274–280.
7. Poewe, W. H., Lees, A. J., and Stern, G. M. (1986) Low-dose L-dopa therapy in Parkinson's disease: a 6-year follow-up study. *Neurology* **36,** 1528–1530.
8. Davis, G. C., Williams, A. C., Markey, S. P., Ebert, M. H., Caine, E. D., Reichert, C. M., et al. (1979) Chronic Parkinsonism secondary to intravenous injection of meperidine analogues. *Psychiatry Res.* **1,** 249–254.
9. Langston, J. W., Ballard, P., Tetrud, J. W., and Irwin, I. (1983) Chronic Parkinsonism in humans due to a product of meperidine-analog synthesis. *Science* **219,** 979–980.
10. Forno, L. S., Langston, J. W., DeLanney, L. E., Irwin, I., and Ricaurte, G. A. (1986) Locus ceruleus lesions and eosinophilic inclusions in MPTP-treated monkeys. *Ann. Neurol.* **20,** 449–455.
11. Burns, R. S., Chiueh, C. C., Markey, S. P., Ebert, M. H., Jacobowitz, D. M., and Kopin, I. J. (1983) A primate model of parkinsonism: selective destruction of dopaminergic neurons in the pars compacta of the substantia nigra by N-methyl-4- phenyl-1,2,3,6-tetrahydropyridine. *Proc. Natl. Acad. Sci. USA* **80,** 4546–4550.
12. Delong, M. R., Georgopoulos, A. P., Crutcher, M. D., Mitchell, S. J., Richardson, R. T., and Alexander, G. E. (1984) Functional organization of the basal ganglia: contributions of single-cell recording studies. In: *Functions of the Basal Ganglia* (Evered, D. and O'Connor, M., eds.), Pitman, London, pp. 64–82.
13. DeLong, M. R. (1990) Primate models of movement disorders of basal ganglia origin. *Trends Neurosci.* **13,** 281–285.
14. Filion, M. and Tremblay, L. (1991) Abnormal spontaneous activity of globus pallidus neurons in monkeys with MPTP-induced parkinsonism. *Brain Res.* **547,** 142–151.
15. Mitchell, I. J., Clarke, C. E., Boyce, S., Robertson, R. G., Peggs, D., Sambrook, M. A., et al. (1989) Neural mechanisms underlying parkinsonian symptoms based upon regional uptake of 2-deoxyglucose in monkeys exposed to 1-methyl-4-phenyl- 1,2,3,6-tetrahydropyridine. *Neuroscience* **32,** 213–226.
16. Bergman, H., Wichmann, T., and DeLong, M. R. (1990) Reversal of experimental parkinsonism by lesions of the subthalamic nucleus. *Science* **249,** 1436–1438.
17. Aziz, T. Z., Peggs, D., Sambrook, M. A., and Crossman, A. R. (1991) Lesion of the subthalamic nucleus for the alleviation of 1-methyl-4-phenyl-1,2,3,6-tetrahydropyridine (MPTP)-induced parkinsonism in the primate. *Mov. Disord.* **6,** 288–292.
18. Benazzouz, A., Gross, C., Feger, J., Boraud, T., and Bioulac, B. (1993) Reversal of rigidity and improvement in motor performance by subthalamic high-frequency stimulation in MPTP-treated monkeys. *Eur. J. Neurosci.* **5,** 382–389.
19. Sellal, F., Hirsch, E., Lisovoski, F., Mutschler, V., Collard, M., and Marescaux, C. (1992) Contralateral disappearance of parkinsonian signs after subthalamic hematoma. *Neurology* **42,** 255–256.
20. Aziz, T. Z., Peggs, D., Agarwal, E., Sambrook, M. A., and Crossman, A. R. (1992) Subthalamic nucleotomy alleviates parkinsonism in the 1-methyl-4-phenyl-1,2,3,6-tetrahydropyridine (MPTP)-exposed primate. *Br. J. Neurosurg.* **6,** 575–582.
21. Robertson, R. G., Clarke, C. A., Boyce, S., Sambrook, M. A., and Crossman, A. R. (1990) The role of striatopallidal neurones utilizing gamma-aminobutyric acid in the pathophysiology of MPTP-induced parkinsonism in the primate: evidence from. *Brain Res.* **531,** 95–104.
22. Laitinen, L. V., Bergenheim, A. T., and Hariz, M. I. (1992) Leksell's posteroventral pallidotomy in the treatment of Parkinson's disease. *J. Neurosurg.* **76,** 53–61.
23. Svennilson, E., Torvik, A., Lowe, R., and Leksell, L. (1960) Treatment of parkinsonism by stereotactic thermolesions in the pallidal region. *Acta Psychiatr. Neurol. Scand.* **35,** 358–377.
24. Sutton, J. P., Couldwell, W., Lew, M. F., Mallory, L., Grafton, S., DeGiorgio, C., et al. (1995) Ventroposterior medial pallidotomy in patients with advanced Parkinson's disease. *Neurosurgery* **36,** 1112–1116; discussion 1116–1117.
25. Iacono, R. P., Lonser, R. R., Oh, A., and Yamada, S. (1995) New pathophysiology of Parkinson's disease revealed by posteroventral pallidotomy. *Neurol. Res.* **17,** 178–180.
26. Baron, M. S., Vitek, J. L., Bakay, R. A., Green, J., Kaneoke, Y., Hashimoto, T., et al. (1996) Treatment of advanced Parkinson's disease by posterior GPi pallidotomy: 1–year results of a pilot study. *Ann. Neurol.* **40,** 355–366.
27. Dalvi, A., Winfield, L., Yu, Q., Cote, L., Goodman, R. R., and Pullman, S. L. (1999) Stereotactic posteroventral pallidotomy: clinical methods and results at 1-year follow up. *Mov. Disord.* **14,** 256–261.
28. de Bie, R. M., de Haan, R. J., Nijssen, P. C., Rutgers, A. W., Beute, G. N., Bosch, D. A., et al. (1999) Unilateral pallidotomy in Parkinson's disease: a randomised, single-blind, multicentre trial. *Lancet* **354,** 1665–1669.
29. Dogali, M., Fazzini, E., Kolodny, E., Eidelberg, D., Sterio, D., Devinsky, O., et al. (1995) Stereotactic ventral pallidotomy for Parkinson's disease. *Neurology* **45,** 753–761.

30. Giller, C. A., Dewey, R. B., Ginsburg, M. I., Mendelsohn, D. B., and Berk, A. M. (1998) Stereotactic pallidotomy and thalamotomy using individual variations of anatomic landmarks for localization. *Neurosurgery* **42,** 56–62; discussion 62–65.
31. Lang, A. E., Lozano, A. M., Montgomery, E., Duff, J., Tasker, R., and Hutchinson, W. (1997) Posteroventral medial pallidotomy in advanced Parkinson's disease. *N. Engl. J. Med.* **337,** 1036–1042.
32. Shannon, K. M., Penn, R. D., Kroin, J. S., Adler, C. H., Janko, K. A., York, M., et al. (1998) Stereotactic pallidotomy for the treatment of Parkinson's disease. Efficacy and adverse effects at 6 months in 26 patients. *Neurology* **50,** 434–438.
33. Jankovic, J., Lai, E., Ben-Arie, L., Krauss, J. K., and Grossman, R. (1999) Levodopa-induced dyskinesias treated by pallidotomy. *J. Neurol. Sci.* **167,** 62–67.
34. Ondo, W. G., Jankovic, J., Lai, E. C., Sankhla, C., Khan, M., Ben-Arie, L., et al. (1998) Assessment of motor function after stereotactic pallidotomy. *Neurology* **50,** 266–270.
35. Samuel, M., Caputo, E., Brooks, D. J., Schrag, A., Scaravilli, T., Branston, N. M., et al. (1998) A study of medial pallidotomy for Parkinson's disease: clinical outcome, MRI location and complications. *Brain* **121(Pt 1),** 59–75.
36. Uitti, R. J., Wharen, R. E. Jr., and Turk, M. F. (1998) Efficacy of levodopa therapy on motor function after posteroventral pallidotomy for Parkinson's disease. *Neurology* **51,** 1755–1757.
37. Alterman, R. L. and Kelly, P. J. (1998) Pallidotomy technique and results: the New York University experience. *Neurosurg. Clin. North Am.* **9,** 337–343.
38. Pollak, P., Benabid, A. L., Gross, C., Gao, D. M., Laurent, A., Benazzouz, A., et al. (1993) [Effects of the stimulation of the subthalamic nucleus in Parkinson disease]. *Rev. Neurol. (Paris)* **149,** 175–176.
39. Limousin, P., Krack, P., Pollak, P., Benazzouz, A., Ardouin, C., Hoffmann, D., et al. (1998) Electrical stimulation of the subthalamic nucleus in advanced Parkinson's disease. *N. Engl. J. Med.* **339,** 1105–1111.
40. Alexander, E. III, Kooy, H. M., van Herk, M., Schwartz, M., Barnes, P. D., Tarbell, N., et al. (1995) Magnetic resonance image-directed stereotactic neurosurgery: use of image fusion with computerized tomography to enhance spatial accuracy. *J. Neurosurg.* **83,** 271–276.
41. Kooy, H. M., van Herk, M., Barnes, P. D., Alexander, E. III, Dunbar, S. F., Tarbell, N. J., et al. (1994) Image fusion for stereotactic radiotherapy and radiosurgery treatment planning. *Int. J. Radiat. Oncol. Biol. Phys.* **28,** 1229–1234.
42. Schaltenbrand, G. and Wahren, W. (eds.) (1977) *Atlas for Stereotaxy of the Human Brain.* Thieme, Stuttgart.
43. Aziz, T. Z. and Bain, P. G. (1996) A multidisciplinary approach to tremor. *Br. J. Neurosurg.* **10,** 435–437.
44. Munro-Davies, L. E., Gregory, R., Squires, W., Radatz, M., Silburn, P., Scott, R., et al. (1999) Lateral pallidotomy exacerbates akinesia in the Parkinsonian patient. *J. Clin. Neurosci.* **6,** 474–476.

44a. Vitek, J., Bakay, R., and DeLong, M. (1997) Microelectrode-guided pallidotomy for medically intractable Parkinson's disease. In: *Advances in Neurology* (Obeso, J., DeLong, M., Ohye, C., and Marsden, C. D., eds.), Lippincott-Raven, Philadelphia, PA, pp. 183–198.

44b. Esklander, E. N., Cosgrove, G. R., Shinobu, L. A., and Penney, J. B. (1998) The importance of accurate lesion placement in posteroventral pallidotomy: report of two cases. *J. Neurosurg.* **89,** 630–634.

44c. Bronte-Stewart, H. M., Hill, B., Molander, M. P., Kaufman, R. L., Pappas, C., Fross, R. D., and Klingman, J. (1998) Lesion location predicts clinical outcome of pallidotomy. *Mov. Disord.* **13(Suppl. 2),** 300.

45. Gibb, W. R. and Lees, A. J. (1988) The relevance of the Lewy body to the pathogenesis of idiopathic Parkinson's disease. *J. Neurol. Neurosurg. Psychiatry* **51,** 745–752.
46. Scott, R., Gregory, R., Hines, N., Carroll, C., Hyman, N., Papanasstasiou, V., et al. (1998) Neuropsychological, neurological and functional outcome following pallidotomy for Parkinson's disease. A consecutive series of eight simultaneous bilateral and twelve unilateral procedures. *Brain* **121(Pt 4),** 659–675.
47. Trepanier, L. L., Saint-Cyr, J. A., Lozano, A. M., and Lang, A. E. (1998) Neuropsychological consequences of posteroventral pallidotomy for the treatment of Parkinson's disease. *Neurology* **51,** 207–215.
48. Lozano, A. M., Kumar, R., Gross, R. E., Giladi, N., Hutchison, W. D., Dostrovsky, J. O., et al. (1997) Globus pallidus internus pallidotomy for generalized dystonia. *Mov. Disord.* **12,** 865–870.
49. Luciana, M. and Nelson, C. A. (1998) The functional emergence of prefrontally-guided working memory systems in four- to eight-year-old children. *Neuropsychologia* **36,** 273–293.
50. Kumar, R., Lozano, A. M., Kim, Y. J., Hutchison, W. D., Sime, E., Halket, E., et al. (1998) Double-blind evaluation of subthalamic nucleus deep brain stimulation in advanced Parkinson's disease. *Neurology* **51,** 850–855.
51. Moro, E., Scerrati, M., Romito, L. M., Roselli, R., Tonali, P., and Albanese, A. (1999) Chronic subthalamic nucleus stimulation reduces medication requirements in Parkinson's disease. *Neurology* **53,** 85–90.
52. Volkmann, J., Sturm, V., Weiss, P., Kappler, J., Voges, J., Koulousakis, A., et al. (1998) Bilateral high-frequency stimulation of the internal globus pallidus in advanced Parkinson's disease. *Ann. Neurol.* **44,** 953–961.
53. Houeto, J. L., Damier, P., Bejjani, P. B., Staedler, C., Bonnet, A. M., Arnulf, I., et al. (2000) Subthalamic stimulation in Parkinson disease: a multidisciplinary approach. *Arch. Neurol.* **57,** 461–465.
54. Carroll, C. B., Scott, R., Davies, L. E., and Aziz, T. (1998) The pallidotomy debate. *Br. J. Neurosurg.* **12,** 146–150.

transient hemiballism in five patients, in no case was it prolonged and the lesions were reported to be otherwise safe. Houdart et al. *(12)* tried a slightly different lesion involving partial destruction of the cerebellorubrothalamic pathway with the lesion placed medial to STN and lateral to the red nucleus, below the nucleus ventrolateralis (VL) of the thalamus. In their series of 47 patients with PD, one developed athetoid movements that appeared 1 mo after surgery and persisted for 10 mo, whereas another developed hemiballism that disappeared with medical treatment. Thus, although confirmation of target accuracy in the pre-MRI era was uncertain, it is not the case that STN ablation is an altogether new procedure.

Stereotactic surgery is sometimes used for treatment of hemiballism. It is intriguing that the effective target appears to be a lesion involving pallidofugal fibers and the zona incerta *(13)*, which lie immediately dorsal to STN. Because it is likely that either lesions or DBS of STN will involve zona incerta and pallidofugal fibers, it is possible that damage to these areas effectively counteracts any prodyskinetic effect of the STN lesion.

By the mid 1980s, with the availability of an animal model of PD—the 1-methyl-4-phenyl-1,2,3,6-tetrahydropyridine (MPTP) lesioned monkey—there developed greater understanding of basal ganglia function and circuitry *(13)* and an appreciation of the pivotal role of the STN within basal ganglia circuitry. Hyperactivity of the STN is now considered a hallmark of the parkinsonian state as demonstrated by microelectrode recordings in MPTP lesioned monkeys *(14)* and in patients undergoing surgery for PD *(15)*. Increased activity in STN leads, through its glutamatergic excitatory effect, to increased activity in the GPi and substantia nigra pars reticulata (SNpr), which in turn overinhibit thalamocortical and brainstem projections. Excitotoxic or thermolytic lesions or STN DBS in MPTP monkeys have been shown to alleviate many parkinsonian symptoms *(16–19)*. Bergman et al. were the first to report improvement in contralateral akinesia, rigidity, and postural tremor after unilateral injection of ibotenic acid into the STN in two MPTP monkeys *(16)*. Both monkeys developed hemichorea which lasted 1 wk in one animal and persisted to the time of sacrifice in the other. Subsequently Aziz et al. *(17)* lesioned the STN in six monkeys with MPTP parkinsonism. In three of these monkeys, hemichorea persisted for up to 8 wk. Guridi and Obeso *(18)* lesioned STN in five monkeys with MPTP parkinsonism, all of which developed hemichorea. Benazzouz et al. reported improvement in motor performance during high-frequency stimulation in the STN in two hemiparkinsonian MPTP monkeys without inducing dyskinesia or hemiballism. Thus, although animal studies suggested that STN appeared to be a rational target for functional surgery in PD, the possibility of hemiballism, based on clinical experience with hemmorhages and infarcts in STN, and reports of hemiballism in STN lesioned monkey models of PD has understandably made surgeons reluctant to consider it as a target for ablation.

Benabid et al. *(20)* observed that chronic DBS in the ventralis intermedius nucleus (Vim) of the thalamus had the same beneficial effect as a lesion for treatment of tremor. They observed that if adverse effects occurred with stimulation these were reversible by adjustment of stimulation parameters. They then carried out STN DBS with the assumption that any involuntary movements produced by stimulation would be reversible *(3–5,21)*. Benabid et al. demonstrated 60% improvement in most aspects of "off" state parkinsonism measured by the Unified Parkinson's Disease Rating Scale (UPDRS), including improvement in gait and axial symptoms *(21)*. Unlike pallidotomy, STN stimulation allows reduction of L-dopa dose by approx 50%, as a consequence of which dyskinesia is significantly reduced *(22)*. Thalamic lesions or DBS effectively reduce tremor but it has been demonstrated that even in tremor-dominant PD, STN stimulation is as effective *(23)* and is actually preferable because it will counter other PD symptoms not dealt with by thalamotomy or thalamic stimulation. Although many investigators consider STN as the optimal target for patients requiring surgery for PD, we will have to wait for the results of randomized trials of STN vs GPi stimulation for PD before final conclusions can be drawn.

DBS is a procedure rapidly gaining favor because of its reversibility and the reduced likelihood of permanent adverse effects compared with ablative surgery of the basal ganglia. DBS also offers the possibility of dose titration and of modifying the target of influence by selecting from among four active contacts. However, there are several drawbacks associated with DBS, such as the need for intensive and specialized medical assistance to obtain optimal clinical benefit as well as periodic surveillance to guarantee the correct functioning of the system. Stimulator units need to be replaced every 3–5 yr. DBS also has unique potential complications including electrode migration, electrode wire fracture, electrical or mechanical problems with the pulse generator, problems of induction by external electromagnetic fields and, as with any implanted device, the risk of infection. Placement and maintenance of stimulators is an expensive option both financially and for the amount of time and effort required to adjust stimulation parameters postoperatively. These problems make implantation of bilateral deep brain stimulators into STN a less practical option for millions of patients suffering from advanced PD worldwide who are in an economic or geographic position that will not accommodate the application of DBS.

In recent years, Alvarez et al. *(24)* reported major clinical benefits in patients with advanced PD who were unilaterally lesioned in STN. The results obtained by this group together with those from our own group in Bristol will be discussed in the remainder of this chapter. We select the dorsolateral portion of STN for lesion placement because this is recognized as the sensorimotor portion of STN. Hamada and DeLong *(25,26)* have shown that a small amount of ibotenic acid injected into STN produces contralateral chorea in normal monkeys. The injections that successfully produced dyskinesia were placed dorsolaterally and posteriorly. This region of the STN receives important cortical motor afferents and has efferent projections to the Gpi and SNpr, thus forming an important component of the basal ganglia "motor" circuit. More medial portions of the STN are associated with nonmotor function and are not considered to play an integral role in the development of parkinsonian motor signs. However, the potential benefit of targeting the dorsolateral STN has to be weighed against the risk of infringing on the internal capsule, which lies immediately adjacent to this region.

3. PATIENT SELECTION FOR SUBTHALAMIC NUCLEOTOMY

We believe that assessment of appropriateness and fitness for functional neurosurgery must be carried out by a team experienced in the task. The minimum infrastructure for preoperative and postoperative care and assessment should be: a neurosurgeon, a neurologist, a neuropsychologist, and a specialist nurse. Ideally, the team should also have ready access to speech therapy, occupational therapy, and physiotherapy.

It is generally agreed that functional neurosurgery in PD should be reserved for those patients who have functionally disabling disease despite best medical therapy. Candidates for surgery with advanced PD and a narrow therapeutic window typically have two unsatisfactory alternatives: either to be "on" but dyskinetic for significant portions of the day or, with less L-dopa, to have less dyskinesia but to be "off" for significant portions of the day. Patients must be fully informed about the procedure and have a realistic understanding of the outcome of surgery. It is very important that patients not expect that their parkinsonism will be cured and are aware that pharmacologic treatment will continue to be necessary after surgery.

There are generally agreed upon contraindications to functional neurosurgery in PD. An important role for the neurologist member of the assessment team is to exclude patients who do not have idiopathic PD. We believe there is no role for functional surgery in atypical parkinsonism or parkinson's plus syndromes. Patients undergoing surgery should be L-dopa responsive. This is important for two reasons. Firstly, the absence of a significant clinical response to L-dopa should raise serious doubts about the diagnosis of idiopathic PD. Secondly, the response to L-dopa is a good indicator of the patient's potential response to surgery. Dementia is an important contraindication, and preoperative neuropsychological assessment is important for patients in whom there is any concern for cognitive impairment.

Preoperatively, the patient should be able to function at a reasonable level of independence for a significant portion of the average day. Patients who are continuously confined to chair or bed due to end stage disease respond less well to surgery. Age is not an absolute selection criterion but analysis suggests that, at least for pallidotomy, older patients do less well *(27,28)*.

If it is decided for a given patient that STN is the appropriate target, then it remains to be determined whether a lesion should be placed or stimulators implanted. Most patients with PD considered for surgery have bilateral and midline symptoms and therefore require bilateral procedures. Procedures that are relatively safe unilaterally may have significant morbidity when carried out bilaterally. It is now clear that bilateral thalamotomy has significant risk for postoperative dysarthria and other adverse effects *(29–31)*. As a result, most centers do not currently contemplate bilateral thalamotomy. Evidence that bilateral pallidotomy carries significant risk is not as well-established. Although some authors have reported few significant postoperative complications after bilateral pallidotomy *(32)* others regard bilateral pallidotomy as carrying too significant a risk to speech or cognitive function for it to be a surgical option for most patients *(27,33)*. The Grenoble group have reported no significant neuropsychological deficits after bilateral STN DBS *(21)* although some patients did experience mood alteration, withdrawal, and hypophonia *(5)*.

4. PRE- AND POSTOPERATIVE ASSESSMENT

Subthalamic lesioning is still at a developmental stage and therefore patients must be rigorously assessed pre- and postoperatively. The Bristol group assesses all patients with the following protocols preoperatively and at least annually postoperatively: UPDRS, Core Assessment Program for Intracerebral Transplantation (CAPIT) *(35)*, neuropsychological testing, Quality of Life Questionnaires, and formal speech assessment.

5. SURGICAL TECHNIQUE

There is no general agreement among neurosurgeons about the safest and most effective way to locate the target nucleus in functional PD surgery. Some centers use magnetic resonance imaging (MRI) and microelectrode recording and regard microelectrode recording as essential for accurate placement *(36)*. Our own view and that of some other centers is that accurate placement is possible with good-quality image guidance and macrostimulation without microelectrode recording, thereby avoiding the additional operative time and potential danger of repeated microelectrode tracks. In Bristol, STN is targeted by an MRI-based direct method with macrostimulation utilized for adjustment. Under general anesthesia, a modified Leksell stereotactic frame is fitted parallel to the orbito-meatal plane and MRI is performed on a 1.5 Tesla scanner (Phillips Gyroscanner ACS-NT). The anterior-posterior commissural (AC-PC) plane is identified on a mid-sagittal T2-weighted planning scan. High-resolution T2-weighted axial images (TR 2,500, TE 150, TSE 11, NSA 12) with 2 mm slice thickness are obtained parallel to the AC-PC plane and coronal images orthogonal to these are then obtained. We have found that these sequences give optimum delineation of STN and related structures.

Using magnified hard copies of the MRI scans and after comparison to the Schaltenbrand atlas *(37)* the boundaries of STN are identified. The boundary of STN is co-registered on the coronal and axial scans giving optimum three-dimensional target definition (Fig. 1). Stereotactic coordinates of the target, which is the dorsolateral portion of STN, are recorded and a trajectory is planned down the long axis of STN. During surgery patients are awake and in an "off" state with antiparkinsonian medications having been stopped 24 h previously. A 1.24-mm diameter electrode with a 2 mm exposed tip (Radionics Inc.) is guided to the dorsolateral STN. Stimulation frequency is 100 Hz, pulse width 1 msec, and voltage between 0.75 and 2 volts. Changes in tremor, rigidity, and bradykinesia are monitored. Because the procedure is relatively short, with the patient being awake in the operating room for only 1–2 h, he/she is not so fatigued as to be unable to cooperate with repeated clinical examination. Probe position is adjusted to gain maximal clinical improvement in the observed parkinsonian signs without the development of adverse effects. At the optimal position, one or two radiofrequency lesions are made, typically at 80°C for 60 s (Fig. 2). The patient undergoes a postoperative high-resolution MRI scan to confirm lesion position. Antiparkinson medication is reintroduced as required.

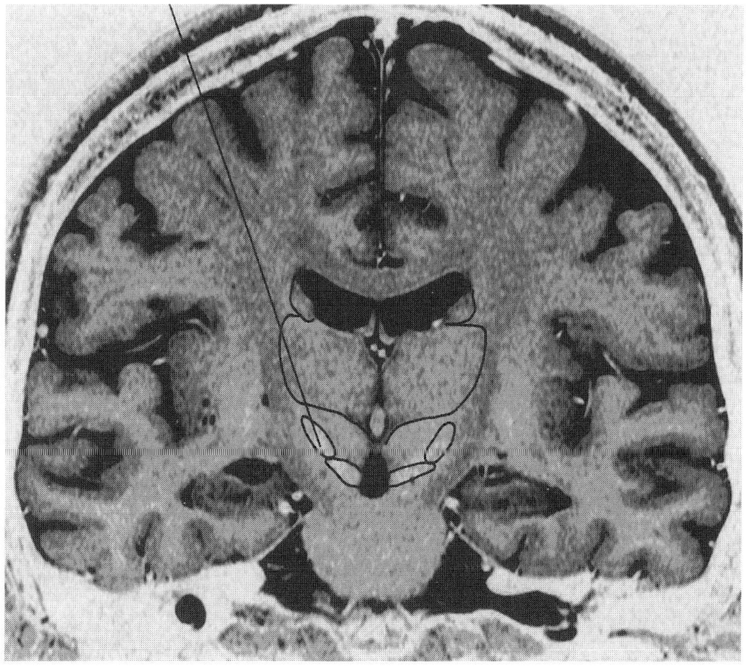

Fig. 1. Inverted coronal T2 weighted MRI scan showing pre-operative planned trajectory.

6. CLINICAL RESULTS OF SUBTHALAMIC NUCLEOTOMY

In recent years, centers in Havana, Cuba *(24,38–41)*, Istanbul, Turkey *(42)*, and Bristol, UK *(43,44)* have reported on results of STN ablative surgery: The Cuban group reported on 11 patients with a minimum of 12 mo follow-up who underwent unilateral subthalamic ablation. STN was localized with CT digitized planning using the Schaltenbrand and Wahren atlas and semi-microelectrode recording *(24)*. Parkinsonian features of all patients were greatly alleviated with a marked effect on axial symptoms, gait, freezing, and parkinsonian signs on the side contralateral to the lesion. There was a significant improvement in UPDRS Part II (activities of daily living) and UPDRS Part III scores (motor examination) in the "off" state, and percentage of daily "off" time at 1-, 6-, and 12-mo follow-up. These improvements were maintained in 4 patients for up to 24 mo. However, the effect was more pronounced on the side contralateral to the lesion while ipsilateral effect disappeared by 12 mo postoperatively. L-dopa equivalents treatment was unchanged during the first 12 mo in all but one patient who discontinued medication. Dyskinesia scores did not change postoperatively. Transient dyskinesias occurred during the lesioning procedure in five patients, which lasted for up to 12 h before abating spontaneously. In another patient, chorea of the leg contralateral to the lesion developed postoperatively, which lasted for 5 d before complete resolution. Dyskinesias were a management problem in only one patient who initially recovered but developed severe contralateral hemiballism 7 d postoperatively associated with a large infarction of the subthalamic region and part of the anterior thalamus. A left pallidotomy was carried out 12 mo later with resolution of the hemiballism.

The Cuban group recently updated their results *(41)*, reporting improvement in motor performance without inducing permanent dyskinesias in 18 patients following bilateral dorsal subthalamotomy, carried out either simultaneously in 11 patients or as a staged procedure in seven patients. Following a mean follow-up period of 16 mo there was a 58% improvement in UPDRS motor score while off medication. Severe generalized chorea occurred in three patients, which improved spontaneously within 6 mo of surgery. These three patients also developed dysarthria and balance instability, that lasted for

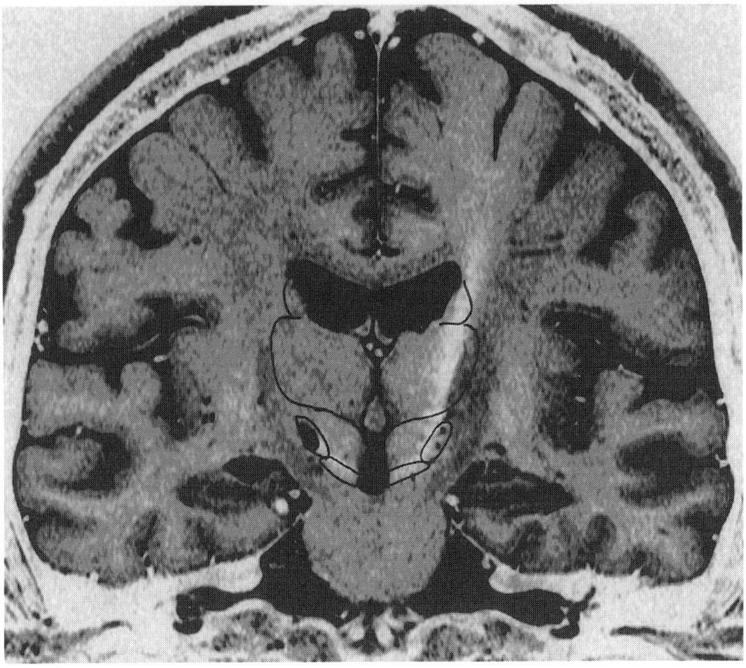

Fig. 2. Postoperative inverted coronal T2 weighted MRI scan showing lesion location (this patient also had an implanted left subthalamic DBS electrode).

6–12 mo postoperatively. No speech or cognitive impairment was observed related to the bilateral procedure.

In a safety study, Barlas et al. *(42)* carried out unilateral subthalamotomy in nine patients with advanced PD and found that no involuntary movements occurred postoperatively in eight patients, whereas one patient developed transient hemiballism lasting for 2 wk followed by mild choreic movements. These authors did not report on the therapeutic outcome of subthalamotomy in their patients.

Our group in Bristol has performed 50 subthalamotomies in 39 patients *(43–45)*. This includes 22 patients with unilateral lesions, 11 patients with bilateral lesions, and six patients with an STN lesion on one side and STN DBS on the contralateral side. We have had two patients with major complications. One patient suffered a superficial intracerebral haemorrhage resulting in hemiparesis from which she partially recovered before expiring from a pulmonary embolus 2 mo later. Another patient with a previous history of seizures had a single intraoperative seizure. Importantly, no major persistent complications have occurred directly attributable to STN lesioning. One patient had significant postoperative hemiballism on the side contralateral to the STN lesion, which persisted for approx 3 wk before gradually subsiding without active treatment. Two other patients displayed minor choreiform movements after bilateral STN lesions that subsided in the immediate postoperative period. None experienced gaze deviation, blepharospasm, or eyelid opening apraxia, which sometimes occur during or following STN DBS. One patient felt that his thinking processes were slow for 6 mo. Two patients had worsening of a preexisting dysarthria.

Following unilateral STN lesions all of our patients showed improvement in contralateral tremor, rigidity, and bradykinesia that persisted for up to 24 mo. Contralateral motor scores (UPDRS Part III) decreased from 16.6 pre-operatively to 8.9 (46.4%). Tremor improved more than other motor signs. Patients still required L-dopa but their overall daily L-dopa dose was reduced by 50%. Associated with this there was a reduction in dyskinesia by approx 70%. UPDRS Part II (activities of daily living) improved from 19.9 pre-operatively to 14.9 (25.1%). Total daily "on" time without significant dyskinesia more than doubled. Neuropsychological testing remained unchanged in all those tested before and after surgery *(45)*. Our 11 patients who underwent bilateral subthalamotomy generally showed striking improvement in motor performance immediately following surgery. However, at 12-mo follow-up motor function declined in these patients, with UPDRS total scores decreased from a pre-operative mean of 92.9 to 66.5 (28.4%) and UPDRS motor scores decreased from 48.3 to 35.1 (27.3%). In general, the lesions made at bilateral surgery were smaller than those carried out at unilateral surgery. The marked improvement observed immediately following surgery may be have been due to the effects of perilesional edema. Alvarez et al. *(24)* showed on postoperative imaging in two patients following unilateral subthalamotomy that the lesion appeared to be correctly placed in the dorsal region of STN with a variable 1–2 mm dorsal extension above the nucleus. In our experience with postoperative imaging, lesions were correctly located in the dorsolateral STN but in a majority of cases the lesion extended to involve fiber tracts within the zona incerta.

In summary, it has been the experience of all groups that STN ablation does not necessarily induce hemiballism and that dyskinesias are not a frequent or significant problem in the majority of operated patients. One explanation concerning why STN lesions do not provoke hemiballism in PD patients is that the lesions also involve pallidofugal fiber tracts within the zona incerta that exert a pallidotomy-like effect *(46)*. It has also been suggested that the dyskinetic threshold to induce hemiballism following STN lesions may be higher in PD than in the normal state *(47)*.

7. CONCLUSIONS

Preliminary results of STN lesioning demonstrate that this procedure can be carried out relatively safely and with good therapeutic effect. Despite this, STN should be regarded as an experimental procedure. As more data accumulate regarding the safety and efficacy of STN lesions it may prove to be a viable alternative to the placement of bilateral deep brain stimulators in STN, especially in patients not suitable for electrode implantation, and may warrant a randomized comparative study between the two treatments.

REFERENCES

1. Laitinen, L. V., Bergenheim, A. T., and Hariz, M. I. (1992) Ventroposterolateral pallidotomy can abolish all parkinsonian symptoms. *Stereotact. Funct. Neurosurg.* **58,** 14–21.
2. Albin, R. L., Young, A. B., and Penney, J. B. (1989) The functional anatomy of basal ganglia disorders. *Trends Neurosci.* **12,** 366–375.
3. Benabid, A. L., Pollak, P., Gross, C., et al. (1994) Acute and long-term effects of subthalamic nucleus stimulation in Parkinson's disease. *Stereotact. Funct. Neurosurg.* **62,** 76–84.
4. Limousin, P., Pollak, P., Benazzouz, A., et al. (1995) Bilateral subthalamic nucleus stimulation for severe Parkinson's disease. *Mov. Disord.* **10,** 672–674.
5. Limousin, P., Krack, P., Pollak, P., et al. (1998) Electrical stimulation of the subthalamic nucleus in advanced Parkinson's disease. *N. Engl. J. Med.* **339,** 1105–1111.
6. Sellal, F., Hirsch, E., Lisovoski, F., Mutschler, V., Collard, M., and Marescaux, C. (1992) Contralateral disappearance of parkinsonian signs after subthalamic hematoma. *Neurology* **42,** 255–256.
7. Vidakovic, A., Dragasevic, N., and Kostic, V. S. (1994) Hemiballism: report of 25 cases. *J. Neurol. Neurosurg. Psychiatry* **57,** 945–949.
8. Mundinger, F. (1968) Results of 500 Subthalamotomies in the region of the zona incerta. Third Symposium on Parkinson's Disease, Livingstone, Edinburgh.
9. Fager, C. A. (1968) Evaluation of thalamic and subthalamic surgical lesions in the alleviation of Parkinson's disease. *J. Neurosurg.* **28,** 145–149.
10. Spiegel, E. A., Wycis, H. T., Szekely, E. G., Adams, J., Flanagan, M., and Baird, H. W. (1963) Campotomy in various extrapyramidal disorders. *J. Neurosurg.* **20,** 871–881.
11. Andy, O. J., Jurko, M. F., and Sias, F. R. (1963) Subthalamotomy in treatment of Parkinsonian tremor. *J. Neurosurg.* **20,** 860–870.
12. Houdart, R., Mamo, H., Dondey, M., and Cophignon, J. (1965) [Results of subthalamic coagulations in Parkinson's disease (apropos of 50 cases)]. *Revue Neurologique* **112,** 521–529.
13. Krauss, J. K. and Mundinger, F. (1996) Functional stereotactic surgery for hemiballism. *J. Neurosurg.* **85,** 278–286.
14. Bergman, H., Wichmann, T., Karmon, B., and DeLong, M. R. (1994) The primate subthalamic nucleus. II. Neuronal activity in the MPTP model of parkinsonism. *J. Neurophysiol.* **72,** 507–520.

15. Hutchison, W. D., Allan, R. J., Opitz, H., et al. (1998) Neurophysiological identification of the subthalamic nucleus in surgery for Parkinson's disease. *Ann. Neurol.* **44,** 622–628.
16. Bergman, H., Wichmann, T., and DeLong, M. R. (1990) Reversal of experimental parkinsonism by lesions of the subthalamic nucleus. *Science* **249,** 1436–1438.
17. Aziz, T. Z., Peggs, D., Agarwal, E., Sambrook, M. A., and Crossman, A. R. (1992) Subthalamic nucleotomy alleviates parkinsonism in the 1-methyl-4-phenyl-1,2,3,6-tetrahydropyridine (MPTP)-exposed primate. *Br. J. Neurosurg.* **6,** 575–582.
18. Guridi, J., Herrero, M. T., Luquin, M. R., et al. (1996) Subthalamotomy in parkinsonian monkeys. Behavioral and biochemical analysis. *Brain* **119,** 1717–1727.
19. Benazzouz, A., Gross, C., Feger, J., Boraud, T., and Bioulac, B. (1993) Reversal of rigidity and improvement in motor performance by subthalamic high-frequency stimulation in MPTP-treated monkeys. *Eur. J. Neurosci.* **5,** 382–389.
20. Benabid, A. L., Pollak, P., Gao, D., et al. (1996) Chronic electrical stimulation of the ventralis intermedius nucleus of the thalamus as a treatment of movement disorders [see comments]. *J. Neurosurg.* **84,** 203–214.
21. Limousin, P., Krack, P., Pollak, P., et al. (1998) Electrical stimulation of the subthalamic nucleus in advanced Parkinson's disease. *N. Engl. J. Med.* **339,** 1105–1111.
22. Krack, P., Pollak, P., Limousin, P., et al. (1998) Subthalamic nucleus or internal pallidal stimulation in young onset Parkinson's disease. *Brain* **121,** 451–457.
23. Krack, P., Benazzouz, A., Pollak, P., et al. (1998) Treatment of tremor in Parkinson's disease by subthalamic nucleus stimulation. *Mov. Disord.* **13,** 907–914.
24. Alvarez, L., Macias, R., Guridi, J., et al. (2001) Dorsal subthalamotomy for Parkinson's disease. *Mov. Disord.* **16,** 72–78.
25. Hamada, I. and DeLong, M. R. (1992) Excitotoxic acid lesions of the primate subthalamic nucleus result in transient dyskinesias of the contralateral limbs. *J. Neurophysiol.* **68,** 1850–1858.
26. Hamada, I. and DeLong, M. R. (1992) Excitotoxic acid lesions of the primate subthalamic nucleus result in reduced pallidal neuronal activity during active holding. *J. Neurophysiol.* **68,** 1859–1866.
27. Lozano, A. M. and Lang, A. E. (1998) Pallidotomy for Parkinson's disease. *Neurosurg. Clin. North Am.* **9,** 325–336.
28. Baron, M. S., Vitek, J. L., Bakay, R. A., et al. (1996) Treatment of advanced Parkinson's disease by posterior GPi pallidotomy: 1-year results of a pilot study. *Ann. Neurol.* **40,** 355–366.
29. Blumetti, A. E. and Modesti, L. M. (1980) Long term cognitive effects of stereotactic thalamotomy on non-parkinsonian dyskinetic patients. *Appl. Neurophysiol.* **43,** 259–262.
30. Kocher, U., Siegfried, J., and Perret, E. (1982) Verbal and nonverbal learning ability of Parkinson patients before and after unilateral ventrolateral thalamotomy. *Appl. Neurophysiol.* **45,** 311–316.
31. Krayenbuhl, H., Wyss, O. A. M., and Yasargil, M. G. (1961) Bilateral thalamotomy and pallidotomy as treatment for bilateral parkinsonism. *J. Neurosurg.* **18,** 429.
32. Iacono, R. P., Shima, F., Lonser, R. R., Kuniyoshi, S., Maeda, G., and Yamada, S. (1995) The results, indications, and physiology of posteroventral pallidotomy for patients with Parkinson's disease [see comments]. *Neurosurgery* **36,** 1118–1125; discussion 1125–1127.
33. Scott, R., Gregory, R., Hines, N., et al. (1998) Neuropsychological, neurological and functional outcome following pallidotomy for Parkinson's disease. A consecutive series of eight simultaneous bilateral and twelve unilateral procedures. *Brain* **121,** 659–675.
34. Krack, P., Gentil, M., Pinto, S., et al. (1999) Effects of subthalamic nucleus stimulation on parkinsonian speech. *Parkinsonism Rel. Disord.* **5,** S106.
35. Langston, J. W., Widner, H., Goetz, C. G., et al. (1992) Core assessment program for intracerebral transplantations (CAPIT). *Mov. Disord.* **7,** 2–13.
36. Vitek, J. L., Bakay, R. A., and DeLong, M. R. (1997) Microelectrode-guided pallidotomy for medically intractable Parkinson's disease. *Adv. Neurol.* **74,** 183–198.
37. Schaltenbrand, G. and Bailey, P. (1959) Einfuhrung in die Stereotaktischen Operationen mit einem Atlas des menschlichen Gehirn. Thieme, Stuttgart.
38. Obeso, J. A., Alvarez, L. M., Macias, R. J., et al. (1997) Lesion of the subthalamic nucleus in Parkinson's disease. *Neurology* **48,** A138.
39. Obeso, J. A., Guridi, J., Alvarez, L., Macias, R., and Linazasoro, G. (1998) Ablataive surgery for Parkinson's disease. In: *Parkinson's Disease and Movement Disorders* (Jankovic, J. and Tolosa, E., eds.), Williams & Wilkins, Baltimore, MD, pp. 1049–1064.
40. Alvarez Gonzalez, L., Macias, J., Guridi, J., et al. (1999) Lesion of the subthalamic nucleus in Parkinson's disease: long-term follow-up. *Ann. Neurol.* **46,** 492.
41. Alvarez, L., Marcias, R., Lopez, G., et al. (2000) Bilateral subthalamotomy in Parkinson's disease. *Mov. Disord.* **15,** 65.
42. Barlas, O., Hanagasi, H. A., Imer, M., Sahin, H. A., Sencer, S., and Emre, M. (2001) Do unilateral ablative lesions of the subthalamic nuclei in parkinsonian patients lead to hemiballism? *Mov. Disord.* **16,** 306–310.
43. Gill, S. S. and Heywood, P. (1997) Bilateral dorsolateral subthalamotomy for advanced Parkinson's disease. *Lancet* **350,** 1224.
44. Gill, S. S. and Heywood, P. (1998) Subthalamotomy can be performed safely. *Mov. Disord.* **13,** 201.
45. McCarter, R. J., Walton, N. H., Rowan, A. F., Gill, S. S., and Palomo, M. (2000) Cognitive functioning after subthalamic nucleotomy for refractory Parkinson's disease. *J. Neurol. Neurosurg. Psychiatry* **69,** 60–66.
46. Lozano, A. M. (2001) The subthalamic nucleus: myth and opportunities. *Mov. Disord.* **16,** 183–184.
47. Guridi, J. and Obeso, J. A. (2001) The subthalamic nucleus, hemiballismus, and Parkinson's disease: reappraisal of a neurosurgical dogma. *Brain* **124,** 5–19.

11

Thalamic Deep Brain Stimulation for Parkinson's Disease and Essential Tremor

Daniel Tarsy, Thorkild Norregaard, and Jean Hubble

1. INTRODUCTION

Discussion of thalamic surgery for treatment of tremor begins with an understanding of anatomic terminology. Several nomenclatures have been used for the nuclei of the human thalamus *(1–4)*. Hassler's terminology *(1)* is the most commonly used in the movement disorders literature and will be used here. The motor thalamus lies ventrally and from front to back consists of lateral polaris (LPo) most anteriorly receiving input from globus pallidus (GPi) and substantia nigra pars reticulata (SNr); ventralis oralis anterior (Voa) and ventralis oralis posterior (Vop) receiving input from GPi; and ventral intermediate nucleus (Vim) receiving input from cerebellum. Ventralis caudalis (Vc) lies posterior to motor thalamus receiving lemniscal and spinothalamic sensory input. In the Anglo-American nomenclature, the ventral anterior nucleus (VA) includes Lpo and Voa, the ventrolateral nucleus (VL) includes Vop and Vim, and the ventral posterior nucleus is equivalent to Vc.

Microelectrode recordings obtained during stereotactic surgery have identified thalamic neurons, which burst spontaneously with a frequency identical to the patient's tremor frequency *(5)*. These are located in the ventral motor thalamus but have also been identified in other thalamic nuclei, globus pallidus, putamen, caudate, and subthalamic nucleus. In the thalamus these have been particularly well-studied in Vc, Vim, Voa, and Vop, where they correlate with electromyographic recordings of tremor. Neuronal bursts also occur in response to active or passive movement of small joints *(7,8)*. Intraoperative identification of these neurons with microelectrode recording has been helpful in locating thalamic sites for optimal placement of surgical lesions or stimulating electrodes for treatment of tremor. Surgical ablation and high-frequency stimulation of the Vim nucleus, which contains "tremor cells," successfully abolishes tremor. However, the etiologic role of these "tremor cells" in generation of tremor is uncertain because similar tremor bursts can be identified in globus pallidus *(9)* and subthalamic nucleus *(10)* and lesions in these areas also abolish tremor.

Thalamotomy was introduced for treatment of tremor in the late 1950s, proved to be very effective, and rapidly became the most commonly performed surgical procedure for the treatment of parkinsonian tremor prior to the introduction of L-dopa therapy. This was mainly because of its reduced morbidity compared with pallidotomy and its particularly striking benefit for tremor, although controlled comparison studies were not carried out. However, despite the availability of emerging pharmacologic treatments for both parkinsonian and essential tremor, medication-resistant tremors continued to provide a valid indication for thalamotomy *(11)*. Although unilateral thalamotomy produces long-term effective treatment of contralateral tremor in up to 85% of patients, there is a high incidence of transient complications lasting up to 3 mo in as many as 60% of patients and a lower but substantial incidence of permanent complications, especially involving speech, in up to 23% of treated patients *(12)*.

From: Contemporary Clinical Neurology: Surgical Treatment of Parkinson's Disease and Other Movement Disorders
Edited by: D. Tarsy, J. L. Vitek, and A. M. Lozano © Humana Press Inc., Totowa, NJ

2. DEEP BRAIN STIMULATION

Deep brain stimulation (DBS) has been a rapidly expanding novel strategy for the treatment of PD *(13,14)*. Three targets have been used in PD: Ventral intermediate nucleus of thalamus (Vim), medial globus pallidus (GPi), and subthalamic nucleus (STN). By the 1960s, the use of intraoperative stimulation of brain targets in preparation for ablative surgery had established the concept that low-frequency Vim stimulation activated or "drove" tremor, whereas high-frequency stimulation in the same location suppressed tremor *(15–17)*. This technique was therefore used at the time of surgery to identify the proper site for thalamic lesioning *(17–19)*. The high frequency of adverse effects associated with bilateral thalamotomy motivated Benabid to carry out the first large-scale permanent implantations of thalamic stimulators for treatment of parkinsonian and essential tremor *(20)*. Because of the reported safety and efficacy of this technique, the use of DBS in other brain targets such as GPi and STN was subsequently explored.

The procedure for Vim thalamic stimulator implantation at our institution (DT,TN) is as follows: Patients are admitted to hospital on the morning of surgery. A stereotactic frame (Radionics Inc.) is attached to the skull under local anesthesia in the operating room. The patient is taken to the radiology suite where a localizing computed tomographic (CT) scan is performed using spiral technique. Axial cuts are made at 1.0-mm intervals through the region of the third ventricle parallel to the anterior commissure-posterior commissure (AC-PC) plane. A target in Vim is selected at the level of the AC-PC line, 25% of the AC-PC distance anterior to PC, and 11.5 mm lateral to the wall of the third ventricle. The target and the fiducial points for the CT localizing frame are recorded from the CT scanner and processed to determine the x, y, and z coordinates for the calculated target. In the operating room a coronal burr hole is placed 3.0 cm lateral to the midline under local anesthesia. Bilateral burr holes are placed when bilateral surgery is done in the same session. We do not routinely use microelectrode recording to identify Vim in patients with PD or essential tremor because the response of tremor to stimulation allows for a clear endpoint. A DBS lead (Medtronic, Inc., Model 3387) with four platinum-iridium contacts, each 1.5 mm long and separated by 1.5 mm, is introduced through the burr hole and advanced towards the target. Test stimulation is performed beginning 8 mm proximal to target and repeated at 2-mm intervals up to a point 6 mm below the AC-PC plane. Stimulation is performed using a hand-held test stimulator (Medtronic, Inc., Model 3625) with electrode 0 (most distal electrode) negative, electrode 1 positive, and electrodes 2 and 3 off (–, +, off, off). Voltage is increased at each stimulation site by 1.0 volt increments to a maximum of 6–8 volts while resting, postural, and action tremor and presence or absence of paresthesias or dysmetria are evaluated. Persistent or excessive paresthesia signifies location is too posterior and, in some cases, dysmetria has signified that location is too anterior. In most cases pulse width is maintained at 60 microseconds and frequency at 140 Hz but these parameters may be adjusted as needed. The electrode tip is implanted at a point where maximal tremor suppression is achieved in several trials with a voltage of 4.0 volts or less while producing no more than transient paresthesia (less than 15 s) in face and/or arm. The final configuration of electrode settings is set with electrode 0 (most distal) off, electrode 1 negative, electrode 2 positive, and electrode 3 (most proximal) off.

In instances when there is inadequate tremor suppression, excessive paresthesia, or dysmetria, additional tracks are carried out spaced 2 mm apart. When tremor control is satisfactory, the DBS lead is anchored to the burr hole using a plastic burr hole ring and cap. Stimulation is repeated to assure that no movement of the lead has occurred. In some centers, lead position is also verified by fluoroscopy at this point. Under general anesthesia a pulse generator (Medtronic, Inc., Model 7424 Itrel II) is implanted in the subclavicular region and connected subcutaneously (Medtronic, Inc., Model 7495) to the DBS lead either during the same operative session or several days later. The pulse generator is turned on several days following surgery and programmed to yield maximal tremor suppression with minimal adverse effects. Stimulation parameters programmed by telemetry (Medtronic, Inc., Model 7432 Console Programmer and Model 745B MemoryMod Software Cartridge) are voltage, pulse width, stimulation frequency, and contact selection. If the patient exhibits a microthalamotomy effect (temporary reduction or disappearance of tremor with stimulator off due to the trauma of electrode placement), programming is delayed until reappearance of baseline tremor. The patient returns for follow-up reprogramming 1 and 3 mo following surgery and at other times as needed. The patient is instructed on how to turn the device on or off with a hand-held magnet and, where tolerated, is encouraged to turn the device off before sleep to conserve battery life and to possibly reduce the likelihood of tolerance.

The potential advantages of thalamic DBS over thalamotomy are several. DBS is reversible and unassociated with significant long-term tissue reaction or damage *(21)*. By contrast to a fixed surgical lesion, DBS therapy can be modified in that several stimulation parameters can be changed as needed following implantation including frequency, amplitude, pulse width, and area of stimulation being delivered to the brain. In studies reported to date, unilateral and bilateral DBS are both associated with fewer adverse effects than ablation. The possibility of bilateral stimulation allows for treatment of bilateral and midline symptoms not treatable with ablation without risking permanent adverse effects on speech and cognitive function. Finally, potential future surgical interventions may be available to a patient following DBS while ablation surgery may possibly prohibit these interventions. Disadvantages of DBS relate to greater cost, need for battery replacement, possible device-related complications such as infection, electrode breakage, or pulse generator failure, and the need for regular follow-up at a center capable of programming the pulse generator.

The mechanism of action of high-frequency DBS is not entirely understood but most commonly it has been assumed to parallel the effects of an ablative lesion. Benabid suggested its effect might be due to "jamming" the targeted nucleus, thereby preventing the relay of excessive or abnormal patterns of neuronal firing *(22)*. He later suggested the term "electrical neuroinhibition" to describe the effect of high-frequency stimulation *(23)*. Although it is assumed that high-frequency stimulation mimics ablation by suppressing abnormal neuronal activity, the situation in GPi and STN, where neurons fire at higher than normal frequency in PD, may be more complex than in thalamus. Whereas thalamic DBS suppresses tremor immediately, the benefit of DBS applied to the GPi and STN DBS in reducing bradykinesia in PD requires a matter of minutes or longer, suggesting a different mechanism of action *(24)*. Laboratory neurophysiologic studies indicate that high-frequency stimulation can either activate or inactivate neurons and nerve fibers, depending on a number of factors *(25,26)*. Effects on nerve fibers may differ anatomically with fiber activation being either orthodromic on cortical structures or antidromic on cerebellar structures *(27)*.

An additional level of complexity is suggested by observations that Vim DBS activates ipsilateral regional motor cortical cerebral blood flow (rCBF), as measured by positron emission tomography (PET) *(28)*, in contrast to thalamotomy, which reduces ipsilateral motor cortical rCBF *(29)*, suggesting that DBS and lesioning may have different mechanisms of action *(28)*. It has also been suggested that thalamic DBS may suppress tremor by activating the thalamic reticular nucleus, which in turn inhibits thalamic relay nuclei such as the Vim nucleus *(30)*. Finally, it is also possible that DBS exerts its effect by causing release of neurotransmitters either locally or in other brain regions receiving input from the targeted nucleus *(24)*.

3. THALAMIC STIMULATION FOR PARKINSONIAN TREMOR

As already discussed, adverse effects on speech and cognitive function that were sometimes associated with thalamotomy, especially when carried out bilaterally, motivated a search for alternative approaches. Historically, chronic thalamic stimulation had already been used for the treatment of chronic pain. Andy *(18)* suggested that chronic thalamic stimulation might be preferable to lesioning for treatment of tremor, especially in elderly, poor-risk patients. He implanted chronic electrodes and stimulated at 50–125 Hz in several thalamic nuclei in nine patients with a variety of motor disorders. He treated five patients with parkinsonian tremor, three of whom were targeted in Vim *(18)*. In most cases, stimulation was limited to 30–60 min, 3 or 4 times daily but three patients underwent continuous stimulation. Results in parkinsonian tremor were "fair to excellent" but duration of follow-up evaluation was unstated. Tasker *(31)* also reported on chronic thalamic stimulation at 60 Hz in a small number of patients, one of whom had parkinsonian tremor, but with poor and short-lived results. Benabid *(20)* pursued Vim stimulation further and concluded that it could be used as chronic adjuvant therapy in patients with contralateral thalamotomy in order to avoid the adverse effects of bilateral thalamotomy. In his initial report, six patients with Parkinson's disease (PD) with previous thalamotomy were implanted in contralateral Vim *(20)* and stimulated at up to 130 Hz. Three patients were greatly improved and were connected to permanent stimulators, thereby inaugurating the era of DBS for the treatment of movement disorders.

In Benabid's early report *(19)* of Vim DBS used as primary treatment for tremor, a total of 26 patients with disabling parkinsonian tremor were implanted, 21 of whom had undergone no previous neurosurgery. Eight patients underwent bilateral Vim DBS implanted at the same time. A Radionics 2.3 mm diameter electrode was used initially and later switched to a Medtronic 1.2 mm diameter electrode. The correct target was determined to be where stimulation at 100 Hz or higher suppressed tremor with the lowest possible voltage. Stimulation at lower frequencies either had no effect or increased tremor. Electrodes were connected to an extension lead externalized over the scalp and test stimulation was carried out over at least 1 wk. Once stimulation effects were deemed satisfactory, a programmable stimulator, the Medtronic Itrel I or Itrel II®, was implanted in the subclavicular region and stimulation was maintained at 130 Hz. Contralateral upper limb tremor was totally suppressed in 23 and markedly improved in nine cases (total of 34 thalami stimulated). Similar to the effects of thalamotomy, rigidity was slightly improved but there was no effect on akinesia. A "microthalamotomy" effect occurred in some patients, whereby tremor was improved postoperatively for 1–10 d (with the device in the "off" mode) owing to reversible electrode induced neuronal injury. Adverse effects in this initial study were mild and stimulation–related. They included limb or face paresthesia, limb dystonia, and dysmetria. Dysarthria and gait dysequilibrium occurred in six patients, five of whom had either bilateral DBS or a previous thalamotomy and could be controlled by reducing the intensity of one or both stimulators.

Subsequent studies by Benabid *(22,32,33)* involving up to 91 patients with PD documented the efficacy of this procedure for up to at least 3–6 mo postoperatively. There was good to excellent tremor suppression in 88% of PD patients. In his experience, resting tremor was better controlled than postural or action tremor, distal better than proximal or axial tremor, and upper better than lower extremity tremor *(23)*. Stimulation voltage had to be increased over the first several weeks following surgery likely owing to increases in tissue impedance. There was a subsequent need to increase stimulus voltage to control action tremor in some patients, more commonly in essential tremor than PD. This was attributed to tolerance, possibly supported by the transient rebound increase in tremor amplitude that occurred in some patients when the stimulator was turned off. However, despite the observation of rebound tremor, tolerance evidenced by reduced clinical effect or need for increased stimulus voltage, has been reported in some *(34)* but not all studies *(35–37)*. More sustained satisfactory benefit of thalamic DBS may be related to lead placement, the use of higher stimulation frequencies, or the more common practice of turning the stimulator off at night *(36)*. Some patients may experience re-emerging or worsening tremor due to unavoidable progression of their underlying disease.

Subsequent studies with more prolonged follow-up have confirmed the remarkable therapeutic effect of Vim DBS in parkinsonian tremor *(36–43)*. In most studies PD patients have had tremor predominant forms of PD. In a North American prospective multicenter trial (four sites), 24 PD patients were implanted with Vim thalamic stimulators and were evaluated using a double-blinded assessment at 3 mo and open follow-up assessments at 6, 9, and 12 mo following surgery *(36)*. There was a statistically significant and clinically clear-cut decrease in contralateral tremor compared to baseline with total resolution of tremor in 14 of 24 PD patients. However, by contrast with essential tremor patients in the same study, functional activities of daily living (ADLs) such as handwriting, dressing, and cutting food were not improved, likely due to lack of improvement in other parkinsonian symptoms. A single center study of 19 patients using similar methodology and examiner-blinded assessment at 3 mo produced similar results with regard to both tremor and ADLs *(41)*. A European prospective multicenter trial (13 sites) in 73 PD patients assessed patients in unblinded fashion for 12 mo following surgery *(42)*. There was a statistically significant decrease in contralateral tremor, which was similar in magnitude to the North American trial. By contrast with the North American trial, ADLs were improved in the European study. Another study also showed that subjective global disability ratings improved similarly in PD patients compared with essential tremor patients *(40)*. Currently bilateral Vim DBS is less frequently carried out in PD than essential tremor because of concerns for aggravating dysarthria and the more recent advent of subthalamic nucleus and pallidal DBS, which also improve tremor while offering more comprehensive control of PD symptoms and drug therapy complications. Despite this, Vim DBS may continue to have a place in the treatment of tremor dominant PD. In our 2-yr follow-up study in which most patients had tremor dominant PD, tremor suppression remained stable for 2 yr without significant increase in akinesia, rigidity, gait disturbance, or dose requirement for antiparkinson medication *(43)*. Longer-term studies will be necessary to support the continued use of Vim DBS in parkinsonian tremor. However, overall it appears that in PD thalamic DBS can improve tremor bilaterally with a lower risk of dysarthria and gait disturbance compared to bilateral thalamotomy *(44)*.

In at least one European trial, Vim nucleus stimulation improved not only tremor but contralateral rigidity and akinesia as well. These signs were mild preoperatively, may have been difficult to assess in the presence of severe tremor, and likely improved postoperatively due to improved tremor. In other studies, rigidity and akinesia have shown little change following Vim DBS *(32,37,39,41)*. Gait and balance in PD patients have shown minor and inconsistent improvement *(45–47)*. In one study, L-dopa dyskinesias were improved following thalamic DBS in five affected patients *(39,48)*, but this has not been a universal finding *(49)*. A subsequent analysis of thalamic stimulation sites concluded that effects on dyskinesia in this study may have been due to more medial and deeper electrode placement closer to centromedian and parafascicular nuclei *(49)*.

Adverse effects associated with Vim DBS are infrequent and related to regional effects of stimulation, foreign body responses, and consequences of intracerebral electrode implantation. In one of Benabid's original reports *(19)*, adverse effects were mild and limited to contralateral paresthesia, limb dystonia, and cerebellar dysmetria all of which were controlled by stimulation adjustment. Dysarthria and gait dysequilibrium were uncommon and nearly always limited to patients receiving bilateral stimulation or who had undergone previous thalamotomy. In a subsequent report by Benabid *(32)*, there were six intracerebral microhematomas in 177 operations, three of which were symptomatic. Other adverse effects included a small number of patients with scalp infections, skin necrosis, or wound granulomas. There were similar stimulation related adverse effects in the North American and European trials while the incidence of documented intracranial hemorrhage was 2% in the North American and 5% in the European trials *(36,42)*. Significant cognitive deficits have not occurred following thalamic stimulation *(39,50)* although mild deficits in verbal fluency have been documented *(32,50)*. In an autopsy study of six PD patients with thalamic DBS, pathological examination up to 70 mo following electrode implantation showed only a thin inner capsule of connective tissue and mild fibrillary gliosis around the lead track and active contact electrode *(21)*. Thus, there is no evidence that thalamic stimulation or the implanted device produce significant or progressive tissue damage.

As already mentioned, speech and cognitive deficits following bilateral as well as unilateral thalamotomy and tremor recurrence rates of 4–22% *(51)* motivated Benabid to initially consider Vim DBS *(32)*. Increasing thalamotomy size to prevent recurrence only served to increase the frequency of neurologic morbidity *(52)*. Direct comparisons of Vim DBS and thalamotomy have been few. In a retrospective study, Tasker *(53)* compared 16 PD patients who underwent Vim DBS with 23 PD patients who underwent thalamotomy in a nonrandomized study (this study also included six patients with essential tremor whose outcomes were not separated from the PD patients). Clinical outcome was similar with contralateral complete abolition of tremor in 42% of both groups and nearly complete abolition of tremor in 79% of DBS patients and 79% of thalamotomy patients. Tremor recurred in 5% of DBS cases and 15% of thalamotomy cases. No DBS case was repeated while 23% of thalamotomy cases had to be repeated in order to achieve a satisfactory response. L-dopa dyskinesia improved in 6 of 16 DBS cases compared with 12 of 23 thalamotomy cases. The major difference between the two groups was in complication rates. Intracerebral hemorrhage occurred in 4% of thalamotomy cases and in none of the DBS cases. Permanent ataxia and paresthesia occurred in 34% of thalamotomy cases. By contrast, stimulation induced ataxia and paresthesia occurred in 5 and 47% of DBS cases, respectively, but could be alleviated by stimulation adjustment. In a prospective, randomized but unblinded study of patients with PD, essential tremor, and multiple sclerosis, 45 patients with PD were assigned to either thalamic DBS or thalamotomy *(54)*. Improvement in PD tremor was similar in the two treatment groups but adverse events were much more common in the thalamotomy group. Tremor was suppressed completely in 20 of 21 DBS cases compared with 20 of 23 thalamotomy cases. Adverse effects were nearly all stimulator related in the DBS cases except for one case each of hematoma, infection at the pulse generator site, and intracerebral hemorrhage. By contrast, permanent adverse effects occurred in 11 of 45 PD patients undergoing thalamotomy including cognitive deterioration, dysarthria, and gait disturbance.

In summary, thalamic DBS is highly effective for treatment of resting or postural parkinsonian tremor. It is safer than thalamotomy and can be carried out bilaterally in either one or two sessions with less risk for speech or gait impairment than thalamotomy. Most adverse effects such as paresthesia, dysmetria, gait disturbance, and dysarthria are related to stimulation and can be easily managed by altering stimulus parameters. Complications such as meningitis and brain abcess are exceedingly rare and there is no long-term tissue damage around the electrodes. Erosion of the extension electrode, scalp infection, or infection at the pulse generator site are uncommon and easily managed. In PD patients, the only indication for thalamic DBS is control of disabling tremor that has failed medical management. Patients with disabling, tremor predominant PD with very slowly progressive akinesia remain potentially good candidates for thalamic DBS. However, improved tremor has not always been associated with reduced disability, likely because of residual bradykinesia or, in some cases, alleviation of a resting rather than postural tremor. If PD appears to be more progressive and disability is owing to bradykinesia, gait disturbance, motor fluctuations, or L-dopa dyskinesia, a pallidal or subthalamic target for DBS is more appropriate.

4. THALAMIC STIMULATION FOR ESSENTIAL TREMOR

Essential tremor is a common disorder that produces various combinations of hand, head, and voice tremor unassociated with other motor symptoms. Because it is primarily a postural or kinetic tremor, it is typically more disabling than parkinsonian tremor, which primarily occurs at rest. Surgical treatment is reserved for those ET patients with severe, disabling hand tremor not responding to medications such as propranolol or primidone. Similar to PD, thalamotomy has also been used for the treatment of severe forms of ET *(55,56)*, but much less extensively and limited in many cases by adverse effects associated with the bilateral surgery often required for meaningful tremor control.

Benabid simultaneously reported his results of Vim DBS in treatment of ET with his reports concerning its effect in parkinsonian tremor *(19,22,32)*. Reporting on findings in 20 ET patients, extremity tremor control was complete or nearly complete in 75% and mild to moderate in 25% in the initial postoperative period, declining to 61 and 39%, respectively, 3–6 mo following surgery *(32)*. Adverse effects were similar to those reported in PD patients. Other single center *(37,39,41,43,51,57)* and multicenter *(36,42)* studies with up to 12 mo follow-up have produced similar results with complete abolition of tremor in 50% of patients, satisfactory results in 90% of patients, lack of tolerance, and very significant improvement in quality of life scales *(58)*. Some longer-term studies indicate that there may be a mild reduction in tremor control over several years of follow-up *(59)*.

Similar to PD, tremor improvement occurs only on the contralateral side with greater improvement in the upper than the less frequently involved lower extremity. For this reason, bilateral Vim DBS, done either as a staged procedure or simultaneously, is currently performed with increasing frequency. Three studies have shown that sequentially or simultaneous bilateral Vim DBS is safe and effective for control of bilateral limb tremor in ET *(60–62)*, confirming Benabid's earlier experience *(32)*. However, dysarthria and gait dysequilibrium are much more frequent following bilateral than unilateral procedures, occurring in 30–50% of cases *(32,60–62)*. In one study, there was no difference in frequency of adverse effects comparing simultaneous with sequential procedures *(62)*. Although these adverse effects usually respond to pulse generator adjustments *(63,64)*, this is sometimes at the expense of satisfactory tremor control *(65)*.

Thalamotomy has been compared with thalamic DBS in some studies *(53,54,66)*. Tasker's retrospective study *(53)* has already been cited but included only a small number of ET patients and did not separate results from those in PD patients. In a retrospective unblinded study, 17 patients who underwent thalamotomy were compared with 17 who underwent thalamic DBS *(66)*. There was no significant difference in several outcome variables in the two groups, but surgical complications were higher in the thalamotomy group including intracranial hemmorhage in six patients, transient cognitive abnormalities in five patients, and transient hemiparesis in two patients. Two patients required repeat thalamotomy due to loss of benefit. There were no surgical complications in the DBS group, but four patients required lead replacements, two had IPG malfunction, and one patient underwent thalamotomy due to lack of benefit. In an unblinded, prospective randomized study that compared thalamic stimulation in seven patients with thalamotomy in six patients *(54)*, there was complete tremor suppression in both groups but fewer adverse effects and better functional improvement following thalamic DBS than thalamotomy.

Response of head and voice tremor following Vim DBS has not been widely studied. In one blinded study of 24 patients, head tremor showed significant improvement in 75% of patients following unilateral Vim DBS *(63)*. In a smaller blinded study of 14 patients, there was a statistically nonsignificant 55% improvement in head tremor *(41)*. In open-label studies, bilateral Vim DBS improved head tremor in 9 of 10 patients in one study *(62)* and head, voice, tongue, face, and trunk tremor among 13 patients in another study *(64)*. Unilateral stimulation failed to improve voice tremor in a blinded study *(61)* and partially improved voice tremor in an unblinded study *(65)*. Based on these results, isolated head and voice tremor are not currently considered indications for Vim DBS although they may improve when the procedure is carried out bilaterally for treatment of limb tremor *(58)*.

In summary, Vim DBS is highly effective for limb tremor in ET, a condition often refractory to pharmacologic treatment. Benefit for head and voice tremor is less well-established and usually requires bilateral Vim DBS to be effective.

REFERENCES

1. Hassler, R. (1959) *Introduction to Stereotaxis with an Atlas of the Human Brain.* Thieme, Stuttgart.
2. Walker, A. E. (1982) Normal and pathological physiology of the human thalamus. In: *Stereotaxy of the Human Brain: Anatomical, Physiological, and Clinical Applications* (Schaltenbrand, G. and Walker, A. E., eds.), Thieme, Stuttgart, pp. 181–217.
3. Jones, E. G. (1990) Correlation and revised nomenclature of ventral nuclei in the thalamus of human and monkey. *Stereotact. Funct. Neurosurg.* **54/55,** 1–20.
4. Hirai, T. and Jones, E. G. (1989) A new parcellation of the human thalamus on the basis of histochemical staining. *Brain Res. Rev.* **14,** 1–34.
5. Albe-Fessard, D., Arfel, G., and Guiot, G. (1962) Activities electriques characteristiques de quelques structures cerebrales chez l'homme. *Ann. Chir.* **17,** 1185–1214.
6. Lenz, F. A., Tasker, R. R., Kwan, H. C., et al. (1988) Single unit analysis of the human ventral thalamic nuclear group: correlation of thalamic "tremor cells" with the 3-6 Hz component of parkinsonian tremor. *J. Neurosci.* **8,** 754–764.
7. Ohye, C. and Narabayashi, H. (1979) Physiological study of presumed ventralis intermedius neurons in the human thalamus. *J. Neurosurg.* **50,** 290–297.

8. Lenz, F. A., Kwan, H. C., Dostrovsky, J. O., Tasker, R. R., Murphy, J. T., and Lenz, Y. E. (1990) Single unit analysis of the human ventral thalamic nuclear group. *Brain* **113,** 1795–1821.
9. Hutchison, W. D., Lozano, A. M., Tasker, R. R., Lang, A. E., and Dostrovsky, J. O. (1997) Identification and characterization of neurons with tremor-frequency activity in human globus pallidus. *Exp. Brain Res.* **113,** 557–563.
10. Bergman, N. H., Wichmann, T., Karmon, B., and DeLong, M. R. (1994) The primate subthalamic nucleus: II. Neuronal activity in the MPTP model of parkinsonism. *J. Neurophysiol.* **72,** 507–520.
11. Kelly, P. J. and Gillingham, F. J. (1980) The long-term results of stereotaxic surgery and L-dopa therapy in patients with Parkinson's disease. *J. Neurosurg.* **53,** 332–337.
12. Hallett, M. and Litvan, I. (1999) A task force on surgery for Parkinson's disease. Evaluation of surgery for Parkinson's disease. *Neurology* **53,** 1910–1921.
13. Starr, P. A., Vitak, J. L., and Bakay, R. A. E. (1998) Deep brain stimulation for movement disorders. *Neurosurg. Clin. North Am.* **9,** 381–402.
14. Obeso, J. A., Benabid, A. L., and Koller, W. C. (2000) Deep brain stimulation for Parkinson's disease and tremor. *Neurology* **55(Suppl. 6),** S1–S66.
15. Hassler, R., Riechart, T., Munginer, F., et al. (1960) Physiological observations in stereotaxic operations in extrapyramidal motor disturbances. *Brain* **83,** 337–350.
16. Ohye, C., Kubota, K., Hooper, H. E., et al. (1964) Ventrolateral and subventrolateral thalamic stimulation. *Arch. Neurol.* **11,** 427–434.
17. Cooper, I. S., Upton, A. R. M., and Amin, I. (1980) Reversibility of chronic neurologic deficits. Some effects of electrical stimulation of the thalamus and internal capsule in man. *Appl. Neurophysiol.* **43,** 244–258.
18. Andy, O. J. (1983) Thalamic stimulation for control of movement disorders. *Appl. Neurophysiol.* **46,** 107–111.
19. Benabid, A. L., Pollak, P., Gervason, C., et al. (1991) Long-term suppression of tremor by chronic stimulation of the ventral intermediate thalamic nucleus. *Lancet* **337,** 403–406.
20. Benabid, A. L., Pollak, P., Loveau, A., Henry, S., and Rougemont, J. (1987) Combined (thalamotomy and stimulation) stereotactic surgery of the VIM thalamic nucleus for bilateral Parkinson disease. *Appl. Neurophysiol.* **50,** 344–346.
21. Haberler, C., Alesch, F., Mazal, P. R., et al. (2000) No tissue damage by chronic deep brain stimulation in Parkinson's disease. *Ann. Neurol.* **48,** 372–376.
22. Benabid, A. L., Pollak, P., Siegneuret, E., Hoffmann, D., Gay, E., and Perret, J. (1993) Chronic VIM thalamic stimulation in Parkinson's disease, essential tremor, and extrapyramidal dyskinesias. *Acta Neurochir.* **58(Suppl.),** 39–44.
23. Benabid, A. L., Benazzouz, A., Hoffmann, D., Limousin, P., Krack, P., and Pollak, P. (1998) Long-term electrical inhibition of deep brain targets in movement disorders. *Mov. Disord.* **13(Suppl. 3),** 119–125.
24. Benazzouz, A. and Hallett, M. (2000) Mechanism of action of deep brain stimulation. *Neurology* **55(Suppl. 6),** S13–S16.
25. Ranck, J. B. (1975) Which elements are excited in electrical stimulation of the mammalian central nervous system: a review. *Brain Res.* **98,** 417–440.
26. Schlag, J. and Villablanca, J. (1967) A quantitative study of temporal and spatial response patterns in a thalamic cell population electrically stimulated. *Brain Res.* **8,** 255–270.
27. Deiber, M. P., Pollak, P., Passingham, R., et al. (1993) Thalamic stimulation and suppression of parkinsonism tremor. Evidence of cerebellar de-activation using positron emission tomography. *Brain* **116,** 267–279.
28. Ceballos-Baumann, A. O., Boecker, H., Fogel, W., et al. (2001) Thalamic stimulation for essential tremor activates motor and deactivates vestibular cortex. *Neurology* **56,** 1347–1354.
29. Boecker, H., Wills, A., Ceballos-Baumann, A. O., et al. (1997) Stereotactic thalamotomy in tremor dominant Parkinson's disease: a H215O PET study of motor activation. *Ann. Neurol.* **41,** 108–111.
30. Ashby, P. and Rothwell, J. C. (2000) Neurophysiologic aspects of deep brain stimulation. *Neurology* **55(Suppl. 6),** S17–S20.
31. Tasker, R. R. (1986) Effets sensitifs et moteurs de la stimulation thalamique chez l'homme. Applications Cliniques. *Rev. Neurol.* **142,** 316–326.
32. Benabid, A. L., Pollak, P., Gao, D., et al. (1996) Chronic electrical stimulation of the ventralis intermedius nucleus of the thalamus as a treatment of movement disorders. *J. Neurosurg.* **84,** 203–214.
33. Benabid, A. L., Benazzouz, A., Gao, D., et al. (1999) Chronic electrical stimulation of the ventralis intermedius nucleus of the thalamus and of other nuclei as a treatment for Parkinson's disease. *Techn. Neurosurg.* **5,** 5–30.
34. Hariz, M. I., Shamsgovara, P., Johansson, F., Hariz, G. M., and Fodstad, H. (1999) Tolerance and tremor rebound fkollowing long-term chronic thalamic stimulation for parkinsonian and essential tremor. *Stereotact. Funct. Neurosurg.* **72,** 208–218.
35. Alesch, F., Pinter, M. M., Helscher, R. J., Fertl, L., Benabid, A. L., and Koos, W. T. (1995) Stimulation of the ventral intermediate thalamic nucleus in tremor dominated Parkinson's disease and essential tremor. *Acta. Neurochir.* **136,** 75–81.
36. Koller, W., Pahwa, R., Busenbark, K., et al. (1997) High-frequency unilateral thalamic stimulation in the treatment of essential and parkinsonian tremor. *Ann. Neurol.* **42,** 292–299.
37. Tarsy, D., Ryan, P., Mechanic, D., and Norregaard, T. (1999) Thalamic deep brain stimulation for Parkinson's and essential tremor. *Parkinsonism Rel. Disord.* **5(Suppl.),** S112.
38. Blond, S. and Siegfried, J. (1991) Thalamic stimulation for the treatment of tremor and other movement disorders. *Acta Neurochirurg.* **52(Suppl.),** 109–111.
39. Blond, S., Caparros-Lefebvre, D., Parker, F., et al. (1992) Control of tremor and involuntary movement disorders by chronic stereotactic stimulation of the ventral intermediate thalamic nucleus. *J. Neurosurg.* **77,** 62–68.

40. Hubble, J. P., Busenbark, K. L., Wilkinson, S., et al. (1997) Effects of thalamic deep brain stimulation based on tremor type and diagnosis. *Mov. Disord.* **12,** 337–341.
41. Ondo, W., Jankovic, J., Schwartz, K., et al. (1998) Unilateral thalamic deep brain stimulation for refractory essential tremor and Parkinson's disease tremor. *Neurology* **51,** 1063–1069.
42. Limousin, P., Speelman, J. D., Gielen, F., et al. (1999) Multicentre European study of thalamic stimulation in parkinsonian and essential tremor. *J. Neurol. Neurosurg. Psychiatry* **66,** 289–296.
43. Apetauerova, D., Ryan, P., Mechanic, D., Norregaard, T., and Tarsy, D. (2001) Parkinson's disease remains stable for two years following thalamic deep brain stimulation for tremor. *Mov. Disord.* **16,** 990–991.
44. Ondo, W., Almaguer, M., Jankovic, J., and Simpson, R. K. (2001) Thalamic deep brain stimulation. Comparison between unilateral and bilateral placement. *Arch. Neurol.* **58,** 218–222.
45. Burleigh, A. L., Horak, F. B., Burchiel, J. K., and Nutt, J. G. (1993) Effects of thalamic stimulation on tremor, balance, and step initiation. A single subject study. *Mov. Disord.* **8,** 519–524.
46. Defebvre, L., Blatt, J. L., Blond, S., et al. (1996) Effect of thalamic stimulation in Parkinson disease. *Arch. Neurol.* **53,** 898–903.
47. Pinter, M. M., Murg, M., Alesch, F., et al. (1999) Does deep brain stimulation of the nucleus ventralis intermedius affect postural control and locomotion in Parkinson's disease? *Mov. Disord.* **6,** 958–963.
48. Caparros-Lefebvre, D., Blond, S., Vermersch, P., et al. (1993) Chronic thalamic stimulation improves tremor and levodopa-induced dyskinesias in Parkinson's disease. *J. Neurol. Neurosurg. Psychiatry* **56,** 268–273.
49. Caparros-Lefebvre, D., Blond, S., Feltin, M. P., Pollak, P., and Benabid, A. L. (1999) Improvement of levodopa induced dyskinesias by thalamic deep brain stimulation as related to slight variation in electrode placement: possible involvement of the centre median and parafascicularis complex. *J. Neurol. Neurosurg. Psychiatry* **67,** 308–314.
50. Troster, A. I., Fields, J. A., Pahwa, R., et al. (1999) Neuropsychological and quality of life outcome after thalamic stimulation for essential tremor. *Neuroloy* **53,** 1174–1780.
51. Hirai, T., Miyazaki, M., Nakajima, H., et al. (1983) The correlation between tremor characteristics and the predicted volume of effective lesions in stereotaxic nucleus ventralis intermedius thalamotomy. *Brain* **106,** 1001–1018.
52. Stellar, S. and Cooper, I. S. (1968) Mortality and morbidity in cryothalamectomy for parkinsonism. A statistical study of 2,868 consecutive operations. *J. Neurosurg.* **28,** 459–467.
53. Tasker, R. R. (1998) Deep brain stimulation is preferable to thalamotomy for tremor suppression. *Surg. Neurol.* **49,** 145–154.
54. Schuurman, P. R., Bosch, D. A., Bossuyt, P. M. N., et al. (2000) A comparison of continuous thalamic stimulation and thalamotomy for suppression of severe tremor. *N. Engl. J. Med.* **342,** 461–468.
55. Goldman, M. S., Ahlskog, J. E., and Kelly, P. J. (1992) The symptomatic and functional outcome of stereotactic thalamotomy for medically intractable essential tremor. *J. Neurosurg.* **76,** 924–928.
56. Jankovic, J., Cardoso, F., Grossman, R. G., and Hamilton, W. J. (1995) Outcome after stereotactic thalamotomy for parkinsonian, essential and other types of tremor. *Neurosurgery* **37,** 680–687.
57. Hubble, J. P., Busenbark, K. L., Wilkinson, S., Penn, R. D., Lyons, K., and Koller, W. C. (1996) Deep brain stimulation for essential tremor. *Neurology* **46,** 1150–1153.
58. Koller, W. C., Pahwa, R., Lyons, K. E., and Wilkinson, S. B. (2000) Deep brain stimulation of the Vim nucleus of the thalamus for the treatment of tremor. *Neurology* **55(Suppl. 6),** S29–S33.
59. Pollak, P., Benabid, A. L., Krack, P., et al. (1998) Deep brain stimulation. In: *Parkinson's Disease and Movement Disorders* (Jankovic, J. and Tolosa, E, eds.), Williams & Wilkins, Baltimore, MD, pp. 1085–1101.
60. Pahwa, R., Lyons, K. L., Wilkinson, S. B., et al. (1999) Bilateral thalamic stimulation for the treatment of essential tremor. *Neurology* **53,** 1447–1450.
61. Ondo, W., Almaguer, M., Jankovic, J., and Simpson, R. K. (2001) Thalamic deep brain stimulation. Comparison between unilateral and bilateral placement. *Arch. Neurol.* **58,** 218–232.
62. Taha, J. M., Janszen, M. A., and Favre, J. (1999) Thalamic deep brain stimulation for the treatment of head, voice, and bilateral limb tremor. *J. Neurosurg.* **91,** 68–72.
63. Koller, W. C., Lyons, K. E., Wilkinson, S. B., and Pahwa, R. (1999) Efficacy of unilateral deep brain stimulation of the VIM nucleus of the thalamus for essential head tremor. *Mov. Disord.* **14,** 847–850.
64. Obwegeser, A. A., Uitti, R. J., Turk, M. F., Strongosky, A. J., and Wharen, R. E. (2000) Thalamic stimulation for the treatment of midline tremors in essential tremor patients. *Neurology* **54,** 2342–2344.
65. Carpenter, M. A., Pahwa, R., Miyawaki, K. L., Wilkinson, S. B., Seral, J. P., and Koller, W. C. (1998) Reduction in voice tremor under thalamic stimulation. *Neurology* **50,** 796–798.
66. Pahwa, R., Lyons, K. E., Wilkinson, S. B., et al. (2001) Comparison of thalamotomy to deep brain stimulation of the thalamus in essential tremor. *Mov. Disord.* **16,** 140–143.

12

Pallidal Deep Brain Stimulation for Parkinson's Disease

Jens Volkmann and Volker Sturm

1. INTRODUCTION

Modern stereotactic surgery extends the previously limited therapeutic options in patients with advanced Parkinson's disease (PD) and side effects of long-term L-dopa treatment. Among those functional neurosurgical procedures, pallidotomy has been the most frequent operation performed in advanced PD after its reintroduction by Laitinen and colleagues in 1992 *(1)*. In the past 10 years, results concerning several hundred successful pallidotomies have been published. The most reliable effect of this procedure is a marked reduction or complete suppression of contralateral L-dopa-induced dyskinesias *(2)*. The amount of improvement of contralateral bradykinesia, rigidity, and tremor differs between studies but is significant in most of them *(2)*. The finding of abnormally increased neuronal activity in the internal segment of the globus pallidus (GPi) in nonhuman primates with N-methyl-4-phenyl-1,2,3,6-tetrahydropyridine (MPTP)-induced-parkinsonism leading to excessive inhibition of downstream thalamocortical motor circuits remains the prevailing pathophysiological basis for pallidal lesioning *(3)*.

High-frequency deep brain stimulation (DBS) is an alternative to ablative surgery, which was first introduced for the treatment of movement disorders in the 1970s *(4,5)* but was not routinely used until the pioneering work of Benabid and colleagues became public in the early 1990s *(6)*. Experience with DBS in the thalamus for the treatment of tremor has been that it is generally safe and effective. There is good evidence that thalamic DBS offers the same symptomatic benefit, but even better functional outcome than thalamotomy *(7)*. For the pallidal target, however, there are still remarkably few studies extending the initial observation of Siegfried and Lippitz *(8)* that chronic high-frequency stimulation of the internal pallidum may have the same clinical effects as pallidotomy, with the advantage of being reversible and adaptable throughout the course of the disease. The most appealing aspect of pallidal stimulation demonstrated in this first report was the possibility of performing safe bilateral procedures. Most patients suffering from advanced stage parkinsonism have bilateral disease with prominent axial symptoms such as gait, balance, or speech deficits, which are not adequately treated by unilateral surgery. However, bilateral pallidotomy is only exceptionally performed in most centers because of concern for increased risk of neuropsychological side effects or speech problems after surgery *(9–11)*. These patients could potentially be good candidates for bilateral pallidal stimulation or unilateral pallidal stimulation and contralateral pallidotomy. However, preliminary reports concerning pallidal DBS involved only small numbers of patients in mostly unblinded studies. Therefore, many claims made about pallidal stimulation still await confirmation in properly designed controlled clinical trials. In this chapter, we present our personal experience with pallidal DBS for advanced Parkinson's disease since 1996 and critically review the current literature.

From: Contemporary Clinical Neurology:
Surgical Treatment of Parkinson's Disease and Other Movement Disorders
Edited by: D. Tarsy, J. L. Vitek, and A. M. Lozano © Humana Press Inc., Totowa, NJ

2. PATIENT SELECTION

Patient selection criteria for pallidal DBS are similar to those for pallidotomy. Ideal candidates have idiopathic PD with a preserved and very good L-dopa response but with side effects of long-term medical treatment such as motor fluctuations or dyskinesias. Dementia, acute psychosis, and depression that persist during "on" periods usually constitute exclusion criteria. The general health of the patient needs to be good enough to withstand the operation and to allow for cooperation during prolonged surgery while awake. In our experience, a presurgical L-dopa test (1–1.5 times the equivalent of the regular morning antiparkinson medication in form of short-acting L-dopa) helps to predict the individual response profile of a patient to bilateral pallidal stimulation. Except for L-dopa dyskinesias, symptoms that persist during the patient's best "on" state after taking a challenge dose of levodopa are less likely to benefit from pallidal DBS.

The treating physician should discuss the patient's personal expectations of surgery and correct any unrealistic perspectives that may exist. The patient needs to understand that the therapeutic benefits of pallidal DBS may not be immediately realized after surgery. Programming the device may be time-consuming and tedious and the patient must be willing and able to cooperate during this process.

3. SURGICAL PROCEDURE

All of our operations for treating advanced PD are planned as simultaneous bilateral lead implantations. We perform stereotactic surgery under local anesthesia after overnight withdrawal of antiparkinson drugs. On the day of surgery, the patient's head is fixed in a modified Riechert-Mundinger stereotactic head ring under brief sedation. After intravenous injection of iodine containing contrast medium (Solutrast®, Byk Gulden, Konstanz, Germany, dose: 1.5 g iopamidol/kg) stereotactic cranial computed tomography (CCT) is performed (SOMATOM PLUS 40, Siemens, Erlangen, FRG) with 2 mm slice thickness, no interslice spacing, and 2-mm table increment. The CT-data are transferred via the hospital's data-net to a workstation (DecWorkstation, Digital Equip., USA) located in the OR. After computerized implementation of a three-dimensional (3D) stereotactic coordinate system, the CCT is used as a distortion-free reference system for magnetic resonance imaging (MRI) and to integrate data provided by teleradiography or ventriculography.

Nonstereotactic MRI is performed the day before surgery. Thin slice axial images (T1- and T2-weighted, 2 mm slice thickness) or coronal images (T2-weighted) are obtained using either a 1.5 Tesla (Philips Gyroscan ACS) or a 1.0 Tesla scanner (Philips Gyroscan T10NT). In the case of T1-weighted axial imaging, data acquisition is done without interslice spacing or interslice overlapping. T2-weighted axial images are obtained with scans of 4 mm slice thickness but 2 mm increment resulting in slices having 2 mm overlap.

MRI data are integrated into the 3D-stereotactic coordinate system using landmark-based image fusion *(12)*. Briefly, a set of corresponding anatomical landmarks such as characteristic vessel branchings, clearly visible on both computed tomography (CT) and MRI, are interactively defined by the neurosurgeon. For each pair of points, the algorithm that is part of the treatment-planning software (STP releases 3.3 and 3.5, Leibinger-Howmedica, Freiburg, FRG) calculates a particular correlation accuracy. Points with a difference exceeding 2 mm are rejected before image fusion. Superimposing the 3D-net of correlation points, the software integrates the MR images into the stereotactic CT-based coordinate system. The fusion result is accepted if the mean deviation is below 1.2 mm. The course of characteristic anatomical contors (large intracranial vessels, ventricular walls, gyri, and/or sulci) in a CT-/MR-spyglass view provides additional visual information about the validity of the fusion process.

A cannula is introduced at a target point immediately above the right foramen of Monro via a right-sided, 8-mm, burr-hole trephination. Positive ventriculography is obtained after intraventricular injection of 10 cc contrast medium (= 5.1 g iopamidol, Solutrast® 250 M, Byk Gulden, Konstanz, Germany). The initial target coordinates for GPi are those reported by Laitinen and colleagues *(1)*. Additionally, the contour of GPi is outlined on the MRI. Stereotactic coordinates obtained from ventriculography are then transferred into the 3D-stereotactic coordinate system and, if necessary, readjusted based on the individual MRI anatomy. In order to minimize operative risks, each trajectory (either planned for ventriculography or electrode implantation) is carefully controlled on MRI. Displays of the trajectories in various reconstruction planes give slice by slice information concerning the position of the probe and surrounding structures in order to avoid crossing of a sulcus, ventricular walls, vessels, if they are visible on the images, and/or larger fiber tracts (e.g., optic tract). Particular attention is paid to the trephination, which is placed over a vessel-free area.

First, a bipolar electrode (TCB013, Howmedica-Leibinger, Freiburg, FRG. OD: 2 mm, distance between the poles: 2 mm,) is introduced stereotactically at a point 4 mm above the target and the position controlled on stereotactic X-rays. If electrode placement is in accordance with the planned trajectory, stepwise macrostimulation (1-mm steps) is performed with a frequency of 130 Hz, and a pulse width of 0.1 ms. The intraoperative improvement of symptoms and possible side effects are evaluated by a neurologist and the electrode position with the optimal clinical effect is documented. Then, the stimulation lead (Medtronic®, model 3387) is introduced under fluoroscopic control at the target point with optimal clinical benefit. The lead is fixed with a suture and additionally stabilized with methylmethacrylate (Palacos®, Merck, Darmstadt, Germany). The correct electrode position is finally documented in the OR with teleradiography.

We recently have started to perform routine microelectrode recordings during surgery; however, based on our experience in more than 100 electrode implantations since 1996, we believe that careful intraoperative neurological examination during macrostimulation is mandatory and probably sufficient to achieve good clinical results. Without microrecording a typical bilateral lead implantation takes approx 6 h in our hands, including time for intraoperative CT scanning. Scientific interest has been the driving force behind establishing microelectrode recordings at our center, but it remains undecided whether better clinical outcomes will justify the extra time and manpower required for microelectrode recording.

During the first 3–4 postoperative days, the leads are connected to percutaneous extensions and the electrode combinations generating good clinical effects are approximated. After that period, the leads are connected to subcutaneously implanted pulse generators (Medtronic®, model ITREL II). Then stimulation parameters are determined by testing the effect of stimulation for each electrode pole in a monopolar mode under controlled medication "off" condition and choosing the contact for chronic stimulation that results in the best clinical effect at lowest stimulation intensity and largest therapeutic range before induction of side effects. During the ensuing months, stimulation parameters and medication are periodically adjusted according to the patient's needs. Usually, only minor changes are necessary after the first 3 mo of follow-up examination.

4. CLINICAL RESULTS

4.1. *Efficacy*

The consistent effect produced by pallidal stimulation in all published reports is a marked reduction of contralateral L-dopa induced dyskinesias *(8,13–25)*. Improvement of "off" period symptoms of parkinsonism is more variable but significant in most studies in the range of 20–30% for unilateral and 30–50% for bilateral stimulation (Table 1). In our own experience, bilateral GPi stimulation ($n = 11$) produced a 54 ± 33.1% (SD) improvement in the "off" period Unified Parkinson's Disease Rating Scale (UPDRS) motor score at 1 yr follow-up (Fig. 1) *(24,25)*. For UPDRS subscores, we found significant improvement for bradykinesia, tremor, posture, and gait, and a tendency towards improvement in rigidity. "On" period motor symptoms did not significantly change after surgery except for dyskinesias, which were reduced by 83% at 1-yr follow-up. The combination of reduced dyskinesias and "off" period motor symptoms led to a significant reduction of self-perceived motor fluctuations in our patients.

Table 1
Literature Review of Pallidal Deep Brain Stimulation for Advanced Parkinson's Disease

					Before surgery		After surgery (Stimulation ON)				
					UPDRS motor score		UPDRS motor score		DRS	LEDD	
Author (year)	Patients n (uni-bilateral)	Age (yr)	Duration of disease (mo)	Duration of follow-up (yr)	Med OFF	% change (Med ON)	% change (Med OFF)	% change (Med ON)	% change	% change	Adverse events[a] (*n*)
Siegfried (1994) *(8)*											
Tronnier (1997) *(23)*	6 (0/6)	61.7	13.8	6.7	36.0	–50.0%	5.6%	55.6%	–77.1%	–6.5%	None
Durif (1999) *(15)*	6 (1/5)	64.0	15.0	6.0	36.0	–75.0%	–36.1%	–44.4%	–50.0%	6.3%	Transient depression (1), hyperthermia (1)
Krack (1998) *(18)*	8 (3/5)	50.9	15.6	6.0	50.0	–62.0%	–32.0%	NA	–72.0%	25.4%	None
Burchiel (1999) *(14)*	4 (0/4)	46.5	10.6	12.0	67.0	–43.3%	–40.2%	–47.4%	–47.4%	5.5%	Lead fracture (1)
Ghika (1998) *(16)*	6 (0/6)	55.0	15.5	24.0	66.0	–42.4%	–50.0%	–26.3%	NA	35.2%	Electrode revision (1)
Gross (1997) *(17)*	7 (7/0)	52.5	11.3	12.0	53.4	–31.6%	–30.7%	–42.5%	NA	NA	None
Pahwa (1997) *(22)*	5 (2/3)	54.8	14.6	3.0	53.4	–17.6%	NA	–60.5%	NA	4.2%	Electrode revision (1), asympt. hemorrhage (1)
Kumar (1998) *(19)*	8 (4/4)	51.5	12.7	5.4	NA	NA	–27.0%	8.0%	–60.0%	NA	Scalp infection (1), electrode explant (1)
Merello (1999) *(21)*	6 (6/0)	55.3	13.5	3.0	29.5	–39.3%	–28.8%	7.5%	–44.3%	NA	Transient crural paresis (1); transient psychosis (1), seroma (1)
Volkmann (2000) *(25)*	11 (0/11)	56.6	10.5	12.0	52.5	–42.5%	–50.5%	–44.0%	–80.0%	–27.6%	Infection (1), lead dislocation (1), scalp erosion (2), transient confusion (3), neuralgia (1), increased falls (1)
DBS for PD Study Group *(20)*	38 (0/38)	55.7	14.5	6.0	50.8	–52.6%	–33.3%	–26.8%	–66.7%	2.8%	Hemorrhage (4), hemiparesis after hemorrhage (3), seizures (1), dysarthria (1), lead dislocation (2), infection (1), lead break (1), seroma (1), dyskinesias (5)

DRS, dystonia rating scale; LEDD, levodopa equivalent daily dose.
[a]Some patients may have had more than one adverse effect.

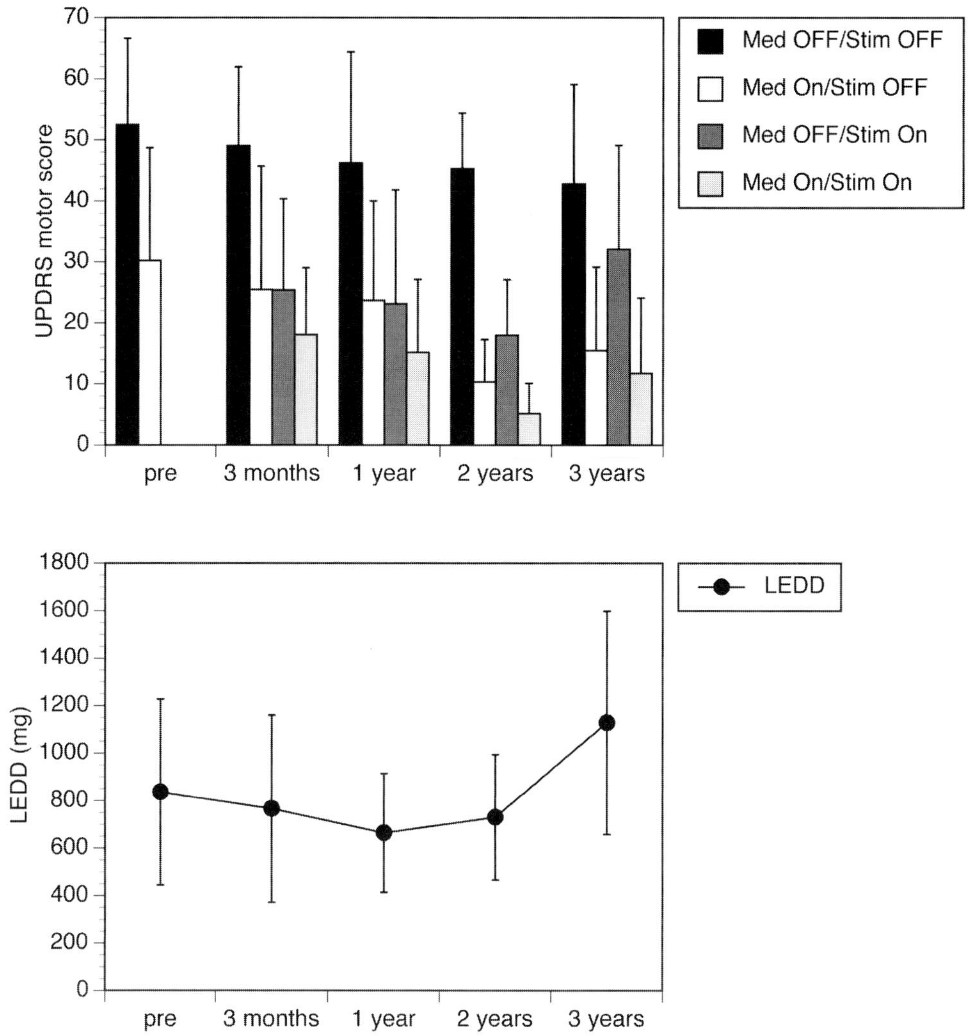

Fig. 1. UPDRS motor scores before surgery (n = 11) and 3 mo (n = 11), 1 yr (n = 9), 2 yr (n = 6), and 3 yr (n = 5) after bilateral pallidal DBS implantation. Bars denote group mean values for the four possible combinations of medication "on" or "off" and stimulation "on" or "off" state. Note a marked reduction in "off" medication UPDRS scores postoperatively produced by pallidal stimulation, which declines at the 3 yr follow-up examination. Below, the group mean LEDD (levodopa equivalent dose) is displayed for the same time points. The decrease in stimulation efficacy at 3 yr is accompanied by an increase in LEDD.

One group reported a reduction of dyskinesias but worsening motor function during the medication "on" period *(23)* after bilateral pallidal stimulation, which stands in contrast to all other published studies. Because the exact position of the stimulating electrodes is uncertain in this and most other studies, it is difficult to discern how much the variable effect of pallidal stimulation is owing to different target locations within GPi. Two preliminary studies *(26,27)* claim that, based on the observation of acute stimulation effects, DBS of the ventral GPi may block dyskinesias but aggravate akinesia, whereas dorsal GPi stimulation ameliorates akinesia while inducing dyskinesia. The importance of these experimental observations for therapeutic long-term stimulation can only be determined in future studies by carefully relating the efficacy of chronic pallidal stimulation to the exact target location within GPi as determined by neuroimaging techniques and microelectrode recordings.

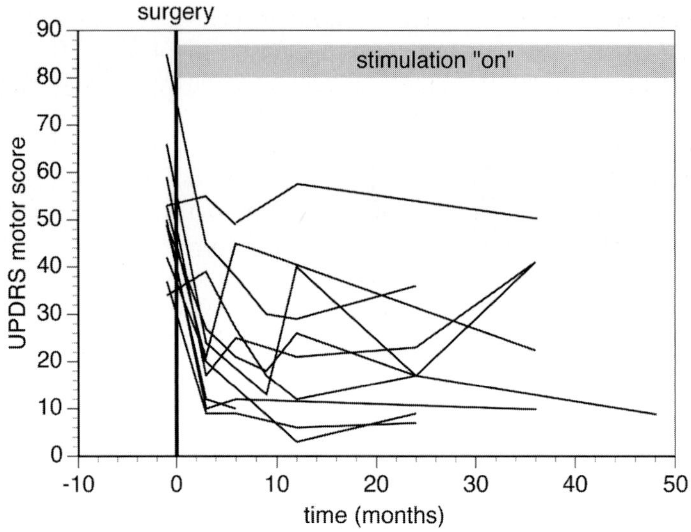

Fig. 2. Individual time course of "off-drug" UPDRS motor scores with pallidal stimulation. Each line represents one of eleven patients treated with bilateral GPi-DBS. Remarkable is the variability of treatment effects during long-term follow-up. Some patients have a stable treatment response over up to 48 mo of follow-up, whereas others show a decline in stimulation efficacy starting around 2 yr after surgery.

Despite the commonly held assumption that DBS is equally effective but safer than lesioning techniques, only one clinical trial has addressed this issue. In a group of 13 patients randomized to either unilateral pallidal DBS or radiofrequency lesioning of the GPi, Merello and colleagues *(21)* found about equal improvement in UPDRS motor score in the two groups after 3 mo follow-up. There was greater reduction of contralateral dyskinesias after pallidotomy whereas bilateral hand tapping scores improved more with DBS. There is no direct comparison of bilateral pallidotomy and bilateral pallidal DBS available so far, but the speech and cognitive problems reported after bilateral pallidal lesioning *(9–11)* have not been encountered in current reports of pallidal stimulation.

So far mainly short-term observations of 1 yr or less following pallidal DBS have been reported. Ghika et al. *(16)* reported persistent improvement in motor scores and activities of daily living 2 yr after pallidal DBS, but noticed some decline in efficacy appearing after 12 mo in their patients. During long-term follow-up of between 2 and 4 yr we also noted some decline in efficacy after 1–2 yr of pallidal stimulation in three of our patients (Figs. 1 and 2). In these patients motor fluctuations returned and did not respond satisfactorily to changes in stimulation parameters or medication. Similar observations of secondary therapeutic failure after pallidal stimulation have been reported in small numbers of patients by other groups *(13,28)*. Similar to the two cases reported by Houeto et al. *(28)*, we have succesfully reimplanted several of our patients in subthalamic nucleus (STN). They had a similar benefit in terms of motor improvement and medication reduction as those patients primarily implanted within STN. These anectodal reports underline the reversability of pallidal stimulation and suggest that the subthalamic target may be preferable to the pallidal target in the treatment of advanced Parkinson's disease. From a group perspective, however, only one comparative study currently supports this conclusion. Krack et al. *(18)* reported a 71% improvement in "off" period UPDRS motor score with STN-stimulation but only 39% with GPi-stimulation in a group of 13 patients with young-onset Parkinson's disease. This significant difference resulted from a greater reduction of akinesia in the STN-stimulated group, whereas other parkinsonian symptoms showed about equal improvement. In contrast, Burchiel et al. *(14)* found no difference in reduction of akinetic-rigid symptoms of PD or dyskinesias between STN- and GPi-stimulated patients in a well designed, but small randomized-prospective trial. In our own retrospective analysis of the initial 11 patients implanted in GPi and 16 patients implanted in

STN, the main finding was a 54 ± 33.1% improvement of "off" period motor symptoms in the GPi group and 67 ± 22.6% improvement in the STN group after 1 yr follow-up *(25)*. The 10–15% difference between the two groups was not significant and power analysis suggested that based on the group variances, a much larger trial including a minimum of 135 patients in each arm would have been needed to prove significance of this possible small difference in favor of STN-stimulation.

The only consistent differences between GPi and STN stimulation reported so far concern medication requirements and stimulation parameters. Patients with GPi-stimulation continue to require preoperative antiparkinson medication doses and, in some cases, even higher doses are introduced postoperatively. By contrast, STN stimulation allows an average reduction of dopaminergic medication in the range of 65% and equivalent improvement of "off" period motor symptoms *(25)*. The energy required for effective GPi stimulation is about two- to threefold higher than values reported for STN or thalamic stimulation *(20,25,29,30)*.

4.2. Safety

In keeping with DBS in other targets, pallidal stimulation carries a low risk of chronic morbidity. Transient morbidity is less exceptional in current studies (Table 1) but most authors acknowledge a learning curve with this procedure, which may expain a higher incidence of technical and minor surgical complications in their initial patients. Pallidal stimulation is adaptable and stimulation parameters can be set to achieve the optimal clinical efficacy in a given patient without inducing permanent stimulation induced side effects. Therefore, visual field disturbances, facial weakness, or dysarthria, characteristic adverse effects of pallidotomy, are rarely encountered after pallidal stimulation unless deliberately accepted by patient and physician because of greater improvement of parkinsonian symptoms.

Global scores of cognitive function exhibit little change after unilateral or bilateral pallidal stimulation *(16,24,31,32)*. However, subtle worsening of frontal lobe scores, including verbal fluency, has been described by several investigators *(24,31,32)*. Although most patients and relatives are unaware of these changes in daily life, behavioral alteration of a frontal nature has been reported in single cases after bilateral pallidal stimulation *(24,33)*. Advanced age and high preoperative doses of L-dopa were found to be predictive factors of postoperative cognitive worsening in one study *(31)*.

5. PHYSIOLOGICAL MECHANISMS

It has been demonstrated that pallidotomy can restore normal levels of activity in thalamocortical motor pathways by decreasing the abnormal inhibitory outflow from the GPi to ventrolateral thalamus. Positron emission tomography (PET) studies after pallidotomy showed increased regional cerebral blood flow (rCBF) *(34,35)* and metabolism *(36)* in ipsilateral supplementary motor cortex (SMA) and dorsolateral prefrontal cortex (DLPFC) of parkinsonian patients after unilateral pallidotomy. These changes in cerebral blood flow were associated with improvements in motor function. Similar reversible changes of rCBF in SMA and DLPFC have been described after high-frequency stimulation of the internal pallidum *(37)*. The effect of pallidal stimulation on the thalamocortical motor network therefore resembles a "functional" lesioning of the GPi. However, it remains uncertain exactly how brain DBS "blocks" neuronal activity on a cellular level. Stimulation at high frequencies (>100 Hz) is necessary to achieve this inactivating effect in all three targets (thalamus, STN, GPi). It has therefore been hypothesized *(38)* that the short interstimulus interval between current pulses may not allow neuronal membranes to recover from depolarization thus inactivating the spike generating mechanism (depolarization block). However, an electrophysiological study in MPTP-monkeys suggests that pallidal stimulation reduces the abnormally increased firing rate of GPi neurons to normal levels rather than silencing cells within GPi *(39)*. The depolarization block theory is not compatible with this observation. Dostrovsky and colleagues examined the effects of microstimulation in GPi on the activity of neurons close to the stimulation site during stereotactic surgery in patients with Parkinson's disease *(40)*. They found inhibition of spontaneous neuronal activity with 10–25 ms duration after single microstimulation pulses. As would be expected from the 20 ms inhibition duration, stimulation at 50 Hz resulted in pronounced but incomplete depression of neuronal firing. The authors conclude that an important effect of stimulation within GPi could be repetitive excitation of inhibitory afferents from putamen and GPe leading to GABA release on GPi neurons. A remaining open question is why the optimal DBS frequency range is between 100 and 200 Hz and not 50–80 Hz as predicted from the time course of single pulse inhibition.

Electrical stimulation is more likely to activate large myelinated fibers before small axons or cell bodies *(41)*. It is therefore possible that macrostimulation within GPi not only stimulates incoming afferents ortho- and antidromically but also the output axons of many GPi neurons. Although high-frequency driving of efferent axons cannot directly reduce inhibition of target neurons in brainstem and thalamus, it may still be important in converting abnormally patterned output that underlies dyskinesias or tremor into a tonic and physiologically meaningless signal.

We still do not know which of the previously proposed mechanisms alone or in combination contribute to the overall effect of pallidal DBS. Based on these experimental observations, however, it is conceivable that the effect of DBS could vary with the predominance of either inibitory or excitatory afferent fibers or efferent axons at different target sites within GPi.

6. ANATOMICAL CONSIDERATIONS

The GPi is a bean-shaped structure surrounded by the external globus pallidus (GPe) dorsolaterally, the internal capsule medially, and the pyramidal tract ventrally. It has a volume of approx 500 mm^2 in humans. Histologically the accessory medullary lamina devides the GPi into an outer segment (GPi,e) and an inner segment (GPi,i). The main afferents to GPi come from GABAergic striatal output neurons ("direct" basal ganglia pathway) and glutamatergic STN neurons ("indirect" basal ganglia pathway). GPe neurons also send GABAergic axon collaterals to GPi. The GPi sends GABAergic efferents to the ventrolateral thalamic complex and the tegmental region *(3)*. Pallidofugal fibers are organized in two distinct bundles, the ansa lenticularis and the lenticular fasciculus. They cross the internal capsule and merge in Forel's Field H. Lesioning and degeneration studies in the monkey suggest that the ansa lenticularis, which runs along the ventral border of GPi, arises from more extensive regions of the medial pallidal segment. The lenticular fasciculus, in contrast, seems to originate predominantly from dorsal and more apical regions of GPi and leaves the nucleus dorsally *(42,43)*.

Current evidence suggests that the basal ganglia are organized into several structurally and functionally distinct cortico-basal ganglia-thalamo-cortical circuits, which are involved in motor, oculomotor, associative, and limbic tasks *(44)*. The motor loop is the most relevant for understanding the cardinal features of PD. The sensorimotor region lies in the ventrolateral aspect of the GPi. Within this subregion, intraoperative microelectrode recordings have revealed a similar somatotopic organization in monkeys and humans with a more dorsal leg area, a ventral face area, and an arm area in between *(45)*. Pallidal areas receiving input from limbic and prefrontal cortex are located more dorsally and medially within GPi *(46)*.

The usual coordinates for pallidotomy are 20–21 mm lateral to the intercommissural line (AC-PC line), 5–6 mm above, and 3 mm anterior to the midcommissural point *(1)*. This corresponds to the ventrolateral aspect of the GPi, where microelectrode recordings demonstrate movement related cells *(47)*. There is a debate as to whether some or all of the pallidotomy effect might result from lesioning of the ansa lenticularis ventral to GPi *(48)*. However, Baron and colleagues *(49)*, using tracer techniques in squirrel monkeys, recently demonstrated that pallidothalamic fibers originating within the sensorimotor region of the GPi project mostly through the lenticular fasciculus and contribute very little to the ansa lenticularis, in contrast with generally accepted schemes *(42,43)*.

To what extent the topography of pallidal stimulation effects is related to the anatomical subdivision of GPi or the anatomy of pallidal fiber tracts remains a matter of speculation. Neither it is known whether the optimal site for pallidal lesioning and stimulation are identical. Two independent acute studies have found evidence for better antiparkinson effects by stimulation through more dorsolateral contacts of the quadrupolar stimulating electrodes *(26,27)*. Stimulation of ventromedial GPi, in contrast, was antidyskinetic but also blocked the beneficial effect of levodopa on akinesia. In our own experience the position of the most beneficial electrode pole used for chronic pallidal stimulation was on average slightly more lateral and dorsal than the standard pallidotomy target (3.5 ± 1.9 mm anterior to the midommissural point, 2.0 ± 2.6 mm below the intercommissural line and 22.5 ± 2.06 lateral to the midline of the third ventricule). This corresponds to a location lateral and dorsal to the optic tract in postoperative MRI controls. Given a current spread of approx 3 mm around the cathode, based on average electrical parameters for pallidal stimulation *(41)*, it is likely that stimulation effects at these coordinates will not remain restricted to the sensorimotor region of GPi, but may also affect the lenticular fasciculus and medial regions of GPe. A possible explanation of why costimulation of GPe may have antiparkinson effects could come from recent physiological observations that pallidal stimulation may block neuronal acitivity within GPi through acitvating inhibitory afferents *(40)*. GPe is one possible source of such GABAergic afferents to GPi. High-frequency stimulation of the lenticular fasciculus on the other hand, could be effective through converting abnormal pallidal output activity into a physiologically meaningless signal to the ventrolateral thalamus. With respect to the functional and anatomical heterogeneity of GPi, it is desirable that future studies on pallidal DBS carefully relate their clinical findings to the final electrode location in order to further optimize the target for pallidal lead implants.

7. CONCLUSIONS

The majority of currently available studies suggest that GPi DBS is highly effective in reducing "off" period motor symptoms, motor fluctuations, and dyskinesias in patients with advanced PD. Bilateral GPi DBS can be safely performed simultaneously, which may be the most relevant advantage over pallidotomy. However, many practical and conceptual questions concerning this therapy remain unanswered. The short duration of follow-up in most studies prevents drawing any conclusion concerning longterm stability of clinical benefit. With respect to the complexity of stimulation effects within subregions of GPi, better documentation of final electrode coordinates and their clinical efficacy is needed in order to determine causes of variable benefits in different reports. Despite the small number of patients treated, the lack of randomized-controlled clinical trials, and very limited comparative studies of bilateral GPi and STN-stimulation *(14,18,25)* the STN target has recently been increasingly favored for treatment of advanced PD. On theoretical grounds, according to current models of basal ganglia circuitry, the STN is in a unique position to influence both output nuclei of the basal ganglia, GPi, and substantia nigra pars reticulata (SNpr) *(3)*. Other reasons for this bias may be the less consistent success rate of pallidal stimulation effects *(23,24,26,27)* and the lack of an incentive for groups successfully performing STN surgery to reconsider their target. Whether a large prospective, randomized, and blinded clinical trial comparing STN and GPi DBS can be organized under these conditions is doubtful. A recent initiative in Germany failed in the initial phase because most centers declined to randomize their patients to either procedure based on their assumption that STN DBS would be superior. GPi DBS may therefore gradually disappear from clinical practice despite never having been properly evaluated. The history of pallidotomy, which was given up on empirical grounds in the 1960s for thalamotomy, followed by a renaissance two decades later, should remind us that a strict adherence to the standards of evidence-based medicine is probably the preferred way for scientific progress to be made in the field of functional neurosurgery.

REFERENCES

1. Laitinen, L. V., Bergenheim, A. T., and Hariz, M. I. (1992) Leksell's posteroventral pallidotomy in the treatment of Parkinson's disease. *J. Neurosurg.* **76(1),** 53–61.
2. Lang, A. E., Duff, J., Saint-Cyr, J. A., et al. (1999) Posteroventral medial pallidotomy in Parkinson's disease. *J. Neurol.* **246(Suppl. 2),** 28–41.

3. DeLong, M. R. (1990) Primate models of movement disorders of basal ganglia origin. *Trends Neurosci.* **13(7),** 281–285.
4. Mundinger, F. (1977) [New stereotactic treatment of spasmodic torticollis with a brain stimulation system (author's transl)]. *Med. Klin.* **72(46),** 1982–1986.
5. Mundinger, F. and Neumuller, H. (1982) Programmed stimulation for control of chronic pain and motor diseases. *Appl. Neurophysiol.* **45(1–2),** 102–111.
6. Benabid, A. L., Pollak, P., Gervason, C., et al. (1991) Long-term suppression of tremor by chronic stimulation of the ventral intermediate thalamic nucleus. *Lancet* **337(8738),** 403–406.
7. Schuurman, P. R., Bosch, D. A., Bossuyt, P. M., et al. (2000) A comparison of continuous thalamic stimulation and thalamotomy for suppression of severe tremor. *N. Engl. J. Med.* **342(7),** 461–468.
8. Siegfried, J. and Lippitz, B. (1994) Bilateral chronic electrostimulation of ventroposterolateral pallidum: a new therapeutic approach for alleviating all parkinsonian symptoms. *Neurosurgery* **35(6),** 1126–1129.
9. Ghika, J., Ghika-Schmid, F., Fankhauser, H., et al. (1999) Bilateral contemporaneous posteroventral pallidotomy for the treatment of Parkinson's disease: neuropsychological and neurological side effects. Report of four cases and review of the literature. *J. Neurosurg.* **91(2),** 313–321.
10. Favre, J., Burchiel, K. J., Taha, J. M., et al. (2000) Outcome of unilateral and bilateral pallidotomy for Parkinson's disease: patient assessment. *Neurosurgery* **46(2),** 344–353.
11. Intemann, P. M., Masterman, D., Subramanian, I., et al. (2001) Staged bilateral pallidotomy for treatment of Parkinson disease. *J. Neurosurg.* **94(3),** 437–444.
12. Ende, G., Treuer, H., and Boesecke, R. (1992) Optimization and evaluation of landmark-based image correlation. *Phys. Med. Biol.* **37(1),** 261–271.
13. Barcia-Salorio, J. L., Roldan, P., Talamantes, F., et al. (1999) Electrical inhibition of basal ganglia nuclei in Parkinson's disease: long-term results. *Stereotact. Funct. Neurosurg.* **72,** 202–207.
14. Burchiel, K. J., Anderson, V. C., Favre, J., et al. (1999) Comparison of pallidal and subthalamic nucleus deep brain stimulation for advanced Parkinson's disease: results of a randomized, blinded pilot study. *Neurosurgery* **45(6),** 1375–1382.
15. Durif, F., Lemaire, J.-J., Debilly, B., et al. (1999) Acute and chronic effects of anteromedial globus pallidus stimulation in Parkinson's disease. *J. Neurol. Neurosurg. Psychiatry* **67,** 315–321.
16. Ghika, J., Villemure, J. G., Fankhauser, H., et al. (1998) Efficiency and safety of bilateral contemporaneous pallidal stimulation (deep brain stimulation) in levodopa-responsive patients with Parkinson's disease with severe motor fluctuations: a 2-year follow-up review. *J. Neurosurg.* **89(5),** 713–718.
17. Gross, C., Rougier, A., Guehl, D., et al. (1997) High-frequency stimulation of the globus pallidus internalis in Parkinson's disease: a study of seven cases. *J. Neurosurg.* **87(4),** 491–498.
18. Krack, P., Pollak, P., Limousin, P., et al. (1998) Subthalamic nucleus or internal pallidum stimulation in young onset Parkinson's disease. *Brain* **121,** 451–457.
19. Kumar, R., Lozano, A. M., Montgomery, E., et al. (1998) Pallidotomy and deep brain stimulation of the pallidum and subthalamic nucleus in advanced Parkinson's disease. *Mov. Disord.* **13(Suppl. 1),** 73–82.
20. The Deep Brain Stimulation for Parkinson's Disease Study Group (2001) Deep brain stimulation of the subthalamic nucleus or the pars interna of the globus pallidus in Parkinson's disease. *N. Engl. J. Med.* **345(13),** 956–963.
21. Merello, M., Nouzeilles, M. I., Kuzis, G., et al. (1999) Unilateral radiofrequency lesion versus electrostimulation of posteroventral pallidum: a prospective randomized comparison. *Mov. Disord.* **14(1),** 50–56.
22. Pahwa, R., Wilkinson, S., Smith, D., et al. (1997) High-frequency stimulation of the globus pallidus for the treatment of Parkinson's disease. *Neurology* **49(1),** 249–253.
23. Tronnier, V. M., Fogel, W., Kronenbuerger, M., et al. (1997) Pallidal stimulation: an alternative to pallidotomy? *J. Neurosurg.* **87(5),** 700–705.
24. Volkmann, J., Sturm, V., Weiss, P., et al. (1998) Bilateral high-frequency stimulation of the internal globus pallidus in advanced Parkinson's disease. *Ann. Neurol.* **44,** 953–961.
25. Volkmann, J., Allert, N., Voges, J., et al. (2001) Safety and efficacy of pallidal or subthalamic nucleus stimulation in advanced PD. *Neurology* **56,** 548–551.
26. Bejjani, B., Damier, P., Arnulf, I., et al. (1997) Pallidal stimulation for Parkinson's disease. Two targets? *Neurology* **49(6),** 1564–1569.
27. Krack, P., Pollak, P., Limousin, P., et al. (1998) Opposite motor effects of pallidal stimulation in Parkinson's disease. *Ann. Neurol.* **43(2),** 180–192.
28. Houeto, J. L., Bejjani, P. B., Damier, P., et al. (2000) Failure of long-term pallidal stimulation corrected by subthalamic nucleus stimulation in PD. *Neurology* **55(5),** 728–730.
29. Benabid, A. L., Pollak, P., Gao, D., et al. (1996) Chronic electrical stimulation of the ventralis intermedius nucleus of the thalamus as a treatment of movement disorders. *J. Neurosurg.* **84(2),** 203–214.
30. Moro, E., Scerrati, M., Romito, L. M., et al. (1999) Chronic subthalamic nucleus stimulation reduces medication requirements in Parkinson's disease. *Neurology* **53(1),** 85–90.
31. Vingerhoets, G., van der Linden, C., Lannoo, E., et al. (1999) Cognitive outcome after unilateral pallidal stimulation in Parkinson's disease. *J. Neurol. Neurosurg. Psychiatry* **66(3),** 297–304.
32. Troster, A. I., Fields, J. A., Wilkinson, S. B., et al. (1997) Unilateral pallidal stimulation for Parkinson's disease: neurobehavioral functioning before and 3 months after electrode implantation. *Neurology* **49(4),** 1078–1083.
33. Dujardin, K., Krystkowiak, P., Defebvre, L., et al. (2000) A case of severe dysexecutive syndrome consecutive to chronic bilateral pallidal stimulation. *Neuropsychologia* **38,** 1305–1315.
34. Ceballos-Baumann, A. O., Obeso, J. A., Vitek, J. L., et al. (1994) Restoration of thalamocortical activity after posteroventral pallidotomy in Parkinson's disease. *Lancet* **344(8925),** 814.

35. Samuel, M., Ceballos-Baumann, A. O., Turjanski, N., et al. (1997) Pallidotomy in Parkinson's disease increases supplementary motor area and prefrontal activation during performance of volitional movements. An $H_2{}^{15}O$ PET study. *Brain* **120,** 1301–1313.
36. Eidelberg, D., Moeller, J. R., Ishikawa, T., et al. (1996) Regional metabolic correlates of surgical outcome following unilateral pallidotomy for Parkinson´s disease. *Ann. Neurol.* **39(1),** 450–459.
37. Davis, K. D., Taub, E., Houle, S., et al. (1997) Globus pallidus stimulation activates the cortical motor system during alleviation of parkinsonian symptoms. *Nature Med.* **3(6),** 671–674.
38. Burbaud, P., Bezard, E., Bioulac, B., et al. (1994) Effect of subthalamic high-frequency stimulation on substantia nigra pars reticulata and globus pallidus neurons in normal rats. *J. Physiol. (Paris)* **88,** 359–361.
39. Boraud, T., Bezard, E., Bioulac, B., et al. (1996) High frequency stimulation of the internal globus pallidus (GPi) simultaneously improves parkinsonian symptoms and reduces firing frequency of GPi neurons in the MPTP-treated monkey. *Neurosci. Lett.* **215,** 17–20.
40. Dostrovsky, J. O., Levy, R., Wu, J. P., et al. (2000) Microstimulation-induced inhibition of neuronal firing in human globus pallidus. *J. Neurophysiol.* **84(1),** 570–574.
41. Ranck, J. B. (1975) Which elements are excited in electrical stimulation of mammalian central nervous system? A review. *Brain Res.* **98,** 417–440.
42. Kuo, J.-S. and Carpenter, M. B. (1973) Organization of pallidothalamic projections in the rhesus monkey. *J. Comp. Neurol.* **151,** 201–236.
43. Gebbink, T. B. (1969) Some remarks on the ansa lenticularis in man. *Psychiatria, Neurolog. Neurochirur.* **72,** 37–43.
44. Alexander, G. E. and Crutcher, M. D. (1990) Functional architecture of basal ganglia circuits: neural substrates of parallel processing. *Trends Neurosci.* **13(7),** 266–271.
45. Sterio, D., Beric, A., Dogali, M., et al. (1994) Neurophysiological properties of pallidal neurons in Parkinson's disease. *Ann. Neurol.* **35(5),** 586–591.
46. Middleton, F. A. and Strick, P. L. (2000) Basal ganglia and cerebellar loops: motor and cognitive circuits. *Brain Res. Rev.* **31(2–3),** 236–250.
47. Lozano, A. M., Lang, A. E., Hutchison, W. D., et al. (1997) Microelectrode recording-guided posteroventral pallidotomy in patients with Parkinson's disease. *Adv. Neurol.* **74,** 167–174.
48. Iacono, R. P., Carlson, J. D., Kuniyoshi, S. M., et al. (1997) Electrophysiologic target localization in posteroventral pallidotomy. *Acta Neurochir.* **139(5),** 433–441.
49. Baron, M. S., Sidibe, M., DeLong, M. R., et al. (2001) Course of motor and associative pallidothalamic projections in monkeys. *J. Comp. Neurol.* **429(3),** 490–501.

13

Subthalamic Deep Brain Stimulation for Parkinson's Disease

Aviva Abosch, Anthony E. Lang,
William D. Hutchison, and Andres M. Lozano

1. INTRODUCTION

An appreciation of the important modulatory role played by the subthalamic nucleus (STN) in regulating basal ganglia projections to the motor thalamus and brainstem, has led to interest in the STN as a target for the treatment of Parkinson's disease (PD). In 1990, DeLong and colleagues first demonstrated the reversal of motor symptoms by lesioning the STN in monkeys with MPTP (1-methyl-4-phenyl-1,2,3,6-tetrahydropyridine)-induced parkinsonism *(1)*. Concern about the possibility of irreversible side effects from the generation of bilateral STN lesions, and experience with the safety *(2)* but limited efficacy of thalamic stimulation, prompted Benabid and colleagues to attempt STN deep brain stimulation (DBS) *(3)*. Recent reports from several centers demonstrating the safety and efficacy of chronic high-frequency STN DBS have generated interest in the STN as a target of choice in the surgical treatment of PD.

Despite its clinical success, the mechanism of action of DBS for the treatment of movement disorders remains unknown. The prevailing theory proposes that DBS causes a blockade of neuronal firing, thereby mimicking the effects of a lesion. The virtue of DBS as opposed to the generation of a lesion is that DBS is reversible and adjustable, allowing for maximal efficacy while minimizing adverse effects.

2. ANATOMY AND PHYSIOLOGY OF THE HUMAN STN

The human STN is composed of approx 300,000 neurons *(4)* and is situated beneath the thalamus, above the substantial nigra, posterior and medial to the pallidum and internal capsule, and anterior to the medial lemniscus. The human STN measures approx 7 mm in medial-lateral, 9 mm in anterior-posterior, and 5 mm in dorsal-ventral dimension *(5,6)*. The STN is ellipsoid in shape, with the rostral end lying superior to the caudal end of the nucleus in the sagittal plain *(5,6)*.

The STN sends projections to both the globus pallidus internus (GPi) and the substantia nigra pars reticulata (SNr) *(7)*, the two output nuclei of the human basal ganglia, as well as to the globus pallidus externa (GPe). Projections from the STN are excitatory and glutamate-secreting *(8)*, whereas the output of GPi and SNr to motor thalamus, the pedunculopontine nucleus (PPN) and the mesencephalic area (MEA) of the brainstem is inhibitory and GABA-secreting. The PPN and MEA are believed to play a role in the control of posture and locomotion. The GPi receives inhibitory projections from the striatum via the direct pathway. The GPe sends inhibitory projections to the STN by means of the indirect pathway.

From: Contemporary Clinical Neurology:
Surgical Treatment of Parkinson's Disease and Other Movement Disorders
Edited by: D. Tarsy, J. L. Vitek, and A. M. Lozano © Humana Press Inc., Totowa, NJ

The substantia nigra pars compacta (SNc) sends dopaminergic projections to the striatum. Striatal output neurons send inhibitory projections to both the GPi and SNr (direct pathway), and to the GPe (indirect pathway). Dopamine released by the nigrostriatal pathway is believed to have opposite effects on the neurons contained within the two different striato-pallidal projections; dopamine inhibits striatal neurons that project to the GPe (largely containing D2 receptors), and excites neurons projecting to the GPi (D1 predominant). In PD, the progressive loss of dopaminergic neurons in the SNc leads to increased activity of the GPi and SNr, secondary to a loss of inhibition from the direct pathway and increased excitation from the indirect pathway *(9)*. The latter derives from hyperactivity of the STN *(10,11)*. This hyperactivity of the GPi/SNr causes an increase in inhibition of thalamocortical activity, and the cardinal symptoms of Parkinson's disease—bradykinesia/akinesia, rigidity, and tremor—become manifest *(9)*. The rationale for surgical targeting of the STN is to block the increased basal ganglia output that leads to inhibition of thalamocortical activity and thereby alleviate the motor signs of Parkinson's disease.

3. PATIENT SELECTION

First, patients being considered for surgery for PD must meet the clinical criteria for this diagnosis. The cardinal signs of PD include tremor, rigidity, and bradykinesia/akinesia. Generally, patients with a diagnosis of a parkinson-plus syndrome or atypical parkinsonism (e.g., multiple system atrophy, progressive supranuclear palsy) are excluded from consideration for STN DBS, based on their usual lack of response to L-dopa treatment and general experience that they respond poorly to surgery. Patients should demonstrate significant disability despite optimization of medications. Advanced age is not necessarily a contraindication for surgery but patients must be able to tolerate a lengthy awake procedure, during which their cooperation and participation is required. Additionally, patients must not have bleeding disorders and must be able to tolerate the general anesthesia required for the internalization of electrode leads and pulse generator placement. Patients who come from remote areas must have ready access to centers with expertise in DBS programming and the resources to deal with possible hardware complications.

All potential surgical candidates are evaluated in the "practical off" (12 h without medication) and "on" state (1 h after the morning dose of medication). The evaluation requires assessment based on objective, standardized PD rating scales, such as the Unified Parkinson's Disease Rating Scale (UPDRS), and the Hoehn and Yahr Scale. Formal neuropsychological testing is useful in assessing cognitive function and motivation and in checking for the presence of significant depression. Major mood disturbances require appropriate therapy before a patient can be considered for surgery. Evidence of dementia is a contraindication to surgery in most centers as this will compromise the likelihood of successful therapy and may even worsen in the postoperative period.

The presence of a complete or near-complete response of parkinsonian symptoms to L-dopa treatment is considered to be predictive of a good response to STN DBS surgery. With the exception of tremor, symptoms that do not respond significantly to L-dopa, are believed unlikely to improve significantly with stimulation *(12,13)*. Tremor, which is sometimes resistant to L-dopa in conventional doses, responds particularly well to STN DBS and is therefore not a contraindication to STN DBS.

4. OPERATIVE TECHNIQUE

4.1. *MRI-Based Anatomical Target Localization*

Patients are admitted to hospital on the morning of surgery, having been off medication the preceding night. Although this may prove difficult for some patients, it allows for the accentuation of both clinical symptoms and microelectrode findings that contribute to intraoperative localization of optimal electrode placement.

The patient is brought to the radiology suite on the morning of surgery, where a stereotactic frame is assembled and affixed to the patient's head. Magnetic resonance (MR) images are then obtained.

We use the following imaging sequence parameters for optimal visualization of the STN: Matrix = 256 × 256, bandwidth = 3.29, FOV = 24, 3 mm-thick slices without skip, TE = 8. The center of the stereotactic frame is determined on an axial MR-image. The x-, y-, and z-coordinates of the patient's anterior commissure (AC), posterior commissure (PC), mid-commissural point (MCP), and targets within each STN are determined relative to the central point of the frame. We favor an initial anatomical target that lies in the ventral and most posterior aspect of the nucleus.

The coordinates of the patient's AC and PC are entered into a computer program that adjusts the 12.0-mm lateral template of the Schaltenbrand-Wahren atlas *(5)* by either shrinking or lengthening the AC-PC distance of the template to fit that of the patient. This adjusted map is then printed out on transparency film, and projected onto a wall chart on which microelectrode data is recorded.

The MRI-based anatomical target coordinates are then compared to calculated coordinates based on the MRI-derived MCP coordinates and standard, atlas-derived coordinates for the STN. We use the following standard, atlas-derived coordinates: 3–4 mm posterior, 5–6 mm inferior, and 12 mm lateral to the MCP. The MRI- and atlas-based coordinates are then averaged to determine the coordinates of the initial target. The coordinates of the final target are determined by subsequent microelectrode recording data.

4.2. *Operative Technique*

Following the MRI, the patient is taken to the operating room, and positioned on the operating room table. Using local anesthetic alone, two paramedian incisions are made lateral to the midline and straddling the coronal suture. Bilateral burr holes are drilled, the underlying dura is coagulated and opened, and the pial surface pierced and coagulated.

4.3. *Physiological Target Localization*

In our experience, physiological localization based on microelectrode recording data is important for target identification. Reliance solely on MRI-based anatomical localization is problematic given the frequent discrepancies between the expected location based on MRI data and the actual location based on microelectrode recording. Given the small size of the STN and the proximity of the internal capsule, medial lemniscus, and substantia nigra (Fig. 1), an error of a couple of millimeters could result in missing the STN entirely and stimulating one of the surrounding structures.

The x-, y-, and z-coordinates of the chosen target are set on the stereotactic frame and arc. A cannula is attached to the arc and lowered into the brain at an acute angle with the horizontal to allow for the longest-possible path through the STN (Fig. 1). A guide tube containing two microelectrodes is carefully inserted into the cannula, and secured to the stereotactic arc. This procedure is described in greater detail elsewhere *(14)*.

Continuous, extracellular recordings begin in the thalamus, 15 mm above target. Single and multi-unit neuronal discharges are amplified, filtered, displayed on an oscilloscope, and fed to an audio monitor. The discharge frequency of neurons, the relative size and shape of the action potentials, and audio monitoring of firing patterns are all recorded.

The electrode trajectory generally passes ventro-caudally through thalamic nucleus reticularis (Rt) and ventralis oralis anterior (Voa) or ventralis oralis posterior (Vop). The identification of cells with bursting activity (15–25 Hz) is viewed as evidence of intra-thalamic location. The other cell type characteristic of the anterior thalamic nuclei, exhibits an irregular firing pattern (15–25 Hz) and no bursting activity. The ventral thalamic border lies approx 3 mm above the STN target. We introduce our electrodes so that the most distal electrode reaches the border between STN and substantia nigra pars reticulata (SNpr), which usually lies 5–7 mm below the intercommissural line.

As the electrode is lowered towards the region of the STN, emergence below the anterior nuclei of the thalamus is characterized by an area relatively devoid of somato dendritic action potentials, spanning several millimeters, which corresponds to the thalamic fasciculus (H1 fields of Forel), and contains mostly pallidofugal fibers and few cells. The zona incerta (ZI) is a thin band of gray matter,

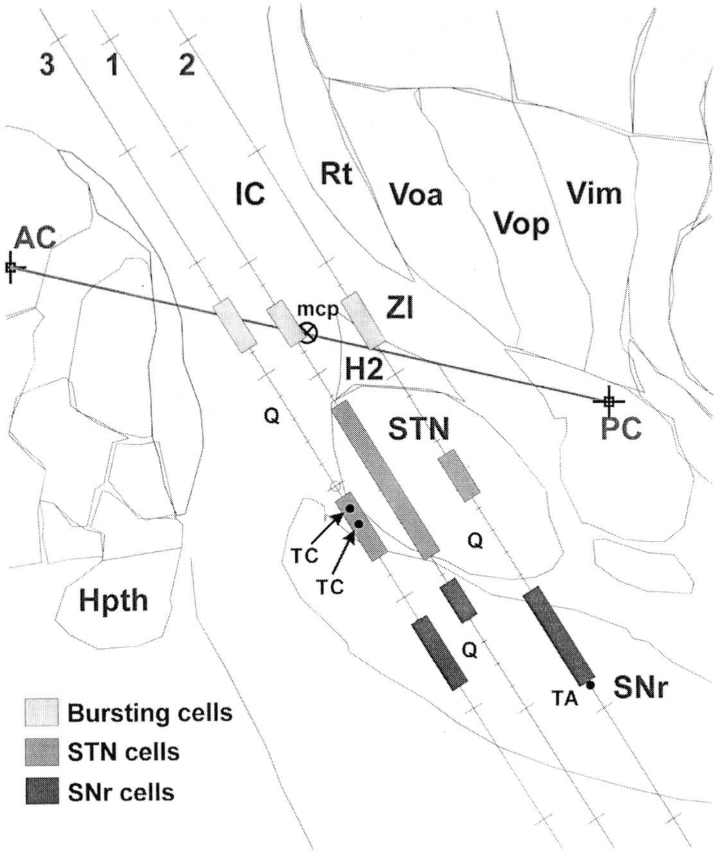

Fig. 1. Sagittal brain map at 12 mm lateral to the midline, depicting the microelectrode trajectory through thalamus, Fields of Forel, zona incerta, STN, and SNr.

lying inferior to the thalamic fasciculus, and containing cells of variable firing patterns. Inferior to ZI is another relatively electrophysiologically quiet region, the lenticular fasciculus (H2 fields of Forel), which also contains pallidofugal fibers.

Entry into the STN is marked by a prominent increase in background activity reflecting the presence of increased cellular density. STN cells are characterized by a firing rate of 25–45 Hz, and the presence of cells with receptive fields that respond to movement. Cells with spontaneous discharge rates that are synchronous with the patient's tremor can sometimes be found in the STN. Occasionally, bursting cells can also be found in the STN.

Another region devoid of somato-dendritic action potentials follows emergence below the ventral border of the STN. This region is briefest at the midsection of the STN and lengthens slightly at both the rounded rostral and caudal ends of the nucleus. Another increase in background activity indicates entry into the substantia nigra, which lies ventral to the STN. The SNr lies anteriorly and the SNc lies more posteriorly. The cells of the SNr are small and characterized by regular, high-frequency firing rates of 60–80 Hz. Occasionally, cells can be found here that respond to saccadic eye movements. Microstimulation of the SNr can cause eye deviation secondary to current spread to the oculomotor fascicles.

High frequency stimulation (0.1–100 μAmps; 1-s train, 300 Hz, 100-μs pulse width) is performed through the same electrode. The elicitation of paresthesias at low thresholds of stimulation is useful in determining proximity to the lemniscal fibers which lie posterior to the STN. The elicitation of muscle contractions at low thresholds of stimulation is useful in determining proximity to the internal capsule which lies anterior and lateral to the STN. Elicitation of eye deviation in response to stimulation results from spread of current to the fibers of the oculomotor nerve which lies medial to the STN.

Typically, three or four electrode tracks are made for the purpose of optimal physiological localization on the first side. In bilateral procedures, the second side may require only one track, which is the mirror image of the optimal track on the first side. One group uses an electrode array that allows for the simultaneous lowering of five microelectrodes, although recordings are only possible from one electrode at a time *(15)*.

4.4. DBS Electrode Placement

The frame and arc are adjusted to the desired target coordinates, the DBS lead is inserted into the cannula, and the passage of the tip of the DBS lead to the intended target is followed by fluoroscopy. Once the distal tip of the DBS lead reaches the target the cannula is withdrawn to expose the electrode contacts.

Ideally, the quadripolar electrode is positioned such that the deepest contact lies immediately inferior to the ventral border of the STN, the next two contacts lie within the body of the STN, and the most superficial contact lies at the anterior-dorsal border of the STN or within the Fields of Forel (H2). This arrangement allows for the greatest flexibility in programming the DBS postoperatively. We use a quadripolar electrode (Medtronic Model 3387), bearing contacts spaced 1.5 mm apart. Electrodes are now available with contacts spaced 0.5 mm apart (Medtronic Model 3389), allowing for more contacts to lie within the target area *(16)*.

For intraoperative DBS electrode screening, one end of a sterile screening cable is then connected to the distal-most external lead contact (contact 0), the other end is connected to an external test stimulator, and intra-operative testing begins. The external test stimulator is set at a frequency of 130 Hz, a pulse width of 60 μs, an amp limit of 10 V. Each contact is tested in series and patient responses determined. Tremor and rigidity are evaluated for each contact as the current is slowly increased. The current threshold for undesirable side effects, such as persistent paresthesias or dysarthria, is determined for each contact. DBS electrode position is considered satisfactory if no undesirable side effects result from stimulation below 4 V.

At the conclusion of intraoperative test stimulation the screening cable is removed. The cannula is then removed and the DBS lead is connected to a percutaneous extension. The extracranial portion of the DBS lead and its connection with the percutaneous extension are inserted into a subgaleal pocket created just lateral to the scalp incision. The incision is then closed, dressings applied, the stereotactic frame removed, and the patient taken to the recovery room. At our institution, a week-long trial of external stimulation ensues. However, at this point, the patient can be placed under general anesthesia, and the DBS lead connected to a subcutaneous lead extension and implanted pulse generator (IPG).

4.5. Implantation of the Pulse Generator

The consequences of obtaining an MR scan on a patient with an IPG in place remain uncertain. Therefore, prior to the implantation of the IPG, we obtain a postoperative MR scan to document DBS lead position. Then, at the culmination of the trial of external stimulation, the patient is brought back to the operating room for placement of the IPG and lead extension. Following the induction of general anesthesia, the IPG is placed in a subcutaneous pocket just caudal to the clavicle. The IPG is connected to a DBS lead extension that is tunneled subcutaneously from the scalp incision, behind the ear, to the infraclavicular incision. Incisions are closed, dressings applied, and the patient awakened from anesthesia and taken to the recovery room.

The IPG is powered by a lithium battery and fully programmable by telemetry. The battery life varies according to the stimulation parameters set for the individual patient but IPGs can be expected to need replacement in approx 3–5 yr.

5. PROGRAMMING OF DBS

In our center, patients are discharged from the hospital approx 5–10 d following DBS lead placement, or 1–2 d after placement of the IPG. The approach to postoperative programming varies greatly from center to center. Due to the potential for considerable micro-lesion effects and profound variability in day-to-day clinical responses, our group generally postpones most of the programming until the patient has fully recovered from the surgery and returned to clinical baseline. Therefore, most patients are discharged with the IPG turned off and return 3–4 wk later for testing, at which time programming commences. This 3–4 wk interval allows for the resolution of postoperative swelling, after which stimulation parameters stabilize.

The goal of DBS programming is to obtain maximal relief of symptoms with minimal side effects at the lowest possible voltage. This goal is attained by varying the parameters of stimulation, which include mode of stimulation, frequency, pulse width, amplitude, and contacts across which stimulation occurs. Each of the four electrode contacts (0, 1, 2, and 3) can be set to positive, negative, or off. Stimulation can be set to a monopolar, bipolar, or multipolar mode. In monopolar stimulation the IPG case serves as the ground. For maximal symptomatic benefit with monopolar stimulation, the best contact across which to stimulate seems to be one located either in the dorsal part of the STN, or immediately dorsal to the nucleus in the region of the ZI. In bipolar mode, current flows from the negative contact (cathode) to the positive contact (anode). Frequency is set at ≥120 Hz in order to achieve a lesion-like effect, but can range up to 185 Hz. Pulse width is generally set at 60–90 μs. The amplitude of stimulation is generally set between 2–3.5 V, but can range from 0.1–10 V. Given the number of parameters involved and the complexity of the clinical syndrome, programming can take many hours and multiple sessions even for experienced practitioners. Programming must be carried out in both the drug-off and drug-on states. STN stimulation may generate or accentuate dyskinesias requiring a reduction in dopaminergic drug dosages. This balancing of stimulation levels and drug doses may take several weeks to optimize. With the Itrel II (Medtronics) IPG, the patient and the patient's family have the ability to turn the IPG off and on by means of a hand-held magnet that is applied to the skin overlying the IPG.

6. OUTCOME

6.1. Overall Effect on Motor Symptoms

Benabid and colleagues first used STN DBS in the treatment of PD in the mid-1990s *(3)*. Since then, a number of other groups have published results concerning the efficacy of STN stimulation (Table 1). Many series have reported STN stimulation-induced improvements in all motor symptoms of PD including tremor, rigidity, bradykinesia, posture, and other axial symptoms of PD, such as rising from a chair, gait, and swallowing. There is, however, considerable range in the degree of improvement in these various categories (Tables 2–6) *(16,17)*. This variation in outcome may be due to differences in study design (blinded vs nonblinded; duration of follow-up), patient selection (age, degree of preoperative impairment in the various categories of the UPDRS, presence of co-morbidities), clinical methods (DBS electrode placement, stimulation parameters, or the use of unilateral versus bilateral electrodes), or the fact that the UPDRS is a subjective rating system.

Kumar et al. compared the effects of unilateral vs bilateral STN DBS in 10 patients *(18)*. These authors found that bilateral stimulation was associated with a much greater improvement in all axial symptoms (postural stability, gait, axial motor features) than unilateral stimulation, and that the improvement in appendicular symptoms was synergistic rather than additive *(18)*. Kumar et al. attributed this synergism to the finding of ipsilateral as well as contralateral effects of STN DBS resulting in the symptoms in each limb improving more with bilateral stimulation than with unilateral stimulation. Thus, most patients with medically refractory symptoms are better served by bilateral STN DBS, although highly asymmetric, tremor-dominant PD may be treated by unilateral STN DBS in an effort to curtail potential morbidity and procedural costs.

Table 1
Summary of Published Series on Outcome from STN DBS

Study	*n*	F/U Mo	% Improved (mUPDRS)	% Mean L-Dopa Reduced
Kumar et al. *(17)* (1998)	7	6	Off meds = 65% On meds = 49%	40%
Limousin et al. *(16)* (1998)	20	12	Off meds = 60% On meds = 10%	50%
Krack et al. *(13)* (1998)	8	6	Off meds = 70% On meds = 19%	56%
Moro et al. *(27)* (1999)	7	12–16	Off meds = 42% On meds = 5% Decline	65%
Burchiel et al. *(19)* (1999)	5	12	Off meds = 44% On meds = 15%	51%
Yokoyama et al. *(24)* (1999)	5	3	Off meds = 44% On meds = Not Significant	0%
Houeto et al. *(40)* (2000)	23	6	Off meds = 66% On meds = 55%	61%
Bejjani et al. *(22)* (2000)	10	6	Off meds = 62% On meds = 80%	62%
Rodriguez-Oroz et al *(41)* (2000)	15 9	12 36	Off meds = 74% On meds = Not Significant Off meds = 61%	55% No further significant change

mUPDRS, motor section of the UPDRS; F/U mo, length of postoperative follow-up in months. Note that all patients in these studies received bilateral STN DBS, except those of Yokoyama et al. *(24)*, who underwent unilateral, right-sided STN DBS implantation.

Table 2
Range of Effect of STN DBS on Tremor

Study	*n*	Mo F/U	% Improved – LD	% Improved + LD
Limousin et al. (1998) *(16)*	20	12	80%	43%
Krack et al. (1998) *(13)*	8	6	88%	57%
Rodriguez et al. (1998) *(20)*	12	3–12	97%	Not recorded
Kumar et al. (1998) *(17)*	7	6	82%	77%
Burchiel et al. (1999) *(19)*	5	12	74%	91%
Yokoyama et al. (1999) *(24)*	5	3	Not significant	Not significant

–LD, off levodopa; + LD, on levodopa.

Table 3
Range of Effect of STN DBS on Rigidity

Study	*n*	Mo F/U	% Improved – LD	% Improved + LD
Limousin et al. (1998) *(16)*	20	12	68%	50%
Krack et al. (1998) *(13)*	8	6	33%	31%
Kumar et al. (1998) *(17)*	7	6	52%	44%
Burchiel et al. (1999) *(19)*	5	12	47%	24%
Yokoyama et al. (1999) *(24)*	5	3	Not significant	Not significant

Table 4
Range of Effect of STN DBS on Bradykinesia/Akinesia

Study	*n*	Mo F/U	% Improved – LD	% Improved + LD
Limousin et al. (1998) *(16)*	20	12	56%	12% Decline
Krack et al. (1998) *(13)*	8	6	71%	5%
Kumar et al. (1998) *(17)*	7	6	57%	53%
Burchiel et al. (1999) *(19)*	5	12	25%	18%
Yokoyama et al. (1999) *(24)*	5	3	33%	Not significant

Table 5
Range of Effect of STN DBS on Levodopa-Induced and Off-State Dyskinesias[a]

Study	*n*	Mo F/U	% Improved – LD	% Improved + LD
Limousin et al. (1998) *(16)*	20	12	Not reported	Nonsignificant reduction
Krack et al. (1998) *(13)*	8	6	Not reported	40%
Kumar et al. (1998) *(17)*	7	6	Not reported	0%
Burchiel et al. (1999) *(19)*	5	12	Not reported	67%
Krack et al. (1999) *(21)*	27	6	90%	50%—diphasic mobile dystonia 30%—peak dose dyskinesias
Krause et al. (2000) *(42)*	12	12	Not reported[b]	58%

[a]Although many authors interchange the terms off-period dyskinesias with off-period dystonia, we assume that they are referring to the phenomenon of off-period dystonia, in the absence of information about postoperative onset of surgically induced abnormal movements.

[b]The UPDRS subscores for dystonia were not reported for the off-medication state, however, the authors noted that stimulation of the STN seemed to result in a reduction in dyskinesias that was secondary to the reduction in medication. These findings for STN DBS were in contrast to their observations for the effect of GPI DBS on dyskinesias, which seemed to reduce dyskinesias directly.

Table 6
Range of Effect of STN DBS on Axial Symptoms (Posture, Gait, and Speech)

Study	*n*	Mo F/U	% Improved – LD	% Improved + LD
Kumar et al. (1998) *(17)*	7	6	49% postural stability + gait	33% postural stability + gait
Krack et al. (1998) *(13)*	8	6	79% gait	Not reported
Yokoyama et al. (1999) *(24)*	5	3	37% gait 39% gait + posture	Not significant Not significant
Bejjani et al. (1999) *(22)*	10	6	69% akinesia + rigidity + tremor 72% axial symptoms:[a] • 77% abnormal posture • 76% postural stability	Not further improved 84% axial symptoms: • 88% abnormal posture • 96% postural stability
Robertson et al. (2001) *(43)*	3	12–30	30% gait 54% up from chair 40% speech	Not reported

[a]Axial categories included speech, neck rigidity, rising from a chair, posture, gait, and postural instability. All of these features—except neck rigidity—were significantly improved by stimulation, but degree of improvement within each individual category was not provided.

Kumar and colleagues also examined the effects of STN DBS in a prospective, randomized, double-blinded fashion *(17)*. These authors found a 65% reduction in off-period motor UPDRS (mUPDRS) scores, a 40% reduction in on-period mUPDRS scores, and an 85% reduction in L-dopa-induced dyskinesias in the seven patients who were evaluated (Table 1). Limousin et al. *(16)* found a 60% improvement in off-period scores, but only a 10% improvement in on-period scores. Of note, the physicians who examined patients in this study were not blinded as to whether the stimulator was on or off. It should be mentioned, though, that attempts to blind investigators and/or patients to turning on or off an effective STN DBS are problematic, as stimulation can induce paresthesias and relatively immediate and visible changes in the patient's tremor. Another important reason for the difference in on-period responses between these two studies is that Kumar et al. *(17)* used the patients' usual dose of medication (which may have been limited by dyskinesias or other side effects), while Limousin and the Grenoble group *(16)* have used a supramaximal dose of levodopa. The latter experience suggests that STN DBS may not result in an improvement in parkinsonian signs to a greater extent than that obtained at the maximal benefit of levodopa.

The relative attributes of STN versus GPi DBS remain unclear. Burchiel and colleagues reported the results of a randomized, blinded comparison between GPi and STN DBS in a small number of patients *(19)*. In their study, four patients received pallidal stimulation and five patients received STN stimulation (Table 1). Both groups demonstrated off-period improvement of approx 40% in mUPDRS at 12 mo. Medication requirements decreased only in the STN group. The GPi group demonstrated a 40% improvement when on levodopa at 12 mo, whereas the STN group improved only 15% during this period. Overall, however, stimulation of either GPi or STN produced little or no additional benefit over that produced by L-dopa alone.

6.2. *Effect on Limb Symptoms*

The reported percentage reduction in tremor brought about by bilateral STN DBS in the absence of L-dopa administration ranges from 74% *(19)* to 97% *(20)* (Table 2). Improvements reported for off-period rigidity in response to bilateral STN DBS range from 33% *(13)* to 68% *(16)* (Table 3). Limousin et al. *(16)* reported a 56% improvement in limb akinesia in response to stimulation alone over untreated baseline, but noted a 12% worsening in akinesia scores when patients were tested with both stimulation and L-dopa. Other reports document improvements in akinesia that range from 25% *(19)* up to 71% *(13)* (Table 4).

L-dopa induces off-period dystonia, end-of-dose and beginning-of-dose dyskinesias, and peak-dose dyskinesias *(21)*. With the benefit of STN DBS, L-dopa induced dyskinesias decreased by 30% in one study *(16)*, likely a consequence of the postoperative reduction in doses of dopaminergic drugs. The authors of this study note, however, that the decrease did not attain significance. Kumar and colleagues reported an 85% reduction in levodopa-induced dyskinesias, but no direct anti-dyskinetic effect of STN stimulation (Table 5) *(17)*. On the other hand, one author reported an anti-dyskinetic effect of STN DBS that was believed to be independent of improvements obtained by medication reduction *(21)*. However, this stimulation-induced improvement in dyskinesias may have related to effects outside of the STN, for example effects on the pallidofugal fibers in the Fields of Forel.

6.3. *Effect on Axial Symptoms*

Bejjani and colleagues *(22)* noted that, consistent with other studies *(16,17)*, limb symptoms (akinesia, rigidity, and tremor) were greatly improved with bilateral STN DBS. Furthermore, these authors noted a dramatic improvement in axial symptoms including posture, postural stability, and gait (Table 6). Dysarthria, swallowing impairment, and neck rigidity were noted to be relatively resistant to both L-dopa therapy and STN stimulation *(22)*. Indeed, some authors have noted that dysarthria may worsen in these patients *(23)*, although this may be a result of L dopa dosage reduction with little beneficial effects of STN stimulation on this feature.

Krack et al. reported a 79% improvement in gait with bilateral STN stimulation in the off-drug state *(13)* and a 70% improvement in gait and posture. In contrast, Yokoyama et al. *(24)* noted only a 37% improvement in gait and a 39% improvement in gait and posture. These authors attribute the discrepancy between their results and those of Krack et al., to the fact that they specifically selected patients with freezing, falling, and akinesia for their study. However, the Yokoyama study differed significantly from other reports in the literature in that the patients underwent exclusively unilateral, right-sided STN DBS, which has been demonstrated to be less effective at reducing symptoms than bilateral STN DBS *(18)*. Furthermore, three of the five patients studied had undergone previous contralateral pallidotomies, no postoperative reduction in L-dopa was implemented, no significant reduction in tremor was noted, and follow-up was only 3 mo.

6.4. Effect on L-dopa Requirements

The decrease in levodopa requirements following stimulation of the STN has been described in numerous publications (Table 1). Reported postoperative L-dopa reductions range from 40% *(17)* to 100%, as some patients have successfully discontinued all dopaminergic drugs following surgery *(25)*. However, the discontinuation of all dopaminergic medications may be associated with a decline in speech as well as profound changes in mood (including anhedonia and depression). Reduction in L-dopa dose, however, is associated with a significant improvement in on-period dyskinesias (Table 5) *(17,26,27)*.

6.5. Effects on Cognition

The current model of the functional anatomy of the basal ganglia includes a "cognitive circuit" comprised of a dorsolateral and lateral orbito-medial prefrontal loop *(28)*. Impairment in the functioning of this circuit has been invoked to explain the cognitive deficits found in PD. The aim of surgical therapies for PD is to ameliorate motor symptoms but it is possible that intervention in the basal ganglia motor loop can affect the functioning of the cognitive circuit in which the basal ganglia are also involved.

From their analysis of 49 patients, Ardouin et al. concluded that bilateral STN DBS did not result in significant impairment of memory or executive function at 3–6 mo following surgery *(29)*. These investigators then studied 48 bilateral STN DBS patients with stimulators turned on and off in a non-blinded fashion *(30)*. They found a significant improvement in psychomotor speed and working memory with the stimulators turned on, but a mild deficit in lexical fluency at 12 mo after surgery. No significant differences between the stimulated and nonstimulated condition were found for the remaining tests of executive function.

Saint-Cyr et al. performed extensive pre- and postoperative neuropsychological evaluations on 11 patients who underwent bilateral STN DBS placement *(31)*. In contrast to the findings of Ardouin et al. *(29)*, Saint-Cyr et al. *(31)*, found that tasks that depended on the integrity of fronto-striatal circuitry were significantly worse at 9–12 mo postoperatively than before surgery. These deficits were more likely to occur in the elderly subgroup (older than 69 yr), as were transient intra-operative and postoperative confusion. All patients were tested exclusively with the stimulators on.Thus, it is not clear whether the observed cognitive deficits were a consequence of the stimulation itself and, if so, whether the deficits were reversible with cessation of stimulation. The mechanism(s) by which STN DBS could cause cognitive dysfunction is not clear but disruption of the widespread influence of the STN within the basal ganglia could possibly have repercussions at the cortical level.

6.6. Effects on Speech

Although patients with PD may show improved speech in response to L-dopa, the improvement is far less than that seen in limb and axial motor performance. Dromey et al. examined the effects of STN DBS on acoustic measures of voice in seven patients with Parkinson's disease *(12)*. These authors noted small but significant increases in vocal intensity and fundamental frequency variability in response to stimulation, when patients were examined on medication 6 mo after surgery. However, the overall impact of these changes was not deemed functionally significant. In contrast, Gentil et al. found improvement in speech in 10 patients when the STN was stimulated *(32)*. However, this latter study reported results for patients only in the off-medication state, without reporting the effects on speech of STN stimulation in patients on medication. Additionally, the patients described in the study by Dromey et al. *(12)*, had only modest speech impairment before and after surgery, whereas the patients included in the study by Gentil et al. *(32)* were specifically chosen for their speech deficits. Thus, the discrepancy in results between these two studies may, in part, reflect significant differences in patient selection.

7. COMPLICATIONS

The surgical complications associated with STN DBS placement are the same as those inherent to stereotactic neurosurgery in general. The intracranial hemorrhage rate reported for DBS varies between 0.6–3.5% *(15,33)*. Deaths are rare, but have occurred as a result of hemorrhage *(16)*.

7.1. *Complications of Hardware*

Infection and/or erosion rates vary between 2.5–23.4% *(15,33)*. Lead fractures, short circuits, and other unspecified hardware malfunctions account for between 5.8–17.7% *(33,34)*. Lead migrations occurred in 14.2% of patients in one series *(33)*, but are not reported in other series.

7.2. *Complications of Stimulation*

Involuntary movements that occur during the initial phase of STN stimulation have been reported frequently, tend to be mild, and generally respond to changing the stimulation parameters and/or contacts being used for stimulation *(18,35)*. These abnormal movements can be ballistic in quality or similar to the patient's preoperative L-dopa-induced dyskinesias *(35)*.

In a retrospective study of the safety and efficacy of GPi vs STN stimulation, Volkmann and colleagues noted similar efficacy with respect to off-period motor symptoms between the two groups *(36)*. However, the authors noted a higher incidence of ongoing adverse events in the STN group (n = 16) at 1 yr after surgery. These adverse events included depression and anhedonia (8.3%), worsening of hypophonia and dysarthria (56.3%), and apraxia of eyelid opening (12.5%). The authors also noted that L-dopa dose was reduced by 65.3 ± 20.2% in the STN group, whereas no significant medication change occurred in the GPi group. L-dopa dose could not be increased in nine of the 16 STN patients owing to dose limiting side effects. The authors concluded that STN stimulation results in a narrowing of the therapeutic window of L-dopa therapy, due to a lower threshold for dyskinesias. Thus, parkinsonian symptoms such as hypophonia, which are less improved by stimulation than by L-dopa therapy, may be unmasked by dose reduction.

7.3. *Acute Cognitive Changes*

Intraoperative and postoperative (lasting 1–2 wk) confusion and agitation are reported as "common" in elderly patients undergoing bilateral STN surgery, whereas patients under the age of 60 seem to tolerate the procedure better and remain lucid throughout the surgery *(17)*. There are also isolated reports of acute onset of both depression *(37,38)* and of laughter *(39)* as a consequence of stimulation, each of which resolved with cessation of stimulation or changing the contacts being stimulated *(18)*.

8. CONCLUSIONS

Bilateral STN DBS greatly improves off-period symptoms of PD, attenuates motor fluctuations, and allows for a reduction in L-dopa dosing, which likely accounts for the decrease in L-dopa-induced dyskinesias. The improvements in L-dopa-sensitive symptoms are sustained at greater than 2 yr of follow-up.

REFERENCES

1. Bergman, H., Wichmann, T., and DeLong, M. R. (1990) Reversal of experimental parkinsonism by lesions of the subthalamic nucleus. *Science* **249,** 1436–1438.
2. Benabid, A. L., Pollak, P., Gervason, C., et al. (1991) Long-term suppression of tremor by chronic stimulation of the ventral intermediate thalamic nucleus. *Lancet* **337,** 403–406.
3. Limousin, P., Pollak, P., Benazzouz, A., et al. (1995) Effect of parkinsonian signs and symptoms of bilateral subthalamic nucleus stimulation. *Lancet* **345,** 91–95.
4. Lange, H., Thorner, G., and Hopf, A. (1976) [Morphometric-statistical structure analysis of human striatum, pallidum and nucleus su-thalamicus. III. Nucleus subthalamicus]. *J. Hirnforsch.* **17,** 31–41.
5. Schaltenbrand, G. and Wahren, W. (1977) Atlas for stereotaxy of the human brain. Architectonic organization of the thalamic nuclei by Rolf Hassler, with an accompanying guide, 2nd ed. Thieme, Stuttgart.
6. Morel, A., Magnin, M., and Jeanmonod, D. (1997) Multiarchitectonic and stereotactic atlas of the human thalamus. *J. Comp. Neurol.* **387,** 588–630.
7. Carpenter, M. B., Baton, R. R., Carleton, S. C., et al. (1981) Interconnections and organization of pallidal and subthalamic nucleus neurons in the monkey. *J. Comp. Neurol.* **197,** 579–603.
8. Smith, Y. and Parent, A. (1988) Neurons of the subthalamic nucleus in primates display glutamate but not GABA immunoreactivity. *Brain Res.* **453,** 353–356.
9. Wichmann, T. and DeLong, M. R. (1996) Functional and pathophysiological models of the basal ganglia. *Curr. Opin. Neurobiol.* **6,** 751–758.
10. Bergman, H., Wichmann, T., Karmon, B., et al. (1994) The primate subthalamic nucleus. II. Neuronal activity in the MPTP model of parkinsonism. *J. Neurophysiol.* **72,** 507–520.
11. Hutchison, W., Allan, R., Optiz, H., et al. (1998) Neurophysiological identification of the subthalamic nucleus in surgery for Parkinson's disease. *Ann. Neurol.* **44,** 622–628.
12. Dromey, C., Kumar, R., Lang, A. E., et al. (2000) An investigation of the effects of subthalamic nucleus stimulation on acoustic measures of voice. *Mov. Disord.* **15,** 1132–1138.
13. Krack, P., Pollak, P., Limousin, P., et al. (1998) Subthalamic nucleus or internal pallidal stimulation in young onset Parkinson's disease. *Brain* **121,** 451–457.
14. Hutchison, W. and Lozano, A. (2000) Microelectrode recordings in movement disorder surgery. In: *Movement Disorder Surgery* (Lozano, A., ed.), Karger, Basel, pp. 103–117.
15. Benabid, A., Benazzouz, A., Hoffmann, D., et al. (1998) Long-term electrical inhibition of deep brain targets in movement disorders. *Mov. Disord.* **13,** 119–125.
16. Limousin, P., Krack, P., Pollack, P., et al. (1998) Electrical stimulation of the subthalamic nucleus in advanced Parkinson's disease. *N. Engl. J. Med.* **339,** 1105–1111.
17. Kumar, R., Lozano, A. M., Kim, Y. J., et al. (1998) Double-blind evaluation of subthalamic nucleus deep brain stimulation in advanced Parkinson's disease. *Neurology* **51,** 850–855.
18. Kumar, R., Lozano, A. M., Sime, E., et al. (1999) Comparative effects of unilateral and bilateral subthalamic nucleus deep brain stimulation. *Neurology* **53,** 561–566.
19. Burchiel, K. J., Anderson, V. C., Favre, J., et al. (1999) Comparison of pallidal and subthalamic nucleus deep brain stimulation for advanced Parkinson's disease: results of a randomized, blinded pilot study. *Neurosurgery* **45,** 1375–1382; discussion 1382–1374.
20. Rodriguez, M. C., Guridi, O. J., Alvarez, L., et al. (1998) The subthalamic nucleus and tremor in Parkinson's disease. *Mov. Disord.* **13,** 111–118.
21. Krack, P., Pollak, P., Limousin, P., et al. (1999) From off-period dystonia to peak-dose chorea. The clinical spectrum of varying subthalamic nucleus activity. *Brain* **122,** 1133–1146.
22. Bejjani, B. P., Gervais, D., Arnulf, I., et al. (2000) Axial parkinsonian symptoms can be improved: the role of levodopa and bilateral subthalamic stimulation. *J. Neurol. Neurosurg. Psychiatry* **68,** 595–600.
23. Hariz, M. I., Johansson, F., Shamsgovara, P., et al. (2000) Bilateral subthalamic nucleus stimulation in a parkinsonian patient with preoperative deficits in speech and cognition: persistent improvement in mobility but increased dependency: a case study. *Mov. Disord.* **15,** 136–139.
24. Yokoyama, T., Sugiyama, K., Nishizawa, S., et al. (1999) Subthalamic nucleus stimulation for gait disturbance in Parkinson's disease. *Neurosurgery* **45,** 41–47; discussion 47–49.
25. Molinuevo, J. L., Valldeoriola, F., Tolosa, E., et al. (2000) Levodopa withdrawal after bilateral subthalamic nucleus stimulation in advanced Parkinson disease. *Arch. Neurol.* **57,** 983–988.
26. Krack, P., Pollak, P., Limousin, P., et al. (1997) Stimulation of subthalamic nucleus alleviates tremor in Parkinson's disease. *Lancet* **350,** 1675.
27. Moro, E., Scerrati, M., Romito, L. M., et al. (1999) Chronic subthalamic nucleus stimulation reduces medication requirements in Parkinson's disease. *Neurology* **53,** 85–90.
28. Alexander, G. E., DeLong, M. R., and Strick, P. L. (1986) Parallel organization of functionally segregated circuits linking basal ganglia and cortex. *Annu. Rev. Neurosci.* **9,** 357–381.
29. Ardouin, C., Pillon, B., Peiffer, E., et al. (1999) Bilateral subthalamic or pallidal stimulation for Parkinson's disease affects neither memory nor executive functions: a consecutive series of 62 patients. *Ann. Neurol.* **46,** 217–223.
30. Pillon, B., Ardouin, C., Damier, P., et al. (2000) Neuropsychological changes between "off" and "on" STN or GPi stimulation in Parkinson's disease. *Neurology* **55,** 411–418.

31. Saint-Cyr, J. A., Trepanier, L. L., Kumar, R., et al. (2000) Neuropsychological consequences of chronic bilateral stimulation of the subthalamic nucleus in Parkinson's disease. *Brain* **123,** 2091–2108.
32. Gentil, M., Garcia-Ruiz, P., Pollak, P., et al. (1999) Effect of stimulation of the subthalamic nucleus on oral control of patients with parkinsonism. *J. Neurol. Neurosurg. Psychiatry* **67,** 329–333.
33. Levy, R., Lamb, S., and Adams, J. (1987) Treatment of chronic pain by deep brain stimulation: long term follow-up and review of the literature. *Neurosurgery* **21,** 885–893.
34. Kumar, K., Toth, C., and Nath, R. (1997) Deep brain stimulation for intractable pain: a 15-year experience. *Neurosurgery* **40,** 736–746.
35. Limousin, P., Pollak, P., Hoffmann, D., et al. (1996) Abnormal involuntary movements induced by subthalamic nucleus stimulation in parkinsonian patients. *Mov. Disord.* **11,** 231–235.
36. Volkmann, J., Allert, N., Voges, J., et al. (2001) Safety and efficacy of pallidal or subthalamic nucleus stimulation in advanced PD. *Neurology* **56,** 548–551.
37. Bejjani, B.-P., Damier, P., Arnulf, I., et al. (1999) Transient acute depression induced by high-frequency deep-brain stimulation. *N. Engl. J. Med.* **340,** 1476–1480.
38. Bezerra, M. L. S., Martinez, J.-V. L., Nasser, J. A., et al. (1999) Transient acute depression induced by high-frequency deep-brain stimulation. *N. Engl. J. Med.* **341,** 1003–1004.
39. Krack, P., Kumar, R., Ardouin, C., et al. (2001) Mirthful laughter induced by subthalamic nucleus stimulation. *Mov. Disord.* **16,** 867–875.
40. Houeto, J., Damier, P., Bejjani, P., et al. (2000) Subthalamic stimulation in Parkinson disease: a multidisciplinary approach. *Arch. Neurol.* **57,** 461–465.
41. Rodriguez-Oroz, M. C., Gorospe, A., Guridi, J., et al. (2000) Bilateral deep brain stimulation of the subthalamic nucleus in Parkinson's disease. *Neurology* **55,** S45–S51.
42. Krause, M., Fogel, W., Heck, A., et al. (2001) Deep brain stimulation for the treatment of Parkinson's disease: subthalamic nucleus versus global pallidus internus. *J. Neurol. Neurosurg. Psychiatry* **70,** 464–470.
43. Robertson, L. T., Horak, F. B., Anderson, V. C., et al. (2001) Assessments of axial motor control during deep brain stimulation in parkinsonian patients. *Neurosurgery* **48,** 544–551; discussion 551–542.

14

Methods of Programming and Patient Management with Deep Brain Stimulation

Rajeev Kumar

1. INTRODUCTION

Deep brain stimulation (DBS) has become a widely performed procedure for the treatment of advanced medication-refractory movement disorders, including Parkinson's disease (PD), dystonia, and various forms of tremor. DBS has been applied to the ventral intermedius (Vim) nucleus of the thalamus, globus pallidus internus (GPi), and subthalamic nucleus (STN). The exact mechanism of action of DBS is unknown, but is consistent with high-frequency stimulation blocking the activity of the target nucleus by direct or indirect means.

Vim DBS has been shown to markedly improve all forms of tremor in a fashion similar to that achieved with thalamotomy but with fewer persistent adverse effects *(1–3)*. Although Vim DBS can markedly improve parkinsonian tremor, this form of therapy does not significantly improve other features of parkinsonism *(2,3)*. However, STN DBS and GPi DBS can markedly improve all levodopa-responsive motor features of parkinsonism *(4–8)*. The practical matter of programming DBS settings in PD patients with electrodes implanted in the GPi or STN is considerably more complex than thalamic DBS and obtaining optimal results is a time-consuming process. In addition, adjustments in stimulation parameters must often be accompanied by alterations in anti-parkinson medication in order to improve both motor fluctuations and levodopa-induced dyskinesias. Although worldwide experience with GPi DBS for dystonia is quite limited and the stimulation parameters used by different investigational groups have been quite variable, the available data provides some useful guidelines for the management of such patients.

We describe our practical approach to postoperative patient management including adjusting stimulation parameters, altering medical therapy, as well as troubleshooting and identifying complications. We propose guidelines based on our clinical experience with variations as suggested by the experience of other groups. These guidelines can only address the most commonly encountered problems and propose the usual solutions to these problems, but cannot possibly address every one of the large variety of clinical problems that may be seen with this therapy. Lastly, we recognize that alternative, equally valid approaches may exist.

2. PATIENT CHARACTERISTICS

Given that the risks of stereotactic surgery include a 2–3% risk of hemorrhage, surgery should generally be restricted to patients who have disabling movement disorders despite maximal medical therapy. Patients and their caregivers must be able to effectively participate in frequent follow-up visits for evaluations and stimulator adjustments.

From: Contemporary Clinical Neurology:
Surgical Treatment of Parkinson's Disease and Other Movement Disorders
Edited by: D. Tarsy, J. L. Vitek, and A. M. Lozano © Humana Press Inc., Totowa, NJ

2.1. *Tremor*

Patients considered for surgery for tremor typically have essential tremor (ET), tremor associated with PD, multiple sclerosis (causing cerebellar tremor), dystonic tremor, or Holmes tremor of midbrain origin (usually due to head trauma or brainstem infarction). The Vim nucleus of the thalamus is usually targeted, though some groups may also target the more anteriorly located Voa/Vop nuclei and the inferiorly located zona incerta (Zi).

2.2. *Parkinson's Disease*

Patients with PD undergoing STN or GPi DBS typically have disabling medication-refractory motor fluctuations and levodopa-induced dyskinesias despite aggressive medical therapy or have marked medication intolerance making medical management unsatisfactory. In general, surgery is restricted to patients without significant cognitive impairment. Our experience suggests that elderly patients with cognitive impairment may be predisposed to aggravation of cognitive deficit especially with bilateral STN surgery *(9)*. We therefore routinely refer all patients for detailed preoperative neuropsychological testing to assess whether patients have the cognitive reserves to withstand surgery. Patients must be motivated and able to actively participate during surgery while awake that may be lengthy, fatiguing, and emotionally stressful. As a result, we commonly exclude patients from surgery if they have active psychiatric symptoms (especially hallucinations due to PD medications) because such patients are commonly cognitive impaired and may become agitated during surgery.

2.3. *Dystonia*

GPi DBS for dystonia is typically restricted to those with severe generalized or segmental dystonia who continue to be disabled despite drug therapy *(10–12)*. Children as well as adults have successfully undergone this therapy. Patients with longstanding dystonia may be improved to the same degree as those with relatively shorter disease duration and improvement in longstanding orthopedic deformities can occur after long-term stimulation *(11)*. More recently, bilateral GPi DBS has also been employed in patients with complex cervical dystonia who have responded inadequately to botulinum toxin injections or have become resistant to botulinum toxin *(13,14)*. The majority of operated patients have had primary dystonia with best results reported in those with mutations in the Torsin A gene (DYT-1) *(10,11)*. However, there are also increasing numbers of reports of significant improvement in patients with secondary dystonia *(15,16)*. The most consistent improvements have occurred in patients with DYT-1 mutations with reduction in Burke-Fahn-Marsden (BFM) rating scale movement scores commonly exceeding 75% *(10)*. GPi DBS may also be valuable in patients with secondary dystonia without focal brain lesions (e.g., post-anoxic states). Recent experience suggests that evaluation of this therapy in individuals with metabolic diseases such as Hallervorden Spatz syndrome (NBIA type 1) and glutaric acidemia is warranted although preliminary results in very small numbers of patients have been highly variable. The value of this therapy in patients with dystonia due to focal lesions (especially symptomatic hemi-dystonia) is less certain and has not been successful in our hands.

3. CLINICAL EFFECTS OF DBS

3.1. *Tremor: Vim DBS*

Thalamic stimulation usually markedly improves most forms of tremor, may reduce dystonia associated with dystonic tremor, but does not improve and may even worsen ataxia in cerebellar tremor *(11,17)*. The clinical effects of Vim DBS in PD are outlined in Table 1: virtually complete suppression of off-period contralateral tremor, mild improvement in rigidity, and no improvement in bradykinesia *(2,3)*. However, electrode placement in the centromedian/ parafascicularis (CM/Pf) nucleus of the thalamus or anterior to the Vim (i.e., in the Voa/Vop) may suppress levodopa-induced dyskinesias *(18, 19)*. Disability as measured by the Unified Parkinson's Disease Rating Scale (UPDRS) is not consistently improved with thalamic stimulation because most disability in PD is due to bradykinesia and gait disorder. By contrast, disability is improved in essential tremor *(2)*.

3.2. *Parkinson's Disease: STN and GPi DBS*

A summary and comparison of the specific clinical effects of STN and GPi DBS in PD is presented in Table 1. The total effect of DBS is achieved as a result of the microlesion caused by electrode implantation (a minor effect) and the direct effect of stimulation (the major effect). The benefit achieved with microlesioning is maximal immediately postoperatively and declines over several weeks as the edema surrounding the implanted electrodes resolves. Nevertheless, some microlesion effects may remain noticeable for at least 6 mo *(20)*. Dramatic and beneficial effects of both STN and GPi DBS has been consistently observed. Both interventions result in significant improvement in motor fluctuations and dyskinesias as measured by patient home diary assessments. In a large multicenter study, on time without dyskinesia during the waking day increased from 25–30% at baseline to 65–75% 6 mo postoperatively *(4)*. In a complementary fashion these interventions markedly decreased off time and on time with dyskinesia *(4)*. Although some preliminary results suggest that STN DBS may be a superior intervention, no large randomized trial of STN and GPi DBS has been conducted and it remains unknown as to whether STN or GPi DBS is more efficacious for the treatment of advanced PD. The most consistent difference between these therapies has been the reduction in antiparkinson medication following STN DBS by contrast with patients undergoing GPi DBS where no significant change in medication doses have been reported *(4)*.

In general, the specific effects of GPi DBS are similar to those seen with pallidotomy; however, the risks to cognitive and bulbar function may be less than with bilateral lesioning *(21)*. As with pallidotomy, GPi DBS may be applied unilaterally or bilaterally depending primarily on the distribution of the patient's symptoms. Although most case series have included only patients who have not undergone prior surgery, our clinical experience suggests that GPi DBS applied contralaterally to a prior unilateral pallidotomy may be an effective strategy in patients who have significant residual disability due to levodopa-induced dyskinesias and parkinsonism ipsilateral to the lesion *(22)*. We have also found that bilateral STN DBS may also be a useful intervention in patients who have previously undergone unilateral pallidotomy or GPi DBS and subsequently present with persistent or recurrent disability.

Two groups have reported on the apparent functional differences between dorsal and ventral globus pallidus stimulation (Fig. 1) *(23,24)*. Dorsal pallidal stimulation produces a marked antiparkinson effect but may induce rather than suppress dyskinesias (similar to STN stimulation), and may possibly be due to stimulation of the globus pallidus externa (GPe) *(25)*. Ventral pallidal stimulation may worsen akinesia and block the beneficial effects of levodopa on bradykinesia and gait, while improving rigidity and markedly suppressing dyskinesias. As a result, the central portion of the pallidum is probably the optimal site for globus pallidus stimulation taking advantage of these two divergent effects.

3.3. *Dystonia: GPi DBS*

As with PD, the clinical effects of GPi DBS in dystonia largely emulate those of pallidotomy. Unlike the rapid improvement seen in PD, GPi stimulation commonly results in delayed and gradual improvement over days to several months. Preliminary observations suggest that more mobile, fluid abnormal posturing may respond more quickly (in seconds to hours) while fixed tonic abnormal posturing may be slower to improve *(10–12)*. GPi DBS may be employed unilaterally or bilaterally depending on the distribution of the patient's dystonia. As with PD, unilateral GPi DBS has been successful when used contralaterally to a prior unilateral pallidotomy *(26)*.

A specific pattern of clinical effects correlating with stimulation in different parts of the GPi has not been described in patients with dystonia. However, empirically many groups have begun with stimulation in the ventral part of the GPi just above the optic tract (since this region has been shown to have anti-dyskinetic effects in PD) with a long pulse width, high frequency, and an amplitude just below

Table 1
Comparison of Clinical Effects of GPi, STN and Vim DBS in Parkinson's Disease

	GPi DBS *(4,7,8)*	STN DBS *(4–9)*	Vim DBS *(1–3)*
Overall clinical effects of bilateral DBS	Mean improvements in rating scales: off-period parkinsonism 30–50%; on-period parkinsonism 0–25%; on-period dyskinesias reduced 66–90%; off-period dystonia usually improved.	Mean improvements in rating scales: off-period parkinsonism 45–65%; on-period parkinsonism improved 10–30%; on-period dyskinesias reduced 67–83%; off-period dystonia usually markedly reduced.	Tremor improved 90%. Minor improvement in rigidity. ADL's not improved.
Overall clinical effects of unilateral DBS	Mean improvements: off-period parkinsonism 10–35%; on-period parkinsonism not improved; on-period dyskinesias reduced 70–80%; off-period dystonia usually reduced.	Mean improvements: off-period parkinsonism 25–30%; effects on on-period parkinsonism and dyskinesias not studied; off-period dystonia usually reduced.	Contralateral limb tremor improved 90%. Minor improvement in axial and ipsilateral tremor. Minor improvement in rigidity. ADL's not improved.
Microlesion effect	Minor beneficial improvement in off-period parkinsonism measurable at least 3 mo; Moderate anti-dyskinetic effect that may last 6 mo or more.	Mild beneficial effects on off-period parkinsonism. Effect on dyskinesias is variable (may be pro-dyskinetic in some and anti-dyskinetic in other patients).	Significant reduction in contra-lateral tremor measurable for at least 3 mo. Occasional patients with marked persistent tremor reduction not requiring stimulation.
Regional stimulation within the nucleus	Dorsal electrodes: greater anti-parkinson effect and can produce contralateral stimulation-induced dyskinesias. Ventral electrodes: greater anti-dyskinetic effect and may block the beneficial effects of levodopa on bradykinesia and gait.	Stimulation-induced laughter and mania due to current spread to limbic portion of STN or adjacent hypothalamus. Acute stimulation-related depression with electrode inferior to STN in SNr.	None.
Mechanism of effects on levodopa-induced dyskinesias	Anti-dyskinetic effect of microlesion and direct anti-dyskinetic effect of stimulation.	Mainly due to reduction in drug dosage. In some patients, microlesion effect directly reduces dyskinesias (possibly due to lesion of lenticular fasciculus). STN stimulation has a pro-dyskinetic effect with no direct anti-dyskinetic effect of stimulation. Stimulation above the STN in the zona incerta or below the STN in the SNr may directly suppress dyskinesias similar to GPi DBS.	Electrodes placed within or adjacent to CM/Pf or Voa/Vop may markedly suppress contralateral dyskinesias.

Stimulation-induced dyskinesias	Onset within 1–2 min. Contralateral. Similar form and distribution to the patients' pre-operative peak dose levodopa-induced dyskinesias (though usually milder). Usually abates in minutes or hours with chronic stimulation.	Onset usually within 5 min, but occasionally delayed onset up to a 2 d with chronic stimulation. Tends to improve with time. Contralateral or even ipsilateral. Two different forms: 1. Hemiballistic/ hemichoreic and sometimes very different from the patient's preoperative peak-dose levodopa-induced dyskinesias (often resembling diphasic dyskinesias); or 2. Dyskinesias resembling the patients pre-operative peak dose dyskinesias. Both types may occur in the same individual; type 1 at low amplitude stimulation and type 2 at high amplitudes. Levodopa and STN DBS have a synergistic effect in promoting dyskinesias, therefore drug reduction is necessary to reduce dyskinesias and allow the use of higher stimulation parameters.	None. Current spread ventrally to the cerebellothalamic fibers may result in stimulation-induced ataxia. Rebound tremor with discontinuing stimulation—physiologic adaptation.
Postoperative drug management	Usually no change. Occasional patients with severe pre-operative dyskinesias may tolerate higher levodopa doses.	Mean reduction in drug dosage 50% (Range 0–100%)	Usually no change. Occasional patients with severe tremor and very mild bradykinesia may reduce anti-parkinson medication.
Timing of anti-parkinson effects	Tremor improvement almost immediate. Most other features of parkinsonism improve within 1 min rapidly escalating to maximal effect in <5 min.	Tremor improvement almost immediate. Other features of parkinsonism improve within 1 min, but slower escalation to maximal benefit compared to GPi DBS and slower offset: perhaps 15 min, but possibly up to several hours (for effects on gait and bradykinesia).	Tremor improvement almost immediate.
Major stimulation-induced adverse effects due to current spread to adjacent structures	Ventrally to optic tract: photopsias and nausea; Posteriorly or medially to internal capsule: tonic contraction or paresthesias.	Anterolaterally to corticospinal tract: tonic contraction; Posteromedially to medial lemniscus: paresthesias; Inferomedially to oculomotor nucleus or its fascicles: diplopia.	Ventrally to cerebellothalamic fibers: ataxia; Laterally to internal capsule: tonic contraction. Posteriorly to VPL nucleus: paresthesias.

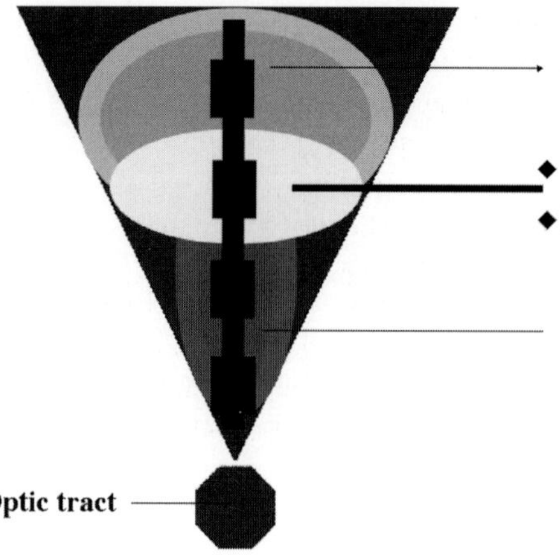

Fig. 1. Diagram of opposing clinical effects of ventral and dorsal globus pallidus simulation in Parkinson's disease.

that which produces adverse effects *(10)*. These groups have then awaited a delayed response before considering a change in choice of electrode stimulation site.

4. PERI-OPERATIVE AND INTRA-OPERATIVE PATIENT MANAGEMENT

Electrode implantation is usually performed with the patient awake in order to facilitate feedback as to the beneficial and adverse clinical effects of microstimulation and macrostimulation. However, in patients with severe generalized dystonia who are unable to tolerate awake surgery and in the case of younger children, electrode implantation is commonly performed under general anesthesia.

In patients with tremor, anti-tremor medications should be tapered and discontinued prior to surgery to maximize tremor during surgery. Similarly, in patients with PD, interventions that maximize off-period parkinsonism and reduce the likelihood of intraoperative confusion may be valuable because they may facilitate detection of improvement in parkinsonian signs during stimulation and validity of patient reports of adverse effects. Preoperative reduction in anti-parkinson medication achieves both of these goals. We therefore usually withhold levodopa and catechol-o-methyl transferase (COMT) inhibitors for 12 h prior to surgery and during surgery. If patients are on high doses of dopamine agonists, it is helpful to discontinue these 24–48 h before surgery because of their long-half life. Lastly, other anti-parkinson medications that have a greater tendency to cause confusion such as anticholinergic drugs and amantadine should be tapered prior to surgery since the adverse cognitive effects of these drugs may take a relatively long time to clear.

Elderly patients sometimes develop postoperative confusion that may last from 1 d to 2 wk following bilateral electrode implantation. In general, only supportive therapy is required and anti-parkinson medication can usually be reinstituted during this period though at a lower dose than preoperatively. In rare cases of prolonged confusion accompanied by psychosis and/or hallucinations, atypical neuroleptics such as clozapine may be useful. Postoperative confusion has been reported much less frequently with GPi electrode implantation than with STN surgery suggesting that this adverse effect may be specific to STN surgery rather than a nonspecific effect caused by antiparkinson drug withdrawal and the rigors and trauma of surgery. If the patient is lucid postoperatively, no change in drug dosage is immediately necessary. As noted earlier, many patients with GPi electrode implantation alone will note improvement in both off-period parkinsonism and dyskinesias as a result of a micropallidotomy effect. STN electrode implantation may reduce dyskinesias possibly due to lesioning of the pallidal outflow (especially the lenticular fasciculus) or more commonly may improve off-period parkinsonism and reduce the threshold for anti-parkinson medication to induce dyskinesias (probably as a result of lesioning the STN itself). In the latter case, it is often necessary to temporarily reduce antiparkinson medication to reduce dyskinesias. Mild chorea occasionally occurs following STN electrode implantation. This usually subsides within 48 h but in our experience, has rarely taken 1–2 mo to resolve. If significant chorea is present, a temporary reduction in levodopa dosage by 50% or more is prudent until the chorea resolves. If the patient is lucid postoperatively and no dyskinesias occur due to electrode insertion, no immediate change in drug dosage is necessary.

Despite the aforementioned measures, patients may become confused or agitated intraoperatively. Care, attention, and reassurance by an individual the patient knows well such as a nurse who helped care for the patient prior to surgery can be helpful since anxiety and fear may underlie the patient's agitation. Where nonpharmacologic measures are insufficient and patient agitation compromises the operative procedure, the use of low-dose, short-acting benzodiazepines such as midazolam may be appropriate. However, these should be used with caution because some patients may be paradoxically further disinhibited by such medications. When patient behavior becomes frankly dangerous (e.g., combative, large amplitude thrashing movements, attempting to leave the operative table while fixed in the stereotactic frame, or persistent reaching movements that may contaminate the operative field), we have found the use of low-dose propafol sedation very useful. In such cases, it is later often possible to terminate sedation and resume the stereotactic procedure with improved patient cooperation. Lastly, patients may complain of neck, head, or back pain due to being fixed in one position for several hours. If adjustment of the relationship between the operating table and the stereotactic frame and additional padding is not sufficient to ease patient discomfort, use of a low-dose, short-acting narcotic such as fentanyl may be helpful.

Where concern exists about the location of the implanted electrode because of inadequate response to intraoperative stimulation or other technical factors, externalization of the DBS electrode via a percutaneous extension may be advisable for a period of test stimulation using an external stimulator. Such test stimulation may be carried out using a hand-held stimulator (Medtronic Model 3625 or 3628) or an electrically isolated constant current stimulator. If acceptable results are obtained from intraoperative stimulation and electrophysiology, no period of test stimulation via a percutaneously externalized electrode is necessary prior to implantation of the permanently implantable pulse generators. We usually allow patients to recover from surgery for about 1–2 wk prior to beginning DBS programming. This allows wounds to heal and some of the more profound microlesion effects to subside, presumably as peri-lesional edema subsides. However, patients with various forms of tremor including tremor-predominant PD patients in whom a significant reduction in tremor was achieved during intraoperative test stimulation may begin chronic stimulation with preliminary DBS parameters, which may be set within a day of surgery and prior to hospital discharge.

5. DBS EQUIPMENT AND STIMULATION PARAMETERS: BASIC PRINCIPLES OF DBS PROGRAMMING

The current most widely used DBS equipment is manufactured by Medtronic, Inc. and consists of a DBS electrode (Medtronic, Inc.) implanted in the brain and fixed in place to the skull. The electrode contains four platinum-iridium contacts each of which is 1.5 mm long and separated by either 1.5 mm (DBS Lead Kit Model 3387) or 0.5 mm (DBS Lead Kit Model 3389). Contacts are numbered 0,1,2,3 with 0 being most distal and 3 most proximal. The shorter electrode is more suitable for STN implantation while the longer electrode continues to be used for Vim and GPi implantation. The electrode is connected to an extension cable (Extension Kit 7495), which is buried underneath the scalp and skin of the neck and attached to an implantable pulse generator (IPG). The stimulation settings are programmed by means of a console programmer (Model 7432, MemoryMod™ HF Software Cartridge Model 7458) attached to a transducer head that is applied over the IPG. The currently available single channel IPGs for movement disorder applications in the United States are the Itrel II and Soletra

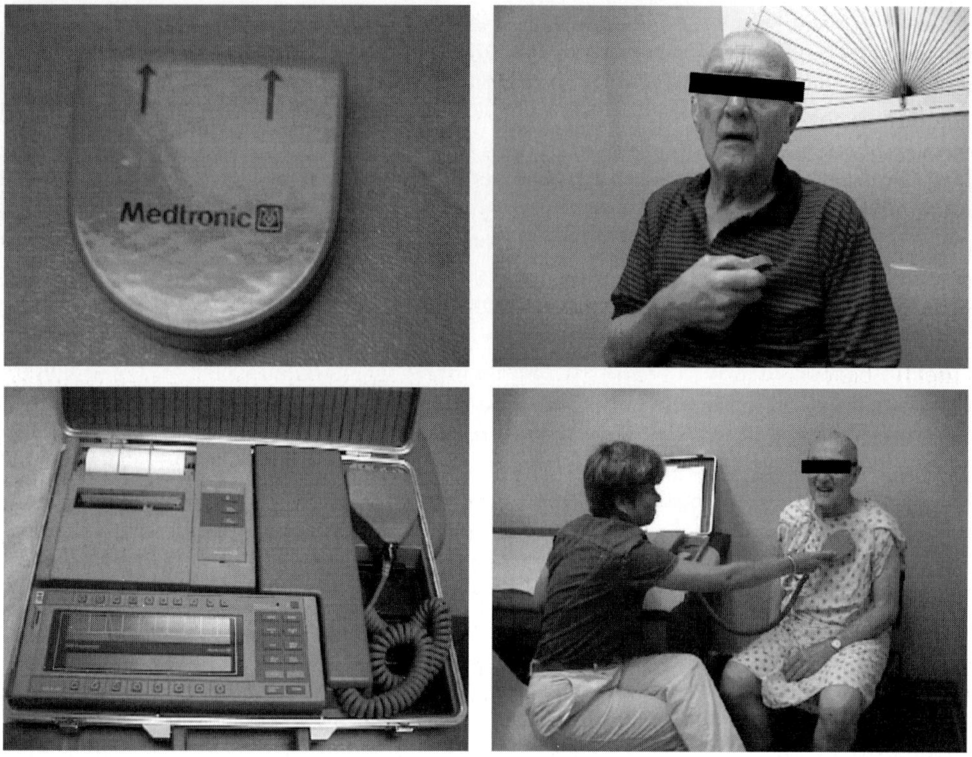

Fig. 2. Control magnet used to turn IPG on and off. Console DBS programmer with programming head applied over the patient's IPG.

(Medtronic, Inc.), while in Europe the Kinetra, a dual channel IPG is also available. With both the Itrel II™ and Soletra™, the patient can be instructed to turn the stimulator on or off using a magnet (Control Magnet Model 7452) applied over the IPG (Fig. 2). The Soletra™ has recently been phased in to replace the Itrel II™ and lacks the "magnet amplitude" feature that allows two different amplitude settings since in practice very few patients use or require two different settings. Application of the magnet over the Itrel II™ for greater than six seconds switches the stimulator from the normal mode to the "magnet amplitude" mode, a second voltage setting, which may be set equal to or less than the normal mode. It is important to set the "magnet amplitude" mode equal to the "normal" mode to prevent patients from accidentally entering a "magnet amplitude" mode set at 0 V (the baseline setting) by applying the magnet over the IPG for too long. In such cases, it is often difficult for patients to turn their stimulator back on. The Kinetra™ allows two quadripolar leads to be connected to one stimulator, each of which can be programmed separately. Kinetra™ comes with an Access Therapy Controller™ that allows the patient to turn the stimulator on and off electronically and also to modify the stimulation amplitude within a given set of parameters determined by the physician.

With the Soletra™ or Kinetra™, a number of stimulation variables must be selected including the following: choice of four active stimulation contacts including monopolar vs bipolar stimulation, frequency, pulse width, and amplitude. Determining the most effective contact(s) for stimulation is the first and most important task during stimulation programming. Monopolar stimulation is always tested first with the pulse generator case itself set as the anode (i.e., +) with a single contact on the lead set as the cathode (i.e., –). Any of the four contacts on the lead may be set as the cathode. For any given stimulation voltage or amplitude, monopolar stimulation results in a wide distribution of current spread of approx 1–1.5 mm diameter per mA *(27)*. Although generally one contact is used as the cathode, it is occasionally useful to activate two adjacent contacts for a broader field of current diffusion. Bipolar stimulation involves using two contacts on the lead: one as the anode and the other as the cathode. This results in a narrower field of current spread compared to monopolar stimulation and thus produces more focused effects. Monopolar stimulation is most commonly used since the greater current spread typically allows lower stimulation settings compared to bipolar stimulation. In contrast, bipolar stimulation may be especially useful when adverse effects due to current spread limit stimulation efficacy. Activating more than two contacts for bipolar stimulation (e.g., "tripolar" stimulation) results in a complex field of current spread. This is only rarely more effective than simple monopolar or bipolar stimulation and results in considerably higher battery drain.

Current spread with an increase in stimulation amplitude increases linearly. However, the Soletra™ and Itrel II™ battery consumption increases abruptly with an increase in stimulation from 3.6 V to 3.7 V due to a "doubling circuit" in which a second capacitor is switched into the system. Similarly, the battery drain also jumps when amplitude is increased above 7.3 V. As a result, efforts should be made to obtain optimal clinical results using an amplitude less than or equal to 3.6 V. If greater current spread and clinical effects are required with a given electrode combination, stimulation pulse width may be increased and voltage reduced to more economically achieve this end. For the Kinetra™, battery consumption is linear across the entire amplitude range.

The Soletra™ and Kinetra™ produce square wave pulses of 60–450 μs duration. Changing stimulation pulse width can alter the neural elements affected by DBS—longer pulse width has a greater effect on cell soma while shorter pulse width preferentially affects axons *(28)*. Typically, a pulse width of 60–120 μs is used in DBS, but much longer pulse widths may be required in patients undergoing GPi stimulation for treatment of dystonia. The Soletra™ is capable of stimulating at 0–185 Hz and the Kinetra™ at rates up to 250 Hz. Vim stimulation has been shown to have frequency dependent effects: tremor improvement begins at approx 100 Hz, plateaus at 130Hz, and only mild additional benefit is obtained in selected cases with increases up to 185 Hz *(17)*. Similar effects on bradykinesia and rigidity have been noted with STN DBS in PD. Increasing stimulation frequency does not increase current spread, but does reduce battery life. Therefore, for Vim and STN stimulation 130 Hz is used initially and frequency is only increased to 185 Hz if suboptimal benefit is achieved and an increase in pulse width or amplitude results in adverse effects due to current spread. Most reports suggest that GPi DBS for PD has the greatest effects at very high stimulation frequencies and so 185 Hz is routinely used *(7, 20,23,24)*. Stimulation at rates greater than 185Hz has not been shown to increase clinical benefit. Stimulation frequencies have been more variable in dystonia, but with few exceptions most groups have employed frequencies similar to those used in PD.

Battery life varies greatly depending on the chronic stimulation settings and hours of average daily use. Battery life also depends on the number of contacts activated and the nature of stimulation—monopolar stimulation is more costly than bipolar stimulation and battery life is also further decreased with the number of contacts activated. Lastly, higher stimulation frequency and pulse width also decreases battery lifespan. Most patients with thalamic DBS for tremor are able to turn stimulation off at night and on only during waking hours in order to reduce battery drain. Most patients undergoing STN or GPi DBS for PD use stimulation 24 h per day since turning the stimulators off at night often compromises nocturnal mobility. As a result, average Soletra™ battery life with STN or GPi DBS is typically 3–5 yr. Many patients with dystonia use the maximum pulse width of the pulse generator, which markedly shortens battery life and necessitates yearly battery replacement. In an individual patient, battery life can be estimated by referring to the Medtronic product literature. Battery replacement can be delayed until the battery has been completely depleted, but this may result in marked worsening of symptoms. In PD patients who have substantially decreased antiparkinson drug dosage, acute deterioration of parkinsonism may occur and there is a theoretical risk of a neuroleptic malignant-like syndrome, which may necessitate a temporary increase in drug dose. Similarly, patients with severe generalized dystonia may develop status dystonicus and rhabdomyolysis. However, unlike PD, acute administration of medications for dystonia is unlikely to quickly resolve this state. Pulse generator batteries typically fail gradually over several days. Therefore patients should be advised to contact their physician if they notice a waning of the effects of stimulation so that this possibility can be evaluated by checking the pulse generator current drain and the battery may be replaced expediently if necessary. In select patients who live far from a tertiary care center, prophylactic battery replacement according to the forecasted lifespan of the battery may be advisable.

Patients without substantial tremor often have difficulty easily determining whether their stimulators are turned on or off. All patients without substantial tremor who have a Soletra™ or Itrel II™ instead of the Kinetra™ pulse generators should be taught how to use a portable AM radio tuned to 530 kHz to verify whether the stimulator is on or off. The pulse generator creates interference heard as a buzz when the radio is held over a stimulator that is on. It is helpful to use a radio with an earphone attachment and without a speaker, since the magnet in the radio's speaker may itself turn the stimulator on or off. Many patients have difficulty mastering the process of turning the IPG on and off by applying a magnet over the pulse generator and verifying its status, so it is often helpful to instruct not only the patient but also a family member or caregiver. Teaching these techniques should occur at the beginning of DBS programming so that patients may easily terminate uncomfortable, delayed-onset adverse effects caused by new stimulation parameters set in the clinic earlier.

In some clinical settings, as an alternative to fully implantable pulse generators, a partially implantable, radio frequency-coupled pulse generator (Extrel™ model 3425), which is predominantly in use for spinal cord stimulation, may be used. With this system, the patient wears a device that is the size of a small portable cassette player on his belt (which includes stimulation controls in addition to a nine volt battery) connected to an antenna that is taped on the skin over the pulse generator. Although the Extrel system is only partially implantable and monopolar stimulation is not possible, this pulse generator has certain advantages: no surgical procedure is required for battery replacement, and higher pulse widths (up to 1000 μs) and stimulation frequencies (up to 1000 Hz) are possible. These features may be especially beneficial in some patients with dystonia who require large pulse widths resulting in more rapid battery depletion. However, because the Extrel™ is used infrequently for DBS the remainder of this paper will focus on the use of fully implantable pulse generators, though most of the principles of DBS programming discussed below may be applied to the use of the Extrel.

6. SCHEDULING DBS PROGRAMMING SESSIONS

The time required to optimally set stimulation parameters may at times be substantial, especially when one is inexperienced or first beginning to learn DBS programming. However, this time typically diminishes as experience in programming is accumulated. Although the amount of time is highly variable between individual patients, several programming sessions are usually required to optimize stimulation settings in all patients with GPi and STN electrodes.

6.1. Tremor: Vim DBS

Patients should withhold anti-tremor and/or anti-parkinson medication at least overnight prior to the initial programming session. Usually a concentrated period of 1–3 h is adequate to determine the most effective anti-tremor settings in the vast majority of patients.

6.2. Parkinson's Disease: GPi or STN DBS

Programming sessions should generally be no more than 2–3 h as longer sessions often result in patient fatigue with variable and unreliable patient performance during tests of bradykinesia. Most DBS programming is performed with patients off medication and ideally sessions should be scheduled in the morning after overnight drug withdrawal. However, in patients with extremely severe off-period immobility or lack of caregiver support this may not be easily accomplished. As a result, a reasonable compromise is to have patients take their first dose of levodopa in the morning allowing them to attend the clinic in a mobile drug-on state; once in the clinic, the effects of antiparkinson medication may be allowed to wear off so that programming can begin in the early afternoon. Patients can then be given levodopa at the conclusion of the session if necessary and sent home. Rare patients may become virtually anarthric and unable to communicate or too disabled to cooperate during programming when completely off medication; such patients may be given just enough antiparkinson medication to induce a suboptimal "on" response without dyskinesias and to allow participation. In such patients, greater emphasis can be placed on the response of rigidity to various DBS settings since testing rigidity requires less active patient cooperation *(29)*. Assessment of the effects of DBS on drug-induced dyskinesias is often best performed in the afternoon once patients have taken more than one dose of levodopa prior to attending the clinic since dyskinesias commonly exhibit a diurnal pattern, mild in the morning with worsening in the afternoon and evening.

6.3. Dystonia: GPi DBS

Because the effects of GPi DBS on dystonia may be delayed and gradual, it is necessary to allow at least 24 h of continuous stimulation on any one setting before assessing the efficacy of stimulation. Therefore, in patients who do not exhibit a relatively quick response, sessions can be relatively brief with assessment of current settings and institution of new settings to be assessed during the next session.

7. ASSESSMENT AND RECORD KEEPING OF CLINICAL EFFECTS OF DBS

Detailed notes are very helpful in allowing a systematic determination of the best stimulation settings. For each electrode combination, it is important to record the stimulation threshold for adverse effects; the nature of the adverse effects (e.g., tonic contraction due to current spread to the corticospinal tract at 4.0 V); a qualitative description of the degree of benefit (e.g., very good benefit for tremor, moderate improvement of arm bradykinesia); and cross-reference the description to the UPDRS, Burke-Fahn-Marsden (BFM) ratings for dystonia, or percentage improvement in tremor obtained at this setting. In patients with tremor, repeated examination of a task that is highly sensitive to tremor such as writing and drawing a spiral may be necessary to differentiate between what may appear to be clinically similar effects achieved by different DBS parameters or electrode contacts. It is valuable to record the severity and distribution of signs and symptoms on both sides of the body (not just contralateral to stimulation) as DBS may have significant ipsilateral effects in individual patients. For patients with PD, a description of the nature, severity, and distribution of off-period dystonia and on-period or stimulation-induced dyskinesias is also important. Use of the Core Assessment Program for Surgical Interventional Therapies in Parkinson's Disease (CAPSIT-PD) scale captures many of these elements and may be especially useful for comparison of the anti-dyskinetic effects of different stimulation settings *(30)*.

8. VIM DBS PROGRAMMING ALGORITHM FOR TREMOR (FIG. 3)

8.1. Initial DBS Programming

1. Before beginning DBS programming it is useful to record the impedance and current drain of monopolar stimulation with each of the four electrode contacts using the following stimulation settings: amplitude 1.0 volts, pulse width 210 µs, and frequency 30 Hz. Being able to refer to the initial impedance and other electrical properties of the system can be helpful in troubleshooting future hardware problems.
2. If two electrodes have been implanted, initially each side should be programmed independently starting with monopolar stimulation.
3. The threshold for persistent adverse effects should be determined with each electrode contact (e.g., case +/1-; case +/2-; etc.). The initial stimulation parameters for Vim DBS should be amplitude 0 V, pulse width 60 µs, and frequency 130 Hz. The amplitude should be gradually increased by 0.5 V every 30–60 s (keeping other stimulation parameters constant) while constantly monitoring the patient for subjective and objective adverse effects. An abrupt increase to high amplitude may cause painful tonic contractions or paresthesias,

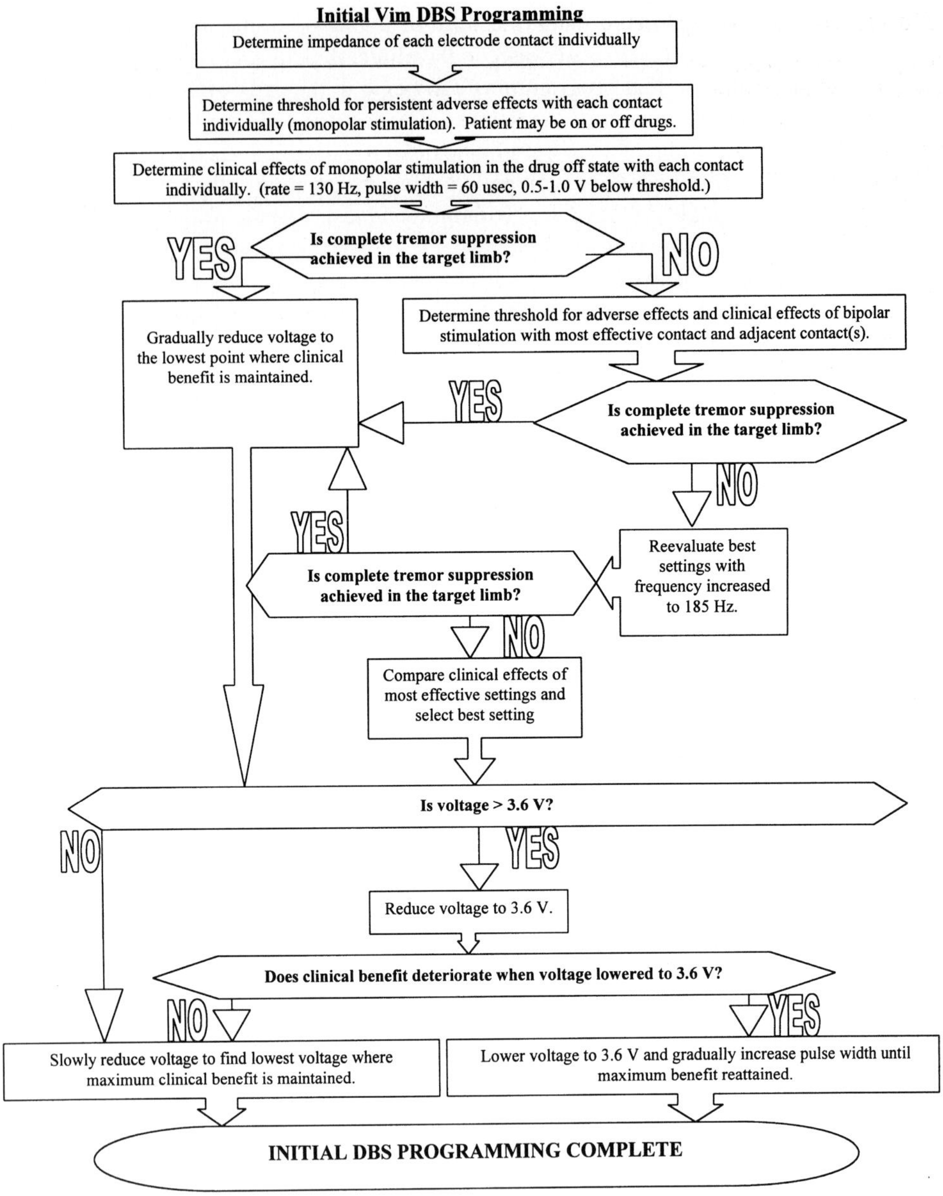

Fig. 3. Algorithm for Vim DBS Programming (see text for details).

but tolerance to these adverse effects (especially paresthesias) commonly develops if the amplitude is increased slowly. The amplitude should be increased until persistent adverse effects occur and then one should note the threshold amplitude and nature of adverse effects. If persistent adverse effects occur at less than 1.0 V that particular electrode contact is probably suboptimally positioned (e.g., tonic contraction at low voltage suggests that the electrode is too close to the corticospinal tract).

Analyzing the threshold and nature of the adverse effects with monopolar stimulation allows one to determine the relative location of each of the contacts to adjacent anatomic structures (*see* Table 1).

8.2. Determination of Efficacy on Tremor

1. First perform a baseline assessment with stimulation off at the beginning of each programming session for assessment of stimulation benefits compared with baseline.
2. The results of monopolar stimulation provide a base of information that allows one to rank bipolar electrode combinations that are more likely to yield good results if necessary.
   a. Using monopolar stimulation for each contact test the effects of stimulation on tremor at an amplitude 0.5–1.0 V below the threshold for persistent adverse effects. Record the clinical benefit noted for each contact. The onset and offset of effect on tremor is virtually immediate so assessments need not be significantly delayed after beginning stimulation with new parameters. If complete tremor suppression can be achieved in the target limb with monopolar stimulation no further electrode combinations need be tested.
   b. For bilaterally stimulated patients repeat the above process using the other side.
3. If complete tremor suppression is not achieved, decide which one (or two) electrodes provide the best anti-tremor effects with monopolar stimulation. Then begin bipolar stimulation by testing the best electrode in combination with those adjacent to it using the same methodology as used for monopolar stimulation, determining the threshold for adverse effects and then efficacy of stimulation. Reversing the polarity of stimulation can also frequently provide superior effects. (For example, if case +/2- is thought to be the best monopolar setting, begin by testing 1-/2+, 1+/2-, 2-/3+, and 2+/3-.)
4. If complete tremor suppression is still not achieved increase frequency to 185 Hz and re-evaluate the best settings thus far determined.
6. If tremor is not completely suppressed with the single monopolar and bipolar electrode combinations, test double monopolar stimulation using the best electrode in combination with those adjacent to it using the same methodology. For example, if case +/2- is thought to be the best monopolar setting, test case +/1-/2-and case +/2-/3-.
6. Rank order the settings which provided the best tremor suppression for each stimulator.
7. Once the best electrode combination has been determined, pulse width and amplitude can be optimized (Fig. 3). Voltage can often be slightly reduced without a reduction in stimulation efficacy. Finally, if voltage is greater than 3.6 V, attempt to increase the pulse width and decrease the voltage to improve the electrical efficiency of stimulation without a reduction in stimulation efficacy. A 30 μs increase in pulse width allows approximately a 0.5 V decrease in amplitude.
8. At the end of each programming session send the patient home on the optimal settings thus far determined.

When evaluating the adverse and beneficial effects of stimulation, one may find that some mild adverse effects cannot be eliminated without significantly reducing the beneficial effects. Therefore, mild adverse effects sometimes must be accepted with chronic stimulation in order to achieve the best overall clinical effect.

8.3. Determination of Efficacy on Drug-Induced Dyskinesias in Parkinson's Disease

In patients with PD and levodopa-induced dyskinesias, current spread to the CM/Pf or Voa/Vop may block dyskinesias. Verifying the presence or absence of this effect with the current anti-tremor stimulation settings after levodopa administration is important since an anti-dyskinetic effect may allow more aggressive drug therapy of off-period bradykinesia and other features of parkinsonism.

8.4. Delayed Stimulation Adjustment and Medication Adjustment

Stimulation parameters become fairly stable by 1 mo postoperatively and only very minor adjustments such as slightly increasing the amplitude may be necessary beyond 3 mo. However, up to 10–25% of patients undergoing long-term Vim DBS for ET may develop tolerance to stimulation requiring progressively higher voltages to maintain the same degree of effectiveness *(31,32)*. Instructing patients to discontinue stimulation at night may reduce the development of tolerance. In those with established tolerance, limiting daytime stimulation to times when optimal fine motor control such as handwriting is required may reduce tolerance. In rare cases where tolerance is severe and markedly limits the usefulness of DBS, radiofrequency lesioning of the thalamus via the DBS electrode may eliminate tremor and tolerance *(33,34)*. Tolerance has not been reported with Vim DBS for PD, but some patients may develop rebound increase in tremor when turning stimulation off at night *(35)*. As a result some PD patients, especially those with prominent resting tremor, must keep stimulation on at night to permit sleep.

Many ET patients with complete or near complete tremor suppression may be able to reduce or discontinue all anti-tremor medications. Although the majority of patients with PD undergoing Vim DBS require little or no change in medication, patients taking large doses of levodopa to suppress tremor may be able to reduce medication *(2,3)*.

9. GPI DBS PROGRAMMING ALGORITHM FOR PARKINSON'S DISEASE (FIG. 4)

9.1. *Initial DBS Programming*

The principles of initial programming are identical to those used for thalamic stimulation except that initial stimulation parameters for GPi DBS should be amplitude 0 V, pulse width 60 μs, and frequency 185 Hz. For patients with PD undergoing GPi or STN DBS, threshold determination may be performed in the medication-on or medication-off state for all electrode combinations, although with the patient on medication detection of mild stimulation-induced dyskinesias may be difficult or impossible. Determining thresholds with the patient on medication can reduce the length of time patients are required to spend off medication as the stimulation amplitude can more quickly be increased to previously determined threshold levels when subsequently testing stimulation efficacy in the medication-off state (see below). This is particularly useful for patients who have great difficulty tolerating being off medication for a significant period of time.

9.2. *Determination of Efficacy on Off-Period Parkinsonism*

1. Baseline assessment and testing of monopolar stimulation is similar to thalamic stimulation.
   a. Allow chronic stimulation for approximately five minutes before rating clinical effects using the UPDRS. Make note of stimulation-induced dyskinesias because they may indicate excessive current spread dorsally. If stimulation-induced dyskinesias are present, rate the improvement in parkinsonism using the UPDRS and then slowly reduce the voltage to identify the largest amplitude that does not induce dyskinesias before again rating the improvement in parkinsonism.
   b. Prior to assessing the effects of stimulation with the next electrode contact, turn the stimulator off and wait for 5–10 min to avoid carry-over effects from the previous setting. Unlike in the thalamus, effects of GPi DBS do not subside immediately after the pulse generator has been turned off and also do not become fully developed immediately after turning the pulse generator on.
   c. For bilaterally stimulated patients repeat the above process using the other side.
2. Decide which one (or two) electrodes provided the best antiparkinson effects with monopolar stimulation, and begin bipolar stimulation by testing the best electrode in combination with those adjacent to it using the same methodology used for monopolar stimulation. If dyskinesias are induced with monopolar stimulation, it may be necessary to use monopolar or bipolar stimulation using more ventrally located electrical contacts.
3. Rank order the settings that provided the best antiparkinson benefit as determined for each stimulator.
4. At the end of each programming session send the patient home on the optimal settings thus far determined.

9.3. *Determination of Efficacy on Drug-induced Dyskinesias*

Once the best parameters to improve off-period parkinsonism have been determined, it is important to verify the absence of a levodopa-blocking effect and presence of adequate dyskinesia suppression. As mentioned earlier, this is often best performed in the afternoon after at least two doses of medication when the patient is fully "on."

1. Assess dyskinesias on the optimal settings which improve off-period parkinsonism (as determined earlier). If dyskinesias are adequately suppressed and there is no worsening of bradykinesia and gait or shortening of the duration of levodopa benefit with stimulation, no further programming is required and current settings are optimal.

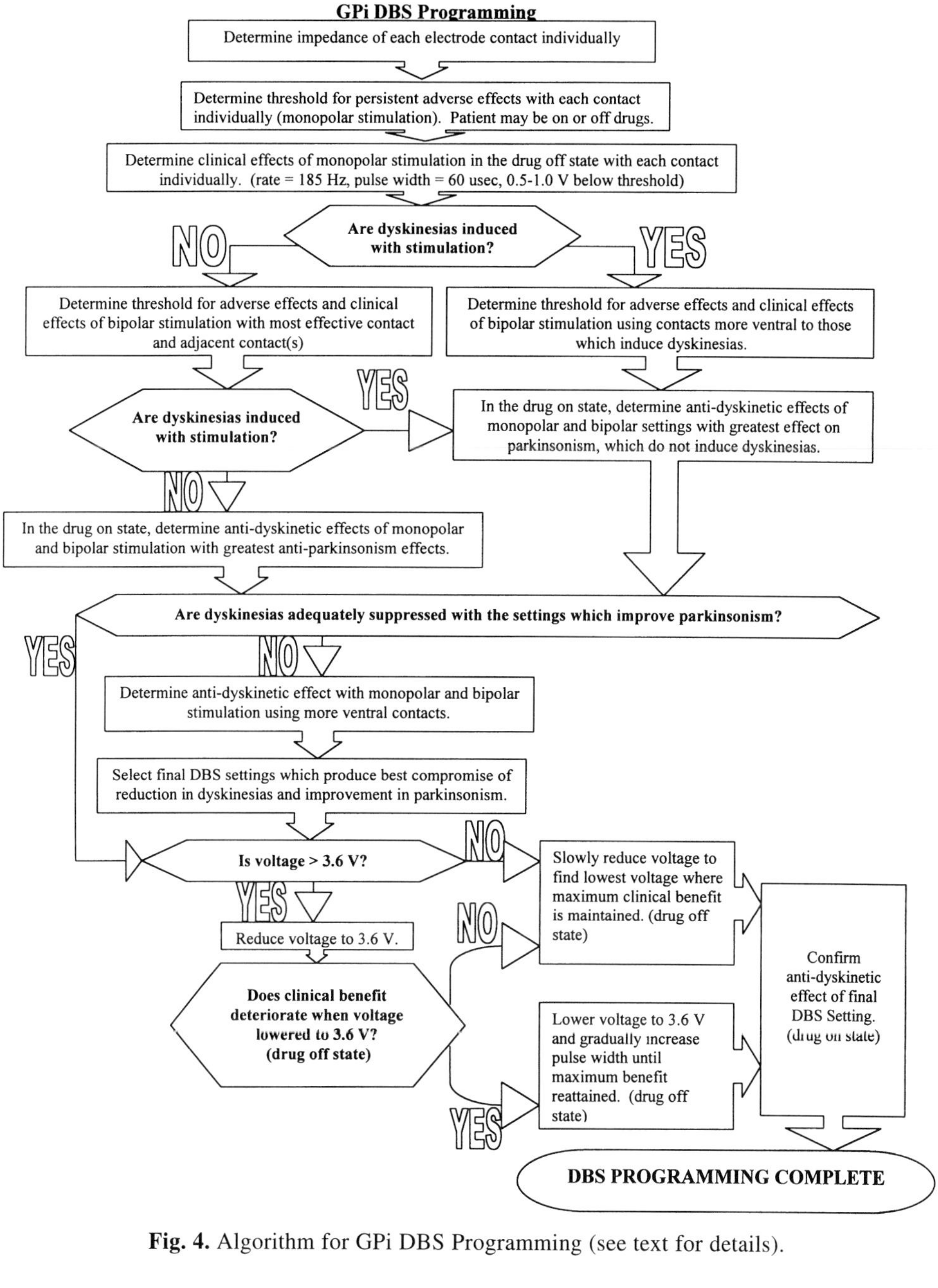

Fig. 4. Algorithm for GPi DBS Programming (see text for details).

2. If dyskinesias are insufficiently suppressed, try to determine the best overall settings for dyskinesia suppression that do not block the beneficial effects of levodopa: examine dyskinesias, bradykinesia, and gait using each of the other two or three settings that provided reasonably good (though not optimal) improvement of off-period parkinsonism. Stimulating with more ventrally located electrodes commonly improves dyskinesia suppression. As a result, the best overall final setting for some patients is a compromise that provides the best combination of improved off-period parkinsonism and on-period dyskinesia suppression, without worsening on-period parkinsonism.
3. Once the best electrode combination has been determined, stimulation pulse width and amplitude can be optimized (Fig. 4) using the same technique as used for thalamic stimulation.

9.4. Delayed Stimulation and Medication Adjustment

As with thalamic stimulation, parameters become fairly stable by 1 mo postoperatively and only very minor adjustments such as slight increases of amplitude may be necessary beyond 3 mo. Unlike thalamic stimulation in essential tremor, tolerance, or habituation has not been observed with GPi DBS in PD. Antiparkinson medication doses and regimen usually do not require significant adjustments with GPi DBS. In patients with marked levodopa sensitivity and disabling dyskinesias preoperatively, the anti-dyskinetic effects of GPi stimulation may allow higher levodopa doses. Patients taking hourly liquid levodopa preparations can usually be converted to a simpler medication regimen.

10. GPI DBS PROGRAMMING FOR DYSTONIA

Worldwide experience with this technique is quite limited in comparison to PD and is marked by considerable heterogeneity with respect to the type of patients operated and the stimulation settings used. As noted earlier, a response to stimulation may occur abruptly within seconds or may be delayed and progressive over weeks or months with mobile forms of dystonia tending to respond more quickly than fixed dystonic postures and gait disorders. Despite this heterogeneity, some useful guidelines can be proposed following many of the same principles used for PD.

1. Determine threshold for adverse effects in a manner similar to that for PD.
2. Initially assess the efficacy of stimulation using high stimulation frequency (130–185 Hz) and low pulse width (60 μs similar to PD) at an amplitude just below threshold using monopolar stimulation for about 1 h with each electrode contact. The best results are typically seen using the lowest contacts. If significant improvement is seen with one or two contacts these are likely to be most efficacious for chronic stimulation. Thereafter the efficacy of bipolar stimulation may be assessed in a similar fashion using contacts adjacent to those that provided significant benefit with monopolar stimulation.
3. If there is no acute benefit with stimulation, then more chronic stimulation for 1–2 d with the monopolar settings should be tested.
4. If no benefit is seen with low pulse width stimulation, it is then helpful to test the effects of high pulse widths (450 microsec) with monopolar stimulation in a similar fashion.
5. Depending on the results with aforementioned test stimulation, it may also be useful to test the effects of double monopolar stimulation in some patients.
6. If no benefit is noted with short-term stimulation, it may be useful to employ the method used almost universally by the Montpelier group. Coubes et al. report stimulating just above the optic tract (usually with electrode 1) at 450 μs, 1–2 V (i.e., just above the adverse effect threshold), and at high frequency. They have seen very delayed and dramatic responses over weeks *(10)*.
7. Consider a trial of low-frequency stimulation at 50 Hz if an inadequate response is obtained, because we have observed a frequency-dependent response in one patient with the best results at this frequency *(12)*.
8. Consider increasing pulse width if promising but suboptimal improvement is noted at lower pulse widths with chronic stimulation.
9. Worsening of dystonia may also be observed in a delayed fashion once stimulation is turned off, with battery failure, or with hardware breakage (which may be more frequent than in PD due to the mechanical stresses of dystonia).
10. Patients with marked improvement in dystonia with GPi DBS are often able to reduce or discontinue anti-dystonia medications such as anticholinergic drugs.

11. STN DBS PROGRAMMING ALGORITHM FOR PARKINSON'S DISEASE (FIG. 5)

11.1. Initial DBS Programming

The initial programming methodology is the same as GPi DBS except that the initial stimulation parameters should be 0 V, 60 μs pulse width, and frequency 130 Hz.

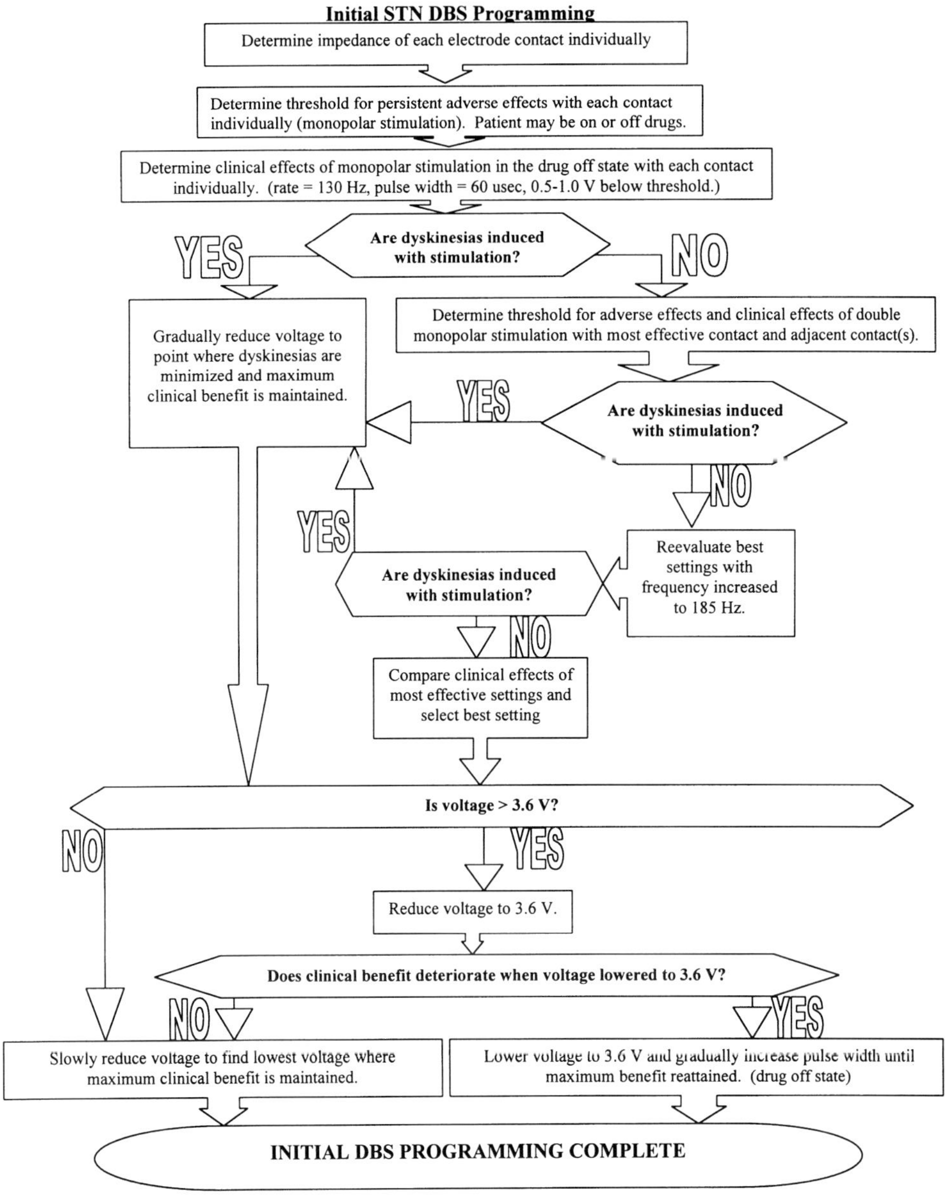

Fig. 5. Algorithm for STN DBS Programming (see text for details).

11.2. Determination of Efficacy on Off-Period Parkinsonism

1. Baseline assessment and testing of monopolar stimulation follows the same principles as GPi DBS.
   a. Allow chronic stimulation for approx 15 min before rating the clinical effect using the UPDRS. STN stimulation generally improves rigidity and tremor in less than 1 min. Although the majority of improvement in bradykinesia gradually builds over several minutes, maximal improvement may take several hours. Off-period dystonia is generally improved within minutes of initiating effective stimulation. Dyskinesias may be induced after minutes to 2 d of chronic STN stimulation in the absence of anti-parkinson medication. The presence of stimulation-induced dyskinesias is an excellent sign and suggests that parkinsonism can be maximally improved *(29,36)*. If stimulation-induced dyskinesias are present rate the improvement

in parkinsonism using the UPDRS and then slowly reduce the voltage to the minimum amplitude that does not induce dyskinesias before rating the improvement in parkinsonism again. The maximal antiparkinson effect of STN stimulation correlates with that achievable by high-dose levodopa therapy, with the exception that tremor may be improved more by stimulation *(5,6)*. Therefore, the pre-operative "best on" can only slightly be improved by the combination of STN stimulation and anti-parkinson drug therapy *(5,29)*.

b. Prior to assessing the effects of stimulation with the next electrode contact, turn the stimulator off and wait for 10–15 min to avoid carry-over effects from the previous setting. If choreiform dyskinesias can be induced with monopolar stimulation, no further electrode combinations need be immediately tested.
c. Repeat the aforementioned process using the other side (for bilaterally stimulated patients).

2. Decide which one (or two) electrodes provide the best antiparkinson effects with monopolar stimulation and then double monopolar stimulation and bipolar stimulation by testing the best electrode(s) in combination with those adjacent to it using the methodology already described.
3. If no dyskinesias have been induced and the benefit achieved has not been at least equal to that seen with levodopa administration. Increase frequency to 185 Hz and re-evaluate the best settings that have thus far been determined
4. Rank order the settings that provided the best antiparkinson benefit as determined earlier for each stimulator.
5. At the end of each programming session, send the patient home on the optimal settings thus far determined. Patients must be warned about the possibility of developing significant delayed-onset dyskinesias and must know how to discontinue stimulation should this occur.
6. Once the best electrode combination has been determined, stimulation pulse width and amplitude can be optimized (Fig. 5).

Identifying the nature of the adverse effects of stimulating the STN region allows one to determine the relative location of each of the contacts to adjacent structures and appropriate management. A large number of adverse effects can be induced by current spread outside of the target (Table 2; Fig. 6). Adverse effects that rapidly habituate (e.g. paresthesias) do not prevent further increase in stimulation if needed, whereas adverse effects that do not habituate (e.g., tonic muscle contraction) require a reduction or change in stimulation *(37)*.

11.3. Determination of Efficacy on Drug-Induced Dyskinesias

STN stimulation and dopaminergic therapy have an additive effect in inducing dyskinesias. Dyskinesia reduction with STN DBS occurs primarily as a result of drug reduction *(38)*. Therefore, we generally reduce antiparkinson medication by one-half when beginning chronic STN stimulation. Periodic "on-drug" examinations are needed to determine the severity of dyskinesias. Antiparkinson medication is usually reduced as stimulation is increased; therefore, the presence of significant on-period dyskinesias usually necessitates further drug reduction (or less commonly reduction of stimulation settings). In contrast, suboptimal effects on parkinsonism without dyskinesias suggest that either anti-parkinson medication or stimulation should be increased. If a direct anti-dyskinetic effect of stimulation is noted, one is likely stimulating the substantia nigra reticulata (SNr) below the STN or zona incerta (Zi) above the STN *(37–39)*.

11.4. Long-Term Stimulation, Medication, and Patient Management

In the first 2–3 mo postoperatively, the effects of STN stimulation may seem to wane as the microlesion associated with surgery diminishes. This can be managed by slightly increasing stimulation. If stimulation-induced adverse effects prevent optimal improvement, then changing stimulation to an adjacent contact or bipolar stimulation should be considered. If optimum improvement is still not achievable, the electrode is likely suboptimally positioned and dopaminergic therapy should be increased. Stimulation settings remain relatively stable in the majority of patients after 3 mo postoperatively. An average reduction of 50% of dopaminergic therapy is achieved at 1-yr follow-up *(5)*. A small minority of patients are able to discontinue all anti-parkinson medication. We prefer to first reduce and discontinue levodopa while maintaining continuous dopaminergic stimulation if needed with long-acting

Table 2
Adverse Effects of Subthalamic Region Stimulation *(37)*

Adverse effect	Habituation	Anatomical location	Mechanism/comments	Management
Weight gain	Months		5–20 kg weight gain is typical. Reduction in dyskinesias and metabolic rate. Possibly also limbic effects of stimulation	Patients should be warned about appropriate diet to prevent excessive weight gain.
Flushing and perspiration	Minutes to hours	Hypothalamus: anterior to STN	Accompanied by feeling of heat.	Change stimulating contact or very slowly increase voltage of most effective contact to allow habituation.
Tonic muscle contraction	None	Corticospinal tract: anteriorly or laterally to STN		Reduce amplitude, change to bipolar stimulation or change stimulating contact.
Dysarthria	None	Corticobulbar tract: lateral to STN		Reduce amplitude, change to bipolar stimulation, or change stimulating contact.
Hypophonia			May be due to excessive levodopa reduction and inadequate effect of stimulation on speech or due to current spread to corticobulbar tract.	Examine speech off stimulation after high-dose levodopa to determine if worsening of speech is due to drug reduction. Then turn stimulation on to determine if current spread to corticolbulbar tract is further worsening hypophonia.
Diplopia	Occasional over days to weeks	Inferomedial: If unilateral ocular deviation then due to current spread to fascicles of oculomotor nerve; if conjugate deviation, then due to supranuclear oculomotor system		Reduce amplitude, change to bipolar stimulation, or change to higher stimulating contact
L-DOPA blocking effect	None	SNr	May be similar to that seen with ventral GPi stimulation with improvement in rigidity and dyskinesias, but worsening of akinesia	Reduce amplitude, change to bipolar stimulation, or change to higher stimulating contact
Paresthesias	Seconds	Medial lemniscus: posterior to STN		May gradually continue to increase voltage if needed and symptoms habituate
Blepharospasm	None Onset over minutes with stimulation	STN	Form of stimulation-induced dystonia and tends to occur as indicator of highly effective stimulation	Botulinum toxin injections to orbicularis oculi.
Dysequilibrium and gait ataxia without limb ataxia	None	Possibly red nucleus: medial to STN		Reduce amplitude, change to bipolar stimulation, or change stimulating contact. Drug increase often also required.

dopamine agonists that are less likely to induce dyskinesias. With drug reduction and continuous STN stimulation, the threshold for induction of dyskinesias gradually increases, allowing a corresponding increase in stimulation. Patients with severe preoperative dyskinesias are more apt to develop severe stimulation-induced dyskinesias or even stimulation-induced dystonia. Stimulation-induced dystonia must be differentiated from tonic muscle contraction (by its development over minutes rather than seconds after starting stimulation) and also from off-period dystonia. As a result, extremely slow increases in stimulation over weeks may be necessary to allow adaptation to stimulation. In the most extreme cases, the therapeutic window between relief of parkinsonism and induction of disabling dyskinesias or dystonia is too narrow to permit effective stimulation. Use of proximal or distal contacts further from the center of the target and often with bipolar stimulation to reduce current diffusion frequently widens the therapeutic window in order to allow a slow increase in stimulation amplitude *(37)*.

Reduction in dopaminergic medication may unmask symptoms of restless legs syndrome (RLS) in patients who have previously never complained of such symptoms *(40)*. More severe cases may be accompanied by dyskinesias during the day resembling periodic limb movements of sleep. Although an increase in stimulation may improve these symptoms, however, in our experience, as following pallidotomy *(41)*, this usually results in inadequate symptom relief and need for additional drug therapy *(40)*. Reintroduction of controlled release levodopa or dopamine agonists may be helpful, but may also significantly increase dyskinesias. In such cases, use of benzodiazepines or opiates can improve RLS symptoms without inducing dyskinesias.

Overly aggressive reduction in antiparkinson medication should be avoided because levodopa also improves non-motor symptoms of PD. A levodopa withdrawal syndrome of abulia, anhedonia, and depression may result *(7)*. Reinstitution of levodopa up to the threshold that produces mild nondisabling dyskinesias usually quickly improves these symptoms. For persistent symptoms or when disabling dyskinesias limit levodopa therapy, the use of selective serotonin reuptake inhibitors can be helpful *(37)*. Depression due to drug withdrawal must be differentiated from acute stimulation-induced depression due to unintentional stimulation of the substantia nigra reticulata (SNr), which lies below the STN *(42)*. In such cases, depression improves immediately with discontinuation of stimulation and greater improvement in parkinsonism is achieved by stimulating through a more proximal contact.

Postoperative hypomania or mania may occur with STN stimulation that is highly effective for the motor features of parkinsonism and mimics the euphoria-inducing effects of levodopa *(43)*. Rapid reduction in dopaminergic therapy and, if necessary, stimulation will commonly improve this behavior. Similarly, laughing spells associated with the appropriate affect have been induced by high-stimulation settings and accompanied by stimulation-induced dyskinesias *(44,45)*.

The anatomy of DBS effects in the STN and surrounding structures has been illustrated by Volkmann et al. *(37)* and is shown in Fig. 6. In their experience, dysesthesias result from stimulation too far posteriorly, which stimulates medial lemniscus; diplopia, conjugate gaze deviation, and mydriasis result from stimulation medial or inferior to STN; and postural disturbance and gait ataxia from stimulation medially in the region of red nucleus. Stimulation ventral to STN in substantia nigra may increase akinesia or inhibit levodopa effect.

Preoperative levodopa refractory postural instability is unlikely to be substantially improved with STN stimulation. As a result of significant improvement in bradykinesia and speed of gait, falls may actually become more frequent postoperatively. Although this may sometimes be improved with physiotherapy, many patients require a walker to prevent falls.

12. TROUBLESHOOTING HARDWARE PROBLEMS WITH DBS PROGRAMMING

Hardware breaks or loose connections may result in lack of stimulation effect, intermittent stimulation, current leak, or short circuit. Neurologists and neurosurgeons must often work together to identify and correct these problems. During the initial programming session, impedance of each electrode should

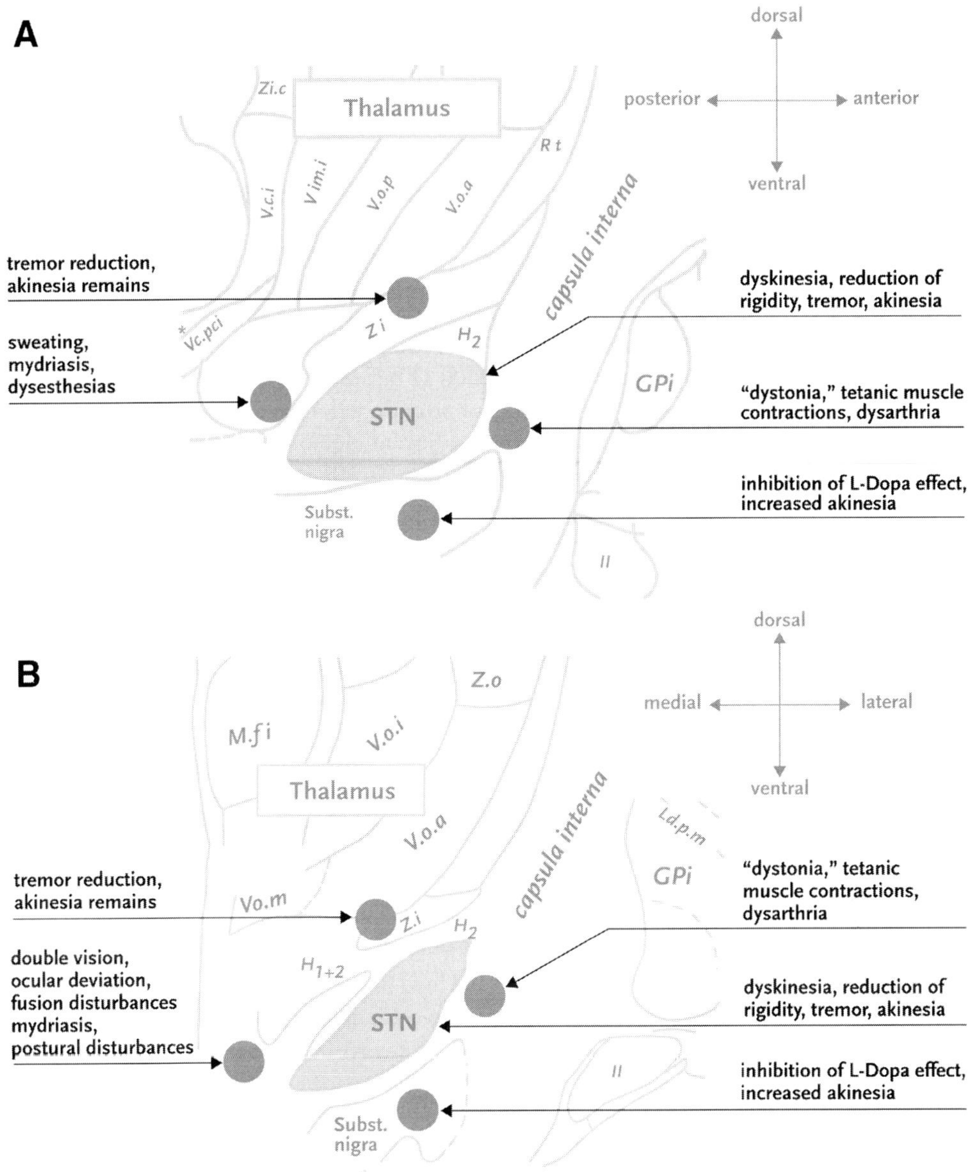

Fig. 6. Stimulation-induced effects and adverse effects with high frequency stimulation of the STN and adjacent structures. (**A**) Sagittal section 12 mm lateral to anterior commissure-posterior commissure line (AC-PC line), and (**B**) Frontal section 1.5 mm behind the midcommissural point (MCP). The anatomic sections were derived with permission from the Schaltenbrand atlas. Reprinted with permission *(37)*.

be checked and recorded to serve as a baseline for comparison should later hardware problems develop. In a normal circuit, impedance is 500–2000 Ω (or greater).

Appropriately functioning stimulators may suddenly stop stimulation because they turn off accidentally or because of hardware failure or trauma (especially falls). The Itrel II and Soletra are quite susceptible to activation of the magnetic read switch by electromagnetic interference including household appliances held close to the IPG such as power tools and mixers, theft and metal detectors in

23. Bejjani, B., Damier, P., Arnulf, I., Bonnet, A. M., Vidailhet, M., Dormont, D., et al. (1997) Pallidal stimulation for Parkinson's disease. Two targets? *Neurology* **49,** 1564–1569.
24. Krack, P., Pollak, P., Limousin, P., Hoffmann, D., Benazzouz, A., Le Bas, J. F., et al. (1998) Opposite motor effects of pallidal stimulation in Parkinson's disease. *Ann. Neurol.* **43,** 180–192.
25. Yelnik, J., Damier, P., Bejjani, B. P., et al. (2000) Functional mapping of the human globus pallidus: contrasting effect of stimulation in the internal and external pallidum in Parkinson's disease. *Neuroscience* **101,** 77–87.
26. Vitek, J. L., Evatt, M., Zhang, J.-Y., et al. (1999) Pallidotomy and deep brain stimulation as a treatment for dystonia. *Neurology* **52(Suppl. 2),** A294.
27. Ashby, P. (2000) What does stimulation in the brain actually do? *Progr. Neurolog. Surg.* **15,** 236–245.
28. Ranck, J. B. (1975) Which elements are excited in electrical stimulation of mammalian central nervous system? A review. *Brain Res.* **98,** 417–440.
29. Pollak, P. (2000) Deep Brain Stimulation. Annual Course of the American Academy of Neurology. Innovative surgical treatment of movement disorders 3AC.0006. San Diego.
30. Defer, G. L., Widner, H., Marie, R. M., Remy, P., and Levivier, M. (1999) Core assessment program for surgical interventional therapies in Parkinson's disease (CAPSIT-PD). *Mov. Disord.* **14,** 572–584.
31. Kumar, R., Lang, A. E., Sime, E., and Lozano, A. M. (1999) Late failure of thalamic deep brain stimulation in Parkinson's disease and essential tremor. *Neurology* **52(Suppl. 2),** A457–A457.
32. Koller, W. C., Lyons, K. E., Wilkinson, S. B., Troster, A. I., and Pahwa, R. (2001) Long-term safety and efficacy of unilateral deep brain stimulation of the thalamus in essential tremor. *Mov. Disord.* **16,** 464–468.
33. Oh, M. Y., Hodaie, M., Kim, S. H., Alkhani, A., Lang, A. E., and Lozano, A. M. (2001) Deep brain stimulator electrodes used for lesioning: proof of principle. *Neurosurgery* **49,** 363–367.
34. Kumar, R. and McVicker, J. M. (2000) Radiofrequency lesioning through an implanted deep brain stimulating electrode: treatment of tolerance to thalamic stimulation in essential tremor. *Mov. Disord.* **15(Suppl. 3),** 69.
35. Hariz, M. I., Shamsgovara, P., Johansson, F., Hariz, G. M., and Fodstad, H. (1999) Tolerance and tremor rebound following long-term thalamic stimulation for parkinsonian and essential tremor. *Sterotact. Funct. Neurosurg.* **72,** 208–218.
36. Limousin, P., Pollak, P., Hoffmann, D., Benazzouz, A., Perret, J., and Benabid, A. L. (1996) Abnormal involuntary movements induced by subthalamic nucleus stimulation. *Mov. Disord.* **11,** 231–235.
37. Volkmann, J., Fogel, W., and Krack, P. (2000) Postoperative neurological management—stimulation of the subthalamic nucleus. *Akt. Neurol.* **27(Suppl. 1),** S23–S39.
38. Fraix, V., Pollak, P., Van Blercom, N., Xie, J., Krack, P., Koudsie, A., and Benabid, A. L. (2000) Effect of subthalamic nucleus stimulation on levodopa-induced dyskinesia in Parkinson's disease. *Neurology* **55,** 1921–1923.
39. Kumar, R., Kedia, S., and McVicker, J. H. (2001) Chronic electrical stimulation of the zona incerta and fields of Forel in Parkinson's disease: implications for the mechanism of deep brain stimulation. *Mov. Disord.* **16,** 991.
40. Kumar, R. and Kramer, R. E. (2001) Emergence of restless legs syndrome (RLS) during subthalamic nucleus deep brain stimulation (STN DBS) for Parkinson's disease (PD). *Parkinsonism Rel. Disord.* **7,** S80.
41. Rye, D. B. and DeLong, M. R. (1999) Amelioration of sensory limb discomfort of restless legs syndrome by pallidotomy. *Ann. Neurol.* **46,** 800–801.
42. Bejjani, B. P., Damier, P., Arnulf, I., Thivard, L., Bonnet, A. M., Dormont, D., et al. (1999) Transient acute depression induced by high-frequency deep-brain stimulation. *N. Engl. J. Med.* **340,** 1476–1480.
43. Ghika, J., Vingerhoets, F., Albanese, A., and Villemure, J. G. (1999) Bipolar swings in mood in patient with bilaterak subthalamic nucleus deeo brain stimulation (DBS) free of antiparkinson medication [abstract]. *Parkinsonism Rel. Disord.* **5(Suppl. 1),** 104.
44. Kumar, R., Krack, P., and Pollak, P. (1999) Transient acute depression-induced by high-frequency deep-brain stimulation [letter]. *N. Engl. J. Med.* **341,** 1003–1004.
45. Krack, P., Kumar, R., Ardouin, C., Limousin-Dowsey, P., McVicker, J. H., Benabid, A.-L., and Pollak, P. (2001) Mirthful laughter induced by subthalamic nucleus stimulation. *Mov. Disord.* **16,** 867–875.
46. Schaltenbrand, G. and Wahren, W. (1977) *Atlas for Stereotaxy of the Human Brain,* 2nd ed. Thieme, Stuttgart.

15

The Role of Neuropsychological Evaluation in the Neurosurgical Treatment of Movement Disorders

Alexander I. Tröster and Julie A. Fields

1. INTRODUCTION

Patients with Parkinson's disease (PD) and their physicians have become increasingly accustomed to treatments having few, if any, or reversible side effects *(1)*. Given the concern about the potential neurobehavioral morbidity associated with movement disorders surgery, particularly in instances of bilateral and ablative surgery, it is important to address neurobehavioral functioning and quality of life outcomes. Consistent with the clinical focus of this volume, this chapter does not delve into the role that movement disorders surgery might have in testing current models of the neurocognitive functions of the basal ganglia (for reviews of this issue see Middleton and Strick *[2,3]*). We focus on neuropsychological evaluation and outcomes in neurosurgery for PD, but also mention the limited literature pertaining to surgery for movement disorders of other conditions (e.g., multiple sclerosis, essential tremor).

2. SYNOPSIS OF THE HISTORY OF NEUROBEHAVIORAL STUDIES OF MOVEMENT DISORDERS SURGERY

Several detailed treatises of the history of movement disorders surgery are available to the interested reader *(4–10)*. Even cursory review of these works reveals that neurobehavioral issues were rarely dealt with in early (pre-levodopa era) studies of movement disorders. Indeed, Gross et al. *(11)* note: "In addition, post-operative complications, that is, mortality, motor abnormalities, dementia, cognitive impairment etc., were often superbly ignored. In the rare cases where they are reported, they are simply noted as risks that had to be taken." (p. 514).

Pioneering neurobehavioral outcome studies were carried out in North America by Cooper and his colleagues Diller, Riklan, and Levita (summarized in Riklan and Levita *[12]*), VanBuren and colleagues *(13,14)*, and by Jurko and Andy *(15,16)*. Ojemann, Ward and colleagues' contributions to understanding thalamic functions via intraoperative stimulation during thalamotomy are widely recognized (for review, *see* Johnson and Ojemann *[17]*). On the other side of the Atlantic, early influential studies were carried out by Almgren et al. *(18,19)*, Asso et al. *(20)*, Christenson and colleagues *(21)*, Fünfgeld *(22)*, McFie *(23)*, and by Vilkki and Laitinen *(24,25)*.

The general neglect of neurobehavioral outcomes in early studies is one of several factors complicating comparisons between current and pre-levodopa era studies. As pointed out by Wilkinson and Tröster *(26)*, several other factors complicate the comparison of early and more recent surgical outcomes: the description in early studies of neurobehavioral outcomes in subjective, inconsistent terms,

From: Contemporary Clinical Neurology: Surgical Treatment of Parkinson's Disease and Other Movement Disorders
Edited by: D. Tarsy, J. L. Vitek, and A. M. Lozano © Humana Press Inc., Totowa, NJ

Table 1
Purposes of Neuropsychological Evaluation

Pre-operative
- Evaluate presence of surgery contra-indications
- Baseline for postoperative comparison
- Differential diagnosis
- Capacity to consent to treatment

Post-operative
- Documentation of surgical outcome
- Rehabilitation planning
- Detection of adverse effects of disease progression, medication, stimulation

and differences in patient characteristics, selection criteria, and surgical methods and targets. Variability in lesion parameters and techniques was also greater in early studies, and chemical lesioning was associated with greater neurobehavioral morbidity than was thermal lesioning *(27)*.

Despite these difficulties in comparing early and more recent neurobehavioral outcomes, some have suggested that neurobehavioral morbidity is lower in modern surgical series *(28)*. In contrast, Laitinen *(29)* noted that neurobehavioral morbidity in Leksell's 1951–1957 pallidotomy series was comparable to that reported by two other centers in the 1990s (although one might counter that the morbidity in the two 1990s studies selected for comparison is higher than that reported in most other pallidotomy studies of the 1990s). Outcomes of modern studies are described in greater detail later on.

3. NEUROPSYCHOLOGICAL EVALUATION: PURPOSES, METHODS, AND INTERPRETATIVE ISSUES

Neuropsychological evaluation is a necessary component of the work-up of movement disorder surgery candidates with PD, a fact highlighted by recent position and guideline papers *(30–32)*. Neuropsychological evaluation in movement disorders has different purposes, depending on whether the evaluation is carried out before or after surgery (Table 1).

3.1. *Purposes of Pre-Operative Neuropsychological Evaluation*

Pre-operative evaluation is typically carried out to determine whether selection and/or exclusion criteria for surgical intervention are met. As reviewed by Fields and Tröster *(33)*, several exclusionary criteria have been advocated in surgical treatment of PD, largely on the basis of anecdotal reports: dementia, significant executive dysfunction, and psychiatric conditions such as major depression, delusions, and hallucinations.

Further reasons for pre-operative evaluation include establishment of a baseline against which potential postoperative changes can be evaluated, and differential diagnosis if a patient meets an exclusionary criterion. For example, if a patient has dementia, is this dementia related to depression or medications and, thus, reversible?

The capacity to consent to treatment, including the ability to perceive a choice to seek and refuse a given treatment, to choose among possible treatments, and the ability to appreciate the possible consequences of each of these courses of action, can be addressed by presurgical evaluation.

All this information can be used by the treatment team to provide the patient and family with tools to make a sound decision regarding the likely outcomes and risks of surgical intervention, or lack thereof. Careful discussion of expectations is indicated, because marital conflict may arise in cases where patient and caregiver expectations of postsurgical improvement and increased functional independence are unmet *(34)*.

3.2. *Purposes of Postoperative Neuropsychological Evaluation*

Postoperative neuropsychological evaluation is not addressed by position papers advocating preoperative evaluation. Postoperative evaluation, nonetheless, is extremely important. Such evaluation objectively describes outcome. In the event that "delayed" complications emerge, it becomes possible to determine whether changes are related to surgical intervention or operative complications, deep brain stimulation (DBS), medications, or disease progression. In the event of significant neurobehavioral changes after surgery, postoperative evaluation can clearly delineate the extent and nature of these changes, thereby facilitating rehabilitation planning. Such intervention is of importance given that neurobehavioral symptoms not only compromise the patient's quality of life, but also that of the caregiver *(35)*.

3.3. *Methods of Neuropsychological Evaluation*

Comprehensive neuropsychological evaluation entails a review of medical records, interviews with patient and family, observation of behavior, and administration and scoring of psychometric test instruments. These sources of information are integrated to arrive at a description of the patient's neurobehavioral strengths and weaknesses, inferences about the etiology of cognitive and emotional dysfunction, and the suitability of surgical intervention for that person. It is important to emphasize that, given the current state of knowledge about the neuropsychological effects of surgical treatments and risk factors for morbidity, prognostic statements are best phrased in terms of broad bands of probability, such as a person being at average, greater than average, or less than average risk of neurobehavioral morbidity.

Several papers recommend specific tests to be employed in the neuropsychological evaluation of surgical candidates with PD *(31,36,37)*, but no papers provide guidance in test selection for the evaluation of persons with other movement disorders who might benefit from surgery. Contents of test batteries for disorders such as multiple sclerosis (MS), essential tremor (ET), and dystonia may ultimately be different than for PD, depending on the neurobehavioral patterns observed in those conditions and test sensitivity. However, until adequate data are available, similar tests might be used in all movement disorders. Such use of similar test batteries would permit comparison of outcomes across disorders.

Specific neuropsychological tests proposed for evaluation of PD by various position and review papers overlap, but are not identical. There is probably less disagreement about which areas of cognition to evaluate than about which specific tests to select. For this reason, we describe the domains of neurobehavioral functioning that need to be evaluated, the criteria that might be considered in test selection and provide a sample rather than a prescriptive list of tests.

3.4. *A Caution About the Core Assessment Program for Surgical Interventional Therapies in Parkinson's Disease (CAPSIT-PD) Neuropsychological Protocol*

The recommendation or prescription of specific test batteries seeks uniformity of approaches across centers and, thus, comparability of outcome data. While such efforts are laudable in intent, their end products are frequently left wanting. One test battery specifically proposed for neuropsychological evaluation in the surgical treatment of movement disorders (as part of the CAPSIT-PD protocol) *(31)* is probably useful for research purposes and group comparisons of average patient and control group scores. Many of the tests included in CAPSIT-PD are tasks sensitive to the neurobehavioral changes of PD. Unfortunately, many of the tests proposed as part of the CAPSIT-PD protocol are now outdated and not informed by recent cognitive psychological theory so as to permit clear delineation of the nature of deficits and their possible amenability to remediation. More importantly, many of the recommended tests are commercially unavailable or difficult to obtain, and lack adequate standardization, normative and other psychometric properties that are requisite to sound clinical decision making in the individual patient's case. In addition, the CAPSIT-PD guidelines on test selection are unnecessarily vague at times: for example, no mention is made of which form of the Auditory Verbal

Table 2
Examples of Standardized Tests Used in the Evaluation of Movement Disorders

Type of test	Specific test
Estimate of premorbid function	North American Adult Reading Test, Barona Demographic Equations
General cognitive functioning	Raven's Progressive Matrices, Wechsler Adult Intelligence Scale (WAIS-R Ward 7-subtest short form, WAIS-III Verbal subtests), Wechsler Abbreviated Scale of Intelligence (WASI), Kaufman Brief Intelligence Test, Mattis Dementia Rating Scale
Language	Controlled Oral Word Association Test, Boston Diagnostic Aphasia Examination's Animal Naming and Boston Naming Tests, Multilingual Aphasia Examination's Sentence Repetition and Token Tests
Attention and working memory	Paced Auditory Serial Attention Test (PASAT), Stroop Color and Word Interference Test, Brief Test of Attention, Digit and Visual Memory Span, WMS-III Letter-Number Sequencing
Executive function	Wisconsin Card Sorting Test (or WCST-64), Cognitive Estimation Test, Booklet Category Test
Memory	Benton Visual Retention Test, Wechsler Memory Scales (revisions) Logical Memory, Rey-Osterreith Complex Figure Test (not for patients with notable motor impairment), Rey Auditory Verbal Learning Test, California Verbal Learning Test-II, Wechsler Memory Scale III Family Pictures and Faces
Motor	Finger Tapping, Grooved Pegboard (for patients with mild movement disorder)
Visuoperceptual-spatial	Benton Judgment of Line Orientation, Benton Facial Recognition Test, Benton Visual Discrimination Test
Mood and personality	Profile of Mood States, Beck Depression Inventory, State-Trait Anxiety Inventory, Zung Depression Index, Beck Anxiety Inventory, Minnesota Multiphasic Personality Inventory (MMPI), Frontal Lobe Personality Scale (FLOPS), Hospital Anxiety and Depression Scale
Quality of life	Sickness Impact Profile (SIP), Parkinson's Disease Questionnaire (PDQ), Nottingham Health Profile
Stressors	Life Stressors and Social Resources Inventory
Coping	Coping Responses Inventory
Experimental tasks	Tower of London (or Hanoi or Toronto), Alternating Fluency, Odd Man Out, 20 Questions, Conditional Associative Learning Test

Learning Test might be used, despite the fact that there are eight alternate forms, many of which are known *not* to be equivalent. Some tests (e.g., the 567-item MMPI-2) included are unduly strenuous for advanced PD patients with fatigability and severe motor problems. For these reasons, we are unable to recommend, and indeed would counsel against, the uncritical adoption of the CAPSIT-PD neuropsychological protocol. Test batteries outlined by Saint-Cyr and Trépanier *(37)* appear to have been selected with careful reasoning, and these batteries permit greater flexibility than the CAPSIT-PD protocol.

3.5. Areas of Functioning Assessed in Neuropsychological Evaluations

The domains of functioning assessed in most evaluations include intelligence or overall level of cognitive functioning, attention and working memory, executive functions, language, visuoperceptual and spatial functions, motor function, memory, mood state, and quality of life. We also recommend a formal assessment of coping responses and stressors. Examples of tests of each of these domains, many of which have been used in published studies of movement disorders surgery, are listed in Table 2.

3.5.1. Intelligence

Except in cases of dementia, intelligence is preserved in PD, ET, and MS. Nonetheless, PD patients may perform poorly on some tests of the Wechsler scales (particularly some of the Performance scale subtests, which are timed and have significant motor demands) due to bradyphrenia and bradykinesia. MS leads to a variable pattern of cognitive impairment but often compromises cognitive functioning in a manner similar to PD. Cognitive impairment in ET and dystonia have not been observed, although in our experience *(38)*, a significant proportion of ET patients evidences impairments in attention, working memory, and/or executive functions.

In practice it is rare that a patient has previously undergone intelligence testing while healthy (i.e., premorbidly). Consequently, indirect methods (such as performance on oral word reading tests resistant to decline subsequent to cerebral dysfunction, or equations utilizing demographic information) are used to estimate premorbid intelligence and infer whether current performance represents a decline from once higher levels.

3.5.2. Cognitive Screening

Brief screening measures, or measures of overall level of cognitive functioning are convenient and inexpensive to use. However, such scales lack sensitivity, meaning that impaired performance is revealing of disease, but intact performance does not imply absence of mild to moderate or selective cognitive deficits. Consequently, use of such a test early in the evaluation process is helpful in sparing the significantly impaired patient further arduous testing for surgical evaluation (although further testing may be indicated for differential diagnosis).

3.5.3. Attention and Working Memory

Working memory is a limited-capacity, multi-component system involved in the temporary storage and manipulation of information. This system, and the allocation of attention resources, is often compromised by PD, some of the medications used to treat the disease *(39,40)*, and by surgical treatments *(41,42)*.

3.5.4. Executive Functions

Executive functions include conceptualization, abstraction, planning, insight, cognitive flexibility, the ability to monitor, regulate, and initiate and inhibit responses. These functions depend, among other factors, on fronto-striatal integrity and are vulnerable to PD and its surgical treatment. Assessment of executive functions is of particular relevance and importance in surgical candidates, because executive deficit in PD is linked to diminution of capacity to consent to medical treatment *(43)*, ability to carry out instrumental activities of daily living *(44)*, and capacity to deploy a range of effective coping strategies *(45)*.

3.5.5. Language

Performance on verbal fluency tasks, requiring oral generation within a time limit of words beginning with a given letter of the alphabet, or belonging to a given semantic category such as animals, is frequently disrupted by neurosurgical interventions. Verbal fluency may or may not be disrupted in PD without dementia, but almost always is disrupted in dementia. Verbal fluency impairments may be a harbinger of incipient dementia in PD *(46,47)*.

In contrast to verbal fluency, other language functions such as repetition, comprehension, word knowledge, and visual confrontation naming are preserved in PD. When impairments are observed in such functions, the diagnostic possibility of a dementia, especially one not due to PD, needs to be considered.

3.5.6. Visuoperceptual Functions

Visuoperceptual deficits have been observed in numerous studies of PD, but not in others, and it is also a matter of debate whether these deficits are true visuoperceptual deficits or secondary to executive deficits (see Tröster, Fields, and Koller *[40]*). Surgical treatment has only rarely been reported to impact these functions.

3.5.7. Memory and Learning

Profound memory impairment is not a hallmark of PD. The ability to recall new information is generally compromised, but recognition is relatively intact. Such a dissociation between recall and recognition has been interpreted as indicating a retrieval deficit in PD. Although this interpretation is probably correct, there is evidence that PD patients also have encoding deficits *(48)*. The exact extent to which encoding and retrieval deficits reflect executive deficits remains debated (*see* Tröster and Fields *[49]*).

Remote memory is preserved in PD, and a retrograde amnesia is typically associated only with dementia *(50)*. Unlike in Alzheimer's disease, the retrograde amnesia in PD with dementia is similar in severity across previous decades, meaning there is not the temporal gradient revealing greater preservation of distant than recent past memories.

Nonverbal memory tests with significant motor components are not recommended in surgical candidates with PD given their severe motor disability (bradykinesia, tremor, dyskinesia) and motor fluctuations. The Wechsler Memory Scale–III includes several visual tasks without motor components (Faces and Family Pictures) that are more appropriate.

3.5.8. Mood State and Behavioral Symptoms

Anxiety and depression symptoms are common in PD: about 50% of persons with PD become depressed at some point during their illness with half of those persons having a dysthymia and the other half a major depression *(40)*. Assessment of depression is of particular relevance in the surgical candidate for at least three reasons: depression exacerbates cognitive impairment in PD *(51–53)*, it may be a harbinger of dementia *(54)*, and it has been associated with poorer surgical outcome *(55)*. Depression also compromises the patient's cooperation during "awake" surgery and reduces resources to cope with peri- and postoperative stressors. It is probably prudent to treat and re-evaluate the patient with depression before making a final decision about the appropriateness of surgical treatment.

Instances of significant postoperative depression have been reported after surgical treatment *(56, 57)*. Although this may relate to misplacement of the lesion or stimulating electrode, depression also has been observed after nonsurgical pallidal lesions *(58)*. Another factor in postoperative depression may relate to patient expectations. It has been suggested that patients with milder disability expect more dramatic improvement *(59)*, thus leading one to hypothesize that such patients may be at greater risk for depression related to unmet expectations.

Assessment of anxiety may also allow a prognosis concerning patient ability to cooperate with an arduous evaluation and surgical procedure. In assessing anxiety by questionnaires, care should be taken to scrutinize items endorsed. Many questionnaires contain symptom items that might reflect symptoms of PD rather than anxiety *(60)*. Patients who report phobic experiences and generalized anxiety may have difficulty tolerating an MRI procedure without sedation. In our experience, patients who have difficulty dealing with the stress of a neuropsychological evaluation prior to surgery are more apt to have difficulty tolerating protracted work-up and surgery. Patient education, including preparation for surgery, can be extremely helpful in this regard.

Because surgical intervention can lead to "frontal" personality changes or exaggeration of presurgical behavioral characteristics and psychopathology *(61)*, evaluation of personality structure by interview or formal assessment is indicated. Measures that have been used in PD include the Neuropsychiatric Inventory *(62)*, the Frontal Lobe Personality Scale *(63)*, and the Minnesota Multiphasic Personality Inventory *(64)*, although the latter is long and difficult to complete for the patient who is easily fatigued and has tremor or dyskinesias.

3.5.9. Stressors and Coping

Informal assessment is frequently made of patients' stressors, resources, and coping mechanisms during the interview. However, self-report questionnaires, permitting a quantitative assessment, are also available. The importance of considering a person's response to stress in predicting outcome was already commented on by Diller et al. in 1956 *(65)*. Stressors can contribute to anxiety and depression, and an assessment of current stressors permits judgments about the timing of surgery. In general, if a patient has numerous other ongoing stressors, one might consider delaying surgery until these stressors are resolved. The evaluation and surgical procedure, as well as the recovery in some instances, are stressful; adding such a significant stressor to an already stressful environment heightens risk for exacerbation of mood disturbance.

The impact that stressors have on a patient is mediated by social resources (such as financial reserves, social support networks) and coping mechanisms. The patient with significant stressors, limited social assets, and restricted coping abilities is likely to be a poorer surgical candidate than one who has significant stressors but a wide range of assets and is able to utilize a diversity of coping strategies. Furthermore, greater social resources and fewer stressors have been associated with a better quality of life after pallidotomy *(66,67)*.

3.5.10. Quality of Life

Adequate definitions and conceptualizations of quality of life are elusive. Pragmatically, health-related quality of life (QOL) is defined as the patient's perception and evaluation of the impact that an illness, its treatment, and its consequences have on his or her life. In general, most agree that physical, psychological, social, economic, vocational, and spiritual factors contribute to overall QOL. Thus, a comprehensive assessment of QOL addresses how an illness and its treatment impacts these areas of a patient's life. QOL is not only becoming an outcome measure of increasing significance in its own right *(68)*, but QOL measures form the basis of modern cost-effectiveness analyses, including of DBS *(69)*. Assessment of QOL is particularly important in movement disorders surgery because the treatment is not curative but designed primarily to improve function and QOL *(70,71)*.

Explicit evaluation of QOL in movement disorders is of recent origin *(66)*. Studies are only beginning to address QOL in surgical candidates *(72)*, and indeed, in neurosurgery more generally *(73)*. Some studies have attempted to quantify QOL outcomes by means of specific psychological or activities of daily living measures *(74)*, but such an approach is too narrow to capture adequately the overall impact of disease and surgery on QOL.

Measures of QOL and functional status fall into two broad categories: generic and disease-specific. The advantage of generic measures is that they permit comparison of QOL across diseases and conditions. Disease-specific measures, in contrast, earn their utility from their sensitivity to issues specific (or at least very important) to individuals with a given disease. In ideal circumstances, assessment should be achieved using both generic and disease-specific measures. No QOL measures have been published that deal specifically with some movement disorders (e.g., ET), but disease-specific measures are now available for PD (*see* Table 2) and MS.

3.6. Interpretative and Practical Considerations for the Neuropsychologist

Several issues need be kept in mind while planning the evaluation of patients with movement disorders and in interpreting pre- and postoperative test results.

3.6.1. Medication Effects

Dopaminergic medications can impact cognitive functions, and in particular working memory and executive functions (although effects on different functions within a given domain of cognition can be heterogeneous; see *[39,75]*). Patients should always be questioned about when they take their medication. Deviations from dosage regimens may result in unpredictable motor fluctuations, thus complicating neuropsychological testing. The complete (neurologic, neuropsychological, neurodiagnostic and neurosurgical) presurgical work-up is time consuming and extensive, often necessitating evaluation over more than one day. Frequently the patient's motor functioning is compared when he/she has and has not taken medication. Patients with PD should be scheduled for neuropsychological evaluation before medication withdrawal, or after sufficient time will have elapsed for the patient to return to the "on" state. The former is preferable as patients on occasion fail to return to the best "on" state in timely fashion after medication withdrawal has ended.

Medication effects also need be considered in comparing pre- and postoperative test performance. Particularly after subthalamic DBS, medication dosage often can be dramatically reduced. Although such effect is expected to be mild, medication reduction can both positively and negatively impact cognitive functions. Of greater complexity is the possibly interactive effect of surgery and medication: it has recently been shown that pallidotomy may alter the effect levodopa has on certain cognitive functions *(76)*.

3.6.2. Motor State and Fluctuations

Neuropsychological evaluation is extremely challenging for the patient with PD and the clinician when the patient is in the "off" state. Not only may the patient be bradykinetic, in a "frozen" state, and bradyphrenic, but speech may become so hypophonic and dysarthric as to be unintelligible. Although comparison of cognitive functioning in the "on" and "off" states is of interest at times, such a comparison is rarely feasible from a practical standpoint. Consequently, it is recommended that patients be tested, as far as possible, within their self-described "on" state. Surgical candidates may have levodopa- or dopamine agonist-induced dyskinesias during portions of the "on" state. The best way to achieve a valid neuropsychological evaluation is to plan ahead: the patient and caregiver should be questioned about duration of "on" state, occurrence and duration of dyskinesias, and duration of "off" state. The rapidly fluctuating patient presents a particular challenge, and testing may have to be interrupted where feasible and spread over several relatively brief sessions.

3.6.3. Practice Effects

When individuals undergo repeated evaluations using the same or similar test instruments, it is conceivable that scores may "improve" not due to an improvement in the function being assessed, but rather because the individual remembers, and has experience with the test. Several strategies are available to minimize practice effects, such as utilizing alternate test forms (i.e., two versions of the test differing in specific content, but not difficulty), maximizing the test-retest interval, or utilizing statistical techniques (*see* Green and Barnhart *[77]* and York et al. *[78]*). Even when alternate test forms are used, a familiarity effect may occur, meaning the individual performs better on tests due to becoming more test sophisticated or "test wise."

An important issue becomes whether comparable test-retest effects observed in normative samples are evident in clinical populations. There is some suggestion that such practice effects may not occur in PD on numerous tests *(79)*. If a practice effect does not occur in PD, then possible score gains after surgery represent improvements rather than practice effects. Conversely, if practice effects are seen in PD, than a lack of gain might actually represent a decline, and a score gain would have to exceed the practice effect before it is considered an "improvement." Of great complexity in interpreting individual patient test score changes is the issue of a possible interaction between surgery, medication, stimulation, and practice effects.

3.6.4. Length and Breadth of Test Battery

Saint-Cyr and Trépanier *(37)*, York and colleagues *(78)*, and Green and Barnhart *(77)* have commented thoughtfully and extensively on the issue of how long a test battery for PD surgery candidates should be, and whether the battery should be broad or narrow in focus. Given the fatigability and motor fluctuations of most PD surgery candidates, the battery should be as short as possible, while still long and broad enough to answer the referral question and to develop clear and valid diagnostic and prognostic impressions.

In clinical endeavors we suggest that the test battery be selected on the basis of: 1) referral question; 2) known neurobehavioral effects of a given disease; 3) known neurobehavioral risks of a given treatment; 4) patient ability to cooperate with tests; and 5) findings uncovered during evaluation (i.e., modification of the test battery according to hypotheses raised during testing). Choice of specific tests is also based on consideration of each test's assets and liabilities (normative data, test-retest data, validity and reliability, availability of alternate forms, sensitivity, and ability of the test to delineate mechanisms underlying deficient task performance).

4. ABLATIVE SURGERY AND NEUROBEHAVIORAL OUTCOMES

4.1. Thalamotomy

4.1.1. Parkinson's Disease

4.1.1.1. Cognition, Memory, and Language

Spiegel et al. *(80)* observed disturbances in memory, orientation, and time sense (i.e., chronotaraxis) after bilateral thalamotomy, and reported this already in 1955, but formal neuropsychological evaluation was not carried out. Niebuhr, a psychologist colleague of Spiegel and Wycis at Temple University, noted in 1962 that among 11 patients undergoing psychological evaluation pre- and post-unilateral thalamotomy, three patients experienced significant cognitive decline, but that these three patients already had marked cognitive impairment prior to surgery *(81)*. However, incidence of cognitive morbidity in early studies is difficult to ascertain. Figures are generally not based on formal neuropsychological evaluation. Some studies combined patients with different diagnoses (e.g., Almgren et al. *[18]*), patients that underwent thalamotomy using different techniques (e.g., Levita et al. *[27]*), or patients that underwent a variety of procedures (thalamotomy, pallidotomy, or combined thalamotomy + pallidotomy). Burchiel *(82)* estimated that up to 39% of individuals undergoing thalamotomy for a movement disorder experienced declines in speech, language, and/or memory, with declines being more common among bilateral than unilateral operates (60% versus 31%), a finding already observed in one early study using formal psychological testing in 8 unilateral and 3 bilateral operates *(83)*.

A detailed review of early thalamotomy studies employing objective neuropsychological evaluation is provided by Wilkinson and Tröster *(26)*. In general, those early studies found that memory, and especially verbal memory declines, occurred after unilateral left and bilateral thalamotomy *(13, 18,20,23,84–87)*. Findings with respect to nonverbal memory (meaning memory for visually presented material) were less consistent. Whereas Riklan et al. *(88)*, Shapiro et al. *(13)*, and Vilkki and Laitinen *(24,25)* observed no changes in nonverbal memory, others reported declines in visual memory after left *(15)* or both left and right thalamotomy *(89)*. Still others reported an improvement in nonverbal memory after right thalamotomy *(90)*. With few exceptions, studies found that deficits typically appeared soon after surgery and resolved in less than 18 mo *(16,19,91)*. In contrast, Perret and Siegfried *(89)* found that memory deficits were still present 18 mo after surgery, and VanBuren et al. *(14)* reported that four left thalamotomy patients, among 78 unilaterally operated on, had sufficiently severe memory problems to preclude independent functioning up to 7 yr after surgery.

Changes in cognition following early thalamotomies were not limited to memory. Several studies reported changes in either Verbal and/or Performance IQ after unilateral, especially left, thalamotomy *(84,89,92,93)*, and one study found that left thalamotomy was associated with slightly greater Verbal IQ losses than was pallidotomy *(23)*. These changes in IQ were short-lived in most studies. Other studies failed to observe changes in IQ *(20,90)*. Attention decreased after left and bilateral thalamotomy in a few studies *(14,94)*.

Numerous early studies examined language and speech. In a controlled study (using a nonoperated PD control group), letter and category fluency decrements were observed soon (about 10 d) after left and bilateral thalamotomy, but these deficits resolved by the time of follow-up testing about 5 mo later *(94, 95)*. Reductions in verbal fluency were also reported by Perret and Siegfried *(89)*, Vilkki and Laitinen *(24)*, and indeed, are concluded by Riklan and Cooper *(96)* to best describe the early consequences of left thalamotomy. In addition to fluency changes, dysnomia occasionally was observed to occur after left but not right thalamotomy *(97,98)*.

One of the most influential early studies of the effects of thalamotomy on language and speech was reported by Samra and colleagues *(99)*. This study related postmortem anatomical findings to formal speech and language findings in 27 patients who had undergone thalamotomy. Interestingly, this study concluded that language and speech outcome was unrelated to lesion size. In contrast to speech changes, language disturbances were typically transient and related to lesion laterality (more common after left thalamotomy). Quaglieri and Celesia found that compared to nonoperated PD patients, a group having had thalamotomy about 8 yr previously performed more poorly in speech but not language *(100)*.

There are few modern studies of thalamotomy in PD. The few reports that do exist, suggest that modern thalamotomy might be much safer than its earlier counterpart. Formal neuropsychological evaluation results in the largest patient series *(101)* show little change in cognition 3 mo after unilateral thalamotomy (28 right and 25 left operations), and, indeed, this study reported mild improvement on one verbal memory (dichotic listening) task. A small sample of 13 patients with PD was also reported to show no deficits on a limited neuropsychological test battery four weeks after unilateral thalamotomy *(102)*, but another study reported side effects (including dysphasia) in 8% of thalamotomy patients *(103)*. Gamma knife thalamotomy and pallidotomy are said to also involve few side effects (1.5–2% complication rate) *(104)*, but formal and detailed neuropsychological data remain to be published. Similarly, neuropsychological results of the recently rediscovered pallidothalamic tractotomy have not been published, but it has been mentioned in passing that some patients experience "slowing" of frontal functions *(105)*.

In a study of particular importance because it involves the only published comparison of thalamotomy and DBS subsequent to random assignment to treatment, Schuurman et al. *(106)* carried out formal neuropsychological evaluation before and 6 mo after surgery. Specific and detailed neuropsychological data were not presented, but it was reported that among 34 patients undergoing thalamotomy, three patients (two PD, one ET) experienced limited cognitive declines (one each in fluency, memory, and initiative). In contrast, none of the DBS patients experienced significant cognitive declines.

4.1.1.2. Mood State and Quality of Life

Detailed studies of QOL and psychiatric complications using formal measures are generally absent in thalamotomy studies. Angelini and colleagues *(107,108)* reported significant depression to occasionally occur after thalamotomy. Hays et al. *(91)* in contrast, using a modified Hamilton rating scale, observed an elevation in mood and decrease in "obsessional symptoms" after unilateral thalamotomy, and suggested that these effects were not placebo effects, a simple reduction in anxiety, or a reaction to improved functioning. Müller and Yasargil *(109)* also observed elevation in mood soon after surgery, but noted that lasting personality changes after a variety of surgical procedures in diagnostically diverese patients were rare. Narabayashi *(64)*, using a translated version of the Minnesota Multiphasic Personality Inventory, found no postoperative changes in test scores among eight thalamotomy patients (although a combined pallidotomy + thalamotomy was associated with reductions in depressive symptoms as measured by the MMPI depression scale), a finding also reported by that group of investigators in a series of 13 patients *(102)*. Jurko and Andy *(110)* described "child-like" behavior, as well as decreased motivation, and schizophrenic-like behavior (including catatonic features and hallucinations) in some bilaterally operated patients up to a year after surgery.

4.1.2. *Essential Tremor, Multiple Sclerosis, and Other Conditions*

Thalamotomy has been undertaken to relieve tremor in a variety of conditions: essential tremor (ET), multiple sclerosis (MS), post-traumatic tremor, and poststroke tremor. As noted earlier, in the study by Schuurman et al. *(106)*, one patient with essential tremor (ET), but none with MS had a cognitive deficit 6 mo after thalamotomy, and none had cognitive deficits after DBS. In a small, nonrandomized study of ET patients undergoing thalamotomy or thalamic DBS, Pahwa et al. *(111)* also found a much lower cognitive complication rate among DBS than thalamotomy patients (0% vs 29%).

Few earlier studies evaluated cognition formally. Blumetti and Modesti *(112)* carried out neuropsychological evaluation in 10 patients (five with familial tremor (ET) and five with MS) before, 3–4 wk, and 12–24 mo after thalamotomy. The group demonstrated declines in attention, verbal skills, and verbal and nonverbal memory. Several other studies have only in passing mentioned speech, language, or cognitive morbidity *(113–118)*.

Rossitch et al. *(119)* specifically attempted to identify risk factors for cognitive decline after thalamotomy. Although results are difficult to interpret given the use of an idiosyncratic neuropsychological evaluation battery, a small (n = 18) and heterogeneous sample (MS, PD, post-traumatic and "post-apoplectic" movement disorders, dystonia), and loosely described criteria for cognitive decline, seven of the eight patients showing significant cognitive decline had MS, and only one had PD. Although formal neuropsychological evaluation was not carried out, Whittle and Hadlow *(120)* in contrast noted a relative absence of morbidity associated with thalamotomy in MS.

Detailed studies of QOL and psychiatric complications using formal measures of these constructs are absent in thalamotomy studies.

4.2. Subthalamotomy

4.2.1. Parkinson's Disease

Early subthalamotomy never gained widespread popularity. It was first reported on by Spiegel et al. *(121)* and Andy et al. *(122)* Spiegel and colleagues preferred interrupting pallidofugal fibers by lesioning Forel's Field H, an operation referred to as campotomy. They, unlike Mundinger, specifically avoided the zona incerta. Spiegel et al. reported, among 33 patients, a 30% incidence of "psycho-organic syndrome." Among 58 patients (six of whom had staged bilateral operations), Andy et al. noted that all bilateral operates developed a lasting (of several years' duration) loss of initiative and spontaneity, and diminished interest in the environment. One patient, after having the second operation, developed a "jovial, carefree attitude" (p. 866). Over one-third of the patients manifested increased desire for food and "some" patients actually became obese.

Mundinger and colleagues *(123)* placed the bulk of the subthalamotomy lesion in the zona incerta. Reporting on outcomes in 456 interventions for PD, Mundinger and colleagues note that 32% of individuals became free of "speech symptoms" postoperatively. Neurobehavioral morbidity data were not reported.

Until recently, subthalamotomy (involving the subthalamic nucleus proper) was avoided given fear of inducing hemiballism. At least two centers have begun performing these operations, and one (at Frenchay Hospital, Bristol, UK) has published detailed neuropsychological findings *(124)*. McCarter et al. *(124)* evaluated neuropsychological functioning in 12 patients undergoing procedures on the dorsolateral portion of the nucleus: two left subthalamic nucleotomy, three right subthalamic nucleotomy, three bilateral subthalamic nucleotomy, and four right subthalamic nucleotomy + left subthalamic deep brain stimulation. Evaluation was carried out about 2 d prior to surgery and 3.5–12 mo (average 6 mo) after surgery.

Poorer average performance was observed after surgery on a complex auditory attention/working memory task (the PASAT), but statistically (albeit probably not clinically) significant gains were observed in Verbal IQ and immediate recall of stories. Thirty-three percent of bilateral subthalamic nucleotomy patients showed reliable decreases in verbal (letter) fluency; no reliable change in fluency was observed in the other groups (unilateral nucleotomy or nucleotomy + contralateral DBS). One-third of the nucleotomy + DBS group showed reliable decrements on several attention measures (PASAT, Stroop, and WMS-R Attention/Concentration Index) and on a list-learning task (RAVLT). None of the right nucleotomy group demonstrated reliable decrements on any measure, while the left operates tended to experience decrements in attention, facial recognition, word list recall, and a version of the Tower of London task (an executive function task) minimizing motor demands (50–100% of patients). Overall, this study suggests that modern subthalamic nucleotomy probably does not lead to global deterioration in cognition. However, mild deficits in select domains of cognition have become apparent, although it remains unknown whether (and when) these deficits resolve. Cognitive changes appear less likely after right than left or bilateral operations. These conclusions must be considered tentative given that they are based on one study with a limited sample size. Psychiatric and QOL issues remain to be investigated.

4.3. *Pallidotomy*

4.3.1. *Parkinson's Disease*

4.3.1.1. Cognition, Memory, and Language

Few formal neuropsychological assessments were undertaken in early studies of pallidotomy. Christensen et al. *(21)*, in a group of patients having undergone either unilateral or bilateral thalamotomy or pallidotomy, found no significant change in IQ, but did note that pallidotomy was associated with "constricted and less active functioning" as indicated by the Rorschach (decreased R). Svennilson and colleagues reported that among 78 unilateral pallidotomy cases, four developed postoperative dementia and 11 a significant memory impairment *(125)*.

The majority of modern studies show that unilateral pallidotomy does not result in significant cognitive morbidity, but laterality specific deficits that are typically mild and transient, are observable. In a recent meta-analysis, Alkhani and Lozano *(126)* estimated that transient memory deficits occur in 1.3% of cases after either unilateral or bilateral pallidotomy, and that persistent memory deficits are seen in less than 1% of cases. These figures might represent under-estimates, however, as not all studies included in the analysis indicate whether memory deficits occurred, and it is improbable that formal neuropsychological evaluation was undertaken in all studies.

The most commonly reported deficits involve verbal fluency, typically observed after left pallidotomy *(41,77,79,127–138)*, but not in combined unilateral right and left pallidotomy groups *(139–141)*. It is unlikely that fluency changes represent a motor speech defect given the laterality effect. Furthermore, speech changes occur less consistently than fluency changes after pallidotomy *(142)*, and they can occur independently of linguistic changes *(143)*. Verbal fluency changes are probably not related to changes in medication, because the decrements are observed in both the "on" and "off" states *(76)*. Indeed, they are probably related to changes in underlying executive mechanisms such as ability to efficiently switch between phonemic or semantic clusters or categories *(41,144)*.

Older patients may be at greater risk for verbal fluency declines *(134,145)*, but pre-operative severity of motor impairment is not predictive *(136)*. In the study by Rettig et al. *(136)*, cognitive outcome also was not different in patients with MMSE scores of 27 and above vs 26 and below (although this might reflect the insensitivity of the MMSE to dementia in PD and the restricted range of MMSE scores in the sample). This supposition is borne out by the findings of Van Horn et al. *(146)*, who found that among 11 unilateral pallidotomy patients not responding to the procedure, seven had pre-operative frontal behavioral syndromes undetected by the MMSE (scores > 25). In the study by Van Horn et al., nonresponders were more likely than responders to have frontal behavioral syndromes prior to surgery, suggesting that such dysfunction might contraindicate pallidotomy.

While some studies reported lesion location as being an important determinant of postoperative cognitive deficits, with anteromedial lesions being associated with greater impairment than posterolateral lesions *(147,148)*, other studies have failed to find a relationship between lesion volumes and/or location on one hand, and outcome on selected cognitive measures on the other hand *(145,149)*. It is possible that studies not finding a relationship between lesion parameters and cognitive outcome include patients with more homogenous lesion characteristics, meaning that a restricted range of values precluded detection of significant effects. However, several studies also report that lesion volumes (thalamic or pallidal) do not correlate with motor outcome *(150–152)*.

A handful of studies have reported more wide-ranging cognitive deficits after pallidotomy *(41, 153)*, or select deficits in domains other than verbal fluency including in verbal and/or nonverbal memory *(41,77,102,127,136,154–156)*, working memory/attention *(41,42,127,132)*, or executive functions, such as categories attained *(77,135)* or perseverative tendency on a card-sorting task *(131,135)*. Other studies have shown mild improvements after right pallidotomy in verbal memory *(41,127,135)* or aspects of nonverbal memory *(127)*. Alterman et al. *(157)* observed progressive dementia in five of 60 unilateral pallidotomy cases, and only one of these five patients had a possible or probable dementia prior to surgery.

Bilateral pallidotomy is assumed to involve greater risk for cognitive dysfunction than unilateral pallidotomy, but the effects are understudied. Findings, based on small samples, are inconsistent. Iacono et al. *(158)* reported that average Wechsler Memory Scale-Revised Index scores improved significantly among 10 bilateral pallidotomy patients. Unfortunately, actual scores were not presented, leaving it unclear whether the reported statistically significant gains approached the sizeable score increases required on these particular measures before they would be considered reliable or clinically meaningful. Scott et al. *(130)* found no significant adverse cognitive effects among eight bilaterally operated patients, other than verbal fluency declines also observed in unilateral operates.

Other studies, in contrast, have reported, at least anecdotally, profound deficits after bilateral pallidotomy. Svennilson et al. *(125)* reported that all three of their bilaterally operated patients had significant memory deficits and dementia after surgery. Among four patients, Ghika et al. *(159)* found no cognitive changes in only one, and either profound overall changes (likely corresponding to dementia), or marked executive or memory impairments in the other two patients. Also, profound changes in personality, depression, and behavior were seen in two of the four patients, and another patient developed obsessive-compulsive features. Trépanier et al. *(137)* reported global cognitive decline after the second operation in two of three bilateral pallidotomy patients who had "atypical" cognitive profiles before surgery. The proportion of patients on whom follow-up neuropsychological data are available is not clear in the report by Intemann et al. *(138)*, but among eight of 12 patients followed-up clinically, four had poorer speech and one had worse memory after staged bilateral surgery.

It is not clear if placing a GPi DBS electrode contralateral to a previous pallidotomy is safer than a bilateral pallidotomy. Gálvez-Jiménez et al. *(160)*, although not reporting detailed data, noted that no overt cognitive changes were observed among four patients undergoing GPi DBS after contralateral pallidotomy.

4.3.1.2. Mood State and Quality of Life

Numerous studies mention psychiatric outcomes anecdotally. Bezerra and colleagues *(161)* reported persistent major depression in five of 41 patients after unilateral pallidotomy. In contrast, several studies employing formal measures of mood state have reported either improvements in depressive symptomatology *(79,127,129,136,138,162,163)*, or no change in mood state *(128,130,134,137,140,164,165)*. Junqué et al. *(166)* reported an improvement in scores on a measure of obsessive-compulsive behavior. In contrast, Trépanier et al. *(41,137)* reported that frontal lobe behavioral syndromes, including lack of insight, lability, impulsivity, poor social judgment, and environmental dependency, are observed on a formal measure (FLOPS) by up to 41% of patients' caregivers after unilateral pallidotomy. In an other study (using the MMPI), Fukuda et al. *(102)* reported that patients reported fewer somatic symptoms and better energy after unilateral pallidotomy.

Studies utilizing formal measures of QOL generally indicate improvements in a wide range of aspects of QOL after unilateral pallidotomy *(130,162–164,167)*. The study by D'Antonio *(167)* is noteworthy for including an unoperated control group. This study shows that QOL improved after 4 mo in the surgical (combined unilateral pallidotomy, bilateral pallidotomy, and pallidotomy + thalamotomy group), but not the medically treated wait-list control group. Unfortunately, the conclusion is weakened by sizeable subject attrition (about 33%). The studies by D'Antonio et al. *(167)* and by Martinez-Martin et al. *(162)* both suggest that improvement in QOL is related to improvement in motor function in the "off" state, and Tröster et al. *(67)* have found that physical aspects of QOL are related to residual motor disability after pallidotomy. Changes in QOL also relate to changes in anxiety *(162)*, depressive symptoms *(163)*, coping method, and social stressors and resources *(67)*. Older individuals may show lesser QOL improvements after pallidotomy *(67)*.

4.3.2. Other Disorders

Formal neuropsychological evaluation results after pallidotomy for other conditions, such as dystonia, have not been published to date.

5. DEEP BRAIN STIMULATION AND NEUROBEHAVIORAL OUTCOMES

5.1. Thalamic Stimulation

5.1.1. Parkinson's Disease

5.1.1.1. Cognition, Language, and Memory

One study mentioned in passing that no significant deficits were observed in the neuropsychological evaluations of 10 PD patients after thalamic DBS *(168)*. Only two studies have reported detailed neuropsychological outcomes after thalamic DBS for PD. Neither Caparros-Lefebvre et al. *(169)* nor Tröster et al. *(170)* found changes in overall level of cognitive functioning in their small samples of nine patients after surgery. In contrast to thalamotomy, thalamic stimulation, at least in PD, seems not to be associated with declines in verbal fluency or memory. Indeed, both studies reported some improvements (possibly practice effects) on certain tasks. Caparros-Lefebvre et al. observed better performance on a card-sorting task 4–10 d after surgery, whereas Tröster et al. found patients to demonstrate improved delayed recall of prose and recognition of a word list, and somewhat better naming, about 4 mo after surgery. In a 12-mo follow-up of five of the patients reported on by Tröster et al. *(170)*, Woods and colleagues *(171)* found that gains in verbal fluency and memory were maintained. Study samples have been too small to elucidate possible material-specific cognitive changes, and this will be of importance to study in the future given the suggestion that left thalamotomy carries a greater risk of cognitive morbidity than does right thalamotomy.

Interpretation of post-DBS changes in cognition is probably even more complex than interpretation of changes after ablation. In addition to medication and/or test practice effects, neurobehavioral changes may reflect a transient microthalamotomy effect. Furthermore, effects on cognition may depend on stimulation parameters (unipolar vs bipolar; amplitude, frequency, pulse width) *(172)*. The importance of considering stimulation parameters is amplified by the findings of Hugdahl and colleagues *(173–175)*. These authors found that intra-operative stimulation (at the typical high frequency of DBS) did not predict the effect on memory of thalamotomy; this is in contrast to the prediction of postthalamotomy memory deficits afforded by low-frequency stimulation *(86)*.

Interpretative complexities of DBS effects on cognition are also illustrated by a case study. Tröster et al. *(176)* evaluated cognitive functioning in a PD patient before surgery, and in four conditions after surgery: with the stimulator turned on when the patient was either on or withdrawn from medication, and again with the stimulator turned off, while the patient was either on or off medication. A postoperative decrement in verbal fluency was observed in that case, but stimulation per se, in both medication conditions, was associated with improved verbal fluency. In essence, surgery and stimulation may have apparently opposite effects on a given function.

5.1.1.2. Mood State and Quality of Life

Caparros-Lefebvre et al. *(169)* found an improvement in mood state (depressive symptoms) 4–10 d after surgery. QOL improvements did not attain statistical significance in the study by Straits-Tröster et al. *(163)*, but this may reflect the fact that a generic QOL measure, probably less sensitive to change than a disease-specific measure was used, and that the sample was small. Indeed, among five patients, QOL gains on the disease-specific PDQ were still observed 12 mo after unilateral thalamic

DBS *(171)*. Alternatively, the lack of significant QOL impact of thalamic DBS (which alleviates predominantly tremor), may reflect the observation that tremor may be a less important determinant of QOL in PD than other symptoms such as bradykinesia, postural instability, and gait difficulties *(177)*.

5.1.2. Essential Tremor, Multiple Sclerosis, and Other Conditions

5.1.2.1. Cognition, Language, and Memory

Detailed neuropsychological data pertaining to unilateral thalamic DBS in ET were presented by Tröster et al. *(178)*. Another study *(168)* mentions in passing that one of four ET patients experienced transient slowing of information processing. Tröster et al. found that among 40 patients with ET the only decrement observed involved lexical verbal fluency (in contrast to the absence of such an effect in PD). Improvements, possibly impacted by test-retest effects, were observed in visuoconstructional skill and visuoperceptual gestalt formation, backward visual span, delayed prose recall, and word list recognition (also seen in PD after thalamic DBS). The effect of stimulation per se in ET was evaluated in a single case study by Lucas and colleagues *(179)*. In that study, no significant effects on cognition of bilateral thalamic DBS were found.

Although thalamic DBS has been used in MS *(180)* formal neuropsychological data have not been reported. Early studies utilizing thalamic stimulation for torticollis *(181,182)*, dystonia, hemiparesis, speech impairment *(181)*, and MS *(183)*, also did not report cognitive outcomes.

5.1.2.2. Mood State and Quality of Life

Tröster and colleagues *(178)* found a reduction in anxiety symptoms 3 mo after unilateral thalamic DBS surgery for ET. QOL, measured with both generic and disease specific measures (a modified PDQ), improved significantly 3 mo after surgery. On the SIP (a generic QOL measure), improvements were found in Total and Psychosocial scores, and on the modified PDQ, significantly increased satisfaction was found for ADLs, communication, emotional functioning, and stigma. Formal assessments of QOL and mood state have not been reported for thalamic DBS in other conditions.

5.2. Pallidal Stimulation

5.2.1. Parkinson's Disease

5.2.1.1. Cognition, Language and Memory

Tröster et al. *(184)*, in nine patients undergoing unilateral pallidal DBS, found that none of the patients experienced significant changes in overall level of cognitive functioning 3 mo after surgery. As a group, the patients demonstrated statistically significant declines in visuoconstructional ability and in verbal fluency, but the changes were rarely of clinical significance.

Subsequent studies yielded similar findings. Vingerhoets et al. *(185)*, in 20 patients, found no statistically significant declines in cognitive functioning after unilateral DBS. These authors also calculated an impairment index (the percentage of measures falling below impairment criterion) for each patient. Using an extremely liberal criterion of impairment (by defining impairment on a test as a score falling 1 SD below the mean of normative samples), they noted that six of the 20 patients showed *any* decrement (i.e., any magnitude increase in percentage of tests in the impaired range). These patients tended to be older and were taking higher medication dosages prior to surgery than patients showing no change or improvement. Merello et al. *(186)*, among six unilateral GPi DBS cases, observed no significant changes in mean scores on neuropsychological tests, but this might reflect the lack of statistical power attributable to the very small sample size.

Safety of bilateral GPi DBS has been addressed in only a few studies, but the majority of these suggest that the procedure is relatively safe from a cognitive standpoint. Ardouin et al. *(187)*, among 13 bilateral GPi DBS cases, found no significant changes in average test scores 3 mo (Grenoble subjects, $n = 8$) or six months (Paris subjects, $n = 5$) after surgery. Pillon et al. *(188)* found no cognitive morbidity, using clinical tests, in a very similar group of patients at 12-mo follow-up. Unlike STN patients, the performance on experimental tasks of five GPi patients at 6 mo was no different on and off levodopa.

Ghika et al. *(189)* found no significant changes in neuropsychological test scores 3 mo after contemporaneous bilateral GPi DBS electrode implantation (n = 6). To determine whether second surgery carries cognitive risks relative to the first surgery, Fields et al. *(190)* examined neuropsychological functioning in six patients undergoing staged bilateral GPi DBS electrode implantation. Patients were evaluated before surgery, 2 mo after the first operation, and again 3 mo after the second operation. No patient experienced significant declines in cognition and delayed recall was improved relative to baseline following the second operation.

Only a single case study with MRI-confirmed electrode location has reported significant executive dysfunction after bilateral GPi DBS *(191)*. Importantly, this study indicates the role stimulation played in this impairment. When the stimulators were turned off, the impairment was partially reversed. Relatively isolated cognitive impairments were reported by the Toronto group *(137)*. Among four patients, there was a significant decrease only in backward digit span. Verbal fluency testing was administered to only one patient, who demonstrated a decline on this task.

Whether unilateral GPi DBS is cognitively safer than pallidotomy has not been adequately addressed, but studies by Merello et al. *(186)* and Fields et al. *(192)* found the cognitive safety of the procedures to be comparable.

5.2.1.2. Mood State and Quality of Life

Vingerhoets et al. *(193)* administered a generic QOL measure (Sickness Impact Profile; SIP) to 20 patients before and 3 mo after unilateral GPi DBS. Significant improvements were evident in the Physical, Psychosocial, and Total scores. Among the 12 subscales, improvements were observed for ambulation, body care and movement, communication, sleep and rest, and eating. Straits-Tröster et al. *(163)*, in their sample of nine unilateral GPi DBS patients, also observed significant improvements in the Physical and Total scales of the SIP, but did not analyze scores on subscales.

Studies employing measures of mood state (Beck Depression Inventory) did not find improvements in depressive symptomatology *(163,185,187,189)*, but Fields et al. *(190)* noted that patients experienced a reduction in anxiety. A single case study has detailed hypomania and manic episodes after unilateral or bilateral GPi DBS *(194)*, but this morbidity may relate to an interaction between stimulation and medication. Higginson and colleagues *(195)* observed improvements in the autonomic, neurophysiologic, and subjective symptoms of anxiety in patients having undergone either unilateral ablative surgery or DBS for PD.

5.2.2. Other Disorders

Formal studies of cognition, mood, and QOL after GPi DBS for treatment of conditions other than PD are lacking. Morrison et al. *(36)* reported minimal cognitive change in two patients with dystonia who underwent right GPi DBS. One patient experienced a decline in verbal fluency, but both patients experienced improvements on some tests of attention and memory.

5.3. Subthalamic Stimulation

5.3.1. Parkinson's Disease

5.3.1.1. Cognition, Language, and Memory

In the largest (n = 49) patient series reported to date, Ardouin et al. *(187)* found few significant groupwise changes in cognition 3–6 mo after bilateral subthalamic nucleus (STN) DBS. Decrements were observed in verbal fluency, but improvements were seen in performance of the Trailmaking test, which requires psychomotor speed and divided visual attention. However, outcome among individual patients was more variable. In a follow-up report with an overlapping patient sample, Pillon et al. *(188)* showed that the 3-mo improvement in Trailmaking A was attributable to stimulation per se.

The decrement in verbal fluency was still evident 12 mo after the operation, but performance was similar with and without stimulation. Somewhat poorer performance on the Stroop was observed 12 mo after surgery. On a more experimental test battery, 6 mo after surgery, STN DBS was associated with improvements on some executive function/working memory tasks. Five other studies with small samples also reported few significant cognitive changes *(196–200)*. The study by Volkmann and colleagues *(200)* is noteworthy for its retrospective comparison of 12-mo outcomes after bilateral pallidal and STN DBS. This comparison suggests that depression, anhedonia, and worsening of speech may occur more frequently after STN than GPi DBS.

STN DBS effects on working memory and executive functions may be quite complex. Just like pharmacotherapy *(75)*, STN DBS may exert heterogeneous effects on different executive function tasks, and indeed, affect performance differently than GPi DBS *(201)*. The findings of nonuniform changes in executive and working memory tasks is also intriguing given a report that at least one physiological index of frontal activity that is related to some cognitive functions (preparation of a response) improves with STN DBS (i.e., the contingent negative variation amplitude increases over the frontal and frontocentral regions with bilateral STN DBS) *(202)*. The observation by the same group of researchers that STN DBS does *not* improve P300 abnormalities *(203)* provides a physiological companion finding to the neuropsychological studies showing a heterogeneity in cognitive functions impacted by STN DBS.

Two groups of researchers have reported more wide-ranging adverse cognitive and behavioral effects in small patient series *(137,204,205)*. Saint-Cyr, Trépanier, and their colleagues found poorer performance on the Trailmaking Test (Part B), poorer delayed recall and recognition of a word list, diminished verbal fluency, and poorer visual memory 3–6 mo after than before bilateral DBS surgery in 11 patients. These deficits were still evident in patients returning for 12-mo follow-up (up to nine patients for some tests). Declines in some other functions were observed at 12 but not 3–6 mo, and these changes, thus, probably relate to disease progression, subject selection bias, and/or attrition. Alegret and co-workers similarly found significant declines in average verbal memory, verbal fluency, complex visual attention, and visuospatial task scores three months after surgery in a group of 15 patients tested off medications. In contrast to Saint-Cyr and colleagues, however, Alegret et al. interpreted the observed cognitive changes *not* to be of clinical significance.

The studies described thus far suggest that neurobehavioral outcomes after bilateral STN DBS might be quite variable across studies and individual patients. Individual patient heterogeneity in outcomes is amplified by the findings of Dujardin and her colleagues *(206)*. Among 9 patients studied on medication 3 mo after surgery, these researchers observed declines in average verbal recall and verbal fluency scores, but gains in reaction time and simple attention (forward digit span). However, when examining change in individual patients, one-third of the patients were deemed to have shown overall declines in cognitive functioning (defined by declines of at least one standard deviation on at least 20% of the tests). On the positive side, among the 6 patients followed to 12 mo, none showed such declines, and importantly, the one patient among the six who had shown significant overall decline at 3 mo, had recovered by 1-yr follow-up.

Morrison et al. *(36)* are the ponly investigators to have published neuropsychological findings pertaining to unilateral STN DBS. In their group of three patients, few cognitive changes were observed. Two of three patients (one left and one right DBS) showed improved category fluency, whereas two (one left, one right DBS) showed decrements in letter verbal fluency. Two patients (both left DBS) also showed poorer performance on the Stroop task and on an alternating fluency task. Although the sample is too small to reliably evaluate laterality effects of STN DBS, it appears changes can occur after both left and right STN DBS.

Speech has been formally evaluated after STN DBS by Dromey et al. *(207)*, and these investigators reported small increases in sound pressure level and fundamental frequency variability after surgery. Gentil et al. *(208)* observed improvements in several speech parameters (longer duration of sustained vowels, shorter sentence duration, more variable fundamental frequency), but unchanged relative speech intensity with STN DBS. Studies with larger samples are needed to determine the reliability and generalizability of these findings.

Risk factors for cognitive deterioration have not been confidently established, given the generally small sample sizes of studies. Nonetheless, more advanced age (greater than 69 years) *(36,137,204)* and pre-existing cognitive deficits *(209)* may predispose to declines. Age also appears to predispose to postoperative confusional episodes *(210)*. The identification of reliable prognostic indicators is of urgency given the heterogeneity of cognitive outcomes among individual patients.

5.3.1.2. Mood State and Quality of Life

Several studies have reported improvement in depressive symptomatology *(187,200,204)* when considering self-report mood state questionnaires. Saint-Cyr et al. *(204)* found worsening on the caregiver-rated version of the FLOPS in 33% of the six patients older than 69 years (37% in all 11 patients). Although the most serious problems were rare, caregiver reports concerned postoperative perseveration, impulsivity, diminished social judgment, diminished insight, lability, and lack of awareness in some patients. Subthalamic DBS has been reported in isolated cases to be associated with laughter and euphoria *(211,212)* and depression *(56,213)*. Depression of likely multifactorial etiology may not be uncommon after STN DBS: Benabid et al. *(212)*, in the largest series of STN DBS to date, observed significant depression in 16 of 137 patients.

Detailed QOL data have not been published for STN DBS. In a group of 25 patients studied by our group four months after surgery, significant improvements were evident on several scales of the disease-specific PDQ-39: mobility, ADL, bodily discomfort, emotional well-being, and stigma. Capus et al. *(214)* noted in passing that QOL (measured by a "PDQ-38" instrument), improved about 50% in seven patients followed an average of 14.5 mo.

6. TRANSPLANTATION

6.1. Adrenal Medullary Autografts

Intrastriatal implantation of autologous adrenal medullary tissue is currently rarely carried out because of lack of lasting benefit. Although the few studies formally evaluating cognition did not report any significant morbidity *(215–217)*, significant psychiatric morbidity was reported *(218,219)*.

6.2. Fetal Mesencephalic Transplants

Intrastriatal grafting of fetal mesencephalic tissue can provide lasting motor benefit in some patients, with clinical benefit predicted by 18 fluorodopa uptake (an index of graft viability) *(220,221)*, but studies differ in tissue preparation, and site (unilateral vs bilateral; caudate and/or putamen) and number of implants. Observed neurobehavioral changes may reflect effects of disease progression, medication, the surgical lesion, or the sprouting of implanted tissue (*see* Diederich and Goetz *[222]*). Transient improvements (up to 2 yr) in memory have been reported *(223)* but cognitive (and speech) outcomes vary across individuals *(224–226)*. While most individuals have not shown significant cognitive changes after surgery, cognitive declines may occur in patients with more than mild pre-operative cognitive deficits *(224,225)*. Psychiatric complications, such as depression, paranoia, and hallucinations, appear more commonly after open *(227,228)* than stereotactic procedures *(229)*. Unfortunately, a recent report *(230)* of a well-controlled study (using a "placebo" or sham surgery control group) did not report neuropsychological or quality of life outcomes, although such data were gathered.

Fetal mesencephalic tissue grafting has recently been attempted in Huntington's disease. Philpott et al. *(231)* reported neuropsychological outcome in three patients. Although none experienced significant changes in overall cognitive function, specific changes were not uniform across patients. Three patients showed better recognition of a word list 4–6 mo after surgery and delayed recall of the word list and of a complex figure was improved in two of three patients. Performance on the WCST (tapping conceptualization) was improved in two of three patients as well. The most consistent decline occurred in verbal fluency, where three of three patients had poorer letter fluency after surgery.

QOL was investigated in detail by Hagell and colleagues *(232)*. Using the Nottingham Health Profile (a generic QOL measure) they observed significant improvements in QOL after bilateral grafting, and particularly in satisfaction with mobility, energy, and emotional well-being.

6.3. Porcine Embryonic Mesencephalic Tissue Xenografts

The recent approach of utilizing porcine xenografts in PD has not been adequately evaluated. Schumacher et al. *(233)* evaluated 12 patients over 12 mo, but neurobehavioral data were not reported.

7. CONCLUSIONS

Levodopa-era surgical interventions for certain movement disorders (PD and ET) appear relatively safe from a cognitive perspective. Surgical interventions appear to involve minimal psychiatric morbidity and, indeed, result, at least in the near term, in significant QOL improvements. When neurocognitive declines are observed, they most often involve verbal fluency, regardless of surgical technique and target. This decline in verbal fluency occurs more often after left-sided operations and may persist for a year or more, independent of motor speech changes. It is usually not of sufficient clinical severity to impact patient satisfaction with communication ability as assessed with disease-specific QOL measures. Other selective changes have been observed in working memory, attention, and episodic memory, but only in a minority of studies and patients.

The relative lack of significant neurobehavioral morbidity demonstrated to date does not imply that surgical interventions do not pose significant risks for some individuals with movement disorders. A small number of studies have, in fact, reported more severe cognitive and psychiatric complications, including severe declines in memory and even dementia in PD and MS.

The obvious question, then, is what are the risk factors that can be identified for such declines? Unfortunately, studies are too few in number and generally have too many significant methodological limitations at this early stage of investigation to permit one to address this issue with confidence. Nonetheless, some preliminary observations are warranted. We believe that the following represent *likely* risk factors for postoperative neurobehavioral morbidity: age (greater than 69 yr), bilateral or language-dominant hemisphere surgery (not necessarily ablative), lesion location in the anteromedial vs posterolateral aspect of the GPi, pre-existing psychiatric disturbance, and pre-existing dementia or marked frontal-subcortical behavioral syndrome. Lesion volume, presumably as long as the lesion is within the intended target site, has not convincingly or consistently been identified as a correlate of cognitive outcome.

Claims that DBS is neuropsychologically safer than ablative surgery are not adequately supported by the literature at this time, although data "favor" such an interpretation. There is also no clear indication at this time that certain targets (thalamus vs GPi vs STN) are preferable from a cognitive or QOL standpoint. Future randomized, preferably blinded, studies are needed to compare interventions (target, treatment method) directly in terms of their effects on neurobehavioral functioning and QOL. Studies are needed in several other areas neglected to date. Recent studies have failed to provide adequate data concerning the neurobehavioral and QOL outcomes of surgical procedures in MS, dystonia, torticollis, and movement disorders of cerebrovascular and post-traumatic etiologies. One might expect patients with disorders of demyelinating, traumatic, and cerebrovascular etiologies to be at risk for postsurgical cognitive morbidity given typically pre-existing cognitive impairments. Studies concerning QOL and cognitive outcomes are also notably lacking and needed in the area of transplantation.

Studies have recently become more sophisticated. For example, effects of DBS on cognition has been assessed by comparing performance during conditions of stimulation and non-stimulation. However, adequately controlled studies continue to be absent from the literature. Furthermore, the need to delineate stimulation effects using different stimulation parameters (*see* Fields and Tröster *[33]*) remains unmet. Until such studies are undertaken, it will be difficult to understand how stimulation affects cognition, and equally difficult to identify the boundary conditions under which stimulation remains safe. The endeavor of understanding effects of stimulation on cognition is especially important in light of the recent study showing that stimulation of STN and thalamus does not cause damage to brain adjacent to the electrode *(234)*, suggesting that cognitive changes with DBS probably reflect effects of stimulation per se rather than of electrode implantation.

Aside from clinical outcomes, neurobehavioral studies might address fruitfully brain-behavior relationship issues and further elucidate the role of subcortical structures in behavior. The availability of functional (vs structural) imaging, cognitive activation paradigms, and neurotransmitter and receptor labeling compounds, together with microelectrode stimulation and single cell recording techniques, offer a new window on the mind that remains to be opened by students of the surgical treatment of movement disorders. Future studies will undoubtedly capitalize on these technical advancements, as well as our improved knowledge of basal ganglia physiology and cognitive neuroscience. Such endeavors would prevent future critics from proclaiming that surgical studies have proved to be a failure in understanding the behavioral functions of the basal ganglia, as stated by Crown *(235)* three decades ago.

REFERENCES

1. Benabid, A. L., Pollak, P., Seigneuret, E., Hoffmann, D., Gay, E., and Perret, J. (1993) Chronic VIM thalamic stimulation in Parkinson's disease, essential tremor and extra-pyramidal dyskinesias. *Acta Neurochir. Suppl.* **58,** 39–44.
2. Middleton, F. A. and Strick, P. L. (2000) Basal ganglia and cerebellar loops: motor and cognitive circuits. *Brain Res. Rev.* **31,** 236–250.
3. Middleton, F. A. and Strick, P. L. (2000) Basal ganglia output and cognition: evidence from anatomical, behavioral, and clinical studies. *Brain Cogn.* **42,** 183–200.
4. Guridi, J. and Lozano, A. M. (1997) A brief history of pallidotomy. *Neurosurgery* **41,** 1169–1180.
5. Ostertag, C. B., Lücking, C. H., Mehdorn, H. M., and Deuschl, G. (1997) Stereotaktische Behandlung der Bewegungstörungen. *Nervenarzt* **68,** 477–484.
6. Siegfried, J. and Blond, S. (1997) *The Neurosurgical Treatment of Parkinson's Disease and Other Movement Disorders.* Williams & Wilkins Europe Ltd., London.
7. Gabriel, E. M. and Nashold, B. S. Jr. (1998) Evolution of neuroablative surgery for involuntary movement disorders: an historical review. *Neurosurgery* **42,** 575–590.
8. Gildenberg, P. L. (1998) The history of surgery for movement disorders. *Neurosurg. Clin. North Am.* **9,** 283–294.
9. Speelman, J. D. and Bosch, D. A. (1998) Resurgence of functional neurosurgery for Parkinson's disease: a historical perspective. *Mov. Disord.* **13,** 582–588.
10. Gildenberg, P. L. (2000) History of movement disorder surgery. In: *Movement Disorder Surgery, Progress in Neurological Surgery,* vol. 15 (Lozano, A. M., ed.), Karger, Basel, pp. 1–20.
11. Gross, C. E., Boraud, T., Guehl, D., Bioulac, B., and Bezard, E. (1999) From experimentation to the surgical treatment of Parkinson's disease: prelude or suite in basal ganglia research? *Prog. Neurobiol.* **59,** 509–532.
12. Riklan, M. and Levita, E. (1969) *Subcortical Correlates of Human Behavior: A Psychological Study of Basal Ganglia and Thalamic Surgery.* Williams and Wilkins, Baltimore, MD.
13. Shapiro, D. Y., Sadowsky, D. A., Henderson, W. G., and Van Buren, J. M. (1973) An assessment of cognitive function in postthalamotomy Parkinson patients. *Confin. Neurol.* **35,** 144–166.
14. Van Buren, J. M., Li, C. L., Shapiro, D. Y., Henderson, W. G., and Sadowsky, D. A. (1973) A qualitative and quantitative evaluation of parkinsonians three to six years following thalamotomy. *Confin. Neurol.* **35,** 202–235.
15. Jurko, M. F. and Andy, O. J. (1964) Psychological aspects of diencephalotomy. *J. Neurol. Neurosurg. Psychiatry* **27,** 516–521.
16. Jurko, M. F. and Andy, O. J. (1973) Psychological changes correlated with thalamotomy site. *J. Neurol. Neurosurg. Psychiatry* **36,** 846–852.
17. Johnson, M. D. and Ojemann, G. A. (2000) The role of the human thalamus in language and memory: evidence from electrophysiological studies. *Brain Cogn.* **42,** 218–230.
18. Almgren, P. E., Andersson, A. L., and Kullberg, G. (1969) Differences in verbally expressed cognition following left and right ventrolateral thalamotomy. *Scand. J. Psychol.* **10,** 243–249.
19. Almgren, P. E., Andersson, A. L., and Kullberg, G. (1972) Long-term effects on verbally expressed cognition following left and right ventrolateral thalamotomy. *Confin. Neurol.* **34,** 162–168.
20. Asso, D., Crown, S., Russell, J. A., and Logue, V. (1969) Psychological aspects of the stereotactic treatment of Parkinsonism. *Br. J. Psychiatry* **115,** 541–553.
21. Christensen, A. L., Juul-Jensen, P., Malmros, R., and Harmsen, A. (1970) Psychological evaluation of intelligence and personality in parkinsonism before and after stereotaxic surgery. *Acta Neurol. Scand.* **46,** 527–537.

22. Fünfgeld, E. W. (1967) *Psychopathologie und Klinik des Parkinsonismus vor und nach stereotaktischen Operationen.* Springer Verlag, Berlin.
23. McFie, J. (1960) Psychological effects of stereotaxic operations for the relief of parkinsonian symptoms. *J. Ment. Sci.* **106,** 1512–1517.
24. Vilkki, J. and Laitinen, L. V. (1974) Differential effects of left and right ventrolateral thalamotomy on receptive and expressive verbal performances and face-matching. *Neuropsychologia* **12,** 11–19.
25. Vilkki, J. and Laitinen, L. V. (1976) Effects of pulvinotomy and ventrolateral thalamotomy on some cognitive functions. *Neuropsychologia* **14,** 67–78.
26. Wilkinson, S. B. and Tröster, A. I. (1998) Surgical interventions in neurodegenerative disease: impact on memory and cognition. In: *Memory in Neurodegenerative Disease: Biological, Cognitive, and Clinical Perspectives* (Tröster, A. I., ed.), Cambridge University Press, Cambridge, UK, pp. 362–376.
27. Levita, E., Riklan, M., and Cooper, I. S. (1964) Verbal and perceptual functions after surgery of subcortical structures. *Percept. Mot. Skills* **18,** 195–202.
28. Koller, W., and Hristova, A. (1996) Efficacy and safety of stereotaxic surgical treatment of tremor disorders. *Eur. J. Neurol.* **3,** 507–514.
29. Laitinen, L. V. (2000) Behavioral complications of early pallidotomy. *Brain Cogn.* **42,** 313–323.
30. Bronstein, J. M., DeSalles, A., and DeLong, M. R. (1999) Stereotactic pallidotomy in the treatment of Parkinson disease: an expert opinion. *Arch. Neurol.* **56,** 1064–1069.
31. Defer, G.-L., Widner, H., Marié, R.-M., Rémy, P., and Levivier, M. (1999) Core assessment program for surgical interventional therapies in Parkinson's disease (CAPSIT-PD). *Mov. Disord.* **14,** 572–584.
32. Hallett, M. and Litvan, I. (1999) Evaluation of surgery for Parkinson's disease: a report of the Therapeutics and Technology Assessment Subcommittee of the American Academy of Neurology. *Neurology* **53,** 1910–1921.
33. Fields, J. A. and Tröster, A. I. (2000) Cognitive outcomes after deep brain stimulation for Parkinson's disease: a review of initial studies and recommendations for future research. *Brain Cogn.* **42,** 268–293.
34. Perozzo, P., Rizzone, M., Bergamasco, B., Castelli, L., Lanotte, M., Tavella, A., et al. (2001) Deep brain stimulation of subthalamic nucleus: behavioural modifications and familiar relations. *Neurol. Sci.* **22,** 81–82.
35. Aarsland, D., Larsen, J. P., Karlsen, K., Lim, N. G., and Tandberg, E. (1999) Mental symptoms in Parkinson's disease are important contributors to caregiver distress. *Int. J. Geriatr. Psychiatry* **14,** 866–874.
36. Morrison, C. E., Borod, J. C., Brin, M. F., Raskin, S. A., Germano, I. M., Weisz, D. J., and Olanow, C. W. (2000) A program for neuropsychological investigation of deep brain stimulation (PNIDBS) in movement disorder patients: development, feasibility, and preliminary data. *Neuropsychiatry Neuropsychol. Behav. Neurol.* **13,** 204–219.
37. Saint-Cyr, J. A. and Trépanier, L. L. (2000) Neuropsychologic assessment of patients for movement disorder surgery. *Mov. Disord.* **15,** 771–783.
38. Tröster, A. I., Woods, S. P., Fields, J. A., Lyons, K. E., Pahwa, R., Higginson, C. I., and Koller, W. C. (2002) Neuropsychological deficits in essential tremor: an expression of cerebello-thalamo-cortical pathophysiology? *Eur. J. Neurol.* **9,** 143–151.
39. Owen, A. M., Sahakian, B. J., Hodges, J. R., Summers, B. A., Polkey, C. E., and Robbins, T. W. (1995) Dopamine-dependent fronto-striatal planning deficits in early Parkinson's disease. *Neuropsychology* **9,** 126–140.
40. Tröster, A. I., Fields, J. A., and Koller, W. C. (2000) Parkinson's disease and parkinsonism. In: *Textbook of Geriatric Neuropsychiatry* (Coffey, C. E. and Cummings, J. L., eds.), American Psychiatric Press, Washington, DC, pp. 559–600.
41. Trépanier, L. L., Saint-Cyr, J. A., Lozano, A. M., and Lang, A. E. (1998) Neuropsychological consequences of posteroventral pallidotomy for the treatment of Parkinson's disease. *Neurology* **51,** 207–215.
42. Stebbins, G. T., Gabrieli, J. D., Shannon, K. M., Penn, R. D., and Goetz, C. G. (2000) Impaired frontostriatal cognitive functioning following posteroventral pallidotomy in advanced Parkinson's disease. *Brain Cogn.* **42,** 348–363.
43. Dymek, M. P., Atchison, P., Harrell, L., and Marson, D. C. (2001) Competency to consent to medical treatment in cognitively impaired patients with Parkinson's disease. *Neurology* **56,** 17–24.
44. Cahn, D. A., Sullivan, E. V., Shear, P. K., Pfefferbaum, A., Heit, G., and Silverberg, G. (1998) Differential contributions of cognitive and motor component processes to physical and instrumental activities of daily living in Parkinson's disease. *Arch. Clin. Neuropsychology* **13,** 575–583.
45. Tröster, A. I., Fields, J. A., Straits-Tröster, A. I., Lyons, K. E., Higginson, C. I., Chmidling, S., et al. (2000) Executive function, coping, mood state, and quality of life in Parkinson's disease patients being evaluated for pallidotomy [abstract]. *J. Int. Neuropsychol. Soc.* **6,** 207.
46. Jacobs, D. M., Marder, K., Cote, L. J., Sano, M., Stern, Y., and Mayeux, R. (1995) Neuropsychological characteristics of preclinical dementia in Parkinson's disease. *Neurology* **45,** 1691–1696.
47. Mahieux, F., Fenelon, G., Flahault, A., Manifacier, M. J., Michelet, D., and Boller, F. (1998) Neuropsychological prediction of dementia in Parkinson's disease. *J. Neurol. Neurosurg. Psychiatry* **64,** 178–183.
48. Buytenhuijs, E. L., Berger, H. J., Van Spaendonck, K. P., Horstink, M. W., Borm, G. F., and Cools, A. R. (1994) Memory and learning strategies in patients with Parkinson's disease. *Neuropsychologia* **32,** 335–342.
49. Tröster, A. I. and Fields, J. A. (1995) Frontal cognitive function and memory in Parkinson's disease: toward a distinction between prospective and declarative memory impairments? *Behav. Neurol.* **8,** 59–74.
50. Huber, S. J., Shuttleworth, E. C., and Paulson, G. W. (1986) Dementia in Parkinson's disease. *Arch. Neurol.* **43,** 987–990.
51. Tröster, A. I., Stalp, L. D., Paolo, A. M., Fields, J. A., and Koller, W. C. (1995) Neuropsychological impairment in Parkinson's disease with and without depression. *Arch. Neurol.* **52,** 1164–1169.

52. Tröster, A. I., Paolo, A. M., Lyons, K. E., Glatt, S. L., Hubble, J. P., and Koller, W. C. (1995) The influence of depression on cognition in Parkinson's disease: a pattern of impairment distinguishable from Alzheimer's disease. *Neurology* **45,** 672–676.
53. Kuzis, G., Sabe, L., Tiberti, C., Leiguarda, R., and Starkstein, S. E. (1997) Cognitive functions in major depression and Parkinson disease. *Arch. Neurol.* **54,** 982–986.
54. Stern, Y., Marder, K., Tang, M. X., and Mayeux, R. (1993) Antecedent clinical features associated with dementia in Parkinson's disease. *Neurology* **43,** 1690–1692.
55. Burchiel, K. J., Taha, J. M., and Favre, J. (1997) Posteroventral pallidotomy for Parkinson's disease patients. In: *Neurosurgical Operative Atlas,* vol. 6 (Rengachary, S. S. and Wilkins, R. H., eds.), Am. Assoc. of Neurol. Surgeons, Park Ridge, IL, pp. 13–26.
56. Bejjani, B. P., Damier, P., Arnulf, I., Thivard, L., Bonnet, A. M., Dormont, D., et al. (1999) Transient acute depression induced by high-frequency deep-brain stimulation. *N. Engl. J. Med.* **340,** 1476–1480.
57. Durif, F., Lemaire, J.-J., Debilly, B., and Dordain, G. (1999) Acute and chronic effects of anteromedial globus pallidus stimulation in Parkinson's disease. *J. Neurol. Neurosurg. Psychiatry* **67,** 315–322.
58. Lauterbach, E. C., Jackson, J. G., Wilson, A. N., Dever, G. E., and Kirsh, A. D. (1997) Major depression after left posterior globus pallidus lesions. *Neuropsychiatry Neuropsychol. Behav. Neurol.* **10,** 9–16.
59. Melnick, M. E., Dowling, G. A., Aminoff, M. J., and Barbaro, N. M. (1999) Effect of pallidotomy on postural control and motor function in Parkinson disease. *Arch. Neurol.* **56,** 1361–1365.
60. Higginson, C. I., Fields, J. A., Koller, W. C., and Tröster, A. I. (2001) Questionnaire assessment potentially overestimates anxiety in Parkinson's disease. *J. Clin. Psychol. Med. Set.* **8,** 95–99.
61. Saint-Cyr, J. A. and Trépanier, L. L. (2000) Neuropsychological considerations in movement disorder surgery. In: *Movement Disorder Surgery, Progress in Neurological Surgery,* vol. 15 (Lozano, A. M., ed.), Karger, Basel, pp. 266–271.
62. Cummings, J. L., Mega, M., Gray, K., Rosenberg-Thompson, S., Carusi, D. A., and Gornbein, J. (1994) The Neuropsychiatric Inventory: comprehensive assessment of psychopathology in dementia. *Neurology* **44,** 2308–2314.
63. Grace, J., Stout, J. C., and Malloy, P. F. (1999) Assessing frontal lobe behavioral syndromes with the frontal lobe personality scale. *Assessment* **6,** 269–284.
64. Narabayashi, H., Miyashita, N., Hattori, Y., Saito, K., and Endo, K. (1997) Posteroventral pallidotomy: its effect on motor symptoms and scores of MMPI test in patients with Parkinson's disease. *Park. Rel. Disord.* **3,** 7–20.
65. Diller, L., Riklan, M., and Cooper, I. S. (1956) Preoperative response to stress as a criterion of the response to neurosurgery in Parkinson's disease. *J. Am. Geriatr. Soc.* **4,** 1301–1308.
66. Tröster, A. I., Lyons, K. E., and Straits-Tröster, K. A. (1999) Determinants of health-related quality of life changes in Parkinson's disease. In: *Quality of Life in Parkinson's Disease* (Martínez-Martín, P. and Koller, W. C., eds.), Masson, Barcelona, pp. 55–77.
67. Tröster, A. I., Fields, J. A., Straits-Tröster, K. A., Lyons, K. E., Miyawaki, E., Wilkinson, S. B., et al. (1998) Motoric and psychosocial correlates of quality of life in Parkinson's disease four months after unilateral pallidotomy [abstract]. *Neurology* **50(Suppl. 4),** A299.
68. Tröster, A. I. (2000) Clinical neuropsychology, functional neurosurgery, and restorative neurology in the next millennium: beyond secondary outcome measures. *Brain Cogn.* **42,** 117–119.
69. Tomaszewski, K. J. and Holloway, R. G. (2001) Deep brain stimulation in the treatment of Parkinson's disease: a cost- effectiveness analysis. *Neurology* **57,** 663–671.
70. Hailey, D. and Harstall, C. (1998) Posteroventral pallidotomy for Parkinson's disease: assessment and policy on a technology in transition. *Health Policy* **43,** 55–64.
71. Thompson, P. D. (2001) Deep brain stimulation is superior to ablative surgery for Parkinson's disease: the case against. *J. Clin. Neurosci.* **8,** 291–292; discussion 293–294.
72. López-Lozano, J. J. and Mata, M. (1999) Surgical treatment for Parkinson's disease: impact on the patient's quality of life. In: *Quality of Life in Parkinson's Disease* (Martínez-Martín, P. and Koller, W. C., eds.), Masson, Barcelona, pp. 107–136.
73. Laing, R. J. (2000) Measuring outcome in neurosurgery [editorial]. *Br. J. Neurosurg.* **14,** 181–184.
74. Iacopino, D. G., Lucerna, S., Giller, C. A., Salpietro, F. M., Lo Presti, R., Sessa, E., et al. (1998) Pallidotomy improves quality of life in selected parkinsonian patients: an Italian report. *Funct. Neurol.* **13,** 105–115.
75. Lange, K. W., Robbins, T. W., Marsden, C. D., James, M., Owen, A. M., and Paul, G. M. (1992) L-dopa withdrawal in Parkinson's disease selectively impairs cognitive performance in tests sensitive to frontal lobe dysfunction. *Psychopharmacology* **107,** 394–404.
76. Alegret, M., Vendrell, P., Junqué, C., Valldeoriola, F., Nobbe, F. A., Rumià, J., and Tolosa, E. (2000) Effects of unilateral posteroventral pallidotomy on 'on-off' cognitive fluctuations in Parkinson's disease. *Neuropsychologia* **38,** 628–633.
77. Green, J. and Barnhart, H. (2000) The impact of lesion laterality on neuropsychological change following posterior pallidotomy: a review of current findings. *Brain Cogn.* **42,** 379–398.
78. York, M. K., Levin, H. S., Grossman, R. G., and Hamilton, W. J. (1999) Neuropsychological outcome following unilateral pallidotomy. *Brain* **122,** 2209–2220.
79. Schmand, B., de Bie, R. M., Koning-Haanstra, M., de Smet, J. S., Speelman, J. D., and van Zomeren, A. H. (2000) Unilateral pallidotomy in PD: a controlled study of cognitive and behavioral effects. The Netherlands Pallidotomy Study (NEPAS) group. *Neurology* **54,** 1058–1064.
80. Spiegel, E., Wycis, H., Orchinik, C., and Freed, H. (1955) Thalamic chronotaraxis. *Arch. Neurol. Psychiatry* **73,** 469–471.

81. Niebuhr, H. Jr. (1962) Some psychological aspects of patients with Parkinson's disease before and after ventrolateral thalamotomy. In: *Stereoencephalotomy. Part II Clinical and Physiological Applications*, vol. II (Spiegel, E. A. and Wycis, H. T., eds.), Grune and Stratton, New York, pp. 349–357.
82. Burchiel, K. J. (1995) Thalamotomy for movement disorders. *Neurosurg. Clin. North Am.* **6,** 55–71.
83. Fünfgeld, E. W. (1961) Die psychischen Hirnfunktionen bei hirnatrophischen Zustandsbildern nach operativer Belastung (stereotaktische Hirnoperationen älterer Parkinsonpatienten). *Acta Neurochir. (Wien)* **7(Suppl.),** 539–544.
84. Riklan, M., Diller, L., Weiner, H., and Cooper, I. S. (1960) Psychological studies on effects of chemosurgery of the basal ganglia in parkinsonism. I. Intellectual functioning. *Arch. Gen. Psychiatry* **2,** 22–31.
85. Krayenbühl, H., Wyss, O. A. M., and Yasargil, M. G. (1961) Bilateral thalamotomy and pallidotomy as treatment for bilateral parkinsonism. *J. Neurosurg.* **18,** 429–444.
86. Ojemann, G. A., Hoyenga, K. B., and Ward, A. A. Jr. (1971) Prediction of short-term verbal memory disturbance after ventrolateral thalamotomy. *J. Neurosurg.* **35,** 203–210.
87. Kocher, U., Siegfried, J., and Perret, E. (1982) Verbal and nonverbal learning ability of Parkinson patients before and after unilateral ventrolateral thalamotomy. *Appl. Neurophysiol.* **45,** 311–316.
88. Riklan, M., Levita, E., and Cooper, I. S. (1966) Psychological effects of bilateral subcortical surgery for Parkinson's disease. *J. Nerv. Ment. Dis.* **141,** 403–409.
89. Perret, E. and Siegfried, J. (1968) Memory and learning performance of Parkinson patients before and after thalamotomy. In: *Third Symposium on Parkinson's Disease* (Gillingham, F. J. and Donaldson, I. M. L., eds.), E. & S. Livingstone Ltd., Edinburgh, UK, pp. 164–168.
90. Krayenbühl, H., Siegfried, J., Kohenof, M., and Yasargil, M. G. (1965) Is there a dominant thalamus? *Confin. Neurol.* **26,** 246–249.
91. Hays, P., Krikler, B., Walsh, L. S., and Woolfson, G. (1966) Psychological changes following surgical treatment of parkinsonism. *Am. J. Psychiatry* **123,** 657–663.
92. Riklan, M., Diller, L., and Weiner, H. (1960) Psychological studies on the effects of chemosurgery of the basal ganglia in parkinsonism. II. Aspects of personality. *Arch. Gen. Psychiatry* **3,** 267–275.
93. Choppy, M., Zimbacca, N., and le Beau, J. (1973) Psychological changes after selective frontal surgery (especially cingulotomy) and after stereotactic surgery of the basal ganglia. In: *Surgical Approaches in Psychiatry* (Laitinen, L. V. and Livingston, K. E., eds.), Medical and Technical Publishing, Lancaster, UK, pp. 175–181.
94. Riklan, M. and Levita, E. (1970) Psychological studies of thalamic lesions in humans. *J. Nerv. Ment. Dis.* **150,** 251–265.
95. Riklan, M., Levita, E., Zimmerman, J., and Cooper, I. S. (1969) Thalamic correlates of language and speech. *J. Neurol. Sci.* **8,** 307–328.
96. Riklan, M. and Cooper, I. S. (1975) Psychometric studies of verbal functions following thalamic lesions in humans. *Brain Lang.* **2,** 45–64.
97. Bell, D. S. (1968) Speech functions of the thalamus inferred from the effects of thalamotomy. *Brain* **91,** 619–638.
98. Petrovici, J. N. (1980) Speech disturbances following stereotaxic surgery in ventrolateral thalamus. *Neurosurg. Rev.* **3,** 189–195.
99. Samra, K., Riklan, M., Levita, E., Zimmerman, J., Waltz, J. M., Bergmann, L., and Cooper, I. S. (1969) Language and speech correlates of anatomically verified lesions in thalamic surgery for parkinsonism. *J. Speech. Hear. Res.* **12,** 510–540.
100. Quaglieri, C. E. and Celesia, G. G. (1977) Effect of thalamotomy and levodopa therapy on the speech of Parkinson patients. *Eur. Neurol.* **15,** 34–39.
101. Lund-Johansen, M., Hugdahl, K., and Wester, K. (1996) Cognitive function in patients with Parkinson's disease undergoing stereotaxic thalamotomy. *J. Neurol. Neurosurg. Psychiatry* **60,** 564–571.
102. Fukuda, M., Kameyama, S., Yoshino, M., Tanaka, R., and Narabayashi, H. (2000) Neuropsychological outcome following pallidotomy and thalamotomy for Parkinson's disease. *Stereotact. Funct. Neurosurg.* **74,** 11–20.
103. Broggi, G., Dones, I., Ferroli, P., Franzini, A., Genitrini, S., and Micon, B. M. (2001) Surgery for movement disorders: complications and complication avoidance. *Semin. Neurosurg.* **12,** 225–231.
104. Young, R. F. (2001) Gamma knife treatment for movement disorders. *Semin. Neurosurg.* **12,** 233–243.
105. Magnin, M., Jeanmonod, D., Morel, A., and Siegemund, M. (2001) Surgical control of the human thalamocortical dysrhythmia: II. Pallidothalamic tractotomy in Parkinson's disease. *Thalamus Rel. Sys.* **1,** 81–89.
106. Schuurman, P. R., Bosch, D. A., Bossuyt, P. M., Bonsel, G. J., van Someren, E. J., de Bie, R. M., et al. (2000) A comparison of continuous thalamic stimulation and thalamotomy for suppression of severe tremor. *N. Engl. J. Med.* **342,** 461–468.
107. Angelini, L., Bono, R., Broggi, G., et al. (1979) Psychological implications of stereotactic thalamotomies for cerebral palsy. *Ital. J. Neurol. Sci.* **1,** 32–36.
108. Angelini, L., Nardocci, N., Bono, R., and Broggi, G. (1982) Depression after stereotactic thalamotomy in patients with abnormal movements. *Ital. J. Neurol. Sci.* **3,** 301–310.
109. Müller, V. C. and Yasargil, M. G. (1959) Zur Psychiatrie der stereotaktischen Hirnoperationen bei extrapyramidalen Erkrankungen. *Schweiz. Arch. Neurol. Neurochirurgie Psychiatrie* **84,** 136–154.
110. Jurko, M. F. and Andy, O. J. (1961) Electrical and behavioral changes following thalamotomy. *Surg. Forum* **12,** 404–406.
111. Pahwa, R., Lyons, K. E., Wilkinson, S. B., Tröster, A. I., Overman, J., Kieltyka, J., and Koller, W. C. (2001) Comparison of thalamotomy to deep brain stimulation of the thalamus in essential tremor. *Mov. Disord.* **16,** 140–143.
112. Blumetti, A. E. and Modesti, L. M. (1980) Long term cognitive effects of stereotactic thalamotomy on non-parkinsonian dyskinetic patients. *Appl. Neurophysiol.* **43,** 259–262.

113. Mohadjer, M., Goerke, H., Milios, E., Etou, A., and Mundinger, F. (1990) Long-term results of stereotaxy in the treatment of essential tremor. *Stereotact. Funct. Neurosurg.* **55,** 125–129.
114. Goldman, M. S. and Kelly, P. J. (1992) Symptomatic and functional outcome of stereotactic ventralis lateralis thalamotomy for intention tremor. *J. Neurosurg.* **77,** 223–229.
115. Goldman, M. S., Ahlskog, J. E., and Kelly, P. J. (1992) The symptomatic and functional outcome of stereotactic thalamotomy for medically intractable essential tremor. *J. Neurosurg.* **76,** 924–928.
116. Jankovic, J., Cardoso, F., Grossman, R. G., and Hamilton, W. J. (1995) Outcome after stereotactic thalamotomy for parkinsonian, essential, and other types of tremor. *Neurosurgery* **37,** 680–686.
117. Shahzadi, S., Tasker, R. R., and Lozano, A. (1995) Thalamotomy for essential and cerebellar tremor. *Stereotact. Funct. Neurosurg.* **65,** 11–17.
118. Critchley, G. R. and Richardson, P. L. (1998) Vim thalamotomy for the relief of the intention tremor of multiple sclerosis. *Br. J. Neurosurg.* **12,** 559–562.
119. Rossitch, E. Jr., Zeidman, S. M., Nashold, B. S. Jr., Horner, J., Walker, J., Osborne, D., and Bullard, D. E. (1988) Evaluation of memory and language function pre- and postthalamotomy with an attempt to define those patients at risk for postoperative dysfunction. *Surg. Neurol.* **29,** 11–16.
120. Whittle, I. R. and Haddow, L. J. (1995) CT guided thalamotomy for movement disorders in multiple sclerosis: problems and paradoxes. *Acta Neurochir. Suppl.* **64,** 13–16.
121. Spiegel, E. A., Wycis, H. T., Szekely, E. G., Adams, J., Flanagan, M., and Baird, H. W., III (1963) Campotomy in various extrapyramidal disorders. *J. Neurosurg.* **20,** 870–884.
122. Andy, O. J., Jurko, M. F., and Sias, F. R. Jr. (1963) Subthalamotomy in treatment of parkinsonian tremor. *J. Neurosurg.* **20,** 861–871.
123. Mundinger, F. (1968) Results of 500 subthalamotomies in the region of the zona incerta. In: *Third Symposium on Parkinson's Disease* (Gillingham, F. J. and Donaldson, I. M. L., eds.), E. & S. Livingstone Ltd., Edinburgh, UK, pp. 261–265.
124. McCarter, R. J., Walton, N. H., Rowan, A. F., Gill, S. S., and Palomo, M. (2000) Cognitive functioning after subthalamic nucleotomy for refractory Parkinson's disease. *J. Neurol. Neurosurg. Psychiatry* **69,** 60–66.
125. Svennilson, E., Torvik, A., Lowe, R., and Leksell, L. (1960) Treatment of Parkinsonism by stereotactic thermolesions in the pallidal region: a clinical evaluation of 83 cases. *Acta Psych. Neurol. Scand.* **35,** 358–377.
126. Alkhani, A. and Lozano, A. M. (2001) Pallidotomy for parkinson disease: a review of contemporary literature. *J. Neurosurg.* **94,** 43–49.
127. Riordan, H. J., Flashman, L. A., and Roberts, D. W. (1997) Neurocognitive and psychosocial correlates of ventroposterolateral pallidotomy surgery in Parkinson's disease [electronic manuscript]. *Neurosurg. Focus* **2(3),** Manuscript 7.
128. Cahn, D. A., Sullivan, E. V., Shear, P. K., Heit, G., Lim, K. O., Marsh, L., et al. (1998) Neuropsychological and motor functioning after unilateral anatomically guided posterior ventral pallidotomy. Preoperative performance and three-month follow-up. *Neuropsychiatry Neuropsychol. Behav. Neurol.* **11,** 136–145.
129. Masterman, D., DeSalles, A., Baloh, R. W., Frysinger, R., Foti, D., Behnke, E., et al. (1998) Motor, cognitive, and behavioral performance following unilateral ventroposterior pallidotomy for Parkinson disease. *Arch. Neurol.* **55,** 1201–1208.
130. Scott, R., Gregory, R., Hines, N., Carroll, C., Hyman, N., Papanasstasiou, V., et al. (1998) Neuropsychological, neurological and functional outcome following pallidotomy for Parkinson's disease. A consecutive series of eight simultaneous bilateral and twelve unilateral procedures. *Brain* **121,** 659–675.
131. Tröster, A. I., Fields, J. A., Wilkinson, S. B., and Koller, W. C. (1998) Neurobehavioral outcome of left and right pallidotomy for Parkinson's disease [abstract]. *Clin. Neuropsychologist* **12,** 268–269.
132. Yokoyama, T., Imamura, Y., Sugiyama, K., Nishizawa, S., Yokota, N., Ohta, S., and Uemura, K. (1999) Prefrontal dysfunction following unilateral posteroventral pallidotomy in Parkinson's disease. *J. Neurosurg.* **90,** 1005–1010.
133. Dewey, R. B. Jr., Giller, C. A., Broline, S. K., Mendelsohn, D. B., Lacritz, L. H., and Cullum, C. M. (2000) Clinical outcome of unilateral stereotactic pallidotomy without microelectroe recording for intractable Parkinson's disease. *Park. Rel. Disord.* **6,** 7–16.
134. Kubu, C. S., Grace, G. M., and Parrent, A. G. (2000) Cognitive outcome following pallidotomy: the influence of side of surgery and age of patient at disease onset. *J. Neurosurg.* **92,** 384–389.
135. Lacritz, L. H., Cullum, C. M., Frol, A. B., Dewey, R. B. Jr., and Giller, C. A. (2000) Neuropsychological outcome following unilateral stereotactic pallidotomy in intractable Parkinson's disease. *Brain Cogn.* **42,** 364–378.
136. Rettig, G. M., York, M. K., Lai, E. C., Jankovic, J., Krauss, J. K., Grossman, R. G., and Levin, H. S. (2000) Neuropsychological outcome after unilateral pallidotomy for the treatment of Parkinson's disease. *J. Neurol. Neurosurg. Psychiatry* **69,** 326–336.
137. Trépanier, L. L., Kumar, R., Lozano, A. M., Lang, A. E., and Saint-Cyr, J. A. (2000) Neuropsychological outcome of GPi pallidotomy and GPi or STN deep brain stimulation in Parkinson's disease. *Brain Cogn.* **42,** 324–347.
138. Intemann, P. M., Masterman, D., Subramanian, I., DeSalles, A., Behnke, E., Frysinger, R., and Bronstein, J. M. (2001) Staged bilateral pallidotomy for treatment of Parkinson disease. *J. Neurosurg.* **94,** 437–444.
139. Soukup, V. M., Ingram, F., Schiess, M. C., Bonnen, J. G., Nauta, H. J., and Calverley, J. R. (1997) Cognitive sequelae of unilateral posteroventral pallidotomy. *Arch. Neurol.* **54,** 947–950.
140. Perrine, K., Dogali, M., Fazzini, E., Sterio, D., Kolodny, E., Eidelberg, D., et al. (1998) Cognitive functioning after pallidotomy for refractory Parkinson's disease. *J. Neurol. Neurosurg. Psychiatry* **65,** 150–154.
141. Kuzis, G., Sabe, L., Tiberti, C., Dorrego, F., and Starkstein, S. (2001) Neuropsychological effects of pallidotomy in patients with Parkinson's disease [letter]. *J. Neurol. Neurosurg. Psychiatry* **71,** 563.

142. Schulz, G. M., Peterson, T., Sapienza, C. M., Greer, M., and Friedman, W. (1999) Voice and speech characteristics of persons with Parkinson's disease pre- and post-pallidotomy surgery: preliminary findings. *J. Speech Lang. Hear. Res.* **42,** 1176–1194.
143. Legg, C. F. and Sonnenberg, B. R. (1998) Changes in aspects of speech and language functioning following unilateral pallidotomy. *Aphasiology* **12,** 257–266.
144. Tröster, A. I., Fields, J. A., Hanisch, C., and Beatty, W. W. (1999) Clustering and switching on semantic verbal fluency in Parkinson's disease after unilateral, microelectrode-guided pallidotomy [abstract]. *J. Int. Neuropsychol. Soc.* **5,** 273.
145. Obwegeser, A. A., Uitti, R. J., Lucas, J. A., Witte, R. J., Turk, M. F., and Wharen, R. E. Jr. (2000) Predictors of neuropsychological outcome in patients following microelectrode-guided pallidotomy for Parkinson's disease. *J. Neurosurg.* **93,** 410–420.
146. Van Horn, G., Hassenbusch, S. J., Zouridakis, G., Mullani, N. A., Wilde, M. C., and Papanicolaou, A. C. (2001) Pallidotomy: a comparison of responders and nonresponders. *Neurosurgery* **48,** 263–271; discussion 271–273.
147. Lombardi, W. J., Gross, R. E., Trépanier, L. L., Lang, A. E., Lozano, A. M., and Saint-Cyr, J. A. (2000) Relationship of lesion location to cognitive outcome following microelectrode-guided pallidotomy for Parkinson's disease: support for the existence of cognitive circuits in the human pallidum. *Brain* **123,** 746–758.
148. Yokochi, F., Okiyama, R., Taniguchi, M., Takahashi, H., Hasegawa, N., and Hamada, I. (2001) Relationship between lesion location and the outcome of pallidotomy for Parkinson's disease. *J. Neurol.* **248(Suppl. 3),** 32–36.
149. Burns, J. M., Wilkinson, S., Kieltyka, J., Overman, J., Lundsgaarde, T., Tollefson, T., et al. (1997) Analysis of pallidotomy lesion positions using three-dimensional reconstruction of pallidal lesions, the basal ganglia, and the optic tract. *Neurosurgery* **41,** 1303–1316.
150. Hariz, M. I. (1990) Correlation between clinical outcome and size and site of the lesion in computed tomography guided thalamotomy and pallidotomy. *Stereotact. Funct. Neurosurg.* **55,** 172–185.
151. Krauss, J. K., Desaloms, J. M., Lai, E. C., King, D. E., Jankovic, J., and Grossman, R. G. (1997) Microelectrode-guided posteroventral pallidotomy for treatment of Parkinson's disease: postoperative magnetic resonance imaging analysis. *J. Neurosurg.* **87,** 358–367.
152. Goodman, S. H., Wilkinson, S., Overman, J., Koller, W. C., Tröster, A., Pahwa, R., et al. (1998) Lesion volume and clinical outcome in stereotactic pallidotomy and thalamotomy. *Stereotact. Funct. Neurosurg.* **71,** 164–172.
153. Shannon, K. M., Penn, R. D., Kroin, J. S., Adler, C. H., Janko, K. A., York, M., and Cox, S. J. (1998) Stereotactic pallidotomy for the treatment of Parkinson's disease. Efficacy and adverse effects at 6 months in 26 patients. *Neurology* **50,** 434–438.
154. Crowe, S. F., O'Sullivan, J. D., Peppard, R. F., McNeill, P. M., Bardenhagen, F., and Bowden, S. (1998) Left posteroventral pallidotomy results in a deficit in verbal memory. *Behav. Neurol.* **11,** 79–84.
155. Rettig, G. M., Lai, E. C., Krauss, J. K., Grossman, R. G., and Jankovic, J. (1998) Neuropsychological evaluation of patients with Parkinson's disease before and after pallidal surgery. In: *Pallidal Surgery for the Treatment of Parkinson's Disease and Movement Disorders* (Krauss, J. K., Grossman, R. G., and Jankovic, J., eds.), Lippincott-Raven, Philadelphia, PA, pp. 211–231.
156. Peppard, R. F., and Crowe, S. F. (1999) Cognitive changes due to neurosurgical ablative and stimulating procedures in PD patients. In: *Mental Dysfunction in Parkinson's Disease II*, vol. 11 (Wolters, E. C., Scheltens, P., and Berendse, H. W., eds.), Academic Pharmaceutical Productions, Utrecht, The Netherlands, pp. 177–188.
157. Alterman, R. L., Kelly, P., Sterio, D., Fazzini, E., Eidelberg, D., Perrine, K., and Beric, A. (1997) Selection criteria for unilateral posteroventral pallidotomy. *Acta Neurochir. Suppl.* **68,** 18–23.
158. Iacono, R. P., Carlson, J. D., Kuniyoshi, S., Mohamed, A., Meltzer, C., and Yamada, S. (1997) Contemporaneous bilateral pallidotomy [electronic manuscript]. *Neurosurg. Focus* **2(3),** Manuscript 5.
159. Ghika, J., Ghika-Schmid, F., Fankhauser, H., Assal, G., Vingerhoets, F., Albanese, A., et al. (1999) Bilateral contemporaneous posteroventral pallidotomy for the treatment of Parkinson's disease: neuropsychological and neurological side effects. Report of four cases and review of the literature. *J. Neurosurg.* **91,** 313–321.
160. Gálvez-Jiménez, N., Lozano, A., Tasker, R., Duff, J., Hutchison, W., and Lang, A. E. (1998) Pallidal stimulation in Parkinson's disease patients with a prior unilateral pallidotomy. *Can. J. Neurol. Sci.* **25,** 300–305.
161. Bezerra, M. L. S., Martinez, J.-V. L., and Nasser, J. A. (1999) Transient acute depresssion induced by high-frequency deep-brain stimulation [correspondence]. *N. Engl. J. Med.* **341,** 1003–1004.
162. Martínez-Martín, P., Valldeoriola, F., Molinuevo, J. L., Nobbe, F. A., Rumia, J., and Tolosa, E. (2000) Pallidotomy and quality of life in patients with Parkinson's disease: an early study. *Mov. Disord.* **15,** 65–70.
163. Straits-Tröster, K., Fields, J. A., Wilkinson, S. B., Pahwa, R., Lyons, K. E., Koller, W. C., and Tröster, A. I. (2000) Health-related quality of life in Parkinson's disease after pallidotomy and deep brain stimulation. *Brain Cogn.* **42,** 399–416.
164. Baron, M. S., Vitek, J. L., Bakay, R. A., Green, J., Kaneoke, Y., Hashimoto, T., et al. (1996) Treatment of advanced Parkinson's disease by posterior GPi pallidotomy: 1-year results of a pilot study. *Ann. Neurol.* **40,** 355–366.
165. Uitti, R. J., Wharen, R. E., Duffy, J. R., Lucas, J. A., Schneider, S. L., Rippeth, J. D., et al. (2000) Unilateral pallidotomy for Parkinson's disease: speech, motor, and neuropsychological outcome measurements. *Park. Rel. Disord.* **6,** 133–143.
166. Junqué, C., Alegret, M., Nobbe, F. A., Valldeoriola, F., Pueyo, R., Vendrell, P., et al. (1999) Cognitive and behavioral changes after unilateral posteroventral pallidotomy: relationship with lesional data from MRI. *Mov. Disord.* **14,** 780–789.
167. D'Antonio, L. L., Zimmerman, G. J., and Iacono, R. P. (2000) Changes in health related quality of life in patients with Parkinson's disease with and without posteroventral pallidotomy. *Acta Neurochir.* **142,** 759–767.

168. Blond, S., Caparros-Lefebvre, D., Parker, F., Assaker, R., Petit, H., Guieu, J.-D., and Christiaens, J.-L. (1992) Control of tremor and involuntary movement disorders by chronic stereotactic stimulation of the ventral intermediate thalamic nucleus. *J. Neurosurg.* **77,** 62–68.
169. Caparros-Lefebvre, D., Blond, S., Pécheux, N., Pasquier, F., and Petit, H. (1992) Evaluation neuropsychologique avant et après stimulation thalamique chez 9 parkinsoniens. *Rev. Neurol.* **148,** 117–122.
170. Tröster, A. I., Fields, J. A., Wilkinson, S. B., Busenbark, K., Miyawaki, E., Overman, J., et al. (1997) Neuropsychological functioning before and after unilateral thalamic stimulating electrode implantation in Parkinson's disease [electronic manuscript]. *Neurosurg. Focus* **2(3),** Article 9.
171. Woods, S. P., Fields, J. A., Lyons, K. E., Koller, W. C., Wilkinson, S. B., Pahwa, R., and Tröster, A. I. (2001) Neuropsychological and quality of life changes following unilateral thalamic deep brain stimulation in Parkinson's disease: a 12-month follow-up. *Acta Neurochir.* **143,** 1273–1278.
172. Tröster, A. I. (2000) Introduction to neurobehavioral issues in the neurosurgical treatment of movement disorders: basic issues, thalamotomy, and nonablative treatments. *Brain Cogn.* **42,** 173–182.
173. Hugdahl, K. and Wester, K. (1997) Lateralized thalamic stimulation: effects on verbal memory. *Neuropsychiatry Neuropsychol. Behav. Neurol.* **10,** 155–161.
174. Wester, K. and Hugdahl, K. (1997) Thalamotomy and thalamic stimulation: effects on cognition. *Stereotact. Funct. Neurosurg.* **69,** 80–85.
175. Hugdahl, K. and Wester, K. (2000) Neurocognitive correlates of stereotactic thalamotomy and thalamic stimulation in Parkinsonian patients. *Brain Cogn.* **42,** 231–252.
176. Tröster, A. I., Wilkinson, S. B., Fields, J. A., Miyawaki, K., and Koller, W. C. (1998) Chronic electrical stimulation of the left ventrointermediate (Vim) thalamic nucleus for the treatment of pharmacotherapy-resistant Parkinson's disease: a differential impact on access to semantic and episodic memory? *Brain Cogn.* **38,** 125–149.
177. Lyons, K. E., Pahwa, R., Tröster, A. I., and Koller, W. C. (1997) A comparison of Parkinson's disease symptoms and self-reported functioning and well-being. *Park. Rel. Disord.* **3,** 207–209.
178. Tröster, A. I., Fields, J. A., Pahwa, R., Wilkinson, S. B., Straits-Tröster, K. A., Lyons, K., et al. (1999) Neuropsychological and quality of life outcome after thalamic stimulation for essential tremor. *Neurology* **53,** 1774–1780.
179. Lucas, J. A., Rippeth, J. D., Uitti, R. J., Shuster, E. A., and Wharen, R. E. (2000) Neuropsychological functioning in a patient with essential tremor with and without bilateral VIM stimulation. *Brain Cogn.* **42,** 253–267.
180. Montgomery, E. B. Jr., Baker, K. B., Kinkel, R. P., and Barnett, G. (1999) Chronic thalamic stimulation for the tremor of multiple sclerosis. *Neurology* **53,** 625–628.
181. Cooper, I. S., Upton, A. R., and Amin, I. (1980) Reversibility of chronic neurologic deficits. Some effects of electrical stimulation of the thalamus and internal capsule in man. *Appl. Neurophysiol.* **43,** 244–258.
182. Andy, O. J. (1983) Thalamic stimulation for control of movement disorders. *Appl. Neurophysiol.* **46,** 107–111.
183. Brice, J. and McLellan, L. (1980) Suppression of intention tremor by contingent deep-brain stimulation. *Lancet* **1,** 1221–1222.
184. Tröster, A. I., Fields, J. A., Wilkinson, S. B., Pahwa, R., Miyawaki, E., Lyons, K. E., and Koller, W. C. (1997) Unilateral pallidal stimulation for Parkinson's disease: neurobehavioral functioning before and 3 months after electrode implantation. *Neurology* **49,** 1078–1083.
185. Vingerhoets, G., van der Linden, C., Lannoo, E., Vandewalle, V., Caemaert, J., Wolters, M., and Van den Abbeele, D. (1999) Cognitive outcome after unilateral pallidal stimulation in Parkinson's disease. *J. Neurol. Neurosurg. Psychiatry* **66,** 297–304.
186. Merello, M., Nouzeilles, M. I., Kuzis, G., Cammarota, A., Sabe, L., Betti, O., et al. (1999) Unilateral radiofrequency lesion versus electrostimulation of posteroventral pallidum: a prospective randomized comparison. *Mov. Disord.* **14,** 50–56.
187. Ardouin, C., Pillon, B., Peiffer, E., Bejjani, P., Limousin, P., Damier, P., et al. (1999) Bilateral subthalamic or pallidal stimulation for Parkinson's disease affects neither memory nor executive functions: a consecutive series of 62 patients. *Ann. Neurol.* **46,** 217–223.
188. Pillon, B., Ardouin, C., Damier, P., Krack, P., Houeto, J. L., Klinger, H., et al. (2000) Neuropsychological changes between "off" and "on" STN or GPi stimulation in Parkinson's disease. *Neurology* **55,** 411–418.
189. Ghika, J., Villemure, J. G., Fankhauser, H., Favre, J., Assal, G., and Ghika-Schmid, F. (1998) Efficiency and safety of bilateral contemporaneous pallidal stimulation (deep brain stimulation) in levodopa-responsive patients with Parkinson's disease with severe motor fluctuations: a 2-year follow-up review. *J. Neurosurg.* **89,** 713–718.
190. Fields, J. A., Tröster, A. I., Wilkinson, S. B., Pahwa, R., and Koller, W. C. (1999) Cognitive outcome following staged bilateral pallidal stimulation for the treatment of Parkinson's disease. *Clin. Neurol. Neurosurg.* **101,** 182–188.
191. Dujardin, K., Krystkowiak, P., Defebvre, L., Blond, S., and Destee, A. (2000) A case of severe dysexecutive syndrome consecutive to chronic bilateral pallidal stimulation. *Neuropsychologia* **38,** 1305–1315.
192. Fields, J. A., Tröster, A. I., Wilkinson, S. B., Lyons, K. E., Miyawaki, E., Pahwa, R., and Koller, W. C. (1998) Comparison of the cognitive safety of unilateral pallidal stimulation and pallidotomy [abstract]. *Neurology* **50(Suppl. 4),** A389.
193. Vingerhoets, G., Lannoo, E., van der Linden, C., Caemaert, J., Vandewalle, V., van den Abbeele, D., and Wolters, M. (1999) Changes in quality of life following unilateral pallidal stimulation in Parkinson's disease. *J. Psychosom. Res.* **46,** 247–255.
194. Miyawaki, E., Perlmutter, J. S., Tröster, A. I., Videen, T. O., and Koller, W. C. (2000) The behavioral complications of pallidal stimulation: a case report. *Brain Cogn.* **42,** 417–434.

195. Higginson, C. I., Fields, J. A., and Tröster, A. I. (2001) Which symptoms of anxiety diminish after surgical interventions for Parkinson's disease? *Neuropsychiatry Neuropsychol. Behav. Neurol.* **14,** 117–121.
196. Moro, E., Scerrati, M., Romito, L. M., Roselli, R., Tonali, P., and Albanese, A. (1999) Chronic subthalamic nucleus stimulation reduces medication requirements in Parkinson's disease. *Neurology* **53,** 85–90.
197. Tröster, A. I., Fields, J. A., and Higginson, C. I. (2000) Near-term cognitive and mood state outcomes after bilateral subthalamic stimulation for Parkinson's disease [abstract]. *J. Int. Neuropsychol. Soc.* **6,** 392–393.
198. Lopiano, L., Rizzone, M., Bergamasco, B., Tavella, A., Torre, E., Perozzo, P., et al. (2001) Deep brain stimulation of the subthalamic nucleus: Clinical effectiveness and safety. *Neurology* **56,** 552–554.
199. Lopiano, L., Rizzone, M., Perozzo, P., Tavella, A., Torre, E., Lanotte, M., and Bergamasco, B. (2001) Deep brain stimulation of the subthalamic nucleus: selection of patients and clinical results. *Neurol. Sci.* **22,** 67–68.
200. Volkmann, J., Allert, N., Voges, J., Weiss, P. H., Freund, H.-J., and Sturm, V. (2001) Safety and efficacy of pallidal or subthalamic nucleus stimulation in advanced PD. *Neurology* **56,** 548–551.
201. Jahanshahi, M., Ardouin, C. M., Brown, R. G., Rothwell, J. C., Obeso, J., Albanese, A., et al. (2000) The impact of deep brain stimulation on executive function in Parkinson's disease. *Brain* **123,** 1142–1154.
202. Gerschlager, W., Alesch, F., Cunnington, R., Deecke, L., Dirnberger, G., Endl, W., et al. (1999) Bilateral subthalamic nucleus stimulation improves frontal cortex function in Parkinson's disease. An electrophysiological study of the contingent negative variation. *Brain* **122,** 2365–2373.
203. Gerschlager, W., Bloem, B. R., Alesch, F., Lang, W., Deecke, L., and Cunnington, R. (2001) Bilateral subthalamic nucleus stimulation does not improve prolonged P300 latencies in Parkinson's disease. *J. Neurol.* **248,** 285–289.
204. Saint-Cyr, J. A., Trépanier, L. L., Kumar, R., Lozano, A. M., and Lang, A. E. (2000) Neuropsychological consequences of chronic bilateral stimulation of the subthalamic nucleus in Parkinson's disease. *Brain* **123,** 2091–2108.
205. Alegret, M., Junqué, C., Valldeoriola, F., Vendrell, P., Pilleri, M., Rumià, J., and Tolosa, E. (2001) Effects of bilateral subthalamic stimulation on cognitive function in Parkinson disease. *Arch. Neurol.* **58,** 1223–1227.
206. Dujardin, K., Defebvre, L., Krystkowiak, P., Blond, S., and Destée, A. (2001) Influence of chronic bilateral stimulation of the subthalamic nucleus on cognitive function in Parkinson's disease. *J. Neurol.* **248,** 603–611.
207. Dromey, C., Kumar, R., Lang, A. E., and Lozano, A. M. (2000) An investigation of the effects of subthalamic nucleus stimulation on acoustic measures of voice. *Mov. Disord.* **15,** 1132–1138.
208. Gentil, M., Chauvin, P., Pinto, S., Pollak, P., and Benabid, A. L. (2001) Effect of bilateral stimulation of the subthalamic nucleus on parkinsonian voice. *Brain Lang.* **78,** 233–240.
209. Hariz, M. I., Johansson, F., Shamsgovara, P., Johansson, E., Hariz, G. M., and Fagerlund, M. (2000) Bilateral subthalamic nucleus stimulation in a parkinsonian patient with preoperative deficits in speech and cognition: persistent improvement in mobility but increased dependency: a case study. *Mov. Disord.* **15,** 136–139.
210. Benabid, A. I., Koudsié, A., Benazzouz, A., Hoffmann, D., Fraix, V., Chabardes, S., et al. (1999) Neurosurgical therapy in Parkinson's disease. In: *Mental Dysfunction in Parkinson's Disease II*, vol. 11 (Wolters, E. C., Scheltens, P., and Berendse, H. W., eds.), Academic Pharmaceutical Productions, Utrecht, The Netherlands, pp. 131–139.
211. Kumar, R., Lozano, A. M., Sime, E., Halket, E., and Lang, A. E. (1999) Comparative effects of unilateral and bilateral subthalamic nucleus deep brain stimulation. *Neurology* **53,** 561–566.
212. Benabid, A. L., Koudsié, A., Benazzouz, A., Vercueil, L., Fraix, V., Chabardes, S., et al. (2001) Deep brain stimulation of the corpus luysi (subthalamic nucleus) and other targets in Parkinson's disease. Extension to new indications such as dystonia and epilepsy. *J. Neurol.* **248(Suppl. 3),** 37–47.
213. Houeto, J. L., Damier, P., Bejjani, P. B., Staedler, C., Bonnet, A. M., Arnulf, I., et al. (2000) Subthalamic stimulation in Parkinson disease: a multidisciplinary approach. *Arch. Neurol.* **57,** 461–465.
214. Capus, L., Melatini, A., Zorzon, M., Torre, P., Carraro, N., Moretti, D., et al. (2001) Chronic bilateral electrical stimulation of the subthalamic nucleus for the treatment of advanced Parkinson's disease. *Neurol. Sci.* **22,** 57–58.
215. Ostrosky-Solis, F., Quintanar, L., Madrazo, I., Drucker-Colin, R., Franco-Bourland, R., and Leon-Meza, V. (1988) Neuropsychological effects of brain autograft of adrenal medullary tissue for the treatment of Parkinson's disease. *Neurology* **38,** 1442–1450.
216. Goetz, C. G., Tanner, C. M., Penn, R. D., Stebbins, G. T., Gilley, D. W., Shannon, K. M., et al. (1990) Adrenal medullary transplant to the striatum of patients with advanced Parkinson's disease: 1-year motor and psychomotor data. *Neurology* **40,** 273–276.
217. Madrazo, I., Franco-Bourland, R., Aguilera, M., Ostrosky-Solis, F., Madrazo, M., Cuevas, C., et al. (1991) Autologous adrenal medullary, fetal mesencephalic, and fetal adrenal brain transplantation in Parkinson's disease: a long-term postoperative follow-up. *J. Neural Transplant. Plast.* **2,** 157–164.
218. Goetz, C. G., Stebbins, G. T., Klawans, H. L., Koller, W. C., Grossman, R. G., Bakay, R. A., and Penn, R. D. (1991) United Parkinson Foundation Neurotransplantation Registry on adrenal medullary transplants: presurgical, and 1- and 2-year follow-up. *Neurology* **41,** 1719–1722.
219. Stebbins, G. T. and Tanner, C. M. (1992) Behavioral effects of intrastriatal adrenal medullary surgery in Parkinson's disease. In: *Parkinson's Disease: Neurobehavioral Aspects* (Huber, S. J. and Cummings, J. L., eds.), Oxford University Press, New York, pp. 328–345.
220. Rehncrona, S. (1997) A critical review of the current status and possible developments in brain transplantation. In: *Advances and Technical Standards in Neurosurgery*, vol. 23 (Cohadon, F., Dolenc, V. V., Lobo Antunes, J., Nornes, H., Pickard, J. D., Reulen, H.-J., et al., eds.), Springer, Vienna, Austria, pp. 3–46.
221. Hagell, P., Schrag, A., Piccini, P., Jahanshahi, M., Brown, R., Rehncrona, S., et al. (1999) Sequential bilateral transplantation in Parkinson's disease: effects of the second graft. *Brain* **122,** 1121–1132.

222. Diederich, N. J. and Goetz, C. G. (2000) Neuropsychological and behavioral aspects of transplants in Parkinson's disease and Huntington's disease. *Brain Cogn.* **42,** 294–306.
223. Sass, K. J., Buchanan, C. P., Westerveld, M., Marek, K. L., Farhi, A., Robbins, R. J., et al. (1995) General cognitive ability following unilateral and bilateral fetal ventral mesencephalic tissue transplantation for treatment of Parkinson's disease. *Arch. Neurol.* **52,** 680–686.
224. Leroy, A., Michelet, D., Mahieux, F., Geny, C., Defer, G., Monfort, J.-C., et al. (1996) Examen neuropsychologique de 5 patients parkinsoniens avant et après greffe neuronale. *Rev. Neurol.* **152,** 158–164.
225. Thompson, L. L., Cullum, C. M., O'Neill, S., and Freed, C. R. (1996) Effects of fetal cell transplantation on cognitive and psychological functioning in Parkinson's disease. Annual Meeting of the National Academy of Neuropsychology, New Orleans.
226. Baker, K. K., Ramig, L. O., Johnson, A. B., and Freed, C. R. (1997) Preliminary voice and speech analysis following fetal dopamine transplants in 5 individuals with Parkinson disease. *J. Speech Lang. Hear. Res.* **40,** 615–626.
227. Molina, H., Quinones, Alvarez, L., et al. (1991) Transplantation of human fetal mesencephalic tissue in caudate nucleus as treatment for Parkinson's disease: the Cuban experience. In: *Intracerebral Transplantation in Movement Disorders: Experimental Basis and Clinical Experiences* (Lindvall, I., Björklund, A., and Widner, H., eds.), Elsevier, Amsterdam, pp. 99–110.
228. Madrazo, I., Franco-Bourland, R. E., Castrejon, H., Cuevas, C., and Ostrosky-Solis, F. (1995) Fetal striatal homotransplantation for Huntington's disease: first two case reports. *Neurol. Res.* **17,** 312–315.
229. Price, L. H., Spencer, D. D., Marek, K. L., Robbins, R. J., Leranth, C., Farhi, A., et al. (1995) Psychiatric status after human fetal mesencephalic tissue transplantation in Parkinson's disease. *Biol. Psychiatry* **38,** 498–505.
230. Freed, C. R., Greene, P. E., Breeze, R. E., Tsai, W.-Y., DuMouchel, W., Kao, R., et al. (2001) Transplantation of embryonic dopamine neurons for severe Parkinson's disease. *N. Engl. J. Med.* **344,** 710–719.
231. Philpott, L. M., Kopyov, O. V., Lee, A. J., Jacques, S., Duma, C. M., Caine, S., et al. (1997) Neuropsychological functioning following fetal striatal transplantation in Huntington's chorea: three case presentations. *Cell Transplant.* **6,** 203–212.
232. Hagell, P., Crabb, L., Pogarell, O., Schrag, A., Widner, H., Brooks, D. J., et al. (2000) Health-related quality of life following bilateral intrastriatal transplantation in Parkinson's disease. *Mov. Disord.* **15,** 224–229.
233. Schumacher, J. M., Ellias, S. A., Palmer, E. P., Kott, H. S., Dinsmore, J., Dempsey, P. K., et al. (2000) Transplantation of embryonic porcine mesencephalic tissue in patients with PD. *Neurology* **54,** 1042–1050.
234. Haberler, C., Alesch, F., Mazal, P. R., Pilz, P., Jellinger, K., Pinter, M. M., et al. (2000) No tissue damage by chronic deep brain stimulation in Parkinson's disease. *Ann. Neurol.* **48,** 372–376.
235. Crown, S. (1971) Psychosomatic aspects of Parkinsonism. *J. Psychosom. Res.* **15,** 451–459.

16
Surgical Treatment of Secondary Tremor

J. Eric Ahlskog, Joseph Y. Matsumoto,
and Dudley H. Davis

1. INTRODUCTION

Disabling tremor occurs in a variety of neurologic disorders. The most common are Parkinson's disease (PD) and essential tremor (ET). Considerable surgical experience in the treatment of tremor associated with these conditions has accumulated over the last few decades and is discussed elsewhere in this volume. Tremor may also occur secondary to one of a variety of brain insults, and in that setting is typically associated with other neurologic deficits. These secondary tremor syndromes also lend themselves to surgical intervention but there has been much less published experience concerning these. Thus, conditions such as multiple sclerosis (MS), traumatic brain injury (TBI), cerebrovascular accidents, perinatal insults/cerebral palsy as well as inborn errors of metabolism (e.g., Wilson's disease) may be associated with tremor, and may be severe and disabling. Surgical treatment of tremor seen in these clinical settings is the subject of this chapter. Because the surgical literature on such secondary tremor syndromes almost exclusively concentrates on upper limb tremor, that will also be the primary focus of this chapter.

2. CHARACTERISTICS OF SECONDARY TREMOR

Tremor secondary to MS, stroke or brain injury may vary in severity from minimal to extremely disabling. Milder cases of tremor are obviously not relevant to this surgical discussion and in fact, may respond to the same medications used to treat ET *(1)*. Severe secondary tremors being evaluated for surgical consideration typically have common clinical characteristics regardless of the underlying cause. The upper limb tremor in these settings is primarily a postural-kinetic tremor; i.e., it is prominent with hands held in a sustained posture or when moving (kinetic). There is often a major proximal arm component of high amplitude and low frequency (e.g., 2.5–7 Hz) *(2)*. Such tremor is occasionally relatively mild with the arms fully extended in front of the patient but severe with the hands held in front of the face, with elbows flexed. In some cases, it may be most severe when bringing a cup or eating utensil to the mouth. In more severe cases, this tremor may preclude meaningful functional use of the upper limbs for any manual tasks. Unfortunately, this severe postural-kinetic tremor is typically refractory to medical therapy. In some cases, a rest tremor may also be present. Such a combined rest-postural-kinetic tremor has been termed Holmes tremor *(3)*. Secondary arm tremor may also be associated with tremor elsewhere, especially axial tremor of trunk, head and/or neck.

The secondary tremor syndromes are associated with other neurological signs and symptoms since brain insults are not typically confined to only tremor circuits. These often make additional major contributions to disability.

From: Contemporary Clinical Neurology:
Surgical Treatment of Parkinson's Disease and Other Movement Disorders
Edited by: D. Tarsy, J. L. Vitek, and A. M. Lozano © Humana Press Inc., Totowa, NJ

Predominant rest tremor may be seen in the context of secondary parkinsonism due to a recognized, localized insult to the nigrostriatal system *(4–6)*. In practice, this type of secondary tremor is distinctly uncommon. Because there is scant literature on its surgical treatment, it will not be considered in this chapter.

2.1. *Neuroanatomic Substrate for Secondary Tremor*

The severe postural-kinetic upper limb tremor seen in surgical clinics typically results from an insult to cerebellothalamic systems *(2,7)*. The specific anatomic substrate includes the superior cerebellar peduncle, with its origins in the deep cerebellar nuclei (especially the dentate), and its projection to the thalamic ventrolateral (VL) nucleus. Midbrain lesions affecting this cerebellar outflow pathway may also damage the substantia nigra/nigrostriatal system resulting in combined rest-postural-kinetic tremor, so-called Holmes tremor *(3)*. The older literature referred to this as rubral tremor, implying pathology to the red nucleus. However, damage to the red nucleus is no longer considered necessary and perhaps not even sufficient to provoke this tremor *(2)*.

2.2. *Cerebellar Outflow Tremor*

2.2.1. *Unique Problems in Patients with Cerebellar Tremor*

Patients with severe secondary tremor syndromes present certain unique challenges to their physicians. First, severe cerebellar outflow tremors are notoriously refractory to pharmacologic therapy. Medications that are effective for either parkinsonian rest tremor or ET typically fail to have any clinically meaningful impact on severe cerebellar outflow tremor. As a result, there is often a nilistic attitude about attempting medical therapy for this type of tremor. Second, other motor deficits typically accompany these secondary tremors, which also are refractory to symptomatic medical therapy. Disability owing to those problems may overshadow that are due to the tremor.

Surgical case selection is especially problematic in cerebellar syndromes where limb ataxia and tremor are both severe. Marked upper limb ataxia may masquerade as tremor during finger-nose assessment or other similar testing *(2)*. A moving ataxic hand typically overshoots the target line, then overshoots in the opposite direction with the corrective movement, and then continues to overshoot with corrective movements until the target is reached. This serial dysmetria has the appearance of tremor *(2)*, but does not respond to surgical treatment because it represents ataxia rather than tremor. The challenge to the examining physician is to distinguish the contribution from serial dysmetria from that due to true tremor. The clinician is often aided by the recognition that true tremor is rhythmic (periodic), whereas serial dysmetria does not display precise and reproducible rhythmicity.

These secondary tremor syndromes also present unique challenges to the stereotactic neurosurgeon. First, the brain insults that cause tremor, such as MS, stroke, or trauma, may have disrupted the anatomic integrity of the brain, as well as possibly altered the thalamic and peri-thalamic architecture. Neuroanatomic and neurophysiologic landmarks employed to target the surgical site are therefore often distorted and less reliable in these cases *(8,9)*. Secondly, patients with secondary tremor already have a burden of central nervous system (CNS) damage. As a result, the addition of a surgical lesion may be less well tolerated. Thirdly, many of these patients have unreasonable surgical expectations. They are often quite severely disabled by the totality of their neurologic problem with tremor making a minor contribution. Despite appropriate physician counseling, they may look to surgery as their last hope for a cure not only for the tremor, but also their underlying neurologic condition. It is not uncommon for such patients to become depressed after surgery, even when successful in relieving the tremor *(10)*. Fourth, there are reimbursement issues. In this era of cost containment, the question is often raised whether the incremental benefit of abolishing tremor in one limb justifies the expense of the surgery in a patient who is otherwise severely disabled.

Of additional note, the academic neurologist/neurosurgeon is confronted with unique problems in assessment of surgical outcome. There is no general consensus about the best method of measuring surgical benefit in this type of patient. Tremor patients severely disabled by their underlying neurologic condition may still experience a very meaningful benefit from surgical tremor relief, despite persisting severe deficits in other motor spheres. In a wheelchair bound patient, severe bilateral tremor may preclude any functional use of the upper extremities, whereas surgical relief, even in one hand, may be very gratifying. However, this benefit may be greatly diluted when assessed using general quality-of-life and activity-of-daily-living scales. Tremor measurement devices may be useful in this situation, but these require special and often expensive equipment that is not universally available. Also, special technical expertise is necessary to employ these techniques, which are usually administered in dedicated motor control laboratories.

2.2.2. *Surgical Technique for Cerebellar Outflow Tremor*

Multiple technical issues are at least partially unique to surgical treatment of severe cerebellar outflow tremor. These include the target location within the thalamus, plus imaging and neurophysiologic methods to assure target precision. In the case of thalamotomy, the size of the lesion must also be considered. The fundamental issue of thalamotomy vs thalamic deep brain stimulation (DBS) must also be considered.

2.2.2.1. Surgical Site

It has long been recognized that lesions in any one of several brain areas will alleviate tremor. These sites are within the cortical-striatal-pallidal-thalamic-cortical loop *(11)*. There is general consensus that the ideal site for surgical treatment of ET or parkinsonian tremor is within Hassler's *(12)* ventralis intermedius nucleus of the thalamus (Vim), which receives projections from the superior cerebellar peduncle *(12)*. In the American terminology *(13)*, this corresponds to the ventral lateral nucleus (VLo) and ventral intermediate nucleus (Vim or VLc with VPLo). There is a general consensus that these nuclei are also the preferred target for treatment of other types of tremor, including the secondary syndromes characterized by severe postural-kinetic tremor, such as that due to MS, stroke, or brain trauma *(14,15)*.

2.2.2.2. Imaging and Neurophysiology

The neuropathologic process causing ET is unknown and does not cause identifiable structural changes within the brain. Therefore, stereotactic localization is not affected by the underlying pathologic process. The same may be said for PD in which pathologic changes are primarily confined to the substantia nigra and certain other brainstem nuclei. Stereotactic surgery for these disorders can therefore be done with good consistency in the stereotactic coordinates measured from the usual landmarks. In contrast, secondary tremor is typically associated with structural changes in the brain, which therefore may produce inconsistencies in stereotactic localization.

Imaging technology to assist the stereotactic neurosurgeon in treatment of secondary tremors includes computed tomography (CT) and magnetic resonance imaging (MRI) compatible head frames with computer-assisted localization as well as ventriculography, which is the older standard *(11,16)*. In the modern era, some surgeons still favor ventriculography for secondary tremor surgery because of the frequent distortion of the ventricles by the underlying pathology *(17)*.

Verification of the surgical target site with intraoperative neurophysiology has been used to a variable extent by stereotactic neurosurgeons treating secondary tremor. Although microelectrode and semimicroelectrode recording are advocated by some as means of neuroanatomic verification *(11,16)*, the literature does not necessarily support one specific strategy. Sensory evoked potential somatotopic localization within the contiguous ventralis posterior thalamic nucleus (VPLc) *(11,16)* is also commonly employed for determining laterality of the target. Surgeons utilizing neurophysiology confront additional special problems in patients with secondary tremors. The primary neuropathologic process responsible for the tremor typically causes more widespread damage outside the target area and hence distortion of the neurophysiology. For example, among poststroke tremor cases, Ohye et al. *(8)* noted that semi-microelectrode-recorded Vim thalamic neuronal activity was much lower than in the typical PD patient and sensory neurons were much less frequently encountered. They also found anatomic reorganization of sensory neuronal distributions. The normal separation of tactile and kinesthetic neurons, which is present in PD, was absent in poststroke tremor cases. Instead, these neurons were intermingled. Among MS tremor cases, there are notorious difficulties in recording sensory-evoked potentials within the VP, which are used for determining laterality *(18)*.

2.2.2.3. Thalamotomy Lesion Size

Some surgeons have found that in secondary tremor cases larger thalamic lesions are required than are employed for PD or ET. Ohye et al. *(19)* retrospectively estimated the volume of effective thalamic lesions for a variety of tremor syndromes, as measured by the number of lesions per operation. They noted that post-traumatic and cerebral palsy related tremor required more lesions than PD. Poststroke tremor required the most lesions of all and was the most difficult to treat. Tremor amplitude may also dictate the optimum lesion size, as higher amplitude tremor requires larger lesions *(15)*. Notably, the amplitude of secondary cerebellar outflow tremor is often much greater than that of PD or ET.

Larger amplitude upper limb tremor usually involves proximal muscles and this proximal-distal factor may also influence optimal lesion size and location. During localization for DBS implantation, Nguyen and Degos *(20)* noted that distal tremor was more effectively treated by stimulation in lower portions of the Vim, whereas proximal tremor responded better to stimulation more superiorly. Geny et al. *(21)* reached similar conclusions, finding that the most effective DBS site for proximal, large-amplitude MS tremor was more dorsal and lateral than for parkinsonian tremor. This somatotopic organization perhaps accounts for the need for larger lesions in treatment of secondary tremor syndromes in which there are often both proximal and distal limb components.

3. SURGICAL TREATMENT OF SECONDARY TREMORS

We will summarize the published experience with stereotactic surgery for secondary tremor syndromes. To compile the series, we sought all published English-language manuscripts reporting outcomes in the surgical treatment of secondary tremor. We initially used the MEDLINE database to identify relevant surgical series published between January 1966 and March 2000. We added additional papers identified from the published reference lists of these manuscripts. Surgical series that are included contained at least three consecutive and previously unreported patients and follow-up was beyond the immediate postoperative period. Patients within the series were categorized in terms of three efficacy categories: (1) number of patients with some sustained benefit; (2); number with post-op tremor no worse than mild; (3) number with tremor essentially abolished. Conditions in which there were at least three published series were subsequently identified for MS, poststroke, post-traumatic, and cerebral palsy-related tremor; these are summarized below. Nearly all of the surgeries cited below were unilateral; less than 10% were bilateral. Because the outcomes concerning efficacy and complications were not separately reported for the bilateral vs unilateral cases, these cases have been lumped together in the compiled series below. Common to all of these secondary tremors is brain pathology that produces other motor and neurologic deficits, which sometimes outweigh the disability from tremor.

3.1. Multiple Sclerosis Tremor

The largest published surgical experience for treatment of secondary tremor is among patients with MS. Many of the issues confronting the surgeon in treating MS tremor have relevance to surgery of other secondary tremors. However, there are also a number of problems or concerns that are unique and especially relevant to the treatment of MS patients:

- Sensory-evoked potentials, which are conventionally used to help confirm the target site, are often poorly developed or unobtainable in MS patients *(18)*. This is the consequence of demyelination affecting central conduction pathways.
- The progression of MS may overshadow any benefit from surgery. The neurologic deficits that occur in most of the other secondary tremor syndromes tend to be stable.
- MS relapse could theoretically be precipitated by brain surgery. This concern has led some surgeons to employ perioperative steroids *(18,22)* or ACTH *(23)*.
- Neurologic deficits wax and wane and sometimes completely remit in MS. Thus, the surgeon must decide how long to observe before concluding that the tremor is unlikely to improve spontaneously. There have been no longitudinal studies on which to base a decision. Haddow et al. *(24)*, in their review of thalamotomy for MS tremor, proposed that the tremor should have been present for at least 1 yr and preferably stable.

The altered neuroanatomy and neurophysiology induced by the demyelinating process plus the superimposed neurologic deficits compromise the surgeon's ability to achieve clinically meaningful efficacy. Surgeons performing thalamotomies typically report better success with treatment of ET or parkinsonian tremor than tremor secondary to MS *(23,25,26)*.

3.1.1. Thalamotomy for MS Tremor

Published series of thalamotomy in MS tremor *(9,11,18,23,25–33)*, which meet the inclusion criteria cited earlier, are summarized in Table 1. At least some anti-tremor efficacy was reported in at least half of the patients in all but one of these 14 surgical series. Of these 14 series, 11 reported that at least two-thirds of patients appreciated at least some sustained benefit. Complete or essentially complete abolition of tremor was reported in anywhere from 0–100% of patients in the 10 series in which this could be ascertained. In four of these 10 series, at least 75% of patients experienced abolition of tremor, whereas in another five series, 20% or fewer patients experienced tremor abolition. Permanent complication rates were highly variable, although relatively few in most series.

Demographic data was inconsistently reported. The mean duration of MS was summarized in six series, where it ranged from 5.5–11 yr *(9,27–31)*. Mean duration of tremor prior to surgery was tabulated in only a few studies, where it ranged from 1.9–8.2 yr *(9,29,31,32)*. Mean ages were specified in eight series *(9,18,22,26–28,31,32)* and ranged from 32–44 yr.

The variable outcomes shown in Table 1 likely reflect a multiplicity of factors including variability of:

- Tremor severity;
- Neurologic deficits and the demyelinating plaque burden from MS;
- Brain atrophy and altered neurophysiology owing to MS, which compromised precise target determination;
- Activity of MS;
- Other medical problems;
- Duration of follow-up (highly variable not only between, but within series);
- Outcome rating schemes and degree of scrutiny.

Although differences in surgical techniques may have accounted for some of the variability, tabulation of these series does not support one surgical approach over another. Unfortunately, only a cursory description of surgical technique was provided in most of these publications.

Outcome rating strategies were also extremely variable among these series and it was apparent in several that the level of assessment was quite superficial. Haddow et al. *(24)*, in their review of thalamotomy for MS tremor, commented that there probably has been a more critical evaluation of patient outcomes in more recent publications.

MS relapse triggered by tremor surgery was addressed in five of these publications *(18,22,23,30,31)*. As shown in Table 1, the relapse risk does not appear to have been great, with approx 7% of patients in these five combined series experiencing MS relapse temporally related to the surgery.

In the aggregate, these published series provide no consensus criteria for patient selection. Haddow et al. *(24)* proposed guidelines that were primarily based on common sense: (1) no other severe medical problems; (2) tremor duration > 1 yr; (3) no severe brain or spinal cord damage; (4) MS quiescent;

Table 1
Thalamotomy for MS Tremor

Thalamotomy series, year	Surgical site, as specified	N	Some sustained benefit	Improvement, with tremor at last F/U mild or absent	% with no tremor[a]	Usual F/U length, years	Permanent complications	# with MS relapse	Death	Imaging used for coordinates	Micro- or semi-microelectrode recording to enhance localization?
Cooper (1967) *(27)*	VL[b]	32	28 of 31 (90%) (plus one death)	28 of 31 (90%) (plus one death)	23 of 31 (74%)	1-8	Unclear if permanent: worsened hemiparesis = 2; dysarthria & dysphagia = 3	?	1 of 32	Ventriculogram	No
Samra et al. (1970) *(32)*	VL (posterior aspect)[b]	25	20 of 25 (80%)	Perhaps 13 of 25 (52%)	?	?	Complications occurred, but details unclear	?	0	Ventriculogram	No
Arsalo et al. (1973) *(28)*	VL	26	At least "three-fourths" (75%)	At least "three-fourths" (75%)	"Three-fourths" (75%)	Mean 3.3	38% with dysarthria; postop hematoma with mental and motor compromise = 1	?	0	Air ventriculogram	No
van Manen (1974) *(33)*	VL	4	No substantial benefit in any of 4 (0%)	0 of 4 (0%)	0 of 4 (0%)	?	"Slight general deterioration"	?	0	?	Probably no
Andrew et al. (1974) *(23)*	Anterior part of ventralis caudalis externus and if necessary in VIM	4	3 of 4 (75%)	?	?	1 to 3	?	?0	0	Presumably ventriculogram	Microelectrode in some cases
Kelly (1980) *(11)*	VL (VOP)	3	3 of 3 (100%)	3 of 3 (100%)	3 of 3 (100%)	?	none	?	0	?	Semi-microelectrode
Speelman & van Manen (1984) *(29)*	Not specified	10	8 of 10 (80%)	?5 of 10 (50%)	0 of 10 (0%)	Mean 4.5	Dysarthria = 1; hemiparesis = 4; slight hypesthesia = 1; urinary dysfunction = 2	?	1 of 11? (after 3 weeks)	?	?
Kandel & Hondcarian (1985) *(30)*	Basal posterior part of VL and sometimes also lesion in subthalamic region (general anesthesia)[b]	20	10 of 14 (71%), plus 2 lost to followup & 2 died of MS	8 of 14 (57%)	?	1 to 10	0	0	0	Ventriculogram	?

Hitchcock et al. (1987) *(25)*	Not specified	30	50% (presumably 15 of 30)	?	?	2	?	?	?	?	?
Goldman & Kelly (1992) *(18)*	VL	5	2 of 3 (67%) plus an additional 2 surgeries aborted	1 of 5 (20%)	1 of 5 (20%)	0.25 to 2.8	Worsened ataxic dysarthria = 1	0	0	CT and/or MRI plus ventriculogram	Semi-microelectrode
Whittle & Haddow (1995) *(9)*	VL	9	9 of 9 (100%)	at least 7 of 9 (78%)	7 of 9 (78%)	1	None	?	0	CT	No
Shahzaki et al. (1995) *(22)*	Not specified	46 (33 with adequate f/u)	22 of 33 (67%)	22 of 33 (67%)	12 of 33 (36%)	0.25 to 10	Subdural hematoma = 1; cognitive disturbance = 2; hemiparesis = 4; dysarthria = 2; arm ataxia = 2; gait disturbance = 1; numbness = 2; meningitis = 1	4	0	?	Micro-electrode in recent cases
Critchley & Richardson (1998) *(31)*	VIM	24	14 of 24 (58%)	12 of 24 (50%)	4 of 24 (17%)	Mean 2.2	Hemiparesis = 1; worsened dysarthria = 1	3	0	Ventriculogram	No
Schuurman et al. (2000) *(26)*	VIM	5	5 of 5 (100%)	4 of 5 (80%)	0 of 5 (0%)	0.5	Severe gait/balance disturbance = 2	?	0	Ventriculogram	Macro-electrode

Abbreviations: Thalamic nuclei, VL, ventralis lateralis; VOP, ventralis oralis posterior; VIM, ventralis intermedius. F/U, follow up.
[a]This category includes cases where the author described tremor that was so minimal that it seemed to be clinically meaningless.
[b]Cryothalamotomy (in all other series, radio frequency electrocoagulation employed).

(5) tremor is the main source of disability; (6) general functional improvement is likely. They also advised against bilateral thalamotomy because of risk for surgical complications.

3.1.2. Thalamic Deep Brain Stimulation (DBS) for MS Tremor

The published surgical experience with thalamic DBS for MS tremor to date is very limited. All three published series reported improvement in the majority of patients, usually with less than 12 mo follow-up (Table 2). Theoretically, thalamic DBS should approximate the efficacy of thalamotomy and offer the potential advantage of bilateral treatment. Bilateral thalamotomy carries a high risk of speech and cognitive complications *(34)*; in fact, Haddow et al. caution against performing bilateral thalamotomy in MS patients *(24)*. Because the effects of DBS are reversible (except for the damage from lead placement), there is less risk associated with this procedure *(35)*.

The results summarized in Table 2 are too limited to draw any conclusions about thalamic DBS for the tremor of MS or how it compares to thalamotomy. The series by Schuurman et al. *(26)*, summarized in Table 2, was part of a randomized prospective trial comparing thalamic DBS to thalamotomy. The thalamotomy series results are shown in Table 1. These authors reported better outcomes with thalamic DBS than thalamotomy for patients with Parkinson's disease or essential tremor. However, the outcomes were similar among the five patients in each treatment arm with MS. Benebid et al. *(37)* commented that, similar to the thalamotomy experience, MS tremor is less consistently or effectively suppressed by thalamic DBS than essential or parkinsonian tremor. One additional series not providing long-term outcomes did report that three of eight patients were not implanted because intraoperative tremor suppression could not be accomplished *(10)*.

Montgomery et al. *(36)* described "tolerance" to the effects of DBS in their MS patients. Benefits could be restored by further readjustment of the pulse generator stimulation parameters. Similarly, Geny et al. *(21)* and Whittle et al. *(10)* also mentioned the need for frequent readjustment of the stimulation parameters among their MS patients. Long-term trends with regard to this "tolerance" effect have yet to be described.

The experience with thalamic DBS for MS tremor is therefore still preliminary. Published series describing outcomes following thalamic DBS for other secondary tremors have not been published with one exception (*see* Subheading 3.3).

3.1.3. Mayo Clinic Experience

Because of the variability in efficacy reported in previous trials, we used a quantitative assessment protocol to evaluate the surgical treatment of MS tremor in our patients *(38)*. The following are preliminary results on nine patients (six female, mean age 42.8 ± 8.8 yr) with clinically definite MS and severe postural-kinetic upper extremity tremor. Patients were excluded if they had arm weakness or numbness. All had serious MS-related disability as judged from the Kurtzke score, mean 7.4 ± 1.4. Patients underwent unilateral Vim thalamotomy (six patients) or thalamic stimulation (three patients). Eight of the procedures were performed on the left side of the brain.

Central to our assessment protocol was a quantitative movement analysis paradigm that provided an objective, instrumental measurement of MS tremor. This technique recorded movement during left-to-right and far-to-near arm reaching movements. Analysis of these data allowed the separation of tremor-related movement from other non-oscillatory movement that may represent dysmetria. In addition, clinical rating scales, disability questionnaires, and a functional upper extremity task (box and blocks test) were performed pre- and postoperatively.

Preliminary results at the 3 mo postoperative assessment are reported in Table 3.

Although this assessment protocol documents a statistically significant group treatment effect in MS tremor, several points need to be emphasized:

1. The measured improvement in disability is small in comparison to the measured improvements in tremor. This presumably reflects the fact that much neurologic disability in MS tremor patients is not attributable to tremor.

Table 2
Thalamic (Vim) Deep Brain Stimulation for MS Tremor

DBS series, year	N	Some sustained benefit	Improvement with tremor at last F/U mild or absent	% with no tremor[a]	Follow-up months	Permanent complications	# with MS relapse	Deaths	Imaging used for coordinates	Micro- or semi-microelectrode recording to enhance localization?
Geny et al. (1996) *(21)*	13	9 of 13 (69.2%)	?1 of 13	0 of 13	Mean, 13.4 (8–26)	None	3 within 12 mo.; thought no different than chance	0	Ventriculogram	Semi-microelectrode
Montgomery et al. (1999) *(36)*	15	14 of 15 = 93% (one not implanted after hematoma)	?	?	<3 to >12	Intracerebral hematoma with stimulator placement aborted; no permanent deficits	1	0	MRI & CT	Micro-electrode
Schuurman et al. (2000) *(26)*	5	3 of 5 (60%)	3 of 5 (60%)	2 of 5 (40%)	6	Dysarthria = 2; severe gait/balance disturbance = 1; arm ataxia = 1	?	0	Ventriculogram	Macro-electrode

[a]This category includes cases where the author described tremor that was so minimal that it seemed to be clinically meaningless.

Table 3
Improvement after Vim Thalamotomy or Thalamic Stimulation in MS Patients (Mayo-Rochester Experience)

Efficacy measures	Mean pre-operative	Mean postoperative (3 mo)	Median % improvement	Significance
Disability Scale	56.6 ± 12.7	52.3 ± 14.6	6.9	$p < .05$[a]
Clinical Tremor Rating Scores	13.0 ± 3.8	5.7 ± 4.6	62.5	$p < .05$[a]
Quantitative Left-Right Tremor	3.7 ± .84	3.1 ± .57	39.4	$p < .05$[a]
Quantitative Far-Near Tremor	4.2 ± .84	3.7 ± .63	63.5	$p < .05$[a]
Box and blocks score	0[b]	17[b]	15 blocks	$p < .05$[c]

$N = 9$ patients.
[a]Student's t-test.
[b]Median.
[c]Wilcoxon signed rank test.

2. Despite the significant group treatment effect, the response to surgery was variable with one-third having marked quantitative improvement, one-third showing no quantitative improvement, and one-third intermediate.

Based on these data we feel that future studies are still needed to address the long-term efficacy of surgical treatment on MS tremor and disability. In addition, the development of pre-operative criteria for prediction of surgical efficacy might allow surgery to be focused on a more select group of MS tremor patients with an increased likelihood of success.

3.2. *Post-Traumatic Tremor*

Traumatic injury to the brainstem including the superior cerebellar peduncles or their connections can result in severe tremor *(38)*. Such post-traumatic tremor may be delayed by weeks to many months following the brain injury *(38,39)*. In some cases, improvement or resolution occurs spontaneously and therefore an observation period of a year has been recommended before considering surgery *(14,18)*.

The published outcomes of thalamotomy for post-traumatic tremor are shown in Table 4. The patients described in these publications *(14,17,18,22,28,32,41,42)* were relatively young, with mean ages 16.9–39.2 yr in these eight series; the mean age was < 20 yr in five series. Duration of tremor was not listed in these articles. As tabulated in Table 4, almost all patients experienced benefit, but complete tremor abolition occurred in only a minority of patients.

The permanent surgical complication rate was higher in this group than among patients with MS tremor. Postoperative dysarthria or worsening of preexisting dysarthria was especially frequent in these studies. Whether this apparently higher complication rate is accurate or reflects differences in levels of scrutiny or reporting is unclear. However, Krauss et al. *(17)* commented that "patients with post-traumatic tremor seem especially prone to persistent postoperative morbidity…." It is not clear from this published literature which patients are at highest risk.

3.3. *Post-Stroke Tremor*

Tremor may occur following infarction or hemorrhage in the brainstem, cerebellum, or thalamus and result in a severe postural and kinetic tremor, which is nearly always refractory to medications. The thalamotomy experience for this type of tremor has been limited but outcomes were generally favorable in the four reported publications *(8,18,41,43)* summarized in Table 5.

Ohye et al. *(8)* described alterations in the intraoperative semi-microelectrode recordings among post-stroke patients, compared to those with PD. They noted reduced background activity and encountered fewer sensory neurons than in PD cases. They commented that in PD a clear topographic separation

Table 4
Thalamotomy for Post-Traumatic Tremor

Series, year[a]	N	Some sustained benefit	Improvement with tremor at last F/U mild or absent	% with no tremor[b]	Follow-up, months	Permanent complications	Deaths	Imaging used for coordinates	Micro- or semi-microelectrode recording to enhance localizatiaon?
Samra et al. (1970) *(32)*	5	5 of 5 (100%)	Perhaps 4 of 5 (80%)	?	?	Complications occurred, but not well-delineated	0	Ventriculogram	No
Andrew et al. (1982) *(14)*	8	8 of 8 (100%)	7 of 8? (86%)?	1 of 8 (13%)	?	Worsened ataxia, dysarthria, gait or hemiparesis in 5; unclear if persistent	0	Ventriculogram	Semi-microelectrode
Bullard & Nashold (1984) *(40)*	7	7 of 7 (100%)	?	probably 0 of 7	3 to 36	Worsened dysarthria = 3; worsened dysphagia = 2	0	Ventriculogram	No
Goldman & Kelly (1992) *(18)*	4	3 of 4 (75%)	3 of 4 (75%)	2 of 4 (50%)	17 to 55	0	0	CT and/or MRI plus ventriculogram	Semi-microelectrode
Marks (1993) *(41)*	7	6 of 7 (86%)	At least 2 of 7 (≥29%)	2 of 7 (29%)	?	Dysarthria = 1	0	Ventriculogram	Probably no
Krauss, et al. (1994) *(17)*	35	28 of 32 (87.5%)	21 of 32 (65.6%)	16 of 32 (50%)	Mean, 126 (3 lost to follow-up)	Of 32 patients, 11 (34%) had increased dysarthria; 3 (9%) had increased truncal ataxia; 2 (6%) had hemiballismus	0	Ventriculogram; CT in many	No
Shahzaki et al. (1995) *(22)*	11	?	?	?	3 to 60	Subdural = 1; hemiparesis = 3; numbness = 2; seizures = 1	0 0	?	Micro-electrode in recent cases
Jankovic et al. (1995) *(42)*	6	6 of 6 (100%)	Probably 1 of 6 (17%)	Probably 1 of 6 (17%)	Mean 47.2	3 of 6 patients with ataxia, dysarthria and/or weakness	0	Ventriculogram and/or CT	No

[a]Surgical sites were specified as VL, VLp, Vim, basal VL, or simply thalamotomy; 12 of Krauss *(17)* cases were targeted to zona incerta.
[b]This category includes cases where the author described tremor that was so minimal that it seemed to be clinically meaningless.

Table 5
Thalamotomy for Tremor Secondary to Stroke [a]

Series, year	N	Some sustained benefit	Improvement, with tremor at last F/U mild or absent	% with no tremor [b]	Usual F/U length, mos.	Deaths	Permanent complications	Imaging used for coordinates	Micro- or semi-microelectrode recording to enhance localizations?
Ohye et al. (1985) *(8)*	7	7 of 7	7 of 7	5 of 7	?	0	?	?	Semi-microelectrode
van Manen & Speelman (1987) *(43)*	3	3 of 3	3 of 3	2 of 3	7–11 yr in two; uncertain in other	0	Dysarthria, dysphagia, hemiparesis with at least partial recovery = 1; dystonia, ataxia of hand = 1	?	?
Goldman & Kelly (1992) *(18)*	5	4 of 5 (one died at 2 wk)	4 of 4 survivors	2 of 4 survivors	3 to 31	1 at 2 wk	Worsened dysarthria	CT and/or MRI plus ventriculogram	Semi-microelectrode
Jankovic et al. (1995) *(42)*	4	3 of 4	3 of 4	Probably 3 of 4	14.8	0	Leg weakness = 1	Ventriculogram and/or CT	No

[a]The etiology of the tremor was listed as stroke, postinfarct, or cerebrovascular accident in these series. Thalamic surgical target was described as VL or Vim.
[b]This category includes cases where the author described tremor that was so minimal that it seemed to be clinically meaningless.

Table 6
Thalamotomy for Tremor among Patients with Cerebral Palsy (CP)

Series, years	Disorder	N	Surgical site, as specified	Some sustained benefit	Improvement, with tremor at last F/U mild or absent	% with no tremor[b]	Usual F/U length, years	Permanent complications	Deaths	Imaging used for coordinates	Micro- or semi-microelectrode recording to enhance localization?
Ohye et al. (1983) *(45)*	CP: neonatal asphyxia or prematurity	8	Vim or VL-Vim; unilateral in 6; staged, bilateral in 2	8 of 8	5 of 8 plus one bilateral with one side nearly completely relieved	5 of 8	Up to 8	Not described	0	?	Semi-microelectrode
Broggi et al. (1983) *(46)*	CP = 27; progressive dystonia = 2; post-traumatic = 2; post embolic = 1; post-brain tumor resection = 1[a]	6 of a larger series which included non-CP patients	Voa, Vop & zona incerta	4 or 5 of 6	"Very good" in 3 of 6	?	1 to >4	Complications not clearly described	0	Ventriculography with air or contrast	No

Abbreviations: Thalamic nuclei, VL, ventralis lateralis; Vim, ventralis intermedius; Voa, ventralis oralis anterior; Vop, ventralis oralis posterior.
[a]CP patients not separately analyzed.
[b]This category includes cases where the author described tremor that was so minimal that it seemed to be clinically meaningless.

was typically found between kinesthetic neurons, which are more rostral, and tactile neurons, which are more caudal. Among poststroke cases, these neuronal types were intermingled, suggesting the possibility that neuronal reorganization had occurred.

Ohye et al. *(8)* also commented that larger lesions were necessary to treat poststroke tremor. They estimated that the coagulation volume necessary for tremor control was on the order of 200–300 mm^3, compared to PD, where coagulation volumes of 40–60 mm^3 were typically sufficient.

One additional series described outcomes of Vim thalamic DBS in nine patients compared to four similar patients treated with epidural cortical stimulation with tremor after brain infarction or hemorrhage *(44)*. Sustained benefit was noted in five of nine patients undergoing thalamic DBS and two of four with cortical (motor, premotor or somatosensory) epidural stimulation. Follow-up was 2–7 yr but few other details were provided in this report.

3.4. *Cerebral Palsy Related Tremor*

Most studies concerning cerebral palsy (CP) *(45,46)* targeted dyskinesias rather than tremor as the problem to be treated surgically. Outcomes of thalamotomy for treatment of CP-related tremor have been reported in two older series, summarized in Table 6. Mean patient age in these two series was 23.6 *(45)* and 16.8 yr *(46)*, respectively.

The results of these two studies suggest at least some sustained benefit in 12 of 14 patients, but the descriptions were limited and it would be premature to draw any firm conclusions about thalamotomy in CP patients. DeSalles *(47)* commented that some CP patients are unable to cooperate during the surgical procedure. This compromises the ability of the surgeon to locate the optimum surgical target and assess the result of test lesions or stimulation on the tremor. Consequently, DeSalles *(47)* performed stereotactic surgery for dyskinesias and tremor in CP patients under general anesthesia.

4. SUMMARY

The general consensus is that thalamotomy for secondary tremor results in less consistently good outcomes than thalamotomy for PD or ET. Nonetheless, the results may be gratifying in many cases. The burden of preoperative neurologic deficits may overshadow benefit from thalamotomy and limit the functional outcomes in these cases. Furthermore, underlying brain damage may distort the anatomic and neurophysiologic landmarks critical for targeting the lesion site.

At this point in time, the published experience with thalamic DBS in secondary tremor is too limited to allow conclusions about how this compares with thalamotomy. However, because of safety issues, if bilateral surgery is necessary, DBS on one or both sides is probably preferable to bilateral thalamotomy.

Although secondary tremor syndromes may also be associated with severe tremor of head, trunk, or lower limbs, published surgical experience has almost exclusively focused on upper limb tremor. Hence, further experience is necessary to address that surgical issue.

REFERENCES

1. Wasielewski, P. G., Burns, J. M., and Koller, W. C. (1998) Pharmacologic treatment of tremor. *Mov. Disord.* **13,** 90–100.
2. Sabra, A. F. and Hallett, M. (1984) Action tremor with alternating activity in antagonist muscles. *Neurology* **34,** 151–156.
3. Deuschl, G., Bain, P., Brin, M., and Committee, A. H. S. (1998) Consensus statement of the Movement Disorder Society on tremor. *Mov. Disord.* **13,** 2–23.
4. Barbosa, E. R., Teixeira, M. J., Chaves, C. J., and Scaff, M. (1991) Parkinson disease associated to a brain tumor. *Arqu. Neuro-Psiquiatria* **49,** 338–341.
5. Chang, D. C., Lin, J. J., and Lin, J. C. (2000) Parkinsonism as an initial manifestation of brain tumor. *Chung Hua i Hsueh Tsa Chih - Chin. Med. J.* **63,** 658–662.
6. Burns, R. S., LeWitt, P. A., Ebert, M. H., Pakkenberg, H., and Kopin, I. J. (1985) The clinical syndrome of striatal dopamine deficiency. Parkinsonism induced by 1-methyl-4-phenyl-1,2,3,6-tetrahydropyridine (MPTP). *N. Engl. J. Med.* **312,** 1418–1421.
7. Vidailhet, M., Jedynak, C.-P., Pollak, P., and Agid, Y. (1998) Pathology of symptomatic tremors. *Mov. Disord.* **13,** 49–54.

8. Ohye, C., Shibazaki, T., Hirai, T., Kawashima, Y., Hirato, M., and Matsumura, M. (1985) Plastic change of thalamic organization in patients with tremor after stroke. *Appl. Neurophysiol.* **48,** 288–292.
9. Whittle, I. R. and Haddow, L. J. (1995) CT guided thalamotomy for movement disorders in multiple sclerosis: problems and paradoxes. *Acta Neurochirurg. Suppl.* **64,** 13–16.
10. Whittle, I. R., Hooper, J., and Pentland, B. (1998) Thalamic deep-brain stimulation for movement disorders due to multiple sclerosis. *Lancet* **351,** 109–110.
11. Kelly, P. J. (1980) Microelectrode recording for the somatotopic placement of stereotactic thalamic lesions in the treatment of parkinsonian and cerebellar intention tremor. *Appl. Neurophysiol.* **43,** 262–266.
12. Hassler, R. (1977) Architectonic organization of the thalamus. In: *Atlas for Stereotaxy of the Human Brain* (Schaltenbrand, G. and Wahren, W, eds.), Thieme, Stuttgart, pp. 23–55.
13. Hirai, T. and Jones, E. G. (1989) A new parcellation of the human thalamus on the basis of histochemical staining. *Brain Res. Rev.* **14,** 1–34.
14. Andrew, J., Fowler, C. J., and Harrison, M. J. (1982) Tremor after head injury and its treatment by stereotaxic surgery. *J. Neurol. Neurosurg. Psychiatry* **45,** 815–819.
15. Hirai, T., Miyazaki, M., Nakajima, H., Shibazaki, T., and Ohye, C. (1983) The correlation between tremor characteristics and the predicted volume of effective lesions in stereotaxic nucleus ventralis intermedius thalamotomy. *Brain* **106,** 1001–1018.
16. Kelly, P. J., Ahlskog, J. E., Goerss, S. J., Daube, J. R., Duffy, J. R., and Kall, B. A. (1987) Computer-assisted stereotactic ventralis lateralis thalamotomy with microelectrode recording control in patients with Parkinson's disease. *Mayo Clin. Proc.* **62,** 655–664.
17. Krauss, J. K., Mohadjer, M., Nobbe, F., and Mundinger, F. (1994) The treatment of posttraumatic tremor by stereotactic surgery. Symptomatic and functional outcome in a series of 35 patients. *J. Neurosurg.* **80,** 810–819.
18. Goldman, M. S. and Kelly, P. J. (1992) Symptomatic and functional outcome of stereotactic ventralis lateralis thalamotomy for intention tremor. *J. Neurosurg.* **77,** 223–229.
19. Ohye, C., Hirai, T., Miyazaki, M., Shibazaki, T., and Nakajima, H. (1982) Vim thalamotomy for the treatment of various kinds of tremor. *Appl. Neurophysiol.* **45,** 275–280.
20. Nguyen, J. P. and Degos, J. D. (1993) Thalamic stimulation and proximal tremor. A specific target in the nucleus ventrointermedius thalami. *Arch. Neurol.* **50,** 498–500.
21. Geny, C., Nguyen, J. P., Pollin, B, et al. (1996) Improvement of severe postural cerebellar tremor in multiple sclerosis by chronic thalamic stimulation. *Mov. Disord.* **11,** 489–494.
22. Shahzadi, S., Tasker, R. R., and Lozano, A. (1995) Thalamotomy for essential and cerebellar tremor. *Stereotact. Funct. Neurosurg.* **65,** 11–17.
23. Andrew, J., Rice Edwards, J. M., and Rudolf, N. D. M. (1974) The placement of stereotaxic lesions for involuntary movements other than in Parkinson's disease. *Acta Neurochirurg.* **Suppl. 21,** 39–47.
24. Haddow, L. J., Mumford, C., and Whittle, I. R. (1997) Stereotactic treatment of tremor due to multiple sclerosis. *Neurosurg. Q.* **7,** 23–34.
25. Hitchcock, E., Flint, G. A., and Gutowski, N. J. (1987) Thalamotomy for movement disorders: a critical appraisal. *Acta Neurochirurg.* **Suppl. 39,** 61–65.
26. Schuurman, P. R., Bosch, D. A., Bossuyt, M. M., et al. (2000) A comparison of continuous thalamic stimulation and thalamotomy for suppression of severe tremor. *NEJM* **342,** 461–468.
27. Cooper, I. S. (1967) Relief of intention tremor of multiple sclerosis by thalamic surgery. *JAMA* **199,** 689–694.
28. Arsalo, A., Hanninen, A., and Laitinen, L. (1973) Functional neurosurgery in the treatment of multiple sclerosis. *Ann. Clin. Res.* **5,** 74–79.
29. Speelman, J. D. and Van Manen, J. (1984) Stereotactic thalamotomy for the relief of intention tremor of multiple sclerosis. *J. Neurol. Neurosurg. Psychiatry* **47,** 596–599.
30. Kandel, E. I. and Hondcarian, O. A. (1985) Surgical treatment of the hyperkinetic form of multiple sclerosis. *Acta Neurol.* **7,** 345–347.
31. Critchley, G. R. and Richardson, P. L. (1998) Vim thalamotomy for the relief of the intention tremor of multiple sclerosis. *Br. J. Neurosurg.* **12,** 559–562.
32. Samra, K., Waltz, J. M., Riklan, M., Koslow, M., and Cooper, I. S. (1970) Relief of intention tremor by thalamic surgery. *J. Neurol. Neurosurg. Psychiatry* **33,** 7–15.
33. van Manen, J. (1974) Stereotaxic operations in cases of hereditary and intention tremor. *Acta Neurochirurg.* **Suppl. 21,** 49–55.
34. Tasker, R. R. (1990) Thalamotomy. *Neurosurg. Clin. North Am.* **1,** 841–864.
35. Pollak, P., Benabid, A. L., Gervason, C. L., Hoffmann, D., Seigneuret, E., and Perret, J. (1993) Long-term effects of chronic stimulation of the ventral intermediate thalamic nucleus in different types of tremor. *Adv. Neurol.* **60,** 408–413.
36. Montgomery, E. B. Jr., Baker, K. B., Kinkel, R. P., and Barnett, G. (1999) Chronic thalamic stimulation for the tremor of multiple sclerosis. *Neurology* **53,** 625–628.
37. Benabid, A. L., Pollak, P., Gao, D., et al. (1996) Chronic electrical stimulation of the ventralis intermedius nucleus of the thalamus as a treatment of movement disorders. *J. Neurosurg.* **84,** 203–214.
38. Matsumoto, J., Morrow, D., Kaufman, K., et al. (2001) Surgical therapy for tremor in multiple sclerosis. An evaluation of outcome measures. *Neurology* **57,** 1876–1882.
39. Krauss, J. K., Wakhloo, A. K., Nobbe, F., Trankle, R., Mundinger, F., and Seeger, W. (1995) Lesions of dentatothalamic pathways in severe post-traumatic tremor. *Neurological Res.* **17,** 409–416.

40. Samie, M. R., Selhorst, J. B., and Koller, W. C. (1990) Post-traumatic midbrain tremors. *Neurology* **40,** 62–66.
41. Bullard, D. E. and Nashold, B. S. J. (1984) Stereotaxic thalamotomy for treatment of posttraumatic movement disorders. *J. Neurosurg.* **61,** 316–321.
42. Marks, P. V. (1993) Stereotactic surgery for post-traumatic cerebellar syndrome: an analysis of seven cases. *Stereotact. Funct. Neurosurg.* **60,** 157–167.
43. Jankovic, J., Cardoso, F., Grossman, R. G., and Hamilton, W. J. (1995) Outcome after stereotactic thalamotomy for parkinsonian, essential, and other types of tremor [see comments]. *Neurosurgery* **37,** 680–686; discussion 686–687.
44. van Manen, J. and Speelman, J. D. (1987) Thalamotomy for tremor after a vascular brain stem lesion. *Acta Neurochirurg. Suppl.* **39,** 70–72.
45. Katayama, Y., Fukaya, C., and Yamamoto, T. (1997) Control of poststroke involuntary and voluntary movement disorders with deep brain or epidural cortical stimulation. *Stereotact. Funct. Neurosurg.* **69,** 73–79.
46. Ohye, C., Miyazaki, M., Hirai, T., Shibazaki, T., and Nagaseki, Y. (1983) Stereotactic selective thalamotomy for the treatment of tremor type cerebral palsy in adolescence. *Childs Brain* **10,** 157–167.
47. Broggi, G., Angelini, L., Bono, R., Giorgi, C., Nardocci, N., and Franzini, A. (1983) Long term results of stereotactic thalamotomy for cerebral palsy. *Neurosurgery* **12,** 195–202.
48. De Salles, A. A. (1996) Role of stereotaxis in the treatment of cerebral palsy. *J. Child Neurol.* **11,** S43–S50.

III Surgical Therapy for Dystonia

17

Thalamotomy for Dystonia

Ronald R. Tasker

1. INTRODUCTION

The terrible disability inflicted by primary and secondary dystonia inspired surgical intervention in attempts to modify the associated movement disorders that strike previously normal patients out of the blue in the case of primary dystonia, or that are superimposed on a pre-existing neurological deficit in the case of secondary dystonia.

Although the work of Russell Meyers *(1)* revolutionized the treatment of movement disorders such as parkinsonian tremor when he showed that destructive lesions made in the basal ganglia could ameliorate these without interruption of the corticospinal tract, the morbidity and mortality of his open operations was not negligible. The application of stereotactic surgery to deep brain structures by Spiegel and Wycis *(2)* allowed Meyers' procedures to be accomplished more safely, thereby leading to worldwide acceptance. Very soon, large numbers of stereotactic pallidotomies were being carried out for Parkinson's disease (PD) as well as for hyperkinetic disorders such as dystonia. Unfortunately only small numbers of published reports dealt with dystonia alone; many dealt with dystonia in combination with other hyperkinetic syndromes. Furthermore, in published series lesions were often made in a variety of brain sites and outcomes in primary and secondary forms of dystonia were often intermingled. Because we are now aware that surgical outcome in the dyskinesias varies with diagnosis and with the targeted brain region, the practice of reporting mixed series containing patients with conditions that either do or do not respond well to surgery at different sites may serve to mask potential beneficial effects. This may account for the fact that this author's previous review of the early pallidotomy literature failed to disclose a clear benefit in dystonia *(3)*. For this reason, when the focus of stereotactic surgery for Parkinson's disease shifted away from globus pallidus (GP) to ventrolateral nucleus (VL) of thalamus (nucleus ventralis intermedius [Vim], ventralis oralis posterior and anterior [Vop, Voa]), and subthalamic region so did the targets for surgical treatment of dystonia. The consensus at that time was that for dystonia results after thalamotomy were superior to those after pallidotomy *(3)*.

Although thalamic nuclei other than VL such as centrum medianum (CM) *(4–6)* and dorsomedian nucleus *(7)* have also been targeted for the treatment of dystonia, these series are small and the benefits less clear. Lesioning the pulvinar appears to benefit chiefly the spasticity that accompanies some cases of secondary dystonia such as cerebral palsy (CP) *(8)*.

This chapter will review published data concerning thalamotomy in VL for the relief of primary and secondary dystonia but not that due to cerebral palsy or other hyperkinetic disorders such as chorea, athetosis and hemiballismus. The pathophysiology of dystonia remains unclear despite the identification of the gene for primary torsion dystonia (DYT1). The mechanism by which thalamotomy influences the disease remains equally uncertain. Recent advances in understanding of the role of the globus

From: Current Clinical Neurology:
Surgical Treatment of Parkinson's Disease and Other Movement Disorders
Edited by: D. Tarsy, J. L. Vitek, and A. M. Lozano © Humana Press Inc., Totowa, NJ

pallidus in parkinsonism have led to concepts of basal ganglia circuitry that might explain the disorder *(9)* while Lenz and his colleagues *(10,11)* have made interesting observations suggesting somatotopographic rearrangements in the thalamus of patients with dystonia.

2. INDICATIONS FOR THALAMOTOMY

Patients being considered for thalamotomy should have failed pharmacologic therapy such as trihexyphenidyl and L-dopa. There should be no contraindication to surgery, the disability should warrant the risk of the procedure, and it should be amenable to modification by the procedure proposed, keeping in mind that thalamotomy usually provides only partial relief of dystonia. In secondary dystonia care must be taken to separate the disability caused by dystonia from that caused by motor deficits secondary to the original neurological insult that cannot be expected to improve following thalamotomy. In all cases, the patient and family should clearly understand the limitations of thalamotomy so far as they can be predicted. Because dystonia is often bilateral and involves axial structures, bilateral surgery will frequently have to be considered. Bilateral thalamotomy is probably no longer an option in contemporary practice because of the high risk of causing speech impairment and, particularly in secondary dystonia, of causing pseudobulbar deficits. Lesions at other sites such as GP or the use of deep brain stimulation (DBS) would then have to be considered for surgery on the contralateral side. At this time it is not possible to offer definitive guidelines concerning the relative roles of ablation and DBS at different brain targets in the various types of dystonia.

3. TECHNIQUE OF THALAMOTOMY

At the Toronto Western Hospital, thalamotomy for dystonia is performed as it would be for Parkinson's disease or essential tremor and has been previously described *(12,13)*. A magnetic resonance imaging (MRI) compatible stereotactic frame is applied to the patient's head using local anesthesia and a stereotactic MRI image is made. From this, the X, Y, and Z coordinates of the anterior and posterior commissures (AC, PC) in stereotactic space are determined. Using a software program based on a personal computer, these coordinates are used to stretch or shrink the sagittal diagrams from a suitable brain atlas until the AC-PC distance matches that of the patient and the program prints out the modified diagrams ruled in 1-mm coordinates corresponding to those of the stereotactic frame as it is applied to the particular patient's head. The lemniscal relay nucleus, ventralis caudalis (Vc), is identified on the diagrams and the site within Vc in the appropriate sagittal plane is identified where tactile neurons related to the body part whose dystonia is to be modified are likely to be found. For upper limb dystonia, attention is directed to the tactile relay for the hand and digits on the same side as the dystonia, usually located in the inferior third of Vc about 15 mm from the midline. In patients with primary dystonia who have normally narrow third ventricles, exploration may have to be directed to a more medial plane, because a radiofrequency (RF) lesion made in a sagittal plane that would be safe in a patient with Parkinson's disease may encroach on the internal capsule and cause hemiparesis *(14)*. The patient is then taken to the operating room where under local anesthesia a twist drill hole is made at or rostral to the coronal suture contralateral to the dystonia and in the same sagittal plane as the intended lesion. A microelectrode capable of identifying and differentiating single cells is introduced through the twist drill hole and through a stab wound in the dura into the brain, directed at the tactile relay for hand and digits (for upper limb dystonia) and advanced by a hydraulic microdrive. Beginning about 10 mm above the target in Vc, continual recording of spontaneous neuronal activity is begun and responses are sought that are evoked by tactile stimuli to the contralateral body.

Receptive fields (RFs) are mapped and the nature of effective stimuli recorded. Recording is continued until arriving at 5–10 mm below the target. At 1-mm intervals, threshold microstimulation is carried out and response threshold and quality and location of the evoked response in the projected field (PF) is noted. RFs and PFs are then mapped on a magnified sagittal brain diagram on which the electrode trajectory is drawn by placing a suitable outline diagram of the body at the appropriate site along the trajectory at which the response is elicited. The appropriate part of the body is then shaded on this diagram and threshold, quality of response, and nature of the effective stimulus are indicated. PFs are displayed along one side and RFs along the other side of the trajectory line. Information concerning spontaneous neuronal activity is also plotted. If facial or trunk and leg RFs and PFs are obtained on the first trajectory instead of the necessary upper extremity fields, then a second trajectory is made 2 mm medially or laterally. If nontactile neurons are found, a new trajectory is made 2 mm removed in a direction dictated by the previous response. If no responsive neurons are found the electrode is usually located too medially. Once suitable tactile neurons are located, a new trajectory is made 2 mm rostrally to identify neurons sensitive to kinesthetic stimuli such as joint bending or muscle squeezing in the upper limb. These are referred to as "kinesthetic cells." Sometimes "voluntary cells" that fire in advance of a discrete contralateral voluntary movement are found rostral to the kinesthetic cells. Microstimulation at kinesthetic cell sites usually produces a feeling of paresthesia. Microstimulation at voluntary cell sites usually produces a muscle twitch in the same part of the body as the RF. Microstimulation amidst kinesthetic and voluntary cells often modifies the dystonia (usually driving it) in the same part of the body as the RFs. Such stimulation usually arrests tremor in patients with Parkinson's disease. Occasionally "dystonia cells" will be identified *(15)* that fire in time with the patient's phasic dystonic movements. If suitable kinesthetic and/or voluntary cells are not located, additional trajectories will be necessary before the target for lesioning is identified.

Once a suitable site is identified, a radiofrequency lesion is made of the same size typically used to control tremor and the effect on the dystonia and any untoward effects are observed. Unlike the tremor of Parkinson's disease or essential temor, dystonia is usually only partially ameliorated by such a lesion and quite often no clinical effect is evident in the operating room because the effect is delayed. For these reasons, thalamic lesions for the treatment of dystonia are often serially enlarged, especially rostrally, but also medially, laterally, and vertically. Cooper *(4–6)* lesioned, "the entire posterior half of ventrolateral nucleus...extending from 1–2 mm into the somesthetic nuclei—the posterior ventrolateral (VPL) and posterior ventromedial (PVM) and often into the centrum medianum." Some surgeons have also included lesions in the subthalamic area.

Postoperative care is similar to that given to patients with Parkinson's disease except that patients with severe disability, especially those with bilateral limb and truncal involvement, major underlying neurological deficits, or pseudobulbar deficits require careful attention to respiratory, nutritional, and cutaneous care as well as an active physiotherapy program.

4. RESULTS OF THALAMOTOMY

Publications concerning patients undergoing thalamotomy for dystonia are few, include small numbers of patients, often report patients with other hyperkinetic disorders, and include thalamic target sites other than VL. In addition, results in primary and secondary forms of dystonia are usually not segregated.

Beneficial results following thalamotomy are sometimes delayed *(8)* and often fade over time *(4–6, 16)*. Cooper found that 67% of his patients did well in the short-term but only 45.2% did well during long-term follow-up *(4–6)*. Cardoso et al. *(16)* reported 47% early and 35% late satisfactory results. Because 12% of their patients reportedly improved gradually over time, length of follow-up is very important in assessing results of thalamotomy in dystonia. Table 1 lists some of the published experiences with thalamotomy in dystonia. Cooper *(4–6)* found that Jewish Ashkenazi patients with a family history of dystonia musculorum deformans, who presumably harbored the DYT 1 gene, showed twice the incidence of marked improvement than other patients with dystonia, especially if operated on between the ages of 11 and 15 yr. In Cooper's series of patients, both limb and truncal dystonia improved. In our own patients with primary dystonia *(17)*, outcome was no different in patients with a family history of dystonia compared to other patients, but none of these were of Jewish Ashkenazi origin. Andrew et al. *(18,19)* reported better results in patients with segmental or focal dystonia compared with those

Table 1
Thalamotomy for Dystonia*

Author/ references	Year	No. of cases	% Bilateral thalamotomy	% Repeated	Outcome: Good	Outcome: Significant improvement	Complication %	Mortality %	Hemiparesis %	Pseudobulbar %	Dysarthria %	Ataxia %	Gait disturbance %	Personality change %	Epilepic seizure %	Comments
Cooper (13–15)	1969 1976	226	54	"Frequent"	25	45	–	2	–	13	18 Of bilateral cases	–	–	–	–	Lesions in VL, CM 35 cases had pulvinar, 2 GP lesions
Andrew et al. (17,18)	1974 1983	55	–	–	– 62 33	–	–	0	16 at 1 yr	15 All bilateral cases	56 Bilateral 11 unilateral	22	–	5	2	All primary dystonia. 3 had pulvinar lesions
Gros et al. (19)	1976	25	–	–	33	18	16	4	–	–	–	–	–	–	–	
Tasker et al. (20)	1988	57	29	45	30–57	14–34	21	2	4	2	7 All bilateral cases	5	4	0	3.5	
Kandel (5)	1989	188	33	7	22	54	10	1.8	2	1	–	–	–	–	–	72 cases VL, 74 VL + ST. VL + ST bilateral best results
Cardoso et al. (16)	1995	17	6	41	47		35	–	–	–	–	–	–	–	–	

*Variability dependent on whether primary, secondary, or atypical.

with hemidystonia or generalized dystonia. Gradual postoperative deterioration after initial improvement characterized two studies *(17,20)*.

Overall, benefit following thalamotomy in dystonia has been modest with good results ranging from 22–34% except for 62% in the focal and segmental cases reported by Andrew et al. *(18,19)* and the small group of seven atypical cases in our own series *(17)*. These results were often achieved by much larger lesions than have been required for treatment of tremor and also often include adjacent thalamic structures not usually lesioned for tremor. Moreover, frequent repetitions of thalamotomy were required in some series *(4–6)*.

The most important observation concerning complications is the frequency with which dysarthria occurred following bilateral thalamotomy. This occurred in 18% of Cooper's bilateral cases *(4–6)*, 56% of the bilateral cases operated by Andrew et al. *(18,19)*, and 7% of our own patients *(17)*, all of which occurred after bilateral lesions. Pseudobulbar deficits were also common following bilateral surgery *(4–6,18,19)*.

A review of our own series *(17)* reveals some interesting observations. Progression of dystonia occurs in both primary and secondary dystonia and, if this is ongoing at the time of surgery, is often associated with a poor result. Moreover, it was sometimes difficult to distinguish postoperative deterioration from continued postoperative progress of the disease. Twenty percent of our 30 secondary dystonia patients and 85% of our primary dystonia patients were progressing at the time of surgery, and 28% of the former and 50% of the latter appeared to still be progressing at latest postoperative follow-up.

Some studies have reported improvement in midline symptoms such as spasmodic torticollis following thalamotomy *(21,22)*. However, in our patients thalamotomy produced little benefit for speech, neck or truncal dystonia, locomotion, or manual dexterity. The apparent differences in outcome for dexterity probably reflect the underlying hemiparesis in secondary cases. Patients with secondary dystonia who were borderline walkers because of additional neurological deficits were at great risk to suffer deterioration in gait postoperatively and to respond poorly to physiotherapy.

In our hands, the chief benefit of thalamotomy occurred in patients with limb dystonia, both phasic and tonic. Upper limb phasic dystonia improved in 53% of patients with primary dystonia and in 52% of those with secondary dystonia. Upper limb tonic dystonia improved in 57% of patients with primary dystonia and 50% of those with secondary dystonia. Lower limb phasic and tonic dystonia showed similar improvement.

5. CONCLUSIONS

Thalamotomy exerts a modest beneficial effect on both the phasic and tonic appendicular features of both primary and secondary dystonia with a tendency towards loss of benefit over time. Some authors *(4–6)* report benefit for axial dystonia whereas others report a preferential effect in focal and segmental primary dystonia *(18,19)*. In many series, multiple thalamotomies were required in order to maintain benefit. Morbidity has generally been high, especially following bilateral thalamotomy, which is often required for treatment of bilateral or axial dystonia.

Although there is more experience with the thalamus as a surgical target for the treatment of dystonia, the internal segment of globus pallidus (GPi) is also being considered. On theoretical grounds GPi has certain advantages. GPi outflow neurons have a dual output to thalamus and to locomotor areas of the brainstem *(23)*. Pallidal interventions thus have the possibililty of direct access to the brainstem as well as through the thalamus to cortical fields, which may be an important advantage. However, no direct comparisons of the effect of lesions in thalamic and pallidal targets are available. In a nonrandomized, historical study of both thalamotomy and pallidotomy in various forms of dystonia, patients with primary dystonia who underwent pallidotomy demonstrated significantly better long-term outcomes than patients who underwent thalamotomy *(24)*. In this study patients with secondary forms of dystonia experienced more modest improvement after either procedure, with little or no difference in outcomes between the two procedures *(24)*.

In view of the increased understanding of the role of GP in movement disorders and the striking benefit of pallidotomy on the dystonia caused by L-dopa, we await accumulating experience so as to be able to construct an algorithm for the use of lesioning as well as deep brain stimulation in thalamus, GP, and possibly subthalamic nucleus for the relief of different types of dystonia.

REFERENCES

1. Meyers, H. R. (1940) Surgical procedures for postencephalitic tremor with notes on the physiology of premotor fibers. *Arch. Neurol. Psychiatry* **44,** 455–459.
2. Spiegel, E. A. and Wycis, H. T. (1950) Pallidothalamotomy in chorea. *Arch. Neurol. Psychiatry* **64,** 295–296.
3. Tasker, R. R. (1998) Surgical treatment of the dystonias. In: *Textbook of Stereotactic and Functional Neurosurgery* (Gildenberg, P. and Tasker, R. R., eds.), McGraw Hill, New York, pp. 1015–1032.
4. Cooper, I. S. (1969) *Involuntary Movement Disorders.* Hoeber, New York, NY.
5. Cooper, I. S. (1976) Surgical approaches to treatment and physiologic implications. In: *The Basal Ganglia* (Yahr, M. D., ed.), Raven, New York, pp. 369–383.
6. Cooper, I. S. (1976) 20-year follow-up study of the neurosurgical treatment of dystonia musculorum deformans. In: *Dystonia: Advances in Neurology*, vol. 14 (Eldridge, R. and Fahn, S., eds.), Raven, New York, pp. 423–452.
7. Spiegel, E. A. and Wycis, H. T. (1962) *Stereoencephalotomy part II. Clinical and physiological applications.* Grune and Stratton, New York.
8. Kandel, E. I. (1989), *Functional and Stereotactic Neurosurgery* (translated by Watts, G.) (Walker, A. E., ed.), Plenum, New York.
9. Vitek, J. L. (1998) Surgery for dystonia. *Neurosurg. Clin. North Am.* **9,** 345–366.
10. Lenz, F. A. and Byl, N. N. (1999) Reorganization in the cutaneous core of the human thalamic principal somatic sensory nucleus (ventral caudal) in patients with dystonia. *J. Neurophysiol.* **82,** 3204–3212.
11. Lenz, F. A., Jaeger, C. V., Seike, M. S., et al. (1999) Thalamic single neuron activity in patients with dystonia: dystonia related activity and somatic sensory reorganization. *J. Neurophysiol.* **82,** 2372–2392.
12. Tasker, R. R., Davis, K. D., Hutchison, W. D., et al. (1998) Subcortical and thalamic mapping in functional neurosurgery. In: *Textbook of Stereotactic and Functional Neurosurgery* (Gildenberg, P. and Tasker, R. R., eds.), McGraw-Hill, New York, pp. 883–909.
13. Tasker, R. R. (1988) Ablative procedures for dystonia. In: *Neurosurgical Treatment of Movement Disorders.* American Association of Neurological Surgeons, Park Ridge, IL, pp. 255–266.
14. Hawrylyshyn, P., Tasker, R. R., and Organ, L. W. (1976) Third ventricular width and the thalamocapsular border. *Appl. Neurophysiol.* **39,** 34–42.
15. Lenz, F. A., Martin, R., Kwan, H. C., et al. (1990) Thalamic single-unit activity occurring in patients with hemidystonia, *Stereotact. Funct. Neurosurg.* **54–55,** 159–162.
16. Cardoso, F., Jankovic, J., Grossman, R. G., et al. (1995) Outcome after stereotactic thalamotomy for dystonia and hemiballismus. *Neurosurgery* **36,** 501–508.
17. Tasker, R. R., Doorly, T., and Yamashiro, K. (1988) Thalamotomy in generalized dystonia. In: *Advances in Neurology*, vol. 50 (Fahn, S., Marsden, C. D., and Calne, D. B., eds.), Raven, New York, pp. 615–631.
18. Andrew, J., Fowler, C. J., and Harrison, M. J. G. (1983) Stereotactic thalamotomy in 55 cases of dystonia. *Brain* **106,** 981–1000.
19. Andrew, J., Rice Edwards, J. M., and Rudolf, N. de M. (1974) Placement of stereotactic lesions for involuntary movements other than in Parkinsons disease. *Acta. Neurochir. Suppl.* **21,** 39–47.
20. Gros, C., Frerebeau, P. H., Perez-Dominquez, E., et al. (1976) Longterm results of stereotactic surgery for infantile dystonia and dyskinesia. *Neurochirurgia* **19,** 171–178.
21. Handa, H., Araki, C., Mori, K., Mizawa, I., and Ito, M. (1962) Spasmodic torticollis treated by chemothalamotomy and chemopallidotomy. *Confin. Neurol.* **22,** 393–396.
22. Von Essen, C., Augustinsson, L. E., and Lindqvist, G. (1980) VOI thalamotomy in spasmodic torticollis. *Appl. Neurophysiol.* **43,** 159–163.
23. Pahapill, P. A. and Lozano, A. M. (2000) The pedunculopontine nucleus and Parkinson's disease. *Brain* **123,** 1767–1783.
24. Yoshor, D., Hamilton, W. J., Ondo, W., Jankovic, J., and Grossman, R. G. (2001) Comparison of thalamotomy and pallidotomy for the treatment of dystonia. *Neurosurgery* **48,** 818–824.

18

Pallidotomy and Pallidal Deep Brain Stimulation for Dystonia

Aviva Abosch, Jerrold L. Vitek, and Andres M. Lozano

1. INTRODUCTION

The progress that has occurred in our understanding of the pathophysiology of idiopathic dystonia, combined with successful surgical treatment of drug-induced dystonia in Parkinson's disease (PD), have led to renewed interest in the surgical treatment of dystonia. The purpose of this review is to summarize the current state of surgery for treatment of dystonia with special emphasis on developments during the last five years. For a comprehensive review of this field prior to 1996, see Lang *(1)*.

1.1. *History of Surgical Approaches*

Myotomy, the sectioning of muscles involved in dystonia, was used as early as 1641, when Isaac Minnius sectioned the sternocleidomastoid muscle in a patient with spasmodic torticollis *(1,2)*. This method was later abandoned in favor of denervation of the involved muscles, which proved to be a more permanent and effective treatment. In addition to myotomy, a variety of peripheral surgeries for dystonia have been attempted over the years (Table 1). Included among the peripheral surgeries for dystonia are intradural sectioning of the cervical anterior nerve roots (rhizotomy), extradural sectioning of the posterior primary divisions of the cervical nerve roots (ramisectomy), epidural cervical cord stimulation, and microvascular decompression of the spinal accessory nerve roots.

1.2. *Central Stereotactic Surgical Procedures for Dystonia*

The latter half of the twentieth century witnessed the use of ablative lesions in a variety of different central nervous system (CNS) sites (Tables 2 and 3), followed by the advent of gamma knife radiosurgery (Table 3) and deep brain stimulation (DBS) (Table 4) for the treatment of dystonia. Included in the list of central targets selected for lesioning have been the globus pallidus *(3–9)*, ansa lenticularis *(3)*, putamen, thalamus *(10,11)*, subthalamic nucleus *(12)*, dentate nucleus *(13,14)*, internal capsule *(15)*, and cerebral cortex *(16)*. The targeting of the globus pallidus in the treatment of dystonia by both pallidotomy and pallidal DBS is reviewed below.

1.3. *Pathophysiology of Dystonia*

Renewed interest in pallidotomy for the treatment of dystonia is based on an improved understanding of the functional organization of basal ganglia and thalamocortical circuits, together with observations in patients undergoing pallidotomy for PD, in whom almost complete amelioration of drug-induced "off" period dystonia has been observed *(17–20)*. Additional factors fueling renewed interest in surgical treatments for dystonia have been the lack of successful pharmacotherapy for generalized dystonia, and the occurrence of immune-mediated resistance to botulinum toxin therapy for the focal dystonias *(21)*.

From: Contemporary Clinical Neurology: Surgical Treatment of Parkinson's Disease and Other Movement Disorders
Edited by: D. Tarsy, J. L. Vitek, and A. M. Lozano © Humana Press Inc., Totowa, NJ

Table 1
Peripheral Surgeries for Cervical Dystonia

Procedure
Myotomies
Spinal Accessory Nerve (SAN) Section
Bilateral Ventral Cervical Rhizotomy + Selective SAN Section
Rhizotomy + Spinal Accessory Nerve Section + Thalamotomy/Pallidotomy
Ramisectomy + Spinal Accessory Nerve Section
Epidural Spinal Cord Stimulation
Microvascular Decompression of Spinal Accessory Nerve Roots

Modified with permission from ref. *(1)*.

Table 2
Central Targets for Generalized Dystonia

Target	References
Cortex	*(16)*
Cerebellum	*(13,14)*
Spinal cord dorsal column	*(47,48)*
Internal Capsule	*(15)*
Thalamus	*(10,11)*
Subthalamic nucleus	*(12)*
Globus pallidus	*(4,7)*

Table 3
Pallidotomy for Dystonia

Study	Diagnosis	Procedure	N	Length F/U	Improvement (Scale)
Lin et al. (1999) *(5)*	2° generalized	Bilat Pallidotomy	1	12 mo	34% (BFMDRS)
Lin et al. (1999) *(6)*	2° generalized	Bilat Pallidotomy	18	12 mo	13% (BFMDRS)
Vitek et al. (1999) *(9)*	1° generalized	Unilat Pallidotomy	3	14, 11, 7 mo	Mean = 56% (BFMDRS)
Ondo et al. (1998) *(8)*	1° & 2° generalized & hemi-dystonia	5 Bilat Pallidotomy 3 L-GPi Pallidotomy	5	Mean = 17.5 wk	Mean = 61% (BFMDRS)
Lozano et al. (1997) *(7)*	Generalized	Bilat GPi Pallidotomy	1	3 mo	79% (BFMDRS)
Iacono et al. (1996) *(3)*	1° generalized	Bilat Pallidoansotomy	1	12 mo	100% (no evidence of dystonia)
Kwon et al. (1995) *(4)*	2° hemidystonia	Gamma Knife R-GPi	1	16 mo	"Improved"

Although the pathophysiologic basis of dystonia remains unclear, electrophysiological data collected during microelectrode-guided pallidotomy in patients with dystonia and other hyperkinetic disorders have led to the development of a working model based on changes in mean neuronal discharge rate, patterns of neuronal activity, degree of synchronization, and somatosensory responsiveness of pallidal neurons *(9,22)*. Early models of hyperkinetic disorders such as dystonia were based on the assumption that changes in neuronal activity in the pallidum would be opposite to those observed in hypokinetic disorders such as Parkinson's disease. Since mean discharge rates were increased in

Table 4
Deep Brain Stimulation for Dystonia

Study	Diagnosis	Procedure	N	Length F/U	Improvement (Scale)
Vercueil et al. (2001) *(46)*	1° & 2°	Uni- and bilateral thalamic and GPi DBS	19	4.5 yr thalamic 14 mo GPi	Thalamic: None GPi: 50% (BFMDRS)
Coubes et al. (2000) *(44)*	1° (DYT1) generalized	Bilateral GPi DBS	7	12 mo	Mean = 90% (BFMDRS)
Tronnier et al. (2000) *(42)*	1° & 2° generalized	Bilateral GPi DBS	3	6 mo	59%, 14%, 34% (BFMDRS)
Loher et al. (2000) *(43)*	2° hemidystonia	R-GPi DBS + Thalamotomy	1	4 yr	"Improved"
Krauss et al. (1999) *(40)*	Cervical dystonia	Bilateral GPi DBS	3	15, 12, 6 mo	80%, 54%, 49% (TWSTRS)
Islekel et al. (1999) *(49)*	Cervical dystonia	R-GPi DBS	1	3 wk	"Improved"
Kumar et al. (1999) *(30)*	1° generalized	Bilateral GPi DBS	1	12 mo	67% (BFMDRS)
Sellal et al. (1993) *(50)*	2° hemidystonia	L-VPL Thalamic DBS	1	8 mo	"Improved"

BFMDRS = Burke-Fahn-Marsden Dystonia Rating Scale.
TWSTRS = Toronto Western Spasmodic Torticollis Rating Scale.

the internal segment of the pallidum (GPi) in the 1-methyl-4-phenyl-1,2,3,6-tetrahydropyridine (MPTP) monkey model of Parkinson's disease, a model was proposed for hyperkinetic disorders based on opposite changes in mean discharge rate in GPi *(23)*. This rate model predicted that a loss or lowering of inhibitory output from GPi would disinhibit the thalamus leading to increased neuronal activity and excessive involuntary movement. Although increases and decreases in mean discharge rate in GPi occur coincident with the development of hypokinetic and hyperkinetic movement disorders respectively, there are several problems with this model. The rate model predicts that pallidotomy should induce excessive involuntary movement and worsen hyperkinetic disorders by further reducing inhibitory output to the thalamus, whereas thalamotomy should induce hypokinetic movements and worsen parkinsonian symptoms by decreasing thalamic output. Contrary to these predictions of the model, however, pallidotomy is very effective in alleviating drug-induced dyskinesias *(24)* as well as dystonia, and thalamotomy does not worsen parkinsonian symptoms. Indeed, thalamotomy is effective in alleviating tremor and improving rigidity in patients with Parkinson's disease.

As a result of these observations, it became clear that changes in mean neuronal discharge rate alone were insufficient to account for the development of hyperkinetic and hypokinetic movement disorders. Subsequent examination of spontaneous neuronal activity in patients with dystonia, however, revealed that in addition to changes in mean discharge rate, there were also changes in the pattern and somatosensory responsiveness of neurons in GPi. Contrary to the tonic pattern of discharge present in normal animals, spontaneous discharge patterns of neurons in GPi occur in irregularly grouped discharges with intermittent pauses *(9)*. In addition, receptive fields of neurons in the sensorimotor portion of the GPi are less specific in patients with dystonia: GPi neurons in normal animals respond to movement in one direction about one joint in the contralateral limb, whereas in patients with dystonia as well as Parkinson's disease, neurons may respond to movement in multiple directions about multiple joints in multiple limbs *(9,25)*. The exact relationship between these changes in neural activity in GPi and the development of dystonia remains unclear. However, because pallidotomy is effective in alleviating dystonia, it seems unlikely that reduction in mean discharge rate alone accounts for the development of dystonia. These observations raise the possibility that primary dystonia occurs as a result of alterations in the pattern and somatosensory responsiveness of neurons in the pallidum and that pallidotomy and pallidal DBS are effective in alleviating dystonia because they serve to remove the abnormal pathological pattern of neuronal activity in the pallidum.

The gradual improvement in symptoms that occurs following surgery for nonparkinsonian dystonia, which requires several weeks to months, might be a consequence of physiological compensation that occurs in structures downstream to the pallidum, relearning of tasks, or of plasticity of the nervous system *(7,8)*. For a more detailed discussion of the pathophysiology of dystonia please see Vitek et al. *(9,22)*.

2. UNILATERAL AND BILATERAL PALLIDOTOMY (TABLE 3)

2.1. *Patient Selection*

Pallidotomy has been used with varying degrees of success to treat primary generalized dystonia *(3,8,9)*, off-period dystonia in Parkinson's disease, and dystonia associated with cerebral palsy (CP) *(5)*, cervical dystonia *(25a)*, Huntington's disease (HD) *(26)*, Hallervordan-Spatz disease *(27)*, and brain injury or structural lesions *(5,6,8)*.

2.2. *Technique*

The following description of operative technique applies to targeting GPi for both pallidotomy and GPi DBS. In our experience, physiological localization based on microelectrode recording data has been extremely important for accurate target identification. Comparison between the accuracy of target localization using conventional radiographic techniques versus microelectrode recording has demonstrated a frequent difference in the final target location from that predicted by brain imaging alone. Thus, reliance solely on magnetic resonance imaging (MRI)-based anatomical localization may be problematic given the frequent discrepancies between expected location based on MRI data and the actual final target location based on microelectrode recording *(28)*.

The technical details of stereotactic pallidal surgery are covered elsewhere in this volume. Briefly, patients undergo stereotactic MR or CT imaging to target GPi directly or indirectly as a function of its relationship to the anterior (AC) and posterior (PC) commissures. The coordinates of the patient's AC and PC are entered into a computer program that then adjusts the 20-mm lateral template of the Schaltenbrand-Wahren atlas *(29)* by either shrinking or lengthening the AC-PC length of the template. Microelectrode data is recorded on this adjusted map.

Following MRI, the patient is taken to the operating room and positioned on the operating room table. Depending on whether bilateral simultaneous or staged unilateral procedures are performed, unilateral or bilateral paramedian incisions are made at the level of the coronal suture. A burr hole is drilled within each incision and the underlying dura is opened. Starting 10–50 mm above GPi, a microelectrode is driven towards the target. Single and multi-unit neuronal discharges are amplified, filtered, displayed on an oscilloscope, and fed to an audio monitor. The discharge frequency of particular neurons, the relative size and shape of the action potentials, and audio monitoring of firing patterns are all determined.

Within the pallidal complex, cells of the GPe are encountered first followed by a region devoid of cells that corresponds to the lamina between GPe and GPi. An increase in background noise precedes entry into GPi. The electrode then passes into another cell-sparse region that overlies the optic tract. Microelectrode recording is used to identify movement-related neurons within the GPi and to determine its borders. Neurons in GPi are examined for their receptive field properties by characterizing their responses to passive and active manipulations of the extremities and orofacial structures. High frequency stimulation (0.1–100 μAmps, one second train, 300 Hz, 100 μs pulse width) is performed through the same electrode. The internal capsule is identified at the posterior border of GPi by the absence of somato-dendritic action potentials and by the production of contralateral muscular contractions with low threshold microstimulation. The optic tract is identified within 2–3 mm of the ventral border of GPi by the production of flash-evoked action potentials in optic tract axons and by the production of contralateral phosphenes in response to microstimulation of the optic tract *(7)*. The location of the structures identified (GPe, GPi, optic tract, and corticospinal tracts) along each track are then plotted together with the location of neurons and their identified receptive fields to develop a physiological map of the pallidum. This map is then aligned with parasagittal planes of the basal ganglia taken from the human atlas.

Firing rates of GPi neurons in dystonia patients have been reported to be in the range of 80–85 Hz and therefore lower than those recorded in Parkinson's disease *(7,30)*, but recording techniques and states of consciousness may have influenced some of these data. For example, intravenous propofol has been shown to decrease neuronal firing rates in locus coeruleus and neocortical neurons, thereby confounding assessments of neuronal firing rate in the dystonic pallidum *(31,32)*. As yet, no studies have been published that correlate specific characteristics of neuronal activity, such as neuronal firing rate and pattern, with surgical outcome.

Once the desired target within GPi has been identified, the microelectrodes are removed and either a lesioning probe or DBS electrode is inserted into the target. A radiofrequency lesion is generated with a thermistor-coupled electrode heating up to 60–90°C for a period of 60–90 s *(33)*, although these lesion parameters may vary somewhat between centers. The technique for placement of DBS electrodes has been described elsewhere *(34)*. In programming DBS stimulators for dystonia patients, a much longer pulse width (>210 μs) is usually required to achieve clinical effects than is typically used for Parkinson's disease (60–90 μs) *(30)*.

2.3. *Outcome of Pallidotomy for Dystonia (Table 3)*

Iacono et al. *(3)* noted that bilateral posteroventral pallidotomy and pallido-ansotomy were effective in alleviating the dystonia and dyskinesias of Parkinson's disease without the high incidence of speech impairment that had been associated with bilateral thalamotomy. They therefore performed simultaneous, bilateral, posteroventral pallidoansotomy on a patient who was severely incapacitated by primary generalized dystonia. The patient's dystonia immediately resolved postoperatively and remained absent at 12 mo of follow-up.

Lozano et al. reported a patient with generalized dystonia treated by simultaneous, bilateral GPi pallidotomy *(7)*. The patient was a 9-yr-old Ashkenazic Jewish boy with severe, juvenile-onset, generalized dystonia of variable distribution, carrying a deletion in the DYT1 gene. Bilateral chronic DBS was considered but decided against in favor of radiofrequency-generated pallidal lesions because of the patient's young age and the possibility of electrode migration with subsequent body and brain growth. Microelectrode recording and stimulation were used to map the location of GPi and its boundaries. The mean firing rates of GPi neurons were markedly reduced (right = 21 ± 2.4; left = 31 ± 2.8) compared with firing rates of GPi neurons in patients with Parkinson's disease. The patient's Burke-Fahn-Marsden Dystonia Rating Scale (BFMDRS) *(35)* improved by 31% 5 d following surgery and 79% 3 mo following surgery. The patient was left with mild persistent hypophonia but axial and appendicular symptoms were both improved.

Vitek et al. reported on three patients with generalized dystonia who underwent unilateral pallidotomy *(9,22)*. All three patients improved following pallidotomy. Improvement on the Burke-Fahn-Marsden motor and disability scales (BFMDRS) shortly following surgery (1–8 wk) was 80 and 72%, respectively. Longer-term follow-up (7–14 mo) revealed sustained improvement in the two patients who had predominately appendicular symptoms. However the patient with predominately axial dystonia regressed over the following year with a return of axial symptoms *(9)*. Subsequent contralateral DBS implantation led to dramatic improvement in axial symptoms with an overall improvement in the BFMDRS of 82%, which has persisted over 4 yr of follow-up (Vitek, unpublished observations). Mean discharge rates in GPi were significantly lower than those reported in patients with Parkinson's disease (50 ± 20 Hz). Somatosensory responses, however, were similar to those reported for Parkinson's disease with neurons responding to movement in multiple directions about multiple joints, often in more than one limb *(9,22,25)*.

Ondo et al. reported results using pallidotomy to treat dystonia in eight patients *(8)*. Five patients underwent bilateral pallidotomy for generalized dystonia and three patients underwent unilateral left-sided pallidotomy for asymmetric symptoms. All patients with oromandibular or axial dystonia underwent bilateral procedures. Four patients had primary and four patients had secondary dystonia. Patients were placed under general anesthesia for the procedures due to the severity of their involuntary movements. Single unit extracellular recordings were used to help localize the target and photic stimulation was used to identify the optic tracts. Lesions were generated by radiofrequency. The mean BFMDRS score improved by 61.2 ± 13.6% ($p < 0.01$), with a mean follow-up of 17.5 wk. The authors noted that the typical pattern of symptom amelioration was a moderate improvement during the immediate postoperative period with continued improvement over the subsequent 1–3 mo. The number of patients was too small to draw conclusions about the response of patients with primary as opposed to secondary dystonia, but the authors point out that the patient who received the least benefit had post-traumatic dystonia. Additionally, no conclusions could be drawn about the efficacy of unilateral versus bilateral pallidotomy in the treatment of dystonia, because the type of procedure was chosen based on preoperative symptom distribution. The authors noted, however, that one patient who underwent a staged bilateral pallidotomy derived predominantly contralateral benefit following the first procedure and axial and bilateral improvement following the second procedure. These observations are consistent with older surgical experience in which axial symptoms were reported to respond better and more consistently following bilateral than unilateral ablative procedures *(36)*.

Lin and colleagues *(5,6)* reported results of bilateral posteroventral pallidotomy in 18 patients with secondary generalized dystonia due to a variety of etiologies. They noted only a 13% improvement in BFMDRS scores 12 mo after surgery, with significant improvement limited to the mouth, neck, speech, and swallowing. These findings are in contrast to those reported by Ondo et al. *(8)* of a 61% improvement in dystonia at follow-up, with greater improvement in appendicular as opposed to axial symptoms. These discrepancies highlight the heterogeneous nature of the dystonias and serve as a cautionary note in any attempt to broadly apply the findings of individual studies.

There is only a very small experience with pallidal radiosurgery for the treatment of dystonia. Kwon and Whang *(4)* published a case report concerning a woman with secondary dystonia who was treated by posteroventral pallidotomy using gamma knife radiosurgery (4 mm collimator; 180 Gy). No standardized outcome rating scale was used in her evaluation but the authors reported sustained improvement in the patient's dystonia 16 mo following treatment. Her post-treatment course was marred by the appearance of a contralateral, homonymous hemianopsia at 6 mo following radiosurgery. Target verification by electrophysiological technique is obviously not possible when using radiosurgery to treat dystonia. Subsequent investigators have recommended limiting the dose to less than 160 Gy in order to minimize complications *(36a)*. The role of radiosurgery in the treatment of dystonia is currently highly uncertain.

3. UNILATERAL AND BILATERAL GP DBS (TABLE 4)

As with DBS for other movement disorders, pallidal DBS for dystonia, by contrast with pallidal ablation, affords the advantages of reversibility and the ability to alter stimulus parameters in order to enhance efficacy or decrease adverse effects of stimulation.

GPi modulates primary and association areas of motor cortex via its projections to the thalamus. Excessive activation of these motor areas has been demonstrated in both idiopathic *(37)* and acquired dystonia *(38)*. Although the exact mechanism of DBS is unknown, the frequency-dependent nature of the response to stimulation suggests that overriding or pacing of abnormally patterned neuronal activity may be important to the mechanism of action of DBS *(30)*.

More recently, the subthalamic nucleus (STN) has become a target for the surgical treatment of Parkinson's disease. High-frequency STN DBS has been noted to immediately suppress off-period dystonia *(12,39)*.

3.1. Indications

The indications for pallidal DBS are the same as for pallidotomy, with the added potential benefit of creating a "lesion" that is both reversible and modifiable. These characteristics seem especially desirable in young patients, such as those with juvenile-onset or secondary dystonia in whom additional lesions may lead to unexpected adverse effects that would be potentially irreversible following a permanent lesion.

3.2. Outcome

The striking benefit of bilateral pallidotomy in patients with dystonia *(7,8)* led Kumar et al. *(30)* to place bilateral GPi DBS electrodes in a single patient with idiopathic generalized dystonia with significant improvement in all aspects of dystonia, which was sustained over a period of 1 yr. This patient underwent PET imaging during a motor task 1 yr postoperatively with and without GPi DBS. In a double-blinded study, GPi stimulation was found, in time-locked fashion, to reduce bilateral PET activation in various motor cortical areas, including primary motor, lateral premotor, supplementary motor, anterior cingulate, prefrontal areas, and the ipsilateral lentiform nucleus. Because GPi is known to modulate primary and association motor cortex activity and excessive activation of these areas is present in primary and secondary dystonia, these authors proposed that the mechanism of GPi DBS might be one of direct suppression of excess motor area activation.

Krauss et al. *(40)* treated three patients with cervical dystonia resistant to medications and unsuitable for peripheral denervation with bilateral GPi DBS. They noted a gradual and significant improvement in symptoms over the first three months postoperatively with further improvement at later follow-up. On a modified version of the Toronto Western Spasmodic Torticollis Rating Scale (TWSTRS) *(41)*, patients demonstrated 80, 54, and 49% improvement in total functional disability at postoperative mo 15, 12, and 6, respectively.

Tronnier and Fogel *(42)* reported two cases of primary and one case of secondary generalized dystonia in young adults refractory to medication, who improved significantly on the BMFDRS 6 mo following bilateral pallidal DBS.

Loher et al. *(43)* reported their long-term results on a single patient with post-traumatic hemidystonia who underwent chronic GPi DBS. Their patient was a 24-yr-old man who developed left-sided hemidystonia, pain, and tremor following a head injury at the age of 15. Previous right-sided thalamotomy improved his tremor but only transiently ameliorated the dystonic symptoms. It was therefore decided to attempt treatment with chronic GPi DBS. A target was chosen in the ventroposterolateral portion of the right GPi, 21 mm lateral to midline, 3 mm below the intercommissural line, and 2 mm anterior to the mid-commissural point. Stimulation parameters were set initially at amplitude 0.75V, pulse width 180 μs, and frequency 130 Hz, resulting in early postoperative improvements in both the patient's dystonia as well as associated pain. Several months later, amplitude was increased to 1 V in an attempt to improve control of the dystonia and pulse width reduced to 150 μs to eliminate stimulation-induced paresthesias that were evoked at the higher amplitude. There was further improvement in the patient's dystonia at 2 yr and sustained improvement at 4 yr after surgery, although no standard rating scale was used in the assessment of outcome.

Coubes et al. *(44)* reported their results of bilateral GPi DBS in seven patients (six children and one adult) with DYT1 generalized dystonia. The patients included six children and one adult, with mean preoperative BFMDRS scores of 62 (out of 120). Surgery was carried out under general anesthesia, using MRI-based stereotactic localization of the posteroventral portion of the globus pallidus internus *(45)* and no microelectrode recording. Improvement occured gradually over the course of 3 mo, with a 90% improvement in BFMDRS scores at 1 yr after surgery. The authors note that although the one adult patient operated on attained a 97% improvement in his dystonia score, secondary skeletal deformities limited full functional recovery in this patient.

Finally, in a large retrospective experience accumulated over 12 yr, Vercouil et al. *(46)* reported on 19 patients (mean age 34.8 yr) treated with unilateral (6 patients) or bilateral (16 patients) DBS. The first 12 consecutive patients (4 with primary and 8 with secondary dystonia) were treated with ventrolateral (VL) thalamic DBS. Three of these patients as well as the next seven consecutive patients (5 primary and 2 secondary dystonia) were treated with GPi DBS, two of whom were not treated chronically because of infection and preliminary negative responses to stimulation. Mean follow-up period was 4.5 yr for VL patients and 14 mo for GPi patients. Mean BFMDRS scores in the seven of 12 VL patients in which they were carried out failed to improve despite good functional results, especially for dystonic tremor, in six of 12 patients. By contrast, mean BFMDRS scores in the 10 GPi patients improved by 50%. The authors concluded that GPi DBS was superior to VL DBS and that patients with primary dystonia improved more than those with secondary dystonia.

3.3. *Complications of DBS Surgery*

The use of preoperative MR-based localization, frame-based stereotaxy, intra-operative microelectrode recording and macrostimulation to assess proximity to the optic tract and the internal capsule have all improved localization in the placement of DBS electrodes. Nonetheless, errant placement of DBS electrodes has been reported despite the use of all of these techniques *(42)*. Although data for surgical intracranial hemmorhage in dystonia patients has not been established, a combined symptomatic and asymptomatic hemmorhage rate of approx 3% should be anticipated as for other stereotactic neurosurgical procedures.

The complication rate for the placement of DBS for movement disorders varies according to institution. Hardware breakage, skin erosion, and infection necessitating removal of hardware have all been reported *(30)*.

4. CONCLUSIONS

The accumulated reports in relatively small numbers of patients indicate that pallidotomy and pallidal DBS may both be safe and effective treatments for dystonia. However, determination of the optimal surgical treatment for dystonia is currently not possible given the variability in types of dystonia, surgical techniques, brain targets, underlying pathophysiological mechanisms, the length and nature of follow-up, and the lack of blinded, prospective trials in larger numbers of patients.

REFERENCES

1. Lang, A. E. (1998) Surgical treatment of dystonia. *Adv. Neurol.* **78,** 185–198.
2. Putnam, T., Herz, E., and Glaser, G. (1949) Spasmodic torticollis. *Arch. Neurol. Psychiatry* **61,** 240–247.
3. Iacono, R., Kuniyoshi, S., Lonser, R., et al. (1996) Simultaneous bilateral pallidoansotomy for idiopathic dystonia musculorum deformans. *Pediatr. Neurol.* **14,** 145–148.
4. Kwon, Y. and Whang, C. (1995) Stereotactic Gamma Knife radiosurgery for the treatment of dystonia. *Stereotact. Funct. Neurosurg.* **64,** 222–227.
5. Lin, J.-J., Lin, G.-Y., Shih, C., et al. (1999) Benefit of bilateral pallidotomy in the treatment of generalized dystonia. *J. Neurosurg.* **90,** 974–976.
6. Lin, J.-J., Lin, S.-Z., and Chang, D.-C. (1999) Pallidotomy and generalized dystonia (Letter to the Editor). *Mov. Disord.* **14,** 1057–1059.
7. Lozano, A., Kumar, R., Gross, R., et al. (1997) Globus pallidus internus pallidotomy for generalized dystonia. *Mov. Disord.* **12,** 865–870.
8. Ondo, W., Desaloms, J., Jankovic, J., et al. (1998) Pallidotomy for generalized dystonia. *Mov. Disord.* **13,** 693–698.
9. Vitek, J., Chockkan, V., Zhang, J., et al. (1999) Neuronal activity in the basal ganglia in patients with generalized dystonia and hemiballismus. *Ann. Neurol.* **46,** 22–35.
10. Cooper, I. (1976) 20-year followup study of the neurosurgical treatment of dystonia musculorum deformans. *Adv. Neurol.* **14,** 423–452.
11. Tasker, R., Doorly, T., and Yamashiro, K. (1988) Thalamotomy in generalized dystonia. *Adv. Neurol.* **50,** 615–631.

12. Krack, P., Pollak, P., Limousin, P., et al. (1999) From off-period dystonia to peak-dose chorea. The clinical spectrum of varying subthalamic nucleus activity. *Brain* **122,** 1133–1146.
13. Manrique, M., Oya, S., Vaquero, J., et al. (1978) Chronic paleocerebellar stimulation for the treatment of neuromuscular disorders. Four case report. *Appl. Neurophysiol.* **41,** 237–247.
14. Zervas, N. T. (1977) Long-term review of dentatectomy in dystonia musculorum and deformans and cerebral palsy. *Acta Neurochir. (Wien)* 49–51.
15. Cooper, I. S., Upton, A. R., and Amin, I. (1980) Reversibility of chronic neurologic deficits. Some effects of electrical stimulation of the thalamus and internal capsule in man. *Appl. Neurophysiol.* **43,** 244–258.
16. Giuffre, R. and Ferrante, L. (1975) [Surgical treatment of spasmodic torticollis. Physiopathological considerations and follow-up of 20 cases (author's transl)]. *Riv. Patol. Nerv. Ment.* **96,** 195–208.
17. Baron, M. S., Vitek, J. L., Bakay, R. A., et al. (1996) Treatment of advanced Parkinson's disease by posterior GPi pallidotomy: 1-year results of a pilot study. *Ann. Neurol.* **40,** 355–366.
18. Dogali, M., Fazzini, E., Kolodny, E., et al. (1995) Stereotactic ventral pallidotomy for Parkinson's disease. *Neurology* **45,** 753–761.
19. Laitinen, L., Bergenheim, A., and Hariz, M. (1992) Leksell's posteroventral pallidotomy in the treatment of Parkinson's disease. *J. Neurosurg.* **76,** 53–61.
20. Lozano, A., Lang, A., Galvez-Jimenez, N., et al. (1995) Effect of GPi pallidotomy on motor function in Parkinson's disease. *Lancet* **346,** 1383–1387.
21. Jankovic, J. (1998) Re-emergence of surgery for dystonia. *J. Neurol. Neurosurg. Psychiatry* **65,** 434.
22. Vitek, J. L. and Giroux, M. (2000) Physiology of hypokinetic and hyperkinetic movement disorders: model for dyskinesia. *Ann. Neurol.* **47,** S131–S140.
23. DeLong, M. R. (1990) Primate models of movement disorders of basal ganglia origin. *Trends Neurosci.* **13,** 281–285.
24. Jankovic, J., Lai, E., Krauss, J., et al. (1997) Surgical treatment of levopoda-induced dyskinesias. *Adv. Neurol.* **80,** 603–609.
25. Vitek, J., Bakay, R. A. E., Hashimoto, T., et al. (1998) Microelectrode-guided pallidotomy: technical approach and its application in medically intractable Parkinson's disease. *J. Neurosurg.* **88,** 1027–1043.

25a. Krauss, J. K., Toups, E. G., Jankovic, J., et al. (1997) Symptomatic and functional outcome of surgical treatment of cervical dystonia. *J. Neurol. Neurosurg. Psychiatry* **63,** 642–648.

26. Cubo, E., Shannon, K., Penn, R., et al. (2000) Internal globus pallidotomy in dystonia secondary to Huntington's disease. *Mov. Disord.* **15,** 1248–1251.
27. Justesen, C., Penn, R., Kroin, J., et al. (1999) Stereotactic pallidotomy in a child with Hallervorden-Spatz disease. Case report. *J. Neurosurg.* **90,** 551–554.
28. Starr, P. A., Vitek, J. L., DeLong, M., et al. (1999) Magnetic resonance imaging-based stereotactic localization of the globus pallidus and subthalamic nucleus. *Neurosurg.* **44,** 303–313; discussion 313–304.
29. Schaltenbrand, G. and Wahren, W. (1977) Atlas for stereotaxy of the human brain/Georges Schaltenbrand and Waldemar Wahren. Architectonic organization of the thalamic nuclei by Rolf Hassler: with an accompanying guide, 2nd ed. Thieme, Stuttgart.
30. Kumar, R., Dagher, A., Hutchison, W., et al. (1999) Globus pallidus deep brain stimulation for generalized dystonia: clinical and PET investigation. *Neurology* **53,** 871–874.
31. Antkowiak, B. (1999) Different actions of general anesthetics on the firing patterns of neocortical neurons mediated by the GABA(A) receptor. *Anesthesiology* **91,** 500–511.
32. Chen, C. L., Yang, Y. R., and Chiu, T. H. (1999) Activation of rat locus coeruleus neuron GABA(A) receptors by propofol and its potentiation by pentobarbital or alphaxalone. *Eur. J. Pharmacol.* **386,** 201–210.
33. Lozano, A., Hutchison, W., Kiss, Z., et al. (1996) Methods for microelectrode-guided posteroventral pallidotomy. *J. Neurosurg.* **84,** 194–202.
34. Galvez-Jimenez, N., Lozano, A., Tasker, R., et al. (1998) Pallidal stimulation in Parkinson's disease patients with a prior unilateral pallidotomy. *Can. J. Neurolog. Sci.* **25,** 300–305.
35. Burke, R., Fahn, S., Marsden, C., et al. (1985) Validity and reliability of a rating scale for the primary torsion dystonias. *Neurology* **35,** 73–77.
36. Vitek, J. L. (1998) Surgery for dystonia. *Neurosurg. Clin. N. Am.* **9,** 345–366.

36a. Friehs, G., Noren, G., Ohye, C., et al. (1996) Lesion size following Gamma Knife treatment for functional disorders. *Stereotact. Funct. Neurosurg.* **66,** 320–328.

37. Ceballos-Baumann, A., Passingham, R., Warner, T., et al. (1995) Overactive prefrontal and underactive motor cortical areas in idiopathic dystonia. *Ann. Neurol.* **37,** 363–372.
38. Ceballos-Baumann, A., Passingham, R., Marsden, C., et al. (1995) Motor reorganization in acquired hemidystonia. *Ann. Neurol.* **37,** 746–757.
39. Limousin, P., Pollak, P., Hoffmann, D., et al. (1996) Abnormal involuntary movements induced by subthalamic nucleus stimulation in parkinsonian patients. *Mov. Disord.* **11,** 231–235.
40. Krauss, J. K., Pohle, T., Weber, S., et al. (1999) Bilateral stimulation of globus pallidus internus for treatment of cervical dystonia. *Lancet* **354,** 837–838.
41. Consky, E. S. and Lang, A. E. (1994) Clinical assessments of patients with cervical dystonia. In: *Therapy with Botulinum Toxin* (Jankovic, J., and Hallett, M., eds.), Marcel Dekker, New York, pp. 2111–2137.
42. Tronnier, V. and Fogel, W. (2000) Pallidal stimulation for generalized dystonia. *J. Neurosurg.* **92,** 453–456.
43. Loher, T., Hasdemir, M., Burgunder, J.-M., et al. (2000) Long-term follow-up study of chronic globus pallidus internus stimulation for posttraumatic hemidystonia. *J. Neurosurg.* **92,** 457–460.

44. Coubes, P., Roubertie, A., Vayssiere, N., et al. (2000) Treatment of DYT1-generalised dystonia by stimulation of the internal globus pallidus. *Lancet* **355,** 2220–2221.
45. Vayssiere, N., Hemm, S., Zanca, M., et al. (2000) Magnetic resonance imaging stereotactic target localization for deep brain stimulation in dystonic children. *J. Neurosurg.* **93,** 784–790.
46. Vercueil, L., Pollak, P., Fraix, V., et al. (2001) Deep brain stimulation in the treatment of severe dystonia. *J. Neurol.* **248,** 695–700.
47. Fahn, S. (1985) Lack of benefit from cervical cord stimulation for dystonia. *N. Engl. J. Med.* **313,** 1229.
48. Gildenberg, P. L. (1977) Treatment of spasmodic torticollis with dorsal column stimulation. *Acta Neurochir. (Wien)* **313,** 65–66.
49. Islekel, S., Zileli, M., and Zileli, B. (1999) Unilateral pallidal stimulation in cervical dystonia. *Stereot. Funct. Neurosurg.* **72,** 248–252.
50. Sellal, I., Hirsch, E., Barth, P., et al. (1993) A case of symptomatic hemidystonia improved by ventroposterolateral thalamic electrostimulation. *Mov. Disord.* **8,** 515–518.

19

Surgical Treatment of Spasmodic Torticollis by Peripheral Denervation

Pedro Molina-Negro and Guy Bouvier

1. INTRODUCTION

Spasmodic torticollis, also known as cervical dystonia, is similar to other forms of dyskinesia in that it was once considered a manifestation of a psychological disturbance rather than an organic disease. Brissaud *(1)* spoke of *torticollis mentalis*. At one time, patients suffering from spasmodic torticollis sometimes received psychiatric treatment based on the opinion of some psychoanalysts that patients were turning their head away because of unresolved psychological conflict.

Following several isolated reports concerning surgical procedures intended to section cervical muscles or nerves *(2)*, Walter Dandy published the first report of a systematized surgical procedure consisting of intradural section of the anterior roots of the upper cervical spinal nerves combined with section of the spinal accessory nerve *(3)*. Foerster and McKenzie *(4,5)* contributed to the further systematization of this surgical approach and also reported satisfactory results. However, it soon became evident that intraspinal section of the cervical spinal roots was accompanied in many cases, by swallowing impairment and a variety of unintended spinal cord lesions.

Following reports by Meyers *(6,7)* of a stereotactic surgical approach to the basal ganglia for the treatment of involuntary movements, attempts were made in several centers to find an appropriate target for treatment of spasmodic torticollis. The contribution of Hassler *(8,9)* was paramount in this regard. At Notre-Dame Hospital, under the guidance of Claude Bertrand, the Canadian pioneer of functional neurosurgery, bilateral thalamotomy became the standard procedure for the treatment of segmental cervical dystonia between 1968 and 1976 until the technique of selective peripheral denervation was offered for the first time.

2. HISTORICAL REVIEW OF PERIPHERAL TECHNIQUES

According to Dandy *(3)*, the first peripheral denervation procedure was carried out by Keen in 1891. In 1930, Dandy published the first series describing surgical treatment of spasmodic torticollis by spinal denervation of cervical muscles in seven patients *(3)*. This publication contained a detailed description of the anatomy of cervical muscles. In 1924, McKenzie *(4)* carried out intradural division of the spinal accessory nerve and the first three anterior and posterior cervical roots on one side in a single patient and subsequently promoted selective posterior intradural rhizotomy for the treatment of torticollis. However, in 1954 McKenzie *(5)* recommended against section of the posterior roots and instead proposed section of the first three or four cervical motor roots combined with section of the spinal accessory nerve. McKenzie observed that the trapezius muscle is seldom involved in the disorder and

From: Contemporary Clinical Neurology:
Surgical Treatment of Parkinson's Disease and Other Movement Disorders
Edited by: D. Tarsy, J. L. Vitek, and A. M. Lozano © Humana Press Inc., Totowa, NJ

made the important recommendation that it should not be denervated *(5)*. In the United States this procedure is called the Foerster-Dandy technique but in most other countries intraspinal section of cervical roots and the accessory nerve is referred to as the Dandy-McKenzie procedure. This technique has been used extensively and currently is still being used in some neurosurgical centers around the world *(10–21)*. Although good results have been obtained with this technique, the significant adverse effect of swallowing difficulty occurs in a considerable proportion of patients. As pointed out by Horner et al. *(20)*, this is because the extrinsic pharyngeal muscles, in particular the geniohyoid, thyrohyoid, homohyoid, sternothyroid, and sternohyoid, are innervated by the anterior branches of C1, C2, and C3, which anastomose with the hypoglossal nerve. Unfortunately, paralysis of muscles that contribute to the late phase of deglutition appears to be unavoidable with the intraspinal approach of the Dandy-McKenzie procedure.

Another concern with intraspinal procedures is the appearance of spinal cord injuries, which have been accompanied by tetraplegia, Brown-Sequard syndrome, or monoplegia. Anatomical studies of the blood supply of the spinal cord blood *(22,23)* have contributed to the understanding of these lesions. The anterior spinal artery has a descending direction of blood flow since the main vascular supply arises from the vertebral arteries. This flow is maintained until the 5th or 6th thoracic segment. The lower thoracic and lumbosacral spinal levels are supplied by the great radicular artery of Adamkiewicz in which blood flow is ascending. Collaterals for the cervical segments of the spinal cord reach the anterior and posterior spinal arteries from several radicular branches originating from the descending vertebral arteries, mainly at the level of C4, C5, and C6 from either side. It is now well-established that the radicular arteries must all be identified carefully and spared during intraspinal rhizotomy in order to prevent spinal cord ischemia *(14)*.

Insufficient denervation results in persistent abnormal movements, usually in the form of retrocollis or laterocollis, while excessive denervation results in pronounced weakness of cervical muscles with the appearance of a floppy neck. For example, postoperatively some patients are able to maintain their head erect only by making a constant voluntary effort in order to prevent the head from dropping and are unable to execute normal rotational movements of the head. However, with experience, some neurosurgeons have reported good results and only minor side effects with this technique. Figure 1 summarizes the different techniques of peripheral denervation.

3. DEVELOPMENT OF SELECTIVE PERIPHERAL DENERVATION AT NOTRE-DAME HOSPITAL

In our institution the development of selective peripheral denervation was initiated by Bertrand in 1976, eight years after the last Dandy-McKenzie procedure had been carried out and after eight years of carrying out stereotactic thalamotomy. From 1970–1976, the surgical treatment of choice for spasmodic torticollis had been unilateral or bilateral stereotactic thalamotomy. Occasionally, it was combined with unilateral pallidotomy. As a rule, we performed unilateral thalamotomy on the side opposite the direction of the most prominent abnormal movement or posture. For example, in a patient with right-sided rotational torticollis a left thalamotomy was performed. If involuntary movements persisted after this procedure a right thalamotomy was performed. Bilateral stereotactic lesions resulted in pseudobulbar symptoms in about 10% of cases and these complications were considered unacceptable for a functional surgical procedure *(13)*.

In 1976, we saw a patient with left rotational torticollis. A right thalamotomy was performed with only slight improvement. We observed that the right sternocleidomastoid muscle was very active and obviously hypertrophic. We therefore denervated the right sternocleidomastoid muscle instead of performing a second thalamotomy. The results were impressive and thereafter a series of patients were treated with a unilateral stereotactic thalamic lesion associated with a peripheral surgical approach *(24)*.

Following the satisfactory results obtained with this combined procedure, it was decided to carry out peripheral denervation of the sternocleidomastoid muscle on the side opposite the rotation as the

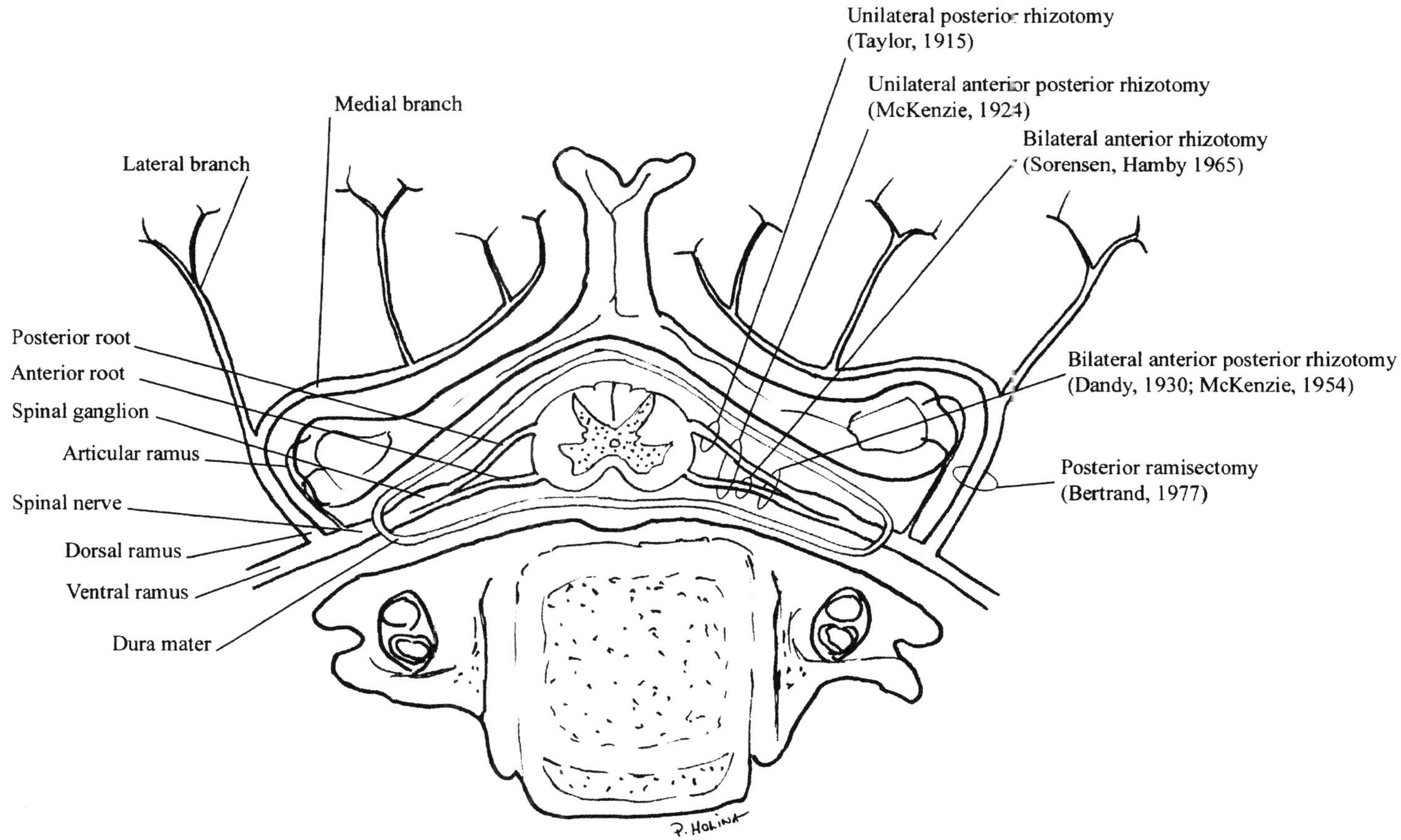

Fig. 1. Historical denervation techniques used for the treatment of spasmodic torticollis.

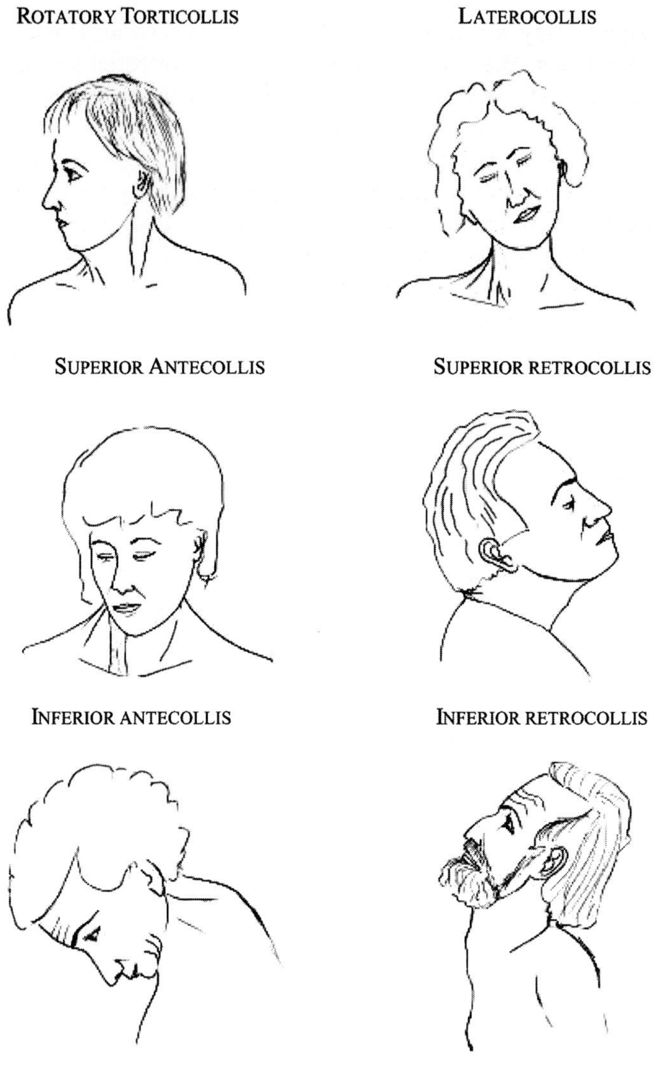

Fig. 2. The six elemental forms of spasmodic torticollis.

initial procedure. Although this produced marked improvement, residual abnormal movements persisted and we added peripheral denervation of the posterior cervical mucles on the side ipsilateral to the rotation. We were sufficiently impressed by our excellent results that this became the procedure of choice for treatment of rotational torticollis at Notre-Dame Hospital between 1976 and 1992. However, during that period of time, other manifestations of cervical dystonia such as laterocollis, retrocollis, or antecollis were considered to be untreatable by this methodology.

The next step was the treatment of retrocollis. We carried out bilateral posterior ramisectomy in our first patient with retrocollis with excellent results. However operations on several more patients with severe retrocollis produced less consistent results. It became apparent to us that there are two types of retrocollis, superior and inferior (Fig. 2). In the superior type, which we call *chin up,* the only active muscles are muscles of the posterior triangle, the recti, and obliques. By contrast, inferior retrocollis is a more complex posture due to extension movements of the lower neck and upper trunk.

Bilateral posterior ramisectomy can achieve excellent relief of superior retrocollis but is much less effective in inferior retrocollis. The main agonists in superior retrocollis are the semispinalis capitis and the superior oblique on the side opposite the rotation. A patient may have left rotational torticollis with right retrocollis or right rotatory torticollis with left retrocollis.

We first began to consider surgical treatment of laterocollis in 1993. We were very reluctant to paralyze the levator scapulae because of concern for possibly creating a sagging shoulder. In a patient with severe laterocollis combined with painful spasms of the levator scapulae, section of the four attachments of the levator scapulae to the transverse processes of C1 to C4 successfully corrected the laterocollis. This procedure was not accompanied by detectable weakness of shoulder elevation. Since then, myectomy of the levator scapulae, combined in some cases with levator scapulae denervation through the anterior ramus of C3 and/or C4, has become our procedure of choice for the treatment of laterocollis.

The surgical technique has remained essentially the same over the last 10 years. During this time, research and experience have permitted a better knowledge and understanding of the anatomy, physiology, and pathophysiology of the musculature of the neck and have influenced and modified the surgical technique. This has led to improved evaluation of the muscles involved and their relative degree of involvement, allowing for a customized peripheral selective denervation procedure properly designed for each patient.

For many years the goal of surgery was to denervate all cervical muscles that appeared to be involved in the dystonia. This aggressive approach gave excellent results but in some patients resulted in markedly limited range of voluntary movement and temporary neck weakness after the procedure. It was thus decided to proceed more prudently in step-wise fashion. The first step was intended to paralyze the agonist and synergist muscles of the the most prominent abnormal movements, even in cases where we expected that some residual abnormal movements would persist. If the result was unsatisfactory, we proceeded with a second operation intended to paralyze the remaining active muscles. This new approach is much more satisfactory. In nearly 50% of patients, the first procedure has been sufficient to control most of the abnormal movements and postures of the neck.

Despite better understanding of the physiology and physiopathology of the cervical musculature, improved patient evaluation, and considerable improvement in surgical technique we still observe residual involuntary movements in 13% of our patients. In some cases, the abnormal movements are sustained by innervation from anterior rami. Our present investigations are focused on the identification of these additional muscles and their innervation.

4. CLINICAL FORMS OF SPASMODIC TORTICOLLIS

The four directions of movement of the head and neck in cervical dystonia are flexion, extension, lateral inclination, and rotation. A distinction should be made between superior flexion and superior extension (chin down and chin up), which produce abnormal postures of the head, and inferior flexion and extension, which produce abnormal postures of the cervical spine as a whole. Superior chin up and chin down movements relate to displacement at the occipito-atlantal joint and, to a lesser extent, the atlanto-axial junction. Inferior antecollis and retrocollis result from movements of all of the cervical intervertebral joints and frequently also include the first two or three dorsal vertebrae. Figure 2 shows an example of each of the six elementary forms of spasmodic torticollis.

Besides these basic types of spasmodic torticollis, there are other clinical forms that represent various combinations of these basic movements. The authors have extensively reviewed these clinical forms of spasmodic torticollis *(25)*. In a recent review of our experience (De Soultrait and Dulou, unpublished observations), analyzing long-term results of selective peripheral denervation, the different types of torticollis were classified according to the axis of movement of the head. In these patients, rotation was the most common direction of head deviation and was present in 75% of cases (Table 1), whereas 50% of patients had abnormal movements in two axes (Table 2).

Table 1
Relative Frequency of Axis of Movement in Spasmodic Torticollis

Axis	Number of cases	Percentage
Rotatory	58	75.3
Laterocollis	15	19.5
Retrocollis	4	5.2
Total	77	100

Table 2
Distribution of Spasmodic Torticollis According to the Number of Axis of Movements Involved

Number of axes	Number of cases	Percentage
1 axis	23	29.9
2 axis	38	49.4
3 axis	16	20.7
Total	77	100

5. PREOPERATIVE EVALUATION

5.1. Clinical Evaluation

A standard medical, neurological, and family history is obtained from each patient. We have found that familial focal or generalized dystonia has sometimes been associated with aggravation or progression of dystonia following selective peripheral denervation. Although possible aggravation of dystonia may not be an absolute contraindication to surgery, we inform the patient of this possibility.

The evaluation protocol includes a careful evaluation of the directions and angles of the abnormal movements, identification of the main agonists for each movement, and identification of the muscles that either contract or are paradoxically inhibited. The Toronto Western Spasmodic Torticollis Rating Scale (TWSTRS) is used preoperatively and postoperatively in order to assess objectively and quantitatively the abnormal movements and their improvement following surgery. This evaluation is combined with a subjective assessment by the patient of his everyday activities of daily living. There are cases in which a patient has not been satisfied after surgery because expectations were excessively high or because of inability to return to a normal life, even if objective assessment of the abnormal movements and postures indicate a good result. The contrary is also true. In some patients in whom the head remains fixed in an abnormal and painful posture after many years of dystonia, pain is relieved. In these cases, the degree of postoperative satisfaction is great even if modification of head posture has not been significant.

5.2. Electromyographic Evaluation

The technique of electromyographic recording (EMG) for evaluation of spasmodic torticollis has been previously described *(25–27)*. In order to obtain accurate information regarding the behavior of dystonic muscles, the electrodes should be inserted into the proper muscles. This is relatively simple in the case of superficial muscles such as the sternocleidomastoid, trapezius, and splenius capitis. However, even the experienced neurophysiologist will frequently replace electrodes several times in order to obtain a proper recording in muscles such as the splenius capitis, semispinalis capitis, and levator scapulae. In some cases it may be necessary to insert the electrodes with the patient reclining in order to avoid a syncopal reaction. However, once the needles are inserted, verification of their position should be assessed in the sitting position in which the anatomy of the muscles is more easily recognized.

Location of electrodes is confirmed in a particular muscle when voluntary contraction of that muscle induces selective EMG recruitment. An exception is the case of paradoxically inhibited muscles that the patient has difficulty activating. For example, in patients with rotational torticollis to the left, there may be inappropriate inhibition of recruitment in left sternomastoid muscle when the patient is asked to turn his head to the right. In this case, application of resistance against the requested movement will usually bring the muscle into action and motor unit recruitment will occur.

We simultaneously record from at least four different muscles, which are the usual major agonists of head movement, in order to obtain clinical correlation between the initiation of abnormal movements and muscle discharge. In most cases of dystonia, practically all muscles will contract at one time or another, either as primary movers or as antagonists responding to the contraction of the agonist. For standard recording, we insert two 20-mm monopolar needles five mm apart in each muscle. This provides a significant sample of activity in the entire muscle. When it becomes evident that deep muscles, such as the superior obliques or semispinalis capitis, play a significant role in the abnormal movements, we use a 40-mm monopolar electrode insulated in its full length except for two mm at the tip. This allows selective recording of deep muscles that can be compared with activity in more superficial muscles in the same trajectory.

For each particular axis of head movement, we analyze voluntary movements performed by the patient at our request. For example, we have the patient rotate the head towards one side, maintain this position for about 5 s, and then bring the head back to the resting position. We then have the patient rotate his head in the opposite direction. Analysis of the EMG recordings permits us to identify muscles that are either paradoxically contracting or paradoxically being inhibited. Following analysis of voluntary movements, we carefully study the pattern of contraction of dystonic muscles. It is important to establish which muscles initiate the abnormal movement and which muscles synergistically contribute to a particular movement.

The analysis of both voluntary and involuntary movements is of major importance in the choice of operative technique. This evaluation also helps determine which muscles should be reeducated during physiotherapy in the postoperative period, because the phenomenon of paradoxical inhibition will remain unchanged even if the agonist muscles responsible for the abnormal movements are completely denervated. In order to obtain full and accurate information about the behavior of different muscles of the neck, electromyographic analysis should be performed at least 4 mo following injections of botulinum toxin, because residual paralytic effects can modify the behavior of injected muscles and provide incorrect information concerning muscle activation.

We often use 5–10 mL of a local anaesthetic agent without epinephrine to assess the role and importance of a particular muscle in producing an abnormal posture of the neck, thereby giving an idea of the eventual result if this muscle is denervated. Effects of anesthetic blocks are particularly useful in evaluating patients who have not responded to botulinum toxin.

6. INDICATION FOR SELECTIVE PERIPHERAL DENERVATION

Selective peripheral denervation is the treatment of choice for patients fulfilling the following criteria:

1. Cervical segmental dystonia present for at least 3 yr and stable for the last year.
2. A well-defined clinical type of torticollis confirmed by a specific pattern of electromyographic activity for voluntary and involuntary movements.
3. Patients having good results with repeated botulinum toxin injections are the best candidates for selective peripheral denervation although, in our experience, unsatisfactory results with botulinum toxin are not necessarily a contraindication.

For many years, we were reluctant to perform this procedure in cases of generalized dystonia. However, this is no longer the case and we have now operated on patients with generalized dystonia with results in cervical spine comparable to those in segmental dystonia. Because surgery is intended to correct segmental and not more generalized dystonia, it is essential that the clinical and electromyographic pattern of simple or combined forms of torticollis is identified. The patient must be advised of the possibility of continued progression and possibly even exacerbation of dystonia following surgery.

In order to diminish the incidence of dystonia exacerbation in the postoperative period, it is important for the patients to remain on their medications for at least 3–6 mo following surgery. Withdrawal of medications such as benzodiazepines may result in exacerbation of anxiety sometimes accompanied by increased manifestations of dystonia. The neurologist and neurosurgeon should discuss with the patient the pros and cons of surgery and establish with the patient reasonable expectations that can be obtained with surgical treatment. Patients responding consistently and repeatedly to botulinum toxin should expect to obtain at least the same result following surgery.

7. SURGICAL TECHNIQUE

We use light general endotracheal anesthesia without paralyzing agents to permit constant intraoperative neurostimulation. Unless there is a specific medical contraindication such as a patent foramen ovale, the patient is placed in a sitting position. The head is lightly flexed and maintained in position by a headrest. This position is comfortable for both the patient and the surgeon and allows access to the sternocleidomastoid muscle and/or the posterior cervical muscles in the same surgical field. Importantly, in the sitting position, the operative field remains dry, permitting safe and easy access to the posterior arches of C1 and C2, the vertebral artery, and the articular facets down to T1.

Electrical stimulation is essential to identify the spinal accessory nerve with its branches to the sternocleidomastoid muscle and trapezius. The trapezius must be spared in order to avoid shoulder elevation weakness. Identification of the anterior branches of the posterior rami of C1 and C2 is achieved through stimulation. It is mandatory to spare these anterior branches in order to avoid swallowing difficulty. Neurostimulation is also very useful to identify all of the posterior rami down to C6. During denervation of the levator scapulae, it is important to spare innervation to muscles other than the levator scapulae such as the diaphragm and trapezius.

7.1. Posterior Ramisectomy

A midline incision is made from the external protuberance to the spinous process of T1. Exposure of the suboccipital region and the posterior arches of C1 and C2 is facilitated by section of the superior nuchal line of the skull and by disinsertion of the minor and major rectus capitis posterior and the obliquus capitis inferior. Dissection is performed in a plane between the semispinalis capitis and the splenius cervicis muscles, which leads directly to the articular facets down to C6-C7. The posterior cervical intertransverse muscles are divided to denude the articular facets. It is thus possible to identify and cut all the posterior rami from C3 to C6. Dissection is pursued anteriorly until there is visualization of the attachments of the levator scapulae to the transverse processes of C1 to C4. We then identifiy the posterior rami of C1 and C2 with their anterior branches that are responsible for swallowing. These anterior branches are stimulated and the posterior ramus of C1 and C2 is cut more laterally in order to spare the anterior branches.

Since 1993 and until recently we use a posterior approach through the same middle line incision employed for the posterior ramicectomy for denervation and myectomy of the levator scapulae. However, in view of the difficulty to perform a selective denervation of this muscle, we have adopted a direct lateral approach. Through a vertical incision between the posterior limit of the sternocleidomastoid and the anterior edge of the levator scapulae the muscle and the terminal nerve branches of the anterior rami are easily attained. The posterior approach of the levator scapulae has thus been abandoned. For denervation and myectomy of the sternocleidomastoid muscle, an incision is made at

Table 3
Patient and Surgeon Degree of Satisfaction Following Surgery

Degree of satisfaction	Patient after surgery	Patient at review	Surgeon at last visit
Very satisfied	29 (37.7%)	22 (28.6%)	29 (37.7%)
Satisfied	37 (48.1%)	36 (46.8%)	24 (31.2%)
Moderately satisfied	3 (3.9%)	6 (7.8%)	6 (7.8%)
Unsatisfied	8 (10.4%)	13 (16.9%)	2 (2.6%)
Total	77 (100%)	77 (100%)	61[a]

[a]We lack medical follow-up in 16 (20.8%) cases.

Table 4
Cumulative Degree of Satisfaction Following Surgery

Degree of satisfaction	Patient after surgery	Patient at review	Surgeon at last visit
Satisfied	66 (85.8%)	58 (75%)	53 (68.9%)
Unsatisfied	11 (14.2%)	19 (25%)	8 (10.4%)

the mastoid process and prolonged posteriorly along the posterior border of the sternocleidomastoid muscle stopping over the trapezius. The spinal accessory nerve is identified at the lower part of the incision. Dissection is carried out upwards and the nerve is followed until its penetration into the base of the skull. All branches leaving the spinal accessory nerve are stimulated and those producing isolated contractions of the sternocleidomastoid muscle are cut and avulsed. Branches to the trapezius are identified and spared. The greater auricular nerve is also identified and spared in order to avoid numbness around the ear. We also carry out sternocleidomastoid myectomy because its clavicular portion is often innervated by anterior rami that have not been sectioned.

8. RESULTS

Our own experience with selective peripheral denervation has been reported previously *(25–30)*. In 1988, Bertrand and Molina-Negro *(26)* analyzed the results of selective peripheral denervation in 111 patients. The follow up was 2 yr in about 80% of cases and more than 5 yr in the remaining cases. Thirty-four (30%) reported an excellent result and 63 (56%) a very good result for a total of 97 (86%) with a favorable response.

In 1996, Bertrand et al. *(27)* reported results of selective peripheral denervation in his most recent 100 consecutive cases operated over 20 years since beginning use of this procedure. Despite improved understanding of the physiology of cervical muscles and a more thorough exposure of posterior rami, the overall results remained almost identical, with 88% reporting good results, although 48% reported excellent responses compared to 30% in the earlier series.

In a current review of our long-term surgical results at Notre-Dame Hospital (De Soultrait and Dulou, unpublished observations), the follow-up period varied between 3 and 16 yr. A questionaire was mailed to our patients and 77 provided sufficient data to complete a statistical analysis. Subjective evaluations made immediately postoperatively and at the time of the survey were compared with our own degree of satisfaction at the time of the patient's last visit (Table 3). Cumulative values of satisfied and unsatisfied responses were also tabulated (Table 4). Long-term results declined from 85% satisfied initially to 75% satisfied long-term. Overall subjective improvement compared favorably with our own evaluation. Persistence of pain following surgery was the most common reason for reported lack of satisfaction. This was followed by disappointment regarding head and neck posture compared with the patient's expectations preoperatively. Reduced satisfaction after prolonged follow-up may also be explained by the progressive nature of dystonia. In this regard, two patients operated several years earlier for simple rotatory torticollis reappeared because of involuntary rotational movements towards the opposite side. Both were treated successfully by standard contralateral selective peripheral denervation.

Results concerning selective peripheral denervation surgery using our methodology have also been reported from other centers *(31–37)*. Arce *(31,32)* has carried out unilateral or bilateral peripheral ramisectomy of C1–C5 with various combinations of sternomastoid denervation or levator scapulae section depending on the pattern of dystonia. Overall results in 145 patients were excellent or very good in 82%, good in 12%, and poor in 6%, with no significant morbidity *(32)*. Patients with laterocollis and retrocollis did as well as those with rotational torticollis, whereas patients with anterocollis had poorer outcomes. Davis *(33)* reported his experience with the same procedure in nine patients, most of whom had rotational torticollis. Over 13–21 mo of follow-up five patients experienced persistent improvement, whereas the other four patients experienced recurrence of symptoms within several months of surgery. Braun *(34)* reported on 50 patients with mean follow-up of 25 mo. Disappearance or significant improvement of dystonia occurred in 76% without major side effects. Responders to botulinum toxin did better than nonresponders.

In recent years more systematic analyses of the response to selective surgery have been carried out. Munchau et al. *(35)* carried out a prospective study in 37 patients with primary or secondary resistance to botulinum toxin. Response was assessed by the TWSTRS at regular intervals for 18 mo. Head tremor, dysphagia, and psychosocial function were also assessed using established rating scales and questionnaires. Using the TWSTRS global score, 68% of patients showed functionally relevant improvement at 12 mo after surgery. There was a mean reduction in total TWSTRS scores and pain, severity, and disability subscores of 20–40%, results that compare favorably with botulinum toxin efficacy. Measures of psychosocial function and quality of life also showed significant improvement. Six patients with primary botulinum toxin treatment failure showed no change following surgery. There were no major complications. Adverse effects included uncomfortable paresthesias in posterior cervical region in seven patients lasting up to 9 mo, transient worsening of pre-existing dysphagia in five of 10 patients, transient new appearance of dysphagia in seven patients, transient balance difficulty in three patients, and worsening of oromandibular dystonia in two patients. Although clinical signs of partial reinnervation appeared in 45% of sternomastoid muscles and 20% of splenius muscles 6–12 mo postoperatively, severity scores did not increase during this time. Two patients with more severe reinnervation who required reoperation had good outcomes

In another prospective study *(36)*, patients with secondary botulinum toxin resistance were assessed by a videotaped modified TWSTRS examination 1–6 mo following selective denervation surgery. Eight of nine patients improved following surgery while total TWSTRS score showed significant improvement. Blair et al. *(37)* carried out a retrospective study of an unselected series of 16 of their patients with primary or secondary botulinum toxin resistance who had undergone selective denervation at three other institutions with a mean follow-up of 5.2 yr. Patients were assessed by structured interview emphasizing functional outcome measures and a videotaped modified TWSTRS examination. Although TWSTRS scores improved in 85.7% of patients, only 37.5% had a moderate or complete return of normal neck function, whereas 62.5% had only minimal relief of dystonia or gain in function. Occupational disability was improved in only one patient.

Approximately 600 patients with cervical dystonia have now undergone peripheral denervation at Notre-Dame Hospital. Pursuing the work initiated by Bertrand, we have developed more precise methods of pre-operative assessment, refined our selection criteria for surgery, and have refined the surgical technique itself. This approach has allowed us to treat certain forms of cervical dystonia that were previously excluded such as retrocollis, laterocollis, and mixed forms of cervical dystonia, without any change in our long-term results.

As already discussed, for a long period of time our understanding of abnormal movements associated with cervical dystonia was very limited. We once attributed a partial clinical response to persistent involuntary movements in denervated muscles. We now believe that some residual movements are due to persistent spasm in muscles that have not been denervated. In rotational torticollis, for example, our attention was initially focused on the sternocleidomastoid muscle contralateral to the direction of rotation and posterior cervical muscles ipsilateral to the rotation while neglecting the occasional presence of mild retrocollis due to actions of the deeper lying oblique and rectus muscles. Recognition of these associated movements has led to complementary denervation, thereby reducing the number of incomplete responses.

The success rate of surgery greatly depends on careful preoperative evaluation, proper selection of patients for surgery, and the quality of postoperative physiotherapy for re-education of neck movement. Adequate denervation and intensive physiotherapy can result in normal or near-normal posture and good range of motion of the neck. Overly aggressive denervation may preclude a good result. Although the combination of selective peripheral denervation and physical rehabilitation can dramatically improve quality of life, the underlying dystonia is not cured. The patient should be aware of the possibility that dystonia may progress and require further treatment in the future. Surgery is intended to help achieve a more normal posture of the neck with improved range of motion. However, it has no direct effect on pain, although pain may be improved if it is due to dystonic muscle contraction. If the patient suffers from severe osteoarthritis of the cervical spine with limited neck movement, selective peripheral denervation may not improve range of motion.

REFERENCES

1. Brissaud, E. (1895) Leçons sur les maladies nerveuses. Recueillies et publiées par H. Meige. Masson X Cie, Paris.
2. Keen, W. W. (1891) A new operation for spasmodic wry neck: namely division or exsection of nerves supplying the posterior rotator muscles of the head. *Ann. Surg.* **13,** 44.
3. Dandy, W. E. (1930) An operation for the treatment of spasmodic torticollis. *Arch. Surg.* **20,** 1021–1032.
4. McKenzie, K. G. (1924) Intrameningeal division of the spinal accessory and root of the upper cervical nerves for the treatment of spasmodic torticollis. *Surg. Gyn. Obstet.* **39,** 5–10.
5. McKenzie, K. G. (1954) The surgical treatment of spasmodic torticollis. *Clin. Neurosurg.* **2,** 37–43.
6. Meyers, R. (1940) A surgical procedure for postencephalitic tremor with notes on the physiopathology of the premotor fibers. *Arch. Neurol. Psychiatry* **44,** 455.
7. Meyers, R. (1941) The modification of alterning tremors, rigidity and festination by surgery of the basal ganglia. *Res. Publ. Ass. Nerv. Ment. Dis.* **21,** 602–665.
8. Hassler, R. (1957/1958) Functional anatomy of the thalamus. *Physiol. Exptl. Med. Sci.* **91,** 56–91.
9. Hassler, R. (1970) Stereotactic treatment of different kinds of spasmodic torticollis. *Confin. Neurol.* **32,** 133–143.
10. Sorensen, B. F. and Hamby, W. B. (1965) Spasmodic torticollis. *JAMA* **194,** 706–708.
11. Hamby, W. B. and Schiffer, S. (1969) Spasmodic torticollis: results after cervical rhizotomy in 50 cases. *J. Neurosurg.* **31,** 323–326.
12. Tasker, R. R. (1976) The treatment of spasmodic torticollis by peripheral denervation: The McKenzie Operation. In: *Current Controversies in Neurosurgery* (Morley, T. P., ed.), pp. 448–454.
13. Molina-Negro, P. (1979) Functional surgery of abnormal movements. In: *Functional Neurosurgery* (Rasmussen, T. and Marino, R., eds.), Raven Press, New York, pp. 25–44.
14. Adams, C. B. T. (1984) Vascular catastrophe following the Dandy-McKenzie operation for spasmodic torticollis. *J. Neurol. Neurosurg. Psychiatry* **47,** 990–994.
15. Freckmann, N., Hagenah, R., and Müller, D. (1986) Bilateral microsurgical lysis of the spinal accessory nerve roots for treatment of spasmodic torticollis. *Acta Neurochirurg.* **83,** 47–53.
16. Speelman, J. D., Van Manen, J., Jacz, K., and Van Beusekom, G. T. (1987) The Foerster-Dandy Operation for the treatment of spasmodic torticollis. *Acta Neurochirurg.* **39(Suppl.),** 85–87.
17. Gauthier, S., Perot, P., and Bertrand, G. (1988) Role of surgical anterior rhizotomies in the management of spasmodic torticollis. In: *Advances in Neurology* (Fahn, S., Marsden, C. D., and Calne, D. B., eds.), Raven Press, New York, pp. 633–635.
18. Hernesniemi, J. and Keränen, T. (1990) Long term outcome after surgery for spasmodic torticollis. *Acta Neurochirurg.* **103,** 128–130.
19. Ojemann, G. A. and Ward, A. A. Jr. (1990) Abnormal movement disorders. In: *Neurological Surgery* (Youmans, J. R., ed.), pp. 4227–4262.
20. Horner, J., Riski, J. E., Ovelman-Levitt, J., and Nashold, B. S. Jr. (1992) Swallowing in torticollis before and after rhizotomy. In: *Dysphagia*. Springer-Verlag, New York, pp. 117–125.
21. Friedman, A. H., Nashold, B. S. Jr., Sharp, R., Caputi, F., and Arruda, J. (1993) Treatment of spasmodic torticollis with intradural selective rhizotomies. *J. Neurosurg.* **78,** 46–53.

22. Lazorthes, G. (1978) Spinal angiomas. In: *Advances in Diagnosis and Therapy* (Pia, H. N. and Djindjian, eds.), Springer Verlag, Berlin, pp. 1–17.
23. Turnbull, I. M., Brieg, A., and Hassler, O. (1966) Blood supply of cervical spinal cord in man. *J. Neurosurg.* **24,** 951–965.
24. Bertrand, C., Molina-Negro, P., and Martinez, S. N. (1978) Combined stereotactic and peripheral surgical approach for spasmodic torticollis. *Appl. Neurophysiol.* **41,** 122–133.
25. Bouvier, G. and Molina-Negro, P. (2002) Surgical treatment of spasmodic torticollis. In: *Neurological Surgery* (Youmans, J. R., ed.), W.B. Saunders, Philadelphia, PA, in press.
26. Bertrand, C. M. and Molina-Negro, P. (1988) Selective peripheral denervation in 111 cases of spasmodic torticollis: rationale and results. In: *Dystonia 2* (Fahn, S., Marsden, C. D., Calne, D. B., eds.), Raven Press, New York, pp. 637–643.
27. Bertrand, C. M., Molina-Negro, P., Bouvier, G., and Benabou, R. (1996) Surgical treatment of spasmodic torticollis. In: *Neurological Surgery,* 4th ed. (Youmans, J. R., ed.), W.B. Saunders, Philadelphia, PA, pp. 3701–3712.
28. Bertrand, C., Molina-Negro, P., and Martinez, S. N. (1982) Technical aspects of selective peripheral denervation for spasmodic torticollis. *Appl. Neurophysiol.* **45,** 326–330.
29. Bertrand, C., Molina-Negro, P., Bouvier, G., and Gorcyca, W. (1987) Observation and analysis of results in 131 cases of spasmodic torticollis after selective denervation. *Appl. Neurophysiol.* **50,** 319–323.
30. Bertrand, C. M. (2002) Surgical management of spasmodic torticollis and adult-onset dystonia with emphasis on selective denervation. In: *Operative Neurosurgical Techniques Indications, Methods and Results,* 2nd ed. (Schmidek, H. H. and Sweet, W. H., eds.),
31. Arce, C. and Russo, L. (1992) Selective peripheral denervation: a surgical alternative in the treatment for spasmodic torticollis. Review of fifty-five patients. *Mov. Disord.* **(Suppl. 1),** 128.
32. Arce, C. (1995) Selective peripheral denervation. Analysis and results in 145 patients. *Mov. Disord.* **10,** 698–699.
33. Davis, D. H., Ahlskog, J. E., Litchy, W. J., and Root, L. M. (1991) Selective peripheral denervation for torticollis: preliminary results. *Mayo Clin. Proc.* **66,** 365–371.
34. Braun, V. and Lichter, H. P. (1994) Selective peripheral denervation for the treatment of spasmodic torticollis. *Neurosurgery* **35,** 58–63.
35. Munchau, A., Palmer, J. D., Dressler, D., et al. (2000) Prospective study of selective peripheral denervation for botulinum toxin-resistant patients with cervical dystonia. *Brain* **124,** 769–783.
36. Comella, C. L., Goetz, C. G., Leurgans, S., and Chmura, T. A. (1998) Selective peripheral denervation surgery in cervical dystonia patients resistant to botulinum toxin injections. *Mov. Disord.* **13(Suppl. 2),** 97.
37. Ford, B., Louis, E. D., Greene, P., and Fahn, S. (1998) Outcome of selective ramisectomy for botulinum toxin resistant torticollis. *J. Neurol. Neurosurg. Psychiatry* **65,** 472–478.

20

Intrathecal Baclofen for Dystonia and Related Motor Disorders

Blair Ford

1. INTRODUCTION

In clinical practice, oral baclofen has long been regarded as a drug of choice for spasticity of spinal origin *(1,2,2a)*. Baclofen has also been considered to be an effective agent for treating dystonia *(3,4)*. However, treatment of dystonia using oral baclofen is often limited due to adverse effects, such as nausea and sedation. Intrathecal catheter systems enable higher concentrations of baclofen to reach the spinal cord than can be safely obtained through purely oral administration of baclofen *(5)*. A subcutaneous reservoir, implanted in the abdominal wall, delivers baclofen directly to the subarachnoid space by a thin catheter. In the treatment of spasticity of spinal origin, this technique has proved to be a safe and effective therapy. Intrathecal delivery enables as much as four times the concentration of baclofen to accumulate at the spinal cord using 1% of the standard oral dosage, thus limiting systemic adverse effects. Because oral baclofen reduces dystonia, clinical investigators considered that intrathecal baclofen (ITB) might benefit dystonia patients, especially for individuals unable to tolerate high oral doses of baclofen.

Although intrathecal baclofen treatment of dystonia has been successful in selected applications, the technique has not found widespread use due to several factors. These include the relative therapeutic resistance of dystonia as compared to spasticity, poorly sustained benefit of ITB therapy, the high incidence of adverse effects, and the emergence of sterotactic neurosurgery (chiefly pallidotomy and deep brain stimulation [DBS]) as potentially more promising treatments for severe generalized dystonia.

In the two largest published series of dystonia treated using ITB *(6,7)*, dystonia rating scale scores were improved by about 30% but patients experienced little functional benefit. Although the technique is not likely to become a primary treatment for dystonia, ITB may hold promise for selected patients, including those with severe tardive dystonia or dystonic storm. It also is useful as palliative treatment for patients with severe secondary or symptomatic dystonia who are not considered candidates for stereotactic neurosurgery.

In addition, ITB has shown dramatic effects in a number of rare motor disorders including stiff-person syndrome, tetanus, and reflex sympathetic dystrophy, which will be discussed later. This chapter reviews the background, pharmacology, and rationale for treating dystonia using ITB and will assess all of the published series and case reports involving this therapy to date.

From: Contemporary Clinical Neurology:
Surgical Treatment of Parkinson's Disease and Other Movement Disorders
Edited by: D. Tarsy, J. L. Vitek, and A. M. Lozano © Humana Press Inc., Totowa, NJ

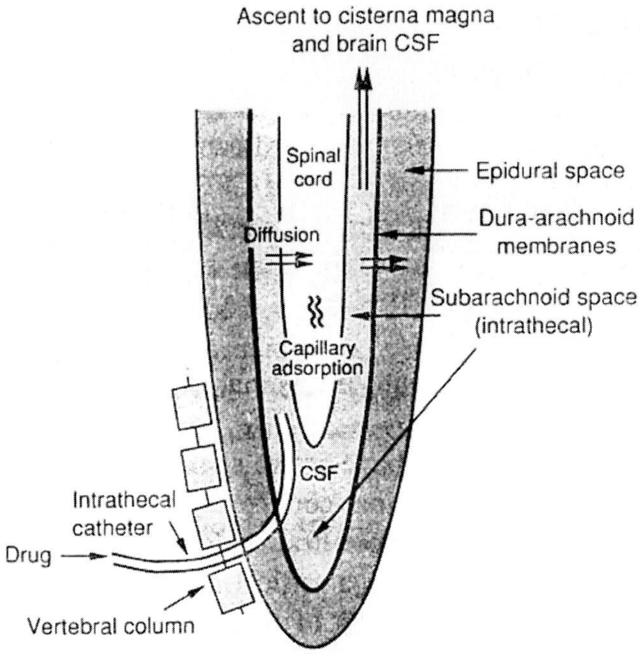

Fig. 1. Diagram of intrathecal catheter system. Reproduced with permission from ref. *(5)*.

2. GENERAL CONSIDERATIONS

2.1. Mechanism of Action and Pharmacokinetics

Intrathecal baclofen (ITB) is a highly effective and reliable treatment for severe spasticity of spinal origin. Baclofen (beta-4-chlorophenyl-gamma-aminobutyric acid) is a synthetic analog of gamma-amino butyric acid or GABA, a ubiquitous inhibitory neurotransmitter in the mammalian central nervous system (CNS) *(2a)*. Acting on presynaptic $GABA_B$ receptors by reducing calcium influx and increasing potassium conductance, baclofen inhibits the release of several neurotransmitters, including the excitatory amino acids glutamate and aspartate *(8)*. $GABA_B$ receptors are distributed throughout the CNS. In the spinal cord, $GABA_B$ receptors are concentrated heavily in superficial layers of the dorsal horn, lamina I, II, III, and IV *(9)*. In the brain, the highest concentration of GABA is in the substantia nigra and putamen *(10)*. Physiologically, baclofen reduces the excitability of spinal cord neurons and interneurons and has many additional effects in the brain that are potentially relevant to its use in disorders of increased muscle tone *(4)*.

Baclofen does not easily cross the blood-brain barrier (BBB), and high systemic doses are required to achieve an effective CNS concentration for disorders of increased muscle tone *(11)*. When administered orally, baclofen is uniformly distributed between the spinal cord and supraspinal centers. When administered intrathecally into the lumbar cistern, baclofen diffuses rostrally with CSF flow, but a concentration gradient is established, giving a lumbar cistern to cisterna magna ratio of approx 4:1 *(5,12)* (Fig. 1). This concentration gradient enables the preferential accumulation of the drug at the spinal site, thereby limiting adverse effects on the brain such as sedation. Onset of action is generally 30–60 min after an intrathecal bolus dose *(13)*. Peak effect occurs about 4 h after a bolus injection, with a gradual waning of effect 6–8 h after the bolus, although some individual variation occurs *(13,14)*.

3. ITB FOR SPASTICITY

3.1. Spasticity of Spinal Origin

ITB has been used in the treatment of spasticity of spinal origin for more than 10 years. It has passed the test of rigorously designed clinical trials *(15)* and its beneficial effect is well-documented in thousands of patients worldwide *(15–24)*. Standard bolus test injections of ITB reliably identify patients with spasticity who will receive long-term benefit from a continuous ITB infusion delivered by implantable pump *(16,21,25)*. Indications for pump implantation exist as well as dosing guidelines for continuous ITB infusion *(18,25)*. ITB is an approved treatment for spasticity of spinal origin of diverse causes, including multiple sclerosis (MS).

In large series of patients with spasticity, the response rate to ITB approaches 100%, even when symptoms are refractory to high doses of oral baclofen *(22)*. In one double-blind, placebo-controlled study of 140 patients with spinal spasticity, all individuals responded to a mean bolus ITB dose of 42.8 μg *(24)*. In spasticity of spinal origin, continuous treatment with ITB provides long-term reduction in motor tone and relief of muscle spasm *(15,18,22)*. In one series, 64 patients implanted with pumps had spasticity rating scale scores that remained constant over a mean follow-up interval of 30 mo *(18)*. A similar result was obtained in a different series of 75 patients followed for 19 mo *(26)*. Sustained functional improvement in a variety of daily living tasks including ability to transfer was described in another report of 18 patients with spinal spasticity *(27)*. To date, the effects of ITB on the functional capacity of patients with spasticity has not been as well-studied as its effect on reducing motor tone *(28)*. Nonetheless, ITB is now regarding as an essential treatment in the armamentarium for treatment of patients with intractable spasticity of spinal origin *(2a)*.

3.2. Spasticity of Cerebral Origin

Increasingly, ITB has been used for spasticity of cerebral origin, including postanoxic encephalopathy, traumatic brain injury (TBI), stroke, and cerebral palsy (CP). In patients with cerebral palsy, chronic ITB predictably improves spasticity rating scores but the effect on motor function is less certain. In a randomized, double-blind, placebo-controlled study *(29)*, 44 of 51 patients (87%) with spastic cerebral palsy responded to ITB test dosing at 50, 75, or 100 μg, thereby justifying the implantation of a permanent pump. Patients had little dystonia or athetosis, however. In a report of chronic ITB treatment for traumatic brain injury *(30)*, 17 patients with "spasticity or dystonia" underwent pump implantation and were followed for 1 yr. Significant reductions in tone were maintained throughout the period of observation, as rated by the Ashworth spasticity scale, but there were no specific measurements of dystonia or motor function.

The effect of ITB on functional capacity in cerebral palsy depends on the severity and distribution of the motor deficit as well as the baseline function. In one series *(31)*, a group of 37 patients was divided into a functional group (n = 25), all capable of self-care, and a dependent group (n = 12), requiring assistance for daily activities. As expected, patients in the functional group showed improvements in spasticity, in addition to fine hand coordination and functional capacity. In the more disabled patients, spasticity also improved, but with no benefit in manual activity or functional capacity. In neither group was the ability to transfer improved. The origin of the spasticity appears less important than its severity. In a group of 17 patients with spastic hypertonia from stroke implanted with ITB pumps and followed for up to 12 mo, reductions in spasticity were documented with some functional gain *(31a)*.

Tolerance to ITB frequently complicates long-term administration *(13,18,22,27–31)*, perhaps owing to downregulation of spinal $GABA_B$ receptors *(32)*. Increasing the infusion rate is often effective in regaining clinical benefit, but this increases the incidence of complications, such as baclofen overdose. Many centers use drug holidays and intermittent intrathecal morphine *(22)* or fentanyl administration *(34)* to de-sensitize patients to ITB. Despite the potential for tolerance, it is rare for ITB to become completely ineffective, and that occurrence should suggest a device malfunction *(33)*.

4. ITB FOR DYSTONIA

The first case report of ITB treatment for dystonia was published in 1991 *(36)*, describing treatment in an 18-yr-old man with severe, predominantly axial dystonia due to birth injury. A report published the same year documented reduced muscle spasms and tone following ITB treatment in a patient with Hallervorden-Spatz disease (*37*; case 3). In a case of postencephalitic dystonia *(38)*, a single test dose of 50 micrograms (µg) ITB appeared to reduce spasticity but increase dystonic movements. A larger series of patients with various motor disturbances included five individuals with dystonia, as well as patients with cerebral palsy with athetosis or spasticity, Wilson's disease, parkinsonism, traumatic brain injury, stiff person syndrome, anoxic encephalopathy, and painful legs/moving toes syndrome *(39)*. Spasticity tended to improve in these patients even when the effect of ITB on dystonia was not marked. Several other reports have been published *(40–46,46a)* and are summarized in Table 1. Although most reports are small retrospective, open-label, nonrandomized series, several important observations have been made.

4.1. Large Series of Primary and Secondary Dystonia

The most detailed information on the treatment of dystonia using ITB is contained in two reports describing 27 patients who underwent implantation of a pump *(6,7)*. The results of these two series are quite similar in terms of outcome and complication rates. In the Columbia series *(6)*, 25 patients with severe segmental or generalized dystonia underwent test doses of ITB in a hospital setting. Whereas the manufacturer's recommendation suggests a series of three bolus doses—50, 75, and 100 µg administered on different days—the clinicians in the Columbia study used test bolus doses ranging from 25–250 µg. There was a trend towards greater test-dose responsiveness among patients with dystonia and spasticity, as opposed to patients with pure dystonia, but this was not statistically significant. Baseline and post-ITB test dose videotapes of 11 individuals were evaluated by blinded observers using the Burke-Fahn-Marsden (BFM) dystonia rating scale *(47)* many months after pump implantation. Although mean rating scale scores improved in 7 of these 11 patients, there was no statistically significant change in scores for the group as a whole (Fig. 2).

Thirteen of the 25 patients who underwent ITB test bolus dosing had subsequent implantation of a permanent ITB delivery system. Follow-up evaluation after a mean interval of 21 mo revealed continuing ITB efficacy in six (55%) implanted patients, based on simple patient self-assessment. Five of 11 patients with implantable pumps who were followed for more than 3 mo were able to reduce or stop their medication for dystonia. The mean daily dose of ITB was 1021.2 µg/d, which is higher than that required for spasticity. Five (38%) patients experienced severe complications of long-term ITB treatment requiring hospitalization. These included baclofen overdose with respiratory depression in four patients and fibrosis of catheter tip requiring replacement, catheter-induced spinal myoclonus and skin erosion requiring pump removal, and acute baclofen withdrawal in one patient each.

The Mt. Sinai Hospital, New York series consisted of 21 patients with dystonia who were screened using test bolus doses of ITB, ranging from 25–75 µg *(7)*. Based on subjective responses to the test dosing, 9 of 14 patients with DYT1 dystonia and 5 of 7 patients with symptomatic dystonia underwent pump implantation to deliver continuous ITB. Baseline dystonia severity ranged from mild to severe (6–90 points on the B-F-M rating scale). The mean treatment interval was 29 mo. The average daily dose of ITB ranged from 50–1000 µg/d. The effect of ITB on dystonia was measured by comparing the BFM rating scale scores obtained at baseline to the scores obtained during the active treatment phase of continuous ITB delivery. The rating scale scores were not improved for the group as a whole but two patients experienced significant reductions in symptoms, including one patient with tardive dystonia. There was a high incidence of complications, including one patient who died of suicide. Four pumps were removed due to lack of benefit and in one patient the pump malfunctioned and had to be replaced. Additional complications included overdosage and underdosage, wound breakdown and dehiscence, catheter fracture, and low-volume alarm failure.

Despite the absence of a controlled randomized trial, the reports to date provide important lessons about the use of ITB in dystonia. When quantified by a blinded videotape reviewer, the effect of ITB bolus doses on dystonia is at best modest (Fig. 2). Unlike ITB for spasticity, the administration of test doses does not predict whether chronic administration will help the dystonia. Higher individual test doses than recommended for spasticity may be needed to determine whether there is any benefit, but this increases the likelihood of toxicity. Moreover, the subjective interpretation of benefit may be confounded by a placebo effect, as noted in the Columbia series *(6)*. To counter these problems, some investigators use a continuous test ITB infusion, gradually increasing the rate until therapeutic effects or adverse effects develop *(42,45)*. The long-term effect on functional capacity of patients with severe generalized dystonia appears limited. There is a high incidence of serious complications including hardware failure, pump dosing errors, infection, skin erosions, and catheter migration, all identical to those reported in the literature on spasticity. Despite the problems with this treatment approach, it remains possible that subgroups of dystonia patients might benefit from ITB therapy. Guidelines for using ITB in patients with dystonia are provided in Table 2.

4.2. *Dystonia and Cerebral Palsy*

It is tempting to speculate that patients with dystonia in combination with spasticity would respond to ITB better than patients with dystonia alone. In patients with cerebral palsy and symptomatic dystonia, investigators have observed disparate effects of ITB on spastic and dystonic elements. In a report of 37 patients with cerebral palsy *(31)*, ranging in age from 5–27 yr, seven patients had “considerable athetosis” in addition to spasticity. The mean daily dose of continuous ITB for the group as a whole did not exceed 325 μg. The authors documented a significant, sustained reduction in spasticity, quantified using the Ashworth scale, but noted no improvement in athetosis. A similar observation was made in a series of patients with motor disorders treated with ITB *(39)*.

In a report of five patients with symptomatic dystonia treated with continuous ITB *(42)*, two individuals had Hallervorden-Spatz disease and one each had dystonia due to an anoxic event in adulthood, postencephalitic dystonia, and cerebral palsy. The ITB testing procedure was accomplished by a short-term continuous infusion rather than by test-bolus doses. Only the adult patient with postanoxic dystonia experienced functional benefit. The individuals with postencephalitic dystonia and cerebral palsy showed improvements in dystonic posturing but this was not quantified. In a follow-up report of 12 patients with “dystonic cerebral palsy” caused by perinatal asphyxia ($n = 10$), perinatal meningitis ($n = 1$), or near drowning ($n = 1$) *(45)* continuous ITB infusion significantly reduced dystonia rating scale scores, according to a blinded videotape reviewer. Ten of 12 patients were improved at infusion rates of 350–750 μg/d, and eight underwent implantation of a permanent pump. After a mean follow-up interval of 16 mo, improvements in dystonia were maintained.

To date, most series of dystonic cerebral palsy have been retrospective, uncontrolled, and unblinded *(47a)*. Nonetheless, improvements in passive motor tone, range of motion, spasms, and orthopedic deformity have been consistently documented *(47a)*. Careful measurements of dystonia and functional capacity in these patients have generally not been performed *(47a)*.

4.3. *Dystonic Storm*

The number of patients with specific forms of dystonia is too small to know whether ITB is useful for special limited indications. There are reports of patients in dystonic storm, an acute, severe life-threatening syndrome of dystonic spasms that may be complicated by respiratory failure or rhabdomyolysis, who were stabilized using ITB *(36,40,44)*. The advantage of using ITB in dystonic storm is that this disorder requires management in an intensive care unit setting, where threatened respiratory depression can be attended carefully.

Table 1
Intrathecal Baclofen for Dystonia: Summary of Reported Cases

Refs.	Study	*n*	Dystonia etiology	Age at ITB treatment	Outcome	F/U (mo)
Narayan *(36)*	Case report	1	Postanoxic birth injury	18	ITB successfully controlled dystonic storm. Sustained improvement in axial spasms and generalized dystonia.	14
Delhaas *(37)*	Case report	1	Hallervorden Spatz (report also describes 4 other pts. with spinal spasticity)	20	Marked improvements in dystonia and axial spasms but treatment was palliative and pt. died.	17
Silbert *(38)*	Case report	1	Post-encephalitic	39	Spastic quadriparesis and athetosis treated with single 50 μg bolus ITB: improved spasticity but increased dystonic movements.	–
Penn *(39)*	Series	18	Various motor disorders, including 5 pts with primary dystonia	36–59	Of the 5 dystonia pts., marked improvement in 3, mild benefit in 1, and worsening in 1 after test dosing. Benefit not sustained in 1 initial responder.	40
Paret *(40)*	Case report	1	DYT1 dystonia	9	Dystonic storm successfully treated in ICU setting.	–
Diederich *(41)*	Case report	1	Primary generalized dystonia	32	Marked improvement in axial and limb dystonia but not cranial dystonia or spasmodic dysphonia. Pt. able to leave wheelchair and ambulate freely.	23
Ford *(6)*					13 pts. underwent pump implantation. Subjective improvements in 6/13 pts. Improvements in dystonia scale scores in 6/10 pts., but not significant for group as a whole. Severe complications in 5 implanted pts.	
Albright *(45)*	Series	5	Cerebral palsy (3), Hallervorden-Spatz (2)	7–36	Functional gain in 1 pt. with postanoxic dystonia during adulthood; improvement in dystonia in 2 patients with cerebral palsy.	13

Dressler *(43)*	Case report	1	tardive dystonia	49	Severe retrocollis and axial dystonia were "substantially" improved by ITB. Previously wheelchair-bound pt. could walk 500 m.	6
Dalvi *(44)*	Case report	1	DYT1 dystonia	16	Dystonic storm successfully treated in ICU setting.	11
Albright *(45)*	Series	12	Cerebral palsy	4–42	Reductions in dystonia rating scale scores in 10/12 pts. after test ITB infusion, according to blinded reviewer.	16
Awaad *(46)*	Case report	1	Dystonia with 18p deletion	15	Marked, sustained improvement.	18
Walker *(7)*	Series	21	Primary and secondary dystonia	19–63	14 of 21 pts. screened with ITB underwent pump implantation. Dystonia rating scale scores dramatically improved in 2 pts., but not for the group overall. High incidence of complication, including 2 deaths (suicide, cardiac) and treatment failure requiring pump removal in 4 pts.	29
Jaffe *(46a)*	Case report	1	Primary	70	Improved dystonia rating scale scores and functional capacity.	3

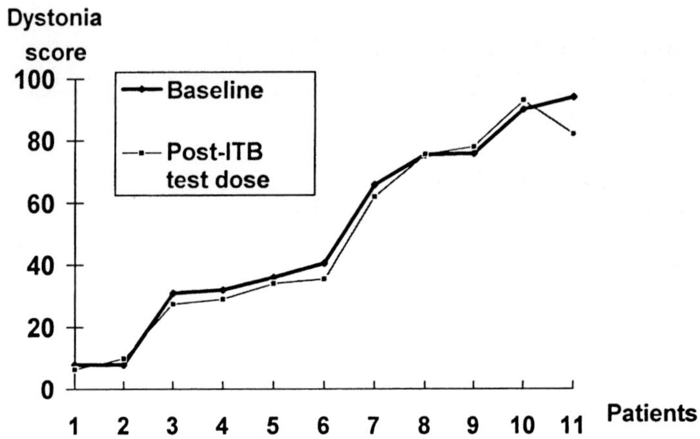

Fig. 2. The effect of ITB on dystonia. Dystonia rating scale scores before and after ITB test bolus dosing. A decrease in score after ITB test dosing represents an improvement and an increase in score denotes a worsening. The patients are arranged in order of increasing severity of dystonia at the baseline (pretest dose) session. In patient 4 with generalized dystonia, due to incomplete videotaping, only cranial dystonia and speech were rated out of a possible maximum score of 24; for all other individuals, the dystonia rating scale maximum score was 120. Reproduced with permission from ref. *(64)*.

5. ITB FOR OTHER MOTOR DISORDERS

5.1. *Stiff Person Syndrome*

Stiff person syndrome is a rare disorder that causes increased tone and paroxysmal muscular spasms. Most patients have antibodies directed against glutamic acid decarboxylase (GAD), the enzyme that catalyzes glutamate to GABA. The proposed pathophysiology involves excessive excitability of spinal motor neurons owing to a lack of GABAergic inhibition. Treatment for this disorder includes oral muscle relaxants and immunotherapy such as corticosteroids, intravenous gamma globulin (IVIG), or plasmapheresis. There are several reports of successful treatment of stiff person syndrome using intrathecal baclofen *(48–50)*. In one report of eight patients with stiff person syndrome or its variant, progressive encephalopathy with rigidity and myoclonus ("interneuronitis"), chronic ITB treatment for up to 6.5 yr reduced muscle spasms and provided functional benefit *(50)*. In theory, ITB is an ideal symptomatic treatment for stiff person syndrome because the medication is delivered to the spinal cord, the putative site of neurochemical abnormality. As with spasticity and dystonia treated with ITB, there is a high complication rate, including fatality from acute baclofen withdrawal *(51)*.

5.2. *Tetanus*

Tetanus, a disorder of painful muscular spasms and rigidity, is caused by a neurotoxin that preferentially accumulates in spinal interneurons and inhibits the release of neurotransmitters glycine and GABA. The treatment of generalized tetanus involves very high doses of muscle relaxants and paralytic agents together with sedation and ventilatory support. Owing to its site and mechanism of action, ITB is a potentially useful adjunctive therapy for tetanus, which may lower requirements for the other agents *(52,53,53a)*. Presumably, ITB could also be potentially helpful in cases of strychnine toxicity, although there have been no published reports to date.

5.3. *Reflex Sympathetic Dystrophy*

Reflex sympathetic dystrophy is a pain syndrome that sometimes follows trauma to a limb and consists of local sensory and autonomic disturbances together with dystonic posturing and tremors, muscle

Table 2
Suggested Guidelines for Use of ITB in Patients with Dystonia, Based on the Experience at the Center for Dystonia, Columbia-Presbyterian Medical Center

A. Candidates for ITB test dosing
  1. Dystonia associated with severe spasticity.
  2. Dystonia with superimposed painful dystonic spasms.
  3. Severe, continuous dystonic movements ("dystonic storm").
  4. Severe tardive dystonia.
  5. Severe dystonia in patients who are not candidates for stereotactic neurosurgery.

B. Procedures for ITB test dose trials
  1. Test doses should be administered in hospital setting on consecutive days.
  2. Make a careful baseline examination.
  3. Quantify the clinical response to each test dose using a dystonia rating scale, Ashworth and spasm scales, pain scales, and measures of activity of daily living capacity.
  4. For ITB test bolus dosing, increase the ITB test doses on consecutive days using increments of no higher than 25%. If ITB test doses greatly exceed 100 μg, or if risk of oversedation and respiratory depression seems present, consider performing the test dosing in an intensive care unit setting.
  5. Consider using a placebo injection, after obtaining informed consent. The effect of a placebo injection may be most clear when it is administered as the first of the series of injections.
  6. For continuous ITB test infusions, begin at a rate of 1000 μg/d and increase by 50 μg/d every 12 h, up to a maximum daily infusion rate in the range of 600–900 μg.

C. Management of suspected drug tolerance during chronic ITB infusion
  1. Ascertain that pump is functioning correctly by checking reservoir and programming features.
  2. Evaluate possible catheter malfunction with X-rays and dye studies.
  3. If tolerance to drug effect appears most likely, increasing the infusion rate may alleviate the problem for a period of time.
  4. Consider addition or increase in oral medications, including baclofen, benzodiazepines, anticholinergics, and dantrolene.
  5. Add ITB morphine to infusion, or replace ITB with intrathecal morphine.
  6. Gradually decrease and discontinue ITB, substituting with oral medications, to provide a drug holiday for several weeks, before gradually reintroducing the treatment at a lower infusion rate.

jerks, and muscle weakness. The disorder is difficult to treat, but in one report seven patients with RSD were given bolus doses of ITB using a double-blind, placebo-controlled design *(54)*. Six patients experienced a marked subjective reduction in dystonia severity and underwent pump implanatation for continuous ITB infusion. Of these, three patients had substantial improvements in dystonia and function, while the other three had worsening and spread of dystonia, after a mean follow-up period of 1.7 yr *(54)*.

6. POTENTIAL COMPLICATIONS OF ITB

Unfortunately, complications appear to be an inevitable part of chronic ITB treatment. Even at specialized centers with broad clinical experience using intrathecal drug-delivery systems, the incidence of severe, life-threatening complications is well-documented *(55,56)*. Complications may result from ITB overdosage or abrupt underdosage of any cause. Pump malfunction, programming error, infection, cerebrospinal fluid (CSF) leaks, headache, and catheter problems have all been reported. In one study, 40% of 102 patients experienced catheter-associated complications at an increasing rate over 80 mo *(57)*. In another series, 26 of 46 (56%) patients required operations to correct complications or pump failure *(55)*. Procedures and algorithms to evaluate suspected pump malfunction are described in the clinical reference manual *(25)* as well as in most published reports. Many complications are not disease-specific but the withdrawal syndromes typically consist of rebound exacerbation of the disorder under treatment *(58)*. Baclofen withdrawal can be severe and even life-threatening. Seizures *(59)*, encephalopathy, hyperthermia *(60)*, and a syndrome resembling neuroleptic malignant syndrome *(61)* have been reported.

In general, adverse events are particularly likely to occur at higher daily doses of ITB, when the margin for error is smaller and a sudden reduction in infusion is more likely to precipitate baclofen withdrawal. This underscores the recommendation that ITB programs be conducted only at centers with adequate clinical experience and resources including intensive care, radiological and neurosurgical support, and outpatient monitoring capacity.

7. CONCLUSION

Intrathecal baclofen is an effective therapy for patients with severe spasticity of spinal cord or cerebral origin. To date, its role as a possible treatment for dystonia has been reported in approx 90 patients with symptomatic dystonia, including two open-label series that retrospectively analyzed the effect of ITB on dystonia rating scales and functional outcome measures *(6,7)*. The main observation is that ITB is not as effective for dystonia, as compared to its effect on spasticity. In patients with severe generalized dystonia, the response rate to test doses of ITB is low, even with doses exceeding the manufacturer's recommended upper limit. ITB has potentially serious adverse effects, so clinicians who apply this treatment for dystonia and conditions other than spasticity should be familiar with the technique, dosing guidelines, and interventions for adverse effects (Table 2).

On the basis of the published experience to date, it would appear that using ITB as a general treatment for medication-refractory dystonia is not warranted. With the rising enthusiasm for stereotactic neurosurgical procedures for dystonia, especially pallidotomy *(62)* and globus pallidus stimulation *(63)*, the role of ITB may be further diminished. However, ITB remains a treatment consideration for selected patients, including those with a combination of dystonia and intractable spasticity. ITB has potential use as a temporizing measure in patients with dystonic storm and as palliative therapy for patients with severe dystonia who are not operative candidates.

REFERENCES

1. Young, R. R. and Delwaide, P. J. (1981) Spasticity (Part I) *N. Engl. J. Med.* **304,** 28–33.
1a. Young, R. R. and Delwaide, P. J. (1981) Spasticity (Part II) *N. Engl. J. Med.* **304,** 96–99.
2. Davidoff, R. A. (1985) Antispasticity drugs: mechanism of action. *Ann. Neurol.* **17,** 107–116.
2a. Kita, M. and Goodkin, D. E. (2000) Drugs used to treat spasticity. *Drugs* **59,** 487–495.
3. Fahn, S. (1987) Systemic therapy of dystonia. *Can. J. Neurol. Sci.* **14,** 528–532.
4. Greene, P. (1992) Baclofen in the treatment of dystonia. *Clin. Neuropharmacol.* **15,** 276–288.
5. Kroin, J. (1992) Intrathecal drug administration: present use and future trends. *Clin. Pharmocokin.* **22(5),** 319–326.
6. Ford, B., Greene, P., Louis, E. D., Petzinger, G., Bressman, S. B., Goodman, R. G., et al. (1996) Treatment of dystonia using intrathecal baclofen. *Arch. Neurol.* **53,** 1241–1246.
7. Walker, R. H., Danisi, F. O., Swope, D. M., Goodman, R. R., Germano, I. M., and Brin, M. F. (2000) Intrathecal baclofen for dystonia: benefits and complications during six years of experience. *Mov. Disord.* **15(6),** 1242–1247.
8. Misgeld, U., Bijak, M., and Jarolimek, W. (1995) A physiological role for $GABA_B$ receptors and the effects of baclofen in the mammalian central nervous system. *Prog. Neurobiol.* **46,** 423–462.
9. Price, G. W., Wilkin, G. P., Turnbull, M. J., and Bowery, N. G. (1984) Are baclofen-sensitive GABAB receptors present on primary afferent terminals of the spinal cord? *Nature* **307,** 71–74.
10. Fahn, S. and Cote, L. J. (1968) Regional distribution of GABA in the brain of the Rhesus monkey. *J. Neurochem.* **15,** 209–213.
11. Knutsson, E., Lindblom, U., Beissinger, R. L., and Martenson, A. (1974) Plasma and cerebrospinal fluid levels of baclofen at optimal therapeutic responses in spastic paresis. *J. Neurol. Sci.* **23,** 473–484.
12. Kroin, J. S., Ali, A., York, M., and Penn, R. D. (1993) The distribution of medication along the spinal canal after chronic intrathecal administration. *Neurosurgery* **33,** 226–230.
13. Sallerin-Caute, B., Lazorthes, Y., Monserrat, B., Cros, J., and Bastide, R. (1991) CSF baclofen levels after intrathecal administration in severe spasticity. *Eur. J. Clin. Pharmacol.* **40,** 363–365.
14. Muller, H., Zierski, J., Dralle, D., Kraub, D., and Mart-Schler, E. (1988) Pharmacokinetics of intrathecal baclofen. In: *Local Spinal Therapy of Spasticity* (Muller, H., Zierski, J., and Penn, R., eds.), Springer, Berlin, pp. 155–214.
15. Penn, R. D., Savoy, S., Corcos, D., et al. (1989) Intrathecal baclofen for severe spinal spasticity: a double blind crossover study. *N. Engl. J. Med.* **320,** 1517–1521.

16. Lazorthes, Y., Sallerin-Caute, B., Verdie, J., Bastide, R., and Carillo, J. (1990) Chronic intrathecal baclofen administration for control of severe spasticity. *J. Neurosurg.* **72,** 393–402.
17. Loubster, P. G., Narayan, R. K., Sandin, K. J., et al. (1991) Continuous infusion of intrathecal baclofen: long-term effects on spasticity in spinal cord injury. *Paraplegia* **29,** 48–64.
18. Penn, R. D. (1992) Intrathecal baclofen for spasticity of spinal origin: seven years of experience. *J. Neurosurg.* **77,** 236–240.
19. Coffey, R. J., Cahill, D., Steers, W., et al. (1993) Intrathecal baclofen for intractable spasticity of spinal origin: results of a long-term multicenter study. *J. Neurosurg.* **78,** 226–232.
20. Ochs, G. A. (1993) Intrathecal baclofen. *Baillieres Clin. Neurol.* **2,** 73–86.
21. Abel, N. A. and Smith, R. A. (1994) Intrathecal baclofen for treatment of intractable spinal spasticity. *Arch. Physical. Med. Rehab.* **75,** 54–58.
22. Lewis, K. S. and Mueller, W. M. (1993) Intrathecal baclofen for severe spasticity secondary to spinal cord injury. *Ann. Pharmacol.* **27,** 767–773.
23. Nance, P., Schryvers, O., Schmidt, B., Dubo, H., Loveridge, B., and Fewer, D. (1995) Intrathecal baclofen therapy for adults with spinal spasticity: therapeutic efficacy and effect on hospital admissions. *Can. J. Neurol. Sci.* **22,** 22–29.
24. Becker, W. J., Harris, C. J., Long, M. L., Ablett, D. P., Klein, G. M., and DeForge, D. A. (1995) Long-term intrathecal baclofen therapy in patients with intractable spasticity. *Can. J. Neurol. Sci.* **22,** 208–217.
25. SynchroMed Infusion System: Clinical Reference Guide. Medtronic, Inc, Minneapolis, MN, 2001.
26. Patterson, V., Watt, M., Byrnes, D., Crowe, D., and Lee, A. (1994) Management of severe spasticity with intrathecal baclofen delivered by a manually operated pump. *J. Neurol. Neurosurg. Psychiatry* **57,** 582–558.
27. Azouvi, P., Mane, M., Thiebaut, J.-B., Denys, P., Remy-Neris, O., and Bussel, B. (1996) Intrathecal baclofen administration for control of severe spinal spasticity: functional improvement and long-term follow-up. *Arch. Phys. Med. Rehab.* **77,** 35–39.
28. Armstrong, R. W. (1992) Intrathecal baclofen and spasticity: what do we know and what do we need to know? *Dev. Med. Child Neurol.* **34,** 739–745.
29. Gilmartin, R., Bruce, D., Storrs, B. B., Abbott, R., Krach, L., Ward, J., et al. (2000) Intrathecal baclofen for management of spastic cerebral palsy: multicenter trial. *Child. Neurol.* **15(2),** 71–77.
30. Meythaler, J. M., Guin-Renfroe, S., Grabb, P., and Hadley, M. N. (1999) Long-term continuously infused intrathecal baclofen for spastic-dystonic hypertonia in traumatic brain injury: 1-year experience. *Arch. Phys. Med. Rehabil.* **80(1),** 13–19.
31. Albright, A. L., Barron, W. B., Fasick, M. P., Polinko, P., and Janosky, J. (1993) Continuous intrathecal baclofen for spasticity of cerebral origin. *JAMA* **270,** 2475–2477.
31a. Meythaler, J. M., Guin-Renfroe, S., Brunner, R. C., and Hadley, M. N. (2001) Intrathecal baclofen for spastic hypertonia from stroke. *Stroke* **32,** 2099–2109.
32. Akman, M. N., Loubser, P. G., Donovan, W. H., O'Neill, R. N., and Rossi, C. D. (1993) Intrathecal baclofen: does tolerance occur? *Paraplegia* **31,** 516–520.
33. Kroin, J. S. and Penn, R. D. (1993) Intrathecal baclofen down-regulates $GABA_B$ receptors in the rat substantia gelatinosa. *J. Neurosurg.* **79,** 544–549.
34. Chabal, C., Jacobson, L., and Terman, G. (1992) Intrathecal fentanyl alleviates spasticity in the presence of tolerance to intrathecal baclofen. *Anesthesiology* **76,** 312–314.
35. Schurch, B. (1993) Errors and limitations of the multimodality checking method of defective spinal intrathecal pump systems. *Paraplegia* **31,** 611–615.
36. Narayan, R. K., Loubster, P. G., Jankovic, J., Donovan, W. H., and Bontke, C. F. (1991) Intrathecal baclofen for intractable axial dystonia. *Neurology* **41,** 1141–1142.
37. Delhaas, E. M. and Brouwers, J. R. B. (1991) Intrathecal baclofen overdose: report of seven events and review of the literature. *Int. J. Clin. Pharmacol. Ther. Toxicol.* **29,** 274–280.
38. Silbert, P. L. and Stewart-Wynne, E. G. (1992) Increased dystonia after intrathecal baclofen [letter] *Neurology* **42,** 1639–1640.
39. Penn, R. D., Gianino, J. M., and York, M. M. (1995) Intrathecal baclofen for motor disorders. *Mov. Disord.* **10,** 675–677.
40. Paret, G., Tirosh, R., Ben Zeev, B., Vardi, A., Brandt, N., and Barzilay, Z. (1996) Intrathecal baclofen for severe torsion dystonia in a child. *Acta. Paediatr.* **85,** 636–637.
41. Diederich, N. J., Comella, C. L., Matge, G., Becker, G., Schiltz, F., and Metz, H. (1997) Sustained effect of high-dose intrathecal baclofen in primary generalized dystonia: a 2-year follow-up study. *Mov. Disord.* **12,** 1100–1102.
42. Albright, A. E. (1996) Baclofen in the treatment of cerebral palsy. *J. Child. Neurol.* **11,** 77–83.
43. Dressler, D., Oeljeschlager, R.-O., and Ruther, E. (1997) Severe tardive dystonia: treatment with continuous intrathecal baclofen administration. *Mov. Disord.* **12,** 585–587.
44. Dalvi, A., Fahn, S., and Ford, B. (1998) Intrathecal baclofen in the treatment of dystonic storm. *Mov. Disord.* **13,** 611–612.
45. Albright, A. L., Barry, M. J., Painter, M. J., and Shultz, B. (1998) Infusion of intrathecal baclofen for generalized dystonia in cerebral palsy. *J. Neurosurg.* **88,** 73–76.
46. Awaad, Y., Munoz, S., and Nigro, M. (1999) Progressive dystonia in a child with chromosome 18p deletion, treated with intrathecal balcofen. *J. Child. Neurol.* **14,** 75–77.
46a. Jaffe, M. S. and Nienstedt, L. J. (2001) Intrathecal baclofen for generalized dystonia: a case report. *Arch. Phys. Med. Rehabil.* **82,** 853–855.

47. Burke, R. E., Fahn, S., Marsden, C. D., Bressman, S. B., Moskowitz, C., and Friedman, J. (1985) Validity and reliability of a rating scale for the primary torsion dystonias. *Neurology* **35,** 73–77.
47a. Butler, C. and Campbell, S. (2000) Evidence of the effects of intrathecal baclofen for spastic and dystonia cerebral palsy. *Dev. Med. Child. Neurol.* **42,** 634–645.
48. Penn, R. D. and Mangieri, E. A. (1993) Stiff-man syndrome treated with intrathecal baclofen. *Neurology* **43,** 2412.
49. Silbert, P. L., Matsumoto, J. Y., McManis, P. G., Stolp-Smith, K. A., Elliott, B. A., and McEvoy, K. M. (1995) Intrathecal baclofen therapy in stiff-man syndrome: a double blind, placebo-controlled trial. *Neurology* **45,** 1893–1897.
50. Stayer, C., Tronnier, V., Dressnandt, J., Mauch, E., Marquardt, G., Rieke, K., et al. (1997). Intrathecal baclofen therapy for stiff-man syndrome and progressive encephalomyelopathy with rigidity and myoclonus. *Neurology* **49,** 1591–1597.
51. Meinck, H. M., Tronnier, V., Rieke, K., Wirtz, C. R., Flugel, D., and Schwab, S. (1994) Intrathecal baclofen treatment for stiff-man syndrome: pump failure may be fatal. *Neurology* **44,** 2209–2210.
52. Brock, H., Moosbauer, W., Gabriel, C., and Necek, S. (1995) Treatment of severe tetanus by continuous intrathecal infusion of baclofen [letter]. *J. Neurol. Neurosurg. Psychiatry* **59,** 193–194.
53. Boots, R. J., Lipman, J., O'Callaghan, J., Scott, P., and Fraser, J. (2000) The treatment of tetanus with intrathecal baclofen. *Anaesth. Intens. Care* **28(4),** 438–442.
53a. Engrand, N. and Benhamou, D. (2001) About intrathecal baclofen in tetanus. *Anaesth. Intens. Care* **29,** 306–307.
54. Van Hilten, B. J., van de Beek, W.-J., Hoff, J. I., Voormolen, J. H. C., and Delhaas, E. M. (2000) Intrathecal baclofen for the treatment of dystonia in patients with reflex sympathetic dystrophy. *N. Engl. J. Med.* **343,** 625–630.
55. Teddy, P., Jamous, A., Gardner, B., Wang, D., and Silver, J. (1992) Complications of intrathecal baclofen delivery. *Br. J. Neurosurg.* **6,** 115–118.
56. Saltuari, L., Kronenberg, M., Marosi, M. J., Kofler, M., Russegger, L., Rifici, C., et al. (1992) Indication, efficiency and complications of intrathecal pump supported baclofen treatmen in spinal spasticity. *Acta. Neurologica.* **14,** 187–194.
57. Penn, R. D., York, M. M., and Paice, J. A. (1995) Catheter systems for intrathecal drug delivery. *J. Neurosurg.* **83,** 215–217.
58. Seigfried, R. N., Jacobson, L., and Chabal, C. (1992) Development of an acute withdrawal syndrome following the cessation of intrathecal baclofen in a patient with spasticity. *Anesthesiology* **5,** 1048–1050.
59. Kofler, M. and Arturo, L. A. (1992) Prolonged seizure activity after baclofen withdrawal. *Neurology* **42,** 697–698.
60. Mandac, B. R., Hurvitz, E. A., and Nelson, V. S. (1993) Hyperthermia associated with baclofen withdrawal and increased spasticity. *Arch. Phys. Med. Rehabil.* **74,** 96–97.
61. Samson-Fang, L., Gooch, J., and Norlin, C. (2000) Intrathecal baclofen withdrawal simulating neuroleptic malignant syndrome in a child with cerebral palsy. *Dev. Med. Child. Neurol.* **42,** 561–565.
62. Lozano, A. M., Kumar, R., Gross, R. E., Giladi, N., Hutchison, W. D., Dostrovsky, J. O., and Lang, A. E. (1997) Globus pallidus internus pallidotomy for generalized dystonia. *Mov. Disord.* **12,** 865–870.
63. Loher, T. J., Hasdemir, M. G., Burgunder, J.-M., and Krauss, J. K. (2000) Long-term follow-up study of chronic globus pallidus internus stimulation for post-traumatic hemidystonia. *J. Neurosurg.* **92,** 457–460.
64. Ford, B., Greene, P. E., Louis, E. D., Bressman, S. B., Goodman, R. R., Brin, M. F., et al. (1998) Intrathecal baclofen in the treatment of dystonia. In: *Advances in Neurology Dystonia* 3 (Fahn, S., Marsden, C. D., and DeLong, M. R., eds.), **78,** 199–210.

IV Miscellaneous

21

Positron Emission Tomography in Surgery for Movement Disorders

Masafumi Fukuda,
Christine Edwards, and David Eidelberg

1. INTRODUCTION

Functional brain imaging with positron emission tomography (PET) has contributed to our understanding of the pathophysiology of Parkinson's disease (PD) and other movement disorders. PET employs small amounts of positron emitting radioligands to produce quantitative measures of physiological and biochemical processes in the brain and other organs. In a PET experiment, a subject is given a compound of biological interest. The spatial and temporal distribution of the radiotracer is measured quantitatively in the course of the PET study, providing a tomographic representation of regional radioactivity concentration. In this chapter, we focus on the potential application of PET in the assessment of surgical interventions such as pallidotomy, thalamotomy, and deep brain stimulation (DBS).

2. BRAIN METABOLISM AND REGIONAL BLOOD FLOW IN PD

Measurements of regional rates of glucose utilization (rCMRGlc) with [^{18}F]-fluorodeoxyglucose (FDG)/PET in PD can be used to quantify the effect of nigrostriatal degeneration on brain regions functionally related to the dopaminergic system. Although the primary pathological abnormality in PD is confined to the substantia nigra, the degeneration of dopaminergic projection neurons from the substantia nigra to the striatum results in widespread alterations in the functional activity of the basal ganglia and motor cortex *(1,2)*. Specifically, the anatomical and functional organization of the basal ganglia *(3)* predicts that the loss of inhibitory dopaminergic input to the striatum results in increased inhibitory output from the putamen to the external globus pallidus (GPe), diminished inhibitory output from the GPe to the subthalamic nucleus (STN), and overactivity of the STN and internal globus pallidus (GPi), resulting in decreased output from the ventrolateral thalamus to the cortex. These functional alterations in basal ganglia activity are accompanied by changes in regional cerebral glucose metabolism and blood flow.

Over the past decade, FDG/PET has been employed to identify alterations in regional brain function in PD patients *(4)*. Parallel efforts have employed [^{15}O] H_2O to identify pathological abnormalities in regional oxygen consumption and cerebral blood flow (rCBF) as additional indices of localized functional pathology in these diseases. In experimental animal models of PD, unilateral nigrostriatal lesions lead to increased regional cerebral glucose metabolism (rCMRGlc) in the ipsilateral globus pallidus *(5)*. Pallidal hypermetabolism is also a consistent feature of PD in human patients *(6,7)*, which may be reversed surgically *(8)* or pharmacologically *(9,10)*. Increased metabolic activity in the

From: Current Clinical Neurology:
Surgical Treatment of Parkinson's Disease and Other Movement Disorders
Edited by: D. Tarsy, J. L. Vitek, and A. M. Lozano © Humana Press Inc., Totowa, NJ

GPi, arising through an increase in synaptic inputs from STN *(6,11)* appears to be a hallmark of idiopathic PD on FDG/PET imaging *(12)*.

FDG/PET can be a powerful tool to differentiate idiopathic PD from atypical parkinsonian syndromes *(13)*. Subjects with atypical parkinsonian syndromes such as striatonigral degeneration (SND), progressive supranuclear palsy (PSP), hemiparkinson-hemiatrophy syndrome (HPHA), and corticobasal ganglionic degeneration (CBGD) often exhibit characteristic patterns of abnormal reductions in regional glucose metabolism. SND, which is typically symmetrical, is characterized by consistent rCMRGlc reductions in the striatum as compared with normal controls as well as duration- and severity-matched PD patients *(14)*. HPHA is a clinically asymmetrical syndrome due to a developmental abnormality in nigrostriatal, and possibly, striatocortical projection systems. In this condition we noted unilateral hypometabolism in the basal ganglia or frontal cortex contralateral to the affected body side, while rCMRGlc measures ipsilateral to the affected body side were normal *(15)*. By contrast, CBGD, an asymmetrically progressive neurodegenerative syndrome is characterized by abnormal metabolic asymmetries in the thalamus and inferior parietal lobes as compared with both normal and hemi-PD controls *(16)*. Thus, FDG/PET can be a helpful adjunct to the clinical examination in the differential diagnosis of parkinsonism *(12)*. This technique may also be utilized in selecting candidates for possible surgical intervention (*8,7,* see below).

3. METABOLIC NETWORK MAPPING IN PD

It is now accepted that while primary abnormalities may be well-localized, focal neurodegeneration results in widespread functional alterations in brain regions spatially removed from the histological or neurochemical locus of pathology. Therefore, the measurement of local rates of metabolism in isolation may not fully describe the complexities of the neural systems involved in neurodegenerative processes. We have developed and applied a statistical modeling approach for the identification and quantification of abnormal metabolic brain networks in PD and related movement disorders *(18)*. This approach, known as the Scaled Subprofile Model (SSM) *(19–21)* is a form of principal component analysis (PCA) and can be applied to identify patterns of regional covariation in brain metabolism data. In SSM, PCA is employed to identify regional covariance patterns (metabolic brain networks) from rCMRGlc data obtained from combined samples of patients and normal controls. This form of analysis is blind to subject class designation and utilizes the variance across the entire population to identify specific patterns associated with the disease state. These patterns reflect covarying regional increases or decreases in brain function relative to a baseline defined by the normal population. SSM/PCA analysis also can be used to measure the expression of the networks in individual subjects (subject scores). In this way, the technique provides a means of comparing network expression across different populations and of examining the relationship of independent clinical descriptors such as disease severity or duration to the network.

In PD, we have identified a reproducible pattern of regional metabolism characterized by increased lentiform and thalamic metabolism associated with metabolic reductions in the lateral frontal and paracentral areas *(6,7,22)*. In addition, the degree of individual expression of this PD-related pattern (PDRP) correlates with independent disease severity ratings *(6,22,23)* and with disease duration *(24)*. These results agree with experimental animal models *(1,2,25)*, in which parkinsonian signs are associated with excessive pallidofugal inhibitory outflow and with concomitant reduction of brain function in primary and association motor cortical regions. Reduced presynaptic nigrostriatal dopaminergic activity leads to increased functional activity in the STN *(2,25,26)*, leading to overactivity of the pallidothalamic pathway and concomitant suppression of thalamocortical excitatory inputs.

SSM/PCA has also been used to identify the network correlates of specific features of PD. Antonini and colleagues studied a cohort of 16 PD patients consisting of individuals with and without appreciable tremor *(27)*. SSM analysis revealed that the tremor-predominant patients expressed a specific brain network. This tremor pattern was characterized by increased expression of a metabolic network comprising the thalamus, pons, and contralateral lateral frontal cortex to tremor side, and was topographically different from the PDRP described earlier. The latter pattern, associated mainly with pallidothalamic output, was expressed equally in tremulous and atremulous patients. The findings suggest that PD patients with tremor are characterized by distinct increases in the functional activity of thalamomotor cortical projections.

4. PALLIDOTOMY/THALAMOTOMY FOR PD

Posterolateral ventral pallidotomy (PVP) has been shown to significantly improve akinetic symptoms in PD as well as to relieve dyskinesia associated with levodopa administration *(28–31)*. The pathophysiology of pallidal ablation for the relief of parkinsonism is not completely understood. The ameliorative effects of PVP have been attributed to the reduction of excessive inhibitory outflow from the GPi *(32)*.

We initially reported findings from eight PD patients undergoing unilateral PVP who were scanned with FDG/PET in the resting state preoperatively and again 6 mo following surgery *(11)*. We found that PVP resulted in a metabolic decline in the thalamus, which occurred in conjunction with a metabolic increase in primary and associative motor cortical regions. Indeed, the improvement in limb performance at 6 mo following surgery was significantly correlated with the operative metabolic decline in the thalamus and with the accompanying increases in lateral premotor cortex (PMC). To quantify potential modulations in the expression of network activity by PVP, we applied network analysis to the operative *changes* in regional glucose metabolism. We found that the postsurgical topography closely resembled the PDRP that we had identified in earlier FDG/PET studies of untreated patients *(8)*. The pattern of operative change subsequent to unilateral PVP was characterized by metabolic decline in the lentiform nucleus and thalamus ipsilateral to the surgery, associated with bilateral metabolic increases in the supplementary motor area. We found that subject scores for this pattern were highly correlated with improvements in both contralateral and ipsilateral limb performance. These findings indicate that metabolic brain networks comprising functionally and anatomically interconnected brain regions remote from the lesion site may be modulated by PVP, including motor cortical regions of the hemisphere contralateral to the surgery. The topography of operative change following pallidal ablation conforms well to that predicted based on the PDRP network.

Because local rates of glucose are a reflection of net afferent synaptic activity *(33)*, it is reasonable to expect a decline in thalamic metabolism subsequent to surgical interference with pallidofugal inhibitory projections to the thalamus. Similarly, the metabolic increases in motor cortical areas occurring with pallidotomy may be related to enhanced cortical afferent synaptic activity from the ventral thalamus following surgical reduction in pallidothalamic inhibitory output *(2)*. Indeed, we have shown that spontaneous GPi single unit activity recorded intraoperatively during pallidotomy correlated significantly with preoperative measures of thalamic glucose utilization obtained in the same patients under comparable behavioral conditions *(11)*. This physiological-metabolic relationship was reproduced in the subgroups of patients scanned on different PET cameras. Moreover, we found that GPi firing rates were also significantly correlated with the expression of an SSM/PCA metabolic network related to the pallidum and its major efferent projections. It is therefore likely that pallidal ablation exerts its primary metabolic effect in spatially distributed projection fields lying in the ventral tier and intralaminar thalamic nuclei as well as the brainstem.

PET activation studies using $[^{15}O]H_2O$ have also supported the notion of modulation of the motor cortico-striato-pallido-thalamo-cortical (CSPTC) motor circuit by postero-ventral pallidotomy. Grafton et al. reported postpallidotomy increases in rCBF in the ipsilateral PMC and in the SMA with movement *(34)*. In another study employing network analysis of motor system connectivity, Grafton and colleagues found significant postoperative reductions in the strength of interactions between the globus pallidus and thalamus, and the thalamus and mesial frontal motor area *(35)*. These activation PET findings, as well as those in the resting state, are consistent with an alteration in the activity of motor CSPTC circuits induced by pallidal ablation.

In addition to improving our understanding of network modulation that occurs following pallidotomy, FDG/PET may be used to select optimal candidates for this procedure. In our original study of 10 patients undergoing pallidotomy, we found that preoperative FDG/PET measurements of lentiform metabolism in the off-state correlated with clinical outcome up to 6 mo following surgery *(8)*. We subsequently studied an additional cohort of 22 PD patients to assess prospectively the usefulness of preoperative FDG/PET as a potential predictor of surgical outcome *(17)*. We found that the pallidotomy lesions were comparable in location and size in all patients, and therefore did not correlate with individual differences in surgical outcome. By contrast, the preoperative measures of lentiform glucose metabolism offered an accurate prediction of ultimate surgical improvement.

We additionally noted that the preoperative levodopa response also correlated with clinical outcome following surgery, albeit to a lesser degree than the PET measure *(17)*. This suggested that the dynamic range of the CSPTC motor loop during pallidal suppression could be estimated clinically with a levodopa challenge. These findings have been supported by FDG/PET experiments in PD patients showing reduction of pallidal hypermetabolism *(9)* and PDRP network expression *(10)* with levodopa infusion. Additionally, the decline in PDRP expression with levodopa correlated significantly with clinical improvement *(10)*. The combination of preoperative FDG/PET measurements of lentiform glucose metabolism and clinical-pharmacological estimates of the patient's capacity for network modulation can provide useful and complementary criteria for patient selection for PVP. Indeed, both measures taken together predicted approx 70% of the response to unilateral PVP *(17)*. The utility of FDG/PET in predicting the outcome of other stereotaxic procedures for PD, such as DBS of GPi or STN, is currently being investigated.

Stereotactic thalamotomy has been shown to significantly improve drug-resistant tremor in Parkinson's disease. The thalamic ventralis intermedius nucleus (Vim) has been targeted in thalamotomy as it relays cerebellar and proprioceptive output to sensorimotor cortical areas. Using [^{15}O]H_2O/PET, Boecker et al. reported significant operative declines in sensorimotor, premotor, and parietal rCBF both at rest and during motor activation in two PD patients who underwent thalamotomy for tremor *(36)*. This supports the notion that parkinsonian tremor arises through the overaction of ventral thalamic projections to cortical motor regions *(27)*. These findings indicate that in relieving PD tremor, thalamotomy may alter functional input from the surgical target to sensorimotor cortical regions. A comprehensive network modeling approach to define the mechanism of surgical improvement using imaging awaits future investigation.

5. DEEP BRAIN STIMULATION FOR PD

Deep brain high-frequency stimulation (DBS) has the advantage of avoiding permanent side effects due to an ablative lesion, therefore allowing for a reversible amelioration of parkinsonian symptoms. In addition, this technique is adaptable to clinical needs as stimulation frequency, intensity, and pulse width can be increased or decreased. High-frequency stimulation of the ventral portion of the thalamus, usually Vim, has been employed originally for the control of parkinsonian resting tremor *(37)*. More recently DBS has been applied to the GPi to improve rigidity and bradykinesia in PD *(38–40)* and to the STN to improve rigidity, akinesia, and tremor *(41–44)*.

Parker et al. investigated the effect of thalamic stimulation with PET. They observed a relative increase in rCBF in the sensorimotor cortex (SMC), PMC, SMA, caudate nucleus and cerebellar vermis during active tremor as compared with DBS-induced tremor arrest *(45)*. Deiber et al. *(46)* observed that suppression of tremor induced by effective stimulation is specifically associated with the reduction of cerebellar rCBF. By contrast, the incomplete arrest of tremor associated with suboptimal stimulation only reduced rCBF in frontal cortex. These observations are consistent with a decline in cerebellar synaptic activity during thalamic stimulation *(46)* occurring either directly, or indirectly through modulation of thalamocortical projections. The results of these studies also suggest that reductions in frontal

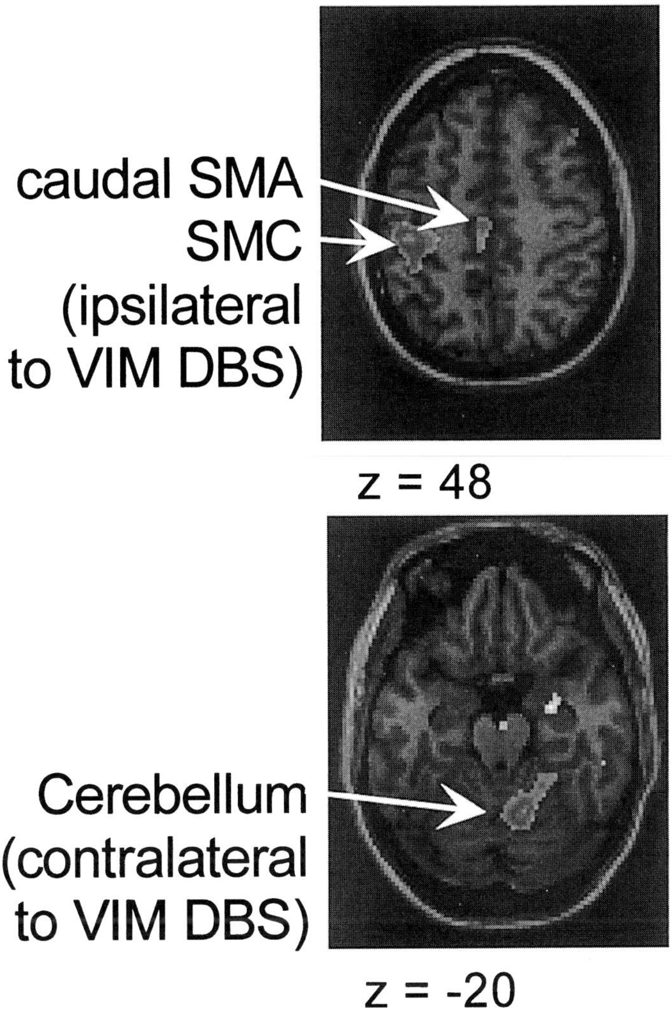

Fig. 1. $H_2{}^{15}O$/PET images of changes in regional cerebral blood flow (rCBF) in six Parkinson's disease patients with intractable tremor undergoing unilateral deep brain stimulation (DBS) of the ventral intermediate (Vim) nucleus. Vim DBS resulted in a significant decrease in rCBF in the sensorimotor area (SMC, BA 4) and the supplementary motor area (SMA, BA 6) ipsilateral to the stimulated hemisphere, and in the cerebellum contralateral to the stimulated side.

activity may be a nonspecific effect of the intervention. Davis et al. *(47)* examined rCBF and parkinsonian symptoms in patients who had Vim DBS implants. Patients were scanned with [^{15}O]H_2O/PET at rest under three stimulation conditions ("off," "sub-optimal," and "optimal" stimulation). During thalamic stimulation, rCBF declined in the ipsilateral sensory association region and in the SMA, cingulate motor area, and cerebellum contralateral to stimulation. rCBF increases were noted in the dorsolateral prefrontal cortex (DLPFC) and in the ipsilateral visual area. We have recently studied six other PD patients with unilateral left Vim DBS for intractable PD tremor. The patients were scanned with [^{15}O]H_2O/PET in three analogous stimulator conditions. We found a significant main effect of tremor characterized by ipsilateral rCBF reductions in SMC and in the contralateral cerebellum (Fig. 1). Additionally, we found that Vim DBS resulted in a localized rCBF increase in the vicinity of the electrode. These findings suggest that Vim DBS modulates the activity of cerebello-thalamocortical projection pathways. Depending on stimulation intensity and electrode placement in the ventral thalamus, it may be possible to alter the functional activity of one or more specific cortical fields.

[^{15}O]H_2O/PET has also been used to study the mechanism of action of GPi stimulation in PD. In their study, Davis et al. measured the effects of unilateral GPi DBS on regional cerebral blood flow. They found increased rCBF in ipsilateral SMA during GPi stimulation, in association with improved rigidity and bradykinesia *(47)*. Comparable rCBF changes with GPi DBS were not evident in the joystick activation study of Limousin et al. *(48)*. Recently, we studied six patients with advanced PD who performed a kinematically controlled motor execution task on and off pallidal stimulation *(49)*. GPi DBS resulted in significant rCBF increases in the SMC contralateral to the moving hand, and bilaterally in SMA (Fig. 2). Motor performance during PET imaging was improved by GPi DBS, especially with regard to movement initiation and spatial accuracy. Improvements in movement onset time also correlated with PET changes in the left (ipsilateral) SMC and ventral thalamus, as well as in the contralateral cerebellum. By contrast, improvements in spatial accuracy correlated with PET changes in both cerebellar hemispheres and in the left SMC.

We also performed adjunctive resting state FDG/PET scans in these patients with stimulation on and off for 12 h in each condition. We found that the expression of the PDRP network described by us previously was reduced significantly with pallidal stimulation. Moreover, the degree of change in this metabolic pattern during stimulation correlated with improvement in UPDRS motor ratings obtained at the time of PET imaging *(50)*. Thus, these findings support our previous observations in PVP. The PET data suggest that as in ablative pallidotomy, GPi DBS acts by suppressing overactive inhibitory pallidal output to the thalamus. Both interventions relieve parkinsonian symptoms by modulating the CSPTC and the cerebello-cortical motor loops.

STN is thought to be more effective than GPi stimulation in that it can influence multiple sources of inhibitory basal ganglia output, i.e., both the GPi and the substantia nigra reticulata. Limousin et al. *(48)* investigated the effect of STN stimulation on rCBF activation during a self-directed joystick task. With effective STN stimulation, there were significant increases in rCBF in SMA, cingulate cortex, and DLPFC. This suggests that STN DBS may play a role in potentiating nonprimary motor cortical areas, especially the DLPFC *(48)*. Ceballos-Baumann et al. *(51)* also demonstrated increases in activation of the rostral SMA and PMC ipsilateral to STN stimulation during joystick movement. Variation in the results of PET studies of STN and GPi DBS may relate to differences in the position of the stimulating electrode as well as the choice of contacts deployed during the different experiments.

6. METABOLIC NETWORK MAPPING IN DYSTONIA

Idiopathic torsion dystonia (ITD) is a common hereditary movement disorder affecting the basal ganglia. Because ITD is genetically mediated, this disorder provides a unique opportunity to assess the complex interrelationship between gene expression and brain network organization. In our first ITD study *(52)*, we identified an abnormal metabolic covariance pattern in dystonia patients with predominantly right-sided signs. This pattern was characterized by relative bilateral lentiform hypermetabolism that was dissociated from metabolic activity in the thalamus. These changes were associated with covariate metabolic increases in primary motor and premotor regions including SMA. Subject scores for this pattern correlated significantly with independent disability ratings for dystonia. We interpreted these results as evidence of resting overactivity of neural networks involving the lentiform nucleus and associative motor regions. Moreover, the dissociation between lentiform and thalamic metabolism in ITD suggested the possibility of functional inhibition of the GP, which has been postulated as a mechanism for hyperkinesia *(25,53,54)*.

Vitek et al. recently demonstrated decreased activity and altered patterns of discharge of neurons in both the GPe and GPi in three dystonia patients using microelectrode recording *(55)*. In this vein,

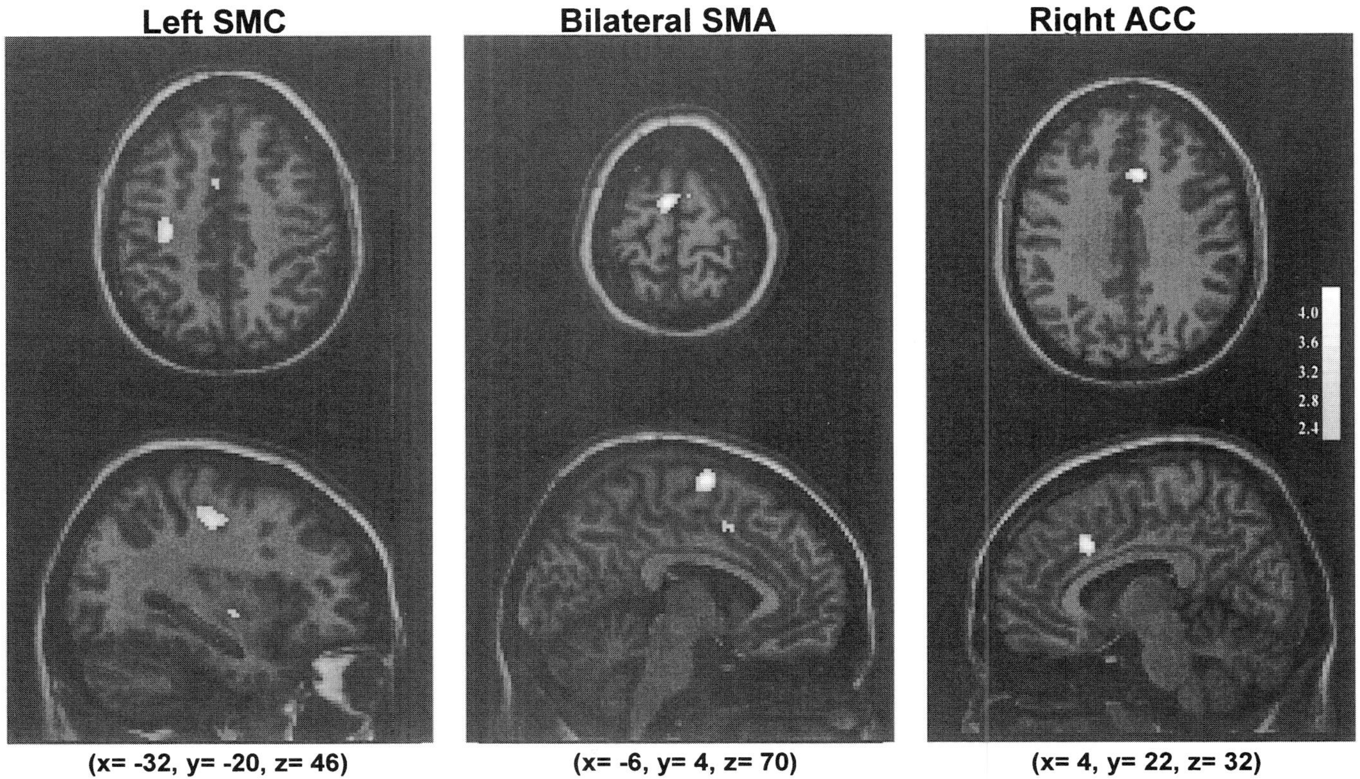

Fig. 2. $H_2{}^{15}O$/PET images of changes in regional cerebral blood flow (rCBF) in six advanced Parkinson's disease patients undergoing unilateral deep brain stimulation (DBS) of the internal pallidum. The patients were scanned in the DBS ON and OFF conditions while performing a kinematically controlled motor execution task using the hand opposite the pallidal stimulator. (The rate and amplitude of movement were controlled across DBS conditions). During task execution, pallidal DBS resulted in a significant increase in rCBF in the sensorimotor area (SMC, BA 4) contralateral to the moving hand, bilaterally in the supplementary motor area (SMA, BA 6), and in the anterior cingulate cortex (ACC, BA 24/32) ipsilateral to the moving hand.

we view the lentiform-thalamic metabolic dissociation present on FDG/PET imaging as consistent with overactivity of direct inhibitory projections from the putamen to GPi, with concomitant release of the ventral tier thalamic nuclei from pallidofugal inhibition *(3,11)*. Thus, the relative lentiform hypermetabolism noted by us may relate to an increase in GPi afferents through the direct striato-pallidal pathway. These findings in the resting state are compatible with the results of motor activation studies of ITD *(56)*, as well as with experimental animal models of dystonia *(25,53)*.

To address the problem of concurrent movement during PET, as well as the genotypic and phenotypic variability inherent in our first study, we subsequently studied a cohort of nonmanifesting carriers of the DYT1 gene for ITD *(57)*. In order to identify metabolic brain networks specifically associated with the DYT1 genotype, we performed network analysis on the combined metabolic dataset for the gene carriers and the normal volunteers, blind to gene status. In this network analysis, we identified a significant covariance pattern, which was topographically similar to that identified in our original ITD study. The DYT1-related pattern was characterized by bilateral lentiform hypermetabolism and thalamo-lentiform dissociation, associated with covarying increases in cerebellar and supplementary motor area (SMA) metabolism. Subject scores for this pattern were abnormally elevated in the nonmanifesting DYT1 carriers, indicating a genotype-related increase in brain network expression in these clinically normal individuals. We prospectively calculated the expression of this pattern in a separate cohort of *affected* DYT1 patients and found an abnormal increase in the expression of this network in the symptomatic patient cohort similar to that found in the nonmanifesting gene carriers. These findings demonstrate that the functional abnormalities of CSPTC motor circuits are associated with the DYT1 genotype and are evident in independent gene-bearing cohorts with and without clinical manifestations of dystonia. Specifically, network-related metabolic overaction of the lentiform nuclei and motor association cortices may be evident in the resting state in both nonmanifesting and affected DYT1 carriers. Similar network-related changes have been recently identified by us in different phenotypes *(58)* and genotypes of ITD *(59)*.

7. PALLIDOTOMY/THALAMOTOMY FOR DYSTONIA

Pallidotomy and thalamotomy may also provide symptom relief for dystonia. Although thalamotomy can alleviate clinical symptoms in some dystonia patients, there are risks of complications such as dysarthria, sensory loss, and gait ataxia, particularly when the surgery is bilateral *(60–62)*. Recently, there have been a few reports showing successful application of pallidotomy *(55,63–65)*. Lozano et al. used the surgery to treat a young boy with severe generalized dystonia. In that case, a 79% improvement in both axial and limb dystonia was noted 3 mo after bilateral pallidotomy *(63)*. Vitek et al. also found marked improvement in motor functioning and dystonic symptoms following GPi pallidotomy in three patients with primary dystonia *(55)*. In regard to neuroimaging studies, the effects of pallidotomy and thalamotomy in dystonia and other movement disorders remain a topic of future investigation.

8. DEEP BRAIN STIMULATION FOR DYSTONIA

DBS may be used as an alternative to pallidotomy and thalamotomy in dystonia and essential tremor *(37,66–68)*. Recent reports of pallidal stimulation describe a marked effect on all dystonic symptoms *(69,70)*. Kumar et al. *(71)* investigated the effect of GPi stimulation on rCBF during a joystick movement task in a patient with severe idiopathic generalized dystonia. Results showed significant decreases bilaterally in primary motor, lateral premotor, SMA, anterior cingulate and prefrontal areas, and ipsilaterally in the lentiform nucleus *(71)*. This suggests that GPi stimulation reverses the overactivity of certain motor cortical areas by indirectly increasing thalamocortical inhibition. It is however unknown whether the effects of DBS in dystonia relate to inhibition or activation of the internal pallidum. It is quite possible that the major role of DBS in dystonia is to reduce the noise that is associated with abnormal pallidal output occurring in the context of overactivity of the direct pathway *(52,57)*. The assessment of the pre- and postoperative effects of DBS in dystonia and other movement disorders using PET awaits confirmation in a larger series.

9. CONCLUSION

Functional brain imaging in conjunction with stereotaxic surgical procedures for PD provide a unique opportunity to study the pathophysiologic basis for clinical benefit following these interventions. Quantitative functional brain imaging markers may also be suitable as outcome measures for assessing the efficacy of surgical interventions for PD and related movement disorders. Lastly, functional brain imaging may serve as a useful tool in predicting optimal candidates for certain surgical interventions.

ACKNOWLEDGMENTS

Supported by NIH RO1 NS 35069, NS 37564, and by K24 NS 02101, as well as grants from the National Parkinson Foundation, the American Parkinson Disease Association, and the Dystonia Medical Research Foundation. Dr. Fukuda is a Veola T. Kerr Fellow of the Parkinson Disease Foundation.

REFERENCES

1. Alexander, G. E., Crutcher, M. D., and DeLong, M. R. (1990) Basal ganglia-thalamocortical circuits: parallel substrates for motor, oculomotor, prefrontal and limbic functions. *Prog. Brain Res.* **85,** 119–146.
2. Wichmann, T. and DeLong, M. R. (1996) Functional and pathophysiological models of the basal ganglia. *Curr. Opin. Neurobiol.* **6(6),** 751–758.
3. Parent, A. and Hazrati, L. N. (1995) Functional anatomy of the basal ganglia. I. The cortico-basal ganglia- thalamocortical loop. *Brain Res. Brain Res. Rev.* **20(1),** 91–127.
4. Eidelberg, D., Edwards, C., Mentis, M., Dhawan, V., and Moeller, J. R. (2000) Movement disorders: Parkinson's Disease. In: *Brain Mapping: The Disorders* (Mazziotta, J. C., Toga, A. W., and Frackowiak, R. S. J., eds.), Academic Press, San Diego, CA, pp. 241–261.
5. Mitchell, I. J., Boyce, S., Sambrook, M. A., and Crossman, A. R. (1992) A 2-deoxyglucose study of the effects of dopamine agonists on the parkinsonian primate brain. Implications for the neural mechanisms that mediate dopamine agonist-induced dyskinesia. *Brain* **115(Pt 3),** 809–824.
6. Eidelberg, D., Moeller, J. R., Dhawan, V., Spetsieris, P., Takikawa, S., Ishikawa, T., et al. (1994) The metabolic topography of parkinsonism. *J. Cereb. Blood Flow Metab.* **14(5),** 783–801.
7. Moeller, J. R., Nakamura, T., Mentis, M. J., Dhawan, V., Spetsieres, P., Antonini, A., et al. (1999) Reproducibility of regional metabolic covariance patterns: comparison of four populations. *J. Nucl. Med.* **40(8),** 1264–1269.
8. Eidelberg, D., Moeller, J. R., Ishikawa, T., Dhawan, V., Spetsieris, P., Silbersweig, D., et al. (1996) Regional metabolic correlates of surgical outcome following unilateral pallidotomy for Parkinson's disease. *Ann. Neurol.* **39(4),** 450–459.
9. Blesa, R., Blin, J., and Miletich, R. (1991) Levodopa-reduced glucose metabolism in striatopallido-thalamocortical circuit in Parkinson's disease. *Neurology* **441(S1),** 359.
10. Feigin, A., Mentis, M., Dhawan, V., Margouleff, C., and Eidelberg, D. (2000) Levodopa infusion reduced the expression of a Parkinson's disease metabolic brain network: A FDG PET study. *Neurology* **54(S3),** A113–A114.
11. Eidelberg, D., Moeller, J. R., Kazumata, K., Antonini, A., Sterio, D., Dhawan, V., et al. (1997) Metabolic correlates of pallidal neuronal activity in Parkinson's disease. *Brain* **120(Pt 8),** 1315–1324.
12. Antonini, A., Kazumata, K., Feigin, A., Mandel, F., Dhawan, V., Margouleff, C., and Eidelberg, D. (1998) Differential diagnosis of parkinsonism with [18F]fluorodeoxyglucose and PET. *Mov. Disord.* **13(2),** 268–274.
13. Antonini, A., Vontobel, P., Psylla, M., Gunther, I., Maguire, P. R., Missimer, J., and Leenders, K. L. (1995) Complementary positron emission tomographic studies of the striatal dopaminergic system in Parkinson's disease. *Arch. Neurol.* **52(12),** 1183–1190.
14. Eidelberg, D., Takikawa, S., Moeller, J. R., Dhawan, V., Redington, K., Chaly, T., et al. (1993) Striatal hypometabolism distinguishes striatonigral degeneration from Parkinson's disease. *Ann. Neurol.* **33(5),** 518–527.
15. Przedborski, S., Giladi, N., Takikawa, S., Ishikawa, T., Dhawan, V., Spetsieris, P., et al. (1994) Metabolic topography of the hemiparkinsonism-hemiatrophy syndrome. *Neurology* **44(9),** 1622–1628.
16. Eidelberg, D., Dhawan, V., Moeller, J. R., Sidtis, J. J., Ginos, J. Z., Strother, S. C., et al. (1991) The metabolic landscape of cortico-basal ganglionic degeneration: regional asymmetries studied with positron emission tomography. *J. Neurol. Neurosurg. Psychiatry* **54(10),** 856–862.
17. Kazumata, K., Antonini, A., Dhawan, V., Moeller, J. R., Alterman, R. L., Kelly, P., et al. (1997) Preoperative indicators of clinical outcome following stereotaxic pallidotomy. *Neurology* **49(4),** 1083–1090.
18. Eidelberg, D. (1998) Functional brain networks in movement disorders. *Curr. Opin. Neurol.* **11(4),** 319–326.

19. Alexander, G. and Moeller, J. (1994) Application of the scaled subprofile model to functional imaging in neuropsychiatric disorders: A principal component approach to modeling brain function in disease. *Hum. Brain Mapp.* **2,** 1–16.
20. Moeller, J. R., Strother, S. C., Sidtis, J. J., and Rottenberg, D. A. (1987) Scaled subprofile model: a statistical approach to the analysis of functional patterns in positron emission tomographic data. *J. Cereb. Blood Flow Metab.* **7(5),** 649–658.
21. Moeller, J. R. and Strother, S. C. (1991) A regional covariance approach to the analysis of functional patterns in positron emission tomographic data. *J. Cereb. Blood Flow Metab.* **11(2),** A121–A135.
22. Eidelberg, D., Moeller, J. R., Dhawan, V., Sidtis, J. J., Ginos, J. Z., Strother, S. C., et al. (1990) The metabolic anatomy of Parkinson's disease: complementary [^{18}F]fluorodeoxyglucose and [^{18}F]fluorodopa positron emission tomographic studies. *Mov. Disord.* **5(3),** 203–213.
23. Eidelberg, D., Moeller, J. R., Ishikawa, T., Dhawan, V., Spetsieris, P., Chaly, T., et al. (1995) Assessment of disease severity in parkinsonism with fluorine-18-fluorodeoxyglucose and PET. *J. Nucl. Med.* **36(3),** 378–383.
24. Moeller, J. R. and Eidelberg, D. (1997) Divergent expression of regional metabolic topographies in Parkinson's disease and normal ageing. *Brain* **120(Pt 12),** 2197–2206.
25. Crossman, A. R. (1990) A hypothesis on the pathophysiological mechanisms that underlie levodopa- or dopamine agonist-induced dyskinesia in Parkinson's disease: implications for future strategies in treatment. *Mov. Disord.* **5(2),** 100–108.
26. Wooten, G. F. and Collins, R. C. (1981) Metabolic effects of unilateral lesion of the substantia nigra. *J. Neurosci.* **1(3),** 285–291.
27. Antonini, A., Moeller, J. R., Nakamura, T., Spetsieris, P., Dhawan, V., and Eidelberg, D. (1998) The metabolic anatomy of tremor in Parkinson's disease. *Neurology* **51(3),** 803–810.
28. Laitinen, L. V., Bergenheim, A. T., and Hariz, M. I. (1992) Leksell's posteroventral pallidotomy in the treatment of Parkinson's disease. *J. Neurosurg.* **76(1),** 53–61.
29. Lozano, A. M., Lang, A. E., Galvez-Jimenez, N., Miyasaki, J., Duff, J., Hutchinson, W. D., and Dostrovsky, J. O. (1995) Effect of GPi pallidotomy on motor function in Parkinson's disease. *Lancet* **346(8987),** 1383–1387.
30. Baron, M. S., Vitek, J. L., Bakay, R. A., Green, J., Kaneoke, Y., Hashimoto, T., et al. (1996) Treatment of advanced Parkinson's disease by posterior GPi pallidotomy: 1-year results of a pilot study. *Ann. Neurol.* **40(3),** 355–366.
31. Dogali, M., Fazzini, E., Kolodny, E., Eidelberg, D., Sterio, D., Devinsky, O., and Beric, A. (1995) Stereotactic ventral pallidotomy for Parkinson's disease. *Neurology* **45(4),** 753–761.
32. Marsden, C. D. and Obeso, J. A. (1994) The functions of the basal ganglia and the paradox of stereotaxic surgery in Parkinson's disease. *Brain* **117(Pt 4),** 877–897.
33. Mata, M., Fink, D. J., Gainer, H., Smith, C. B., Davidsen, L., Savaki, H., et al. (1980) Activity-dependent energy metabolism in rat posterior pituitary primarily reflects sodium pump activity. *J. Neurochem.* **34(1),** 213–215.
34. Grafton, S. T., Waters, C., Sutton, J., Lew, M. F., and Couldwell, W. (1995) Pallidotomy increases activity of motor association cortex in Parkinson's disease: a positron emission tomographic study. *Ann. Neurol.* **37(6),** 776–783.
35. Grafton, S., Sutton, J., Couldwell, W., Lew, M., and Waters, C. (1994) Network analysis of motor system connectivity in Parkinson's disease: Modulation of thalamocortical interactions after pallidotomy. *Hum. Brain Mapp.* **2,** 45–55.
36. Boecker, H., Wills, A. J., Ceballos-Baumann, A., Samuel, M., Thomas, D. G., Marsden, C. D., and Brooks, D. J. (1997) Stereotactic thalamotomy in tremor-dominant Parkinson's disease: an H2(15)O PET motor activation study. *Ann. Neurol.* **41(1),** 108–111.
37. Benabid, A. L., Pollak, P., Gao, D., Hoffmann, D., Limousin, P., Gay, E., et al. (1996) Chronic electrical stimulation of the ventralis intermedius nucleus of the thalamus as a treatment of movement disorders. *J. Neurosurg.* **84(2),** 203–214.
38. Gross, C., Rougier, A., Guehl, D., Boraud, T., Julien, J., and Bioulac, B. (1997) High-frequency stimulation of the globus pallidus internalis in Parkinson's disease: a study of seven cases. *J. Neurosurg.* **87(4),** 491–498.
39. Pahwa, R., Wilkinson, S., Smith, D., Lyons, K., Miyawaki, E., and Koller, W. C. (1997) High-frequency stimulation of the globus pallidus for the treatment of Parkinson's disease. *Neurology* **49(1),** 249–253.
40. Tronnier, V. M., Fogel, W., Kronenbuerger, M., and Steinvorth, S. (1997) Pallidal stimulation: an alternative to pallidotomy? *J. Neurosurg.* **87(5),** 700–705.
41. Limousin, P., Pollak, P., Benazzouz, A., Hoffmann, D., Broussolle, E., Perret, J. E., and Benabid, A. L. (1995) Bilateral subthalamic nucleus stimulation for severe Parkinson's disease. *Mov. Disord.* **10(5),** 672–674.
42. Limousin, P., Krack, P., Pollak, P., Benazzouz, A., Ardouin, C., Hoffmann, D., and Benabid, A. L. (1998) Electrical stimulation of the subthalamic nucleus in advanced Parkinson's disease. *N. Engl. J. Med.* **339(16),** 1105–1111.
43. Kumar, R., Lozano, A. M., Kim, Y. J., Hutchison, W. D., Sime, E., Halket, E., and Lang, A. E. (1998) Double-blind evaluation of subthalamic nucleus deep brain stimulation in advanced Parkinson's disease. *Neurology* **51(3),** 850–855.
44. Kumar, R., Lozano, A. M., Sime, E., Halket, E., and Lang, A. E. (1999) Comparative effects of unilateral and bilateral subthalamic nucleus deep brain stimulation. *Neurology* **53(3),** 561–566.
45. Parker, F., Tzourio, N., Blond, S., Petit, H., and Mazoyer, B. (1992) Evidence for a common network of brain structures involved in parkinsonian tremor and voluntary repetitive movement. *Brain Res.* **584(1–2),** 11–17.
46. Deiber, M. P., Pollak, P., Passingham, R., Landais, P., Gervason, C., Cinotti, L., et al. (1993) Thalamic stimulation and suppression of parkinsonian tremor. Evidence of a cerebellar deactivation using positron emission tomography. *Brain* **116(Pt 1),** 267–279.
47. Davis, K. D., Taub, E., Houle, S., Lang, A. E., Dostrovsky, J. O., Tasker, R. R., and Lozano, A. M. (1997) Globus pallidus stimulation activates the cortical motor system during alleviation of parkinsonian symptoms. *Nat. Med.* **3(6),** 671–674.

48. Limousin, P., Greene, J., Pollak, P., Rothwell, J., Benabid, A. L., and Frackowiak, R. (1997) Changes in cerebral activity pattern due to subthalamic nucleus or internal pallidum stimulation in Parkinson's disease. *Ann. Neurol.* **42(3),** 283–291.
49. Fukuda, M., Ghilardi, M., Mentis, M., Nakamura, T., Dhawan, V., Antonini, A., et al. (2001) Functional correlates of pallidal stimulation for Parkinson's disease. *Ann. Neurol.* **49,** 135–165.
50. Fukuda, M., Mentis, M., Dhawan, V., Lyons, K., Koller, W., and Eidelberg, D. (2000) Metabolic correlates of clinical outcome with pallidal deep brain stimulation for Parkinson's disease. *Neurology* **54(S3),** A283.
51. Ceballos-Baumann, A. O., Boecker, H., Bartenstein, P., von Falkenhayn, I., Riescher, H., Conrad, B., et al. (1999) A positron emission tomographic study of subthalamic nucleus stimulation in Parkinson disease: enhanced movement-related activity of motor-association cortex and decreased motor cortex resting activity. *Arch. Neurol.* **56(8),** 997–1003.
52. Eidelberg, D., Moeller, J. R., Ishikawa, T., Dhawan, V., Spetsieris, P., Przedborski, S., and Fahn, S. (1995) The metabolic topography of idiopathic torsion dystonia. *Brain* **118(Pt 6),** 1473–1484.
53. Mitchell, I. J., Luquin, R., Boyce, S., Clarke, C. E., Robertson, R. G., Sambrook, M. A., and Crossman, A. R. (1990) Neural mechanisms of dystonia: evidence from a 2-deoxyglucose uptake study in a primate model of dopamine agonist-induced dystonia. *Mov. Disord.* **5(1),** 49–54.
54. Hallett, M. (1993) Physiology of basal ganglia disorders: an overview. *Can. J. Neurol. Sci.* **20(3),** 177–183.
55. Vitek, J. L., Chockkan, V., Zhang, J. Y., Kaneoke, Y., Evatt, M., DeLong, M. R., et al. (1999) Neuronal activity in the basal ganglia in patients with generalized dystonia and hemiballismus. *Ann. Neurol.* **46(1),** 22–35.
56. Ceballos-Baumann, A. O., Passingham, R. E., Warner, T., Playford, E. D., Marsden, C. D., and Brooks, D. J. (1995) Overactive prefrontal and underactive motor cortical areas in idiopathic dystonia. *Ann. Neurol.* **37(3),** 363–372.
57. Eidelberg, D., Moeller, J. R., Antonini, A., Kazumata, K., Nakamura, T., Dhawan, V., et al. (1998) Functional brain networks in DYT1 dystonia. *Ann. Neurol.* **44(3),** 303–312.
58. Hutchinson, M., Nakamura, T., Moeller, J. R., Antonini, A., Belakhlef, A., Dhawan, V., and Eidelberg, D. (2000) The metabolic topography of essential blepharospasm: a focal dystonia with general implications. *Neurology* **55(5),** 673–677.
59. Edwards, C., Raymond, D., Saunders-Pullman, R., Mentis, M. J., Bressman, S., and Eidelberg, D. (2000) Abnormal expression in non-DYT1 dystonia. *Neurology* **54,** A196.
60. Tasker, R. R., Doorly, T., and Yamashiro, K. (1988) Thalamotomy in generalized dystonia. *Adv. Neurol.* **50,** 615–631.
61. Andrew, J., Fowler, C. J., and Harrison, M. J. (1983) Stereotaxic thalamotomy in 55 cases of dystonia. *Brain* **106 (Pt 4),** 981–1000.
62. Cardoso, F., Jankovic, J., Grossman, R. G., and Hamilton, W. J. (1995) Outcome after stereotactic thalamotomy for dystonia and hemiballismus. *Neurosurgery* **36(3),** 501–507; discussion 507–508.
63. Lozano, A. M., Kumar, R., Gross, R. E., Giladi, N., Hutchison, W. D., Dostrovsky, J. O., and Lang, A. E. (1997) Globus pallidus internus pallidotomy for generalized dystonia. *Mov. Disord.* **12(6),** 865–870.
64. Ondo, W. G., Desaloms, J. M., Jankovic, J., and Grossman, R. G. (1998) Pallidotomy for generalized dystonia. *Mov. Disord.* **13(4),** 693–698.
65. Lin, J. J., Lin, G. Y., Shih, C., Lin, S. Z., Chang, D. C., and Lee, C. C. (1999) Benefit of bilateral pallidotomy in the treatment of generalized dystonia. Case report. *J. Neurosurg.* **90(5),** 974–976.
66. Blond, S. and Siegfried, J. (1991) Thalamic stimulation for the treatment of tremor and other movement disorders. *Acta Neurochir. Suppl. (Wien)* **52,** 109–111.
67. Benabid, A. L., Pollak, P., Seigneuret, E., Hoffmann, D., Gay, E., and Perret, J. (1993) Chronic VIM thalamic stimulation in Parkinson's disease, essential tremor and extra-pyramidal dyskinesias. *Acta Neurochir. Suppl. (Wien)* **58,** 39–44.
68. Sellal, F., Hirsch, E., Barth, P., Blond, S., and Marescaux, C. (1993) A case of symptomatic hemidystonia improved by ventroposterolateral thalamic electrostimulation. *Mov. Disord.* **8(4),** 515–518.
69. Tronnier, V. M. and Fogel, W. (2000) Pallidal stimulation for generalized dystonia. Report of three cases. *J. Neurosurg.* **92(3),** 453–456.
70. Coubes, P., Roubertie, A., Vayssiere, N., Hemm, S., and Echenne, B. (2000) Treatment of DYT1-generalized dystonia by stimulation of the internal globus pallidus. *Lancet* **355(9222),** 2220–2221.
71. Kumar, R., Dagher, A., Hutchison, W. D., Lang, A. E., and Lozano, A. M. (1999) Globus pallidus deep brain stimulation for generalized dystonia: clinical and PET investigation. *Neurology* **53(4),** 871–874.

22

Fetal Tissue Transplantation for the Treatment of Parkinson's Disease

Paul Greene and Stanley Fahn

1. HISTORICAL BACKGROUND

Current attempts to treat idiopathic Parkinson's disease (PD) and parkinsonism with transplants of dopaminergic tissue began in the 1970s, with the grafting of tissue into animal models of parkinsonism. The history of brain transplantation, however, is over a century old, dating at least back to the unsuccessful attempts by W.G. Thompson in 1890 to transplant adult cortex to adult cortex in cats and dogs *(1)*. Table 1 lists some of the research precursors of modern fetal tissue efforts.

The first transplants into the brain of patients with PD happened almost exactly one century after the earliest brain transplant attempts. Transplants into human beings were attempted after extensive reports in animals indicated that grafted tissue could partially reverse the biochemical, physiological, and behavioral manifestations of experimental parkinsonism. Transplantation into humans was then required to answer basic questions about the possibility of neural transplantation for clinical use: what is the optimal tissue to transplant; will grafts survive in the human brain and for how long; what kind of immunosuppression, if any, will be necessary for graft survival; what are the risks of neural grafting; will grafts release dopamine and/or innervate host striatal cells; will grafts have a sufficient impact on the symptoms of parkinsonism to justify the surgical risks? In addition to general questions relating to any attempt to replace nonfunctioning nerve cells with neural grafts, there are questions peculiar to PD:

1. Will transplanted dopaminergic cells degenerate from whatever process is responsible for the underlying PD?
2. Will transplanted cells change the natural history of PD by providing trophic factors or by providing a more "natural" release of dopamine?
3. Will grafts improve presumed nondopaminergic symptoms such as "on" freezing and loss of postural reflexes?
4. Will grafts influence the development of dementia?
5. Will dopamine released by the graft produce psychosis?
6. Will grafts innervate enough of the striatum to reduce or eliminate the need for exogenous medication?
7. Will grafts provide uniform dopaminergic stimulation that will influence all body regions?
8. How will antiparkinson medications influence functioning of the neural grafts?
9. Will grafts exert effects on extrastriatal dopaminergic targets?

Some of these questions have been answered by the ongoing use of fetal transplants to treat PD, but many questions remain. Before considering the use of fetal mesencephalic tissue transplantation in treating parkinsonism, we review some of the preclinical data in animals and some of the relevant lessons from the experience in autografts of adrenal medullary tissue to treat PD.

From: Contemporary Clinical Neurology:
Surgical Treatment of Parkinson's Disease and Other Movement Disorders
Edited by: D. Tarsy, J. L. Vitek, and A. M. Lozano © Humana Press Inc., Totowa, NJ

Table 1
Initial Transplant Attempts

Date	Description	Ref.
1890	Graft of adult cat cortex to canine brain (unsuccessful)	*(1)*
1917	Graft of neonatal rat cortex to rat brain (successful demonstration that grafted cells could survive)	*(2)*
1962	Demonstration of functional connection between graft tissue and host brain (graft of pituitary tissue into the hypothalamus of rats)	*(3)*
1976	Survival of monoaminergic neurons transplanted in animals (graft of rat fetal tissue into rat adult brain)	*(4)*
1979	Fetal mesencephalic tissue reduces experimental parkinsonism in animals (graft of rat fetal tissue into rat striatum in the 6-hydroxydopamine [6-OHDA] model of parkinsonism)	*(5,6)*
1982	Fetal mesencephalic tissue reduces experimental parkinsonism in animals (graft of rat fetal tissue into rat striatum in the 6-OHDA model of parkinsonism)	*(7)*
1987	Fetal mesencephalic tissue grafted into the striatum in a patient with PD	*(8)*

Table 2
Behavioral Effects of Unilateral 6-OHDA Lesion

Persistent rotation ipsilateral to the lesion
Sensory inattention contralateral to the lesion
Enhanced ipsilateral rotation with dopamine releasing agents (e.g., amphetamine)
Decreased ipsilateral and enhanced contralateral rotation with dopamine agonists (e.g., apomorphine)

Table 3
Behavioral Effects of Fetal Mesencephalic Implantation after a 6-OHDA Lesion in Rodents

Reduced spontaneous rotation with implanted tissue
Reversed apomorphine induced asymmetry with implanted tissue
Reversed amphetamine induced asymmetry with implanted tissue
Implanted tissue reverses some nonrotational behavioral deficits (e.g., impaired response to stimuli contralateral to the 6-OHDA lesion)

2. ANIMAL STUDIES

Neural transplantation has been extensively studied in animal models of parkinsonism *(9,10)*. The most extensive animal testing has been carried out using 6-hydroxydopamine (6-OHDA) to lesion the nigrostriatal tract in rats. Injection of 6-OHDA causes selective damage to catecholaminergic neurons, resulting in depletion of dopamine. If the dopaminergic lesion is substantial the behavioral manifestations of the lesion are persistent. Severe bilateral lesions cause aphagia and adipsia, so that unilateral 6-OHDA lesions are more commonly used. Rats with unilateral 6-OHDA lesions exhibit the behaviors listed in Table 2 *(9)*.

Contralateral rotation following administration of dopamine agonists presumably occurs because of ipsilateral dopamine receptor supersensitivity. The behavioral changes after implantation of fetal mesencephalic tissue into rats with unilateral 6-OHDA lesions are listed in Table 3 *(9)*.

Many of these behavioral improvements can be achieved by implanting either rat or human fetal dopaminergic tissue into 6-OHDA rats. In some experiments, the degree of reversal of 6-OHDA induced behaviors correlates with the number of surviving neurons, amount of neuronal outgrowth, and amount

Table 4
Physiologic and Biochemical Effects of Fetal Mesencephalic Transplantation after a 6-OHDA Lesion in Rodents

Grafted neurons fire and release dopamine spontaneously
Grafted neurons develop axonal projections preferentially into normal dopaminergic target areas
Grafted neurons synapse primarily on host dendrites
Host brain synapses on grafted neurons have been identified
Striatal dopamine levels are restored towards normal (reaching 10–30% of normal)
Some other changes in the striatum are also corrected by grafting (correction of increased striatal firing, return of enkephalin and D2 binding levels towards normal, return of striatal cholinergic activity towards normal, return towards normal of GABAergic neuron activity)

Table 5
Effects of Fetal Mesencephalic Transplantation after a 6-OHDA Lesion in Primates

Increased spontaneous activity in some animals
Decreased rotational effects of amphetamine/apomorphine as in rodents
Increased manual dexterity after grafting: this has been inconsistent, incomplete, and sometimes short-lived
Neglect was not improved after grafting in marmosets

of dopamine released by the transplanted cells. Other biochemical, physiological, and anatomic observations indicate that grafts reverse the effects of dopaminergic lesions at least in part by specific dopaminergic release onto normal dopaminergic target cells in the striatum. Some of these observations are listed in Table 4 *(9,11)*.

Experiments in animals have also indicated that neuronal grafts in the striatum may actually be subject to some feedback control *(11)*. Application of dopamine agonists to grafts causes a decrease in firing rate, application of amphetamine causes increased dopamine release, and intrastriatal grafts have been shown to respond to cortical or striatal stimulation.

The success of neural grafting in rodent models of PD inevitably led to trials of similar grafting in nonhuman primates. A variety of monkeys have been used, including macaques, rhesus monkeys, marmosets, African green monkeys, bonnet monkeys, vervet monkeys, and Macaca fuscata monkeys. Unilateral and bilateral 6-OHDA lesions also provided a primate model to test the results of dopaminergic grafting. In addition, unilateral and bilateral 1-methyl-4-phenyl-1,2,3,6-tetrahydropyridine (MPTP) intoxication provided a model for PD that was pathologically and physiologically closer to PD than the 6-OHDA model. The behavioral effects of 6-OHDA and MPTP lesions in monkeys are similar to effects of 6-OHDA in rodents. The results of fetal mesencephalic grafting was also similar, although far fewer experiments have been reported using primates than rodents. Some results of fetal mesencephalic grafting in primate models of PD are listed in Table 5 *(12)*.

The beneficial effects of grafting in primates has been less consistent than benefits seen in rodents, possibly because of the smaller number of animals involved. In addition, there is some suggestion that benefit in primates may not exclusively be due to dopamine release by the graft. In the monkey, grafts of nondopaminergic tissue (cerebellum, spinal cord) induced sprouting of host dopaminergic fibers and showed beneficial effects in some experiments, suggesting that specific dopaminergic effects might not account for all the effects of grafting *(13)*. Some findings in primates have direct implications for grafting techniques in humans. For instance, in marmosets, rotational activity was reduced by caudate but not putaminal grafts, whereas other behaviors were reduced by putaminal grafts *(12)*. Taken together, the results of transplant studies in rodents and nonhuman primates were sufficiently promising that the stage was set for attempting transplantation in humans.

Table 6
Adrenal Medulla Autograft for PD

Center	# Pts	Description	Ref.
Capital Institute of Medicine, Beijing, China	4	6 mo follow-up: improvement in bradykinesia, rigidity, tremor, posture, speech, gait while taking amantadine and Chinese traditional treatments	*(19)*
Vanderbilt University Medical Center, Nashville, TN	12	1 yr follow-up: mean improvement in modified Unified Parkinson Disease Rating Scale (UPDRS) of 16%, slight reduction in mean levodopa usage: overall improvement in 9/12, 4 with "distinct" improvement	*(20)*
Rush-Presbyterian-St. Luke's Medical Center, Chicago, IL	7	1 yr follow-up: increase in time "on" from 61 to 83%; increase in "on" time without dyskinesias from 22 to 61%; increase from 34 to 60% of normal functioning while "off"	*(21)*
Hospital General de Mexico, National Medical Center, Mexico	10	1 year follow-up: minimal to modest decrease in tremor, rigidity, "on" time, and Hoehn & Yahr stage in some patients; no improvement in bradykinesia, quantitative motor tasks, or overall improvement	*(22)*

3. HUMAN STUDIES

3.1. *Adrenal Medullary Autografts*

Before turning to the results of fetal tissue transplantation in humans, it would be useful to review lessons learned from attempts in the early 1980s to treat PD by transplantation of autologous adrenal medullary cells. These attempts predate the use of fetal mesencephalic tissue for grafting and highlight the problems which arise in evaluating clinical outcomes after grafting for PD.

Normally, the adrenal medulla produces dopamine as an intermediate in the synthesis of epinephrine. When adrenal medullary cells are removed from the influence of cortisol, under some circumstances they release increased amounts of dopamine and develop neuron-like processes *(14)*. In animals, transplantation of adult adrenal medullary tissue into the striatum resulted in poor graft survival except when nerve growth factor was added *(9)*. Transplanted adult adrenal tissue did not show significant fiber outgrowth and, although tyrosine hydroxylase (TH) positive staining was occasionally present in surviving grafts, most surviving cells did not show evidence of dopamine production *(15,16)*.

Despite this, in the early 1980s several patients with PD received implants of their own adrenal medullary tissue. None of these patients experienced dramatic or long-lasting improvement. It is unlikely that this technique for neural grafting would have received much more attention if not for the report in 1987 by Madrazo et al. that two patients improved dramatically after adrenal medullary autografts *(17)*. Within a year, at least 135 additional patients with PD received adrenal medullary autografts *(18)*. Initial reports were interpreted as promising. Some examples are listed in Table 6.

By the early 1990s, it was apparent that, as experience with adrenal medullary transplantation grew results seemed less impressive. In 1991, Goetz et al. summarized the results of adrenal medullary grafting in 61 Canadian and US patients operated in 13 centers *(23)*. After 2 yr of follow-up relatively few features of PD had improved significantly. For example, mean "off" ADL went from 28 to 24%; percent time "off" went from 50 to 39%; percent time "on" without dyskinesias went from 24 to 42%; "off" Hoehn & Yahr stage went from 4.18 to 3.74; "off" functioning went from 35 to 44% of normal. There was a slight (but not statistically significant) increase in medication dosage over that time, and many other measures of PD severity, including all "objective" measures, showed no significant improvement. Overall (including patients who died or were lost to follow-up), only 19% of patients were considered improved at 2 yr. The authors felt this was comparable to benefits reported from treatment with

Table 7
Autopsy Results after Adrenal Medulla Autografting for PD

Duration of implant	Duration of benefit	Description	Ref.
Improved at time of death			
1 yr	NA	No adrenal medulla cells; received RT for glioblastoma multiforme 9 mo after transplantation	*(32)*
8 mo	NA	No adrenal medulla cells, no TH staining	*(33)*
Unimproved at time of death			
4 mo	2 wk	No viable adrenal medulla cells, no TH staining	*(24)*
1 yr	None	No viable adrenal medulla cells	*(25)*
4 mo	None	No viable adrenal medulla cells, no TH/THmRNA staining in graft; increased TH, low-affinity nerve growth factor receptor staining in host striatum	*(26,27)*
4 mo	None	Few adrenal medulla cells with no neurites, no TH staining	*(28)*
30 mo	6 mo	Few nests of TH staining cells with TH staining processes that did not reach the host striatum	*(29)*
35 d	None	No identifiable adrenal medulla cells	*(22)*
69 d	None	No identifiable adrenal medulla cells	*(22)*
6 wk	None	Minimal viable adrenal medulla cells, no evidence of graft to host striatal tissue outgrowth	*(30)*
121 d	None	No identifiable adrenal medulla cells	*(31)*

TH, tyrosine hydroxylase.
NA, not applicable.

dopamine agonists. However, there was considerable short-term morbidity and 11/56 of the patients died in the two years following transplantation. The authors estimated that six of these deaths (11% of 56 patients) were possibly related to surgery. After balancing the therapeutic benefit with morbidity and mortality, all 13 of the groups participating in this report discontinued adrenal medullary transplantation.

Moreover, human autopsy data from patients receiving adrenal medullary grafts also gave little reason for optimism. Autopsy data is summarized in Table 7.

In summary, in most centers, adrenal medullary autografting resulted in questionable clinical outcome but was associated with considerable morbidity and some mortality. Improvement was most marked in the earliest trials, with decreased benefit appearing in subsequent larger trials. Despite the questionable preclinical basis for this type of grafting, initial enthusiasm was maintained for several years. The lack of consistent post-transplantation patient evaluation, coupled with the large variation in techniques of transplantation made it difficult to assess the true value of the procedure.

3.2. Ventral Mesencephalic Grafts into Patients with Parkinsonism

The initial report of fetal tissue implantation for PD came from China in 1987 *(8)* and was followed a year later by reports from Sweden *(34)* and Mexico *(35)*. By 1998 over 200 patients throughout the world had received fetal mesencephalic grafts for parkinsonism *(36)*. By 1999 the figure had climbed to 300 patients *(37)*. Based on animal data and the small number of autopsies in PD patients receiving fetal grafts, it seems likely that at least some effects of fetal grafts come about because of specific neural connections that release dopamine. However, other modes of action have been proposed, including nonspecific release of dopamine, release of trophic factors, other nonspecific effects that might also result from implantation of nondopaminergic tissue, and nonspecific surgical effects such as breakdown of blood-brain barrier (BBB) and the effects of lesions in the caudate and/or putamen. Techniques for fetal tissue implantation in humans have been adapted from techniques used in animals but in most cases optimal techniques in humans have yet to be established. Most groups attempting implantation surgery have developed their own techniques and there remain wide variations in various aspects of the procedure that may significantly affect the outcome.

3.2.1. Fetal Tissue Preparation

Gestational age of the transplanted fetal tissue affects neuronal survival following implantation. The optimal donor age of transplants from human fetal tissue to human adult brain is not known. The optimal survival of human fetal tissue implants into adult rat brain occurs when fetal age is approx 5.5–8 wk gestational age for cell suspensions or 6.5–9 wk gestational age for solid grafts *(38)*. This roughly corresponds to the time of the first appearance of tyrosine hydoxylase containing neurons to the beginning of the outgrowth of neuronal processes *(39,40)*. The optimal technique for fetal tissue preparation is not known. All groups test maternal blood and/or fetal tissue for a panel of antibodies and/or antigens, including HIV1 and 2, hepatitis A, B, and C, cytomegalovirus, toxoplasma, syphilis, and herpes simplex virus. Some groups also culture fetal tissue for bacteria and yeast and screen for viability and for presence of tyrosine hydroxylase *(41)* or production of dopamine metabolites *(42)*. In an attempt to maximize cell survival, most groups have performed transplantation surgery within hours of collection of fetal tissue. This is practical in only a small number of procedures. Some groups have stored the tissue prior to implantation, either for several days *(43)*, cultured for many days *(42)*, or frozen *(41)*. The form of tissue implantation has been about evenly divided between groups using cell suspensions and those using solid fragments of tissue, including one group that uses a strand of tissue *(42)*. Each technique has possible advantages such as more even distribution of cells for suspensions and preserved relationship between neurons and glia for fragments but they have not been directly compared.

The optimal number of cells required for fetal cell implantation is unknown. Both human substantia nigra together have about 550,000 neurons with only about 120,000 projecting to the putamena. *(44,45)*. Animal studies suggest that with current techniques, about 5% of transplanted dopaminergic neurons survive *(46)*. This estimate has been confirmed in an autopsy of a patient with PD who received a fetal tissue implant *(47)*. This would suggest that a relatively small number of fetuses would be adequate to restore dopamine to the putamena. However, neuronal processes from grafts are relatively short, which limits the maximum volume of putamen that can be reinnervated, and there is wide variation in neuronal survival in the same patient in different needle tracks *(47)*. In practice, fetal tissue implantation in PD patients has been carried out using from one to six fetuses per striatum.

3.2.2. Surgical Technique

Several early fetal tissue transplantation attempts implanted tissue unilaterally in the brain. Although bilateral effects were observed, contralateral improvement was greater than ipsilateral benefit *(48)*. Most recent efforts have used bilateral transplantation. There is still controversy about the ideal target for fetal tissue transplantation. The posterior putamen is most severely affected in PD. However, some animal experiments indicated benefit from caudate grafting and patients with early PD who were given caudate fetal tissue implants seemed to improve. Because there have been no definitive studies, most recent transplants have used the posterior putamen as the primary target although sometimes using the caudate as an auxiliary target.

Three groups implanted tissue in a cavity in the caudate nucleus during open craniotomy *(49–51)*. All other groups used stereotactic implantation under magnetic resonance imaging (MRI) guidance. In order to deposit tissue in the putamen, they have used multiple needle passes on each side of the brain from a crown approach. They have attempted to balance the need to maximize the volume of putamen receiving fetal tissue with the risk of hemorrhage, which increases with the number of needle passes. Recently, one group has begun approaching the putamen along its long axis using frontal incisions in order to minimize the number of needle passes *(52)*. Other aspects of the surgical technique including the size of the cannula containing tissue and the exact method for depositing tissue may affect outcome but the optimal procedures are currently unknown.

All groups except two *(42,53)* have used postoperative immunosuppression, although the duration of immunosuppression and exact regimen have differed. Immune cells have been demonstrated surrounding the graft in patients with PD after fetal cell implantation but the functional significance of these cells is not clear *(54)*. It has been demonstrated that tyrosine hydroxylase positive neurons can survive after fetal cell implantation without immunosuppression *(52)*.

3.2.3. Patient Selection

Almost all groups have operated on patients with a complicated response to medications or motor problems that could not be solved with currently available medications. This has been sensible because the procedure is experimental, has potentially serious surgical risk, and there are excellent nonsurgical alternatives for most patients with mild PD. However, because of this patients receiving fetal tissue transplants have almost all had symptoms of PD for many years. The short-term and long-term consequences of transplantation strategies in newly diagnosed patients with mild symptoms is not known. There has been no serious attempt to identify characteristics of fetal tissue-graft recipients that might predict better outcome. Results of a recent controlled study suggest that young patients may be more likely to improve than older patients *(52)*.

3.2.4. Patient Evaluation

There have been a variety of techniques for evaluating patients after transplantation. In recent years, the Core Assessment Program for Intracerebral Transplantation (CAPIT) has become a widely used protocol because it evaluates both the "on" and "off" states in a standardized way *(55)*. More recently, this has been updated to the Core Assessment Program for Surgical Interventional therapies in Parkinson's disease (CAPSIT-PD) *(55a)*. There has also been a consensus that fluorodopa PET is necessary to directly evaluate the status of grafts in addition to any clinical evaluations.

3.2.5. Clinical Outcomes: Literature Review

Table 8 summarizes outcomes in some of the larger reported series. Several groups have reported the same patients multiple times. In that case, we have summarized only the most recent report. All patients in these studies received at least temporary immunosuppression except for the patients of Henderson et al. *(53)* and some of the patients of Freed et al. *(42,52)*. Most underwent stereotactic graft implantation except for the patients of Madrazo et al. *(49)*, Molina et al. *(50)*, and Lopez-Lozano et al. *(51)* who underwent open implantation after craniotomy. Only the patients of Spencer et al. *(41)* received cryopreserved fetal tissue. In addition to these relatively large series, there have been several smaller case series that are difficult to interpret because of the small number of patients involved *(8,62–65)*.

Overall, the reported adverse effects of fetal mesencephalic transplantation have been modest, at least in the short term. The risk of perioperative intracerebral hemorrhage during stereotactic tissue implantation is difficult to estimate directly from the published literature. Few such hemorrhages have been reported but many groups have not published data about all of their transplanted patients. It is likely that the risk is comparable to the risk of stereotactic deep brain stimulation (DBS), which is approx 3–4% *(66)*. Some hemorrhages have been asymptomatic hemorrhages into a needle track *(43, 52)*. Changes in mental status immediately after grafting has been reported, which usually resolves spontaneously. There have been a number of reports of persistent or progressive mental deterioration after grafting but it is not clear whether this is attributable to the transplant procedure. A small number of seizures have been reported. There have been reports of opportunistic infections presumably related to immunosuppression *(51)*. Other perioperative complications such as brain abscess and other infections have only rarely been reported. There were two troubling reports concerning uncontrolled growth of non neuronal tissue, presumably introduced during transplantation, which caused serious morbidity and mortality. In one case, branchial arch tissue introduced into the ventricle proliferated as cartilage,

Table 8
Results of Fetal Mesencephalic Grafting in PD

Ref.	# Pts	F/U Mo	Type of graft	Unilateral/ bilateral	Site	# fetus per side/ fetal age in wk	PET	Comments
(57)	6	10–72	Susp	Uni-4, Bi-2	2-C+P, 4-P	3–4/6–10	+68% in P, no change in C	In patients with PD, there was significant improvement in "off"time, "off" UPDRS motor score, duration "on" after a single dose of levodopa, rigidity, and motor timed tests. One patient was able to stop levodopa entirely.
(56)	2 MPTP	22–24	Susp	Bi	C+P	3–4/6–8	+50% to +100%	The authors felt that 4 of the 6 patients received functionally significant benefit. No group statistics were presented. There was similar, but more dramatic, improvement in the two patients with MPTP-induced parkinsonism, including dramatic reduction in dyskinesias and increased independence.
(49)	4	6–19	Solid	Uni	P	2–4/6–8	NR	No statistics were presented. There was improvement in both "on" and "off" total UPDRS and decrease in requirement for levodopa. Three of the four patients returned to work.
(53)	9	12	Susp	Uni	C	1/11–19	NR	There was initial statistically significant improvement in motor score and disability in the "off" and "on" states that was lost by 12 mo. Only reduction in levodopa dosage and performance on some (not all) timed motor tests significantly improved at 12 mo. The authors conclude that 2 patients were doing very well, with markedly reduced need for levodopa, 4 others moderately well, and the remaining 3 patients poorly at 1 yr.
(50)	30	Up to 24	Solid	Uni	C	?/6–12	NR	There was significant improvement in total "on" and "off" UPDRS, UPDRS motor scores, UPDRS ADL scores, bradykinesia, rigidity and posture at 6 mo. Improvement in tremor was statistically significant at 1 mo. It is stated that improvement was maintained after 6 mo, but was not statistically significant. Mean levodopa dose was reduced from 984 mg/d prior to surgery to 350 mg/d after surgery. At 24 mo, less than 20% of patients had any "off" periods (almost all had "off" periods before transplantation). Patients over age 45 had the same degree of improvement as patients under 45-yr-old.
(42)	7	11–46	Solid	Uni-2, Bi-5	2-C+P, 5-P	1/6–15	++ in 1 patient, no change in 1 patient	Patients had statistically significant 1.2 drop in Hoehn-Yahr stage and 39% reduction in levodopa requirements. Total UPDRS scores did not improve significantly, but bradykinesia and "postural control" did improve significantly as rated by videotape. Four out of the 7 patients were felt to have functionally significant benefit.
(41)	4	4–18	Solid	Uni	C	1/7–11	++	One patient died at 4 mo. At 18 mo, the remaining 3 patients required less medication. They had significant improvements in UPDRS, ADL, and Schwab-England scores compared to baseline, but not compared to a randomly selected, open control group of three candidates for the transplant operation. This was due to improvement in the control group in many of the same measures.
(58)	6	12–24	Solid	Bi	P	3–4/6–9	+61%	Patients had significant improvement of 32% in "off" UPDRS total score, 34.6% in UPDRS ADL, and 174.3% improvement in time "on" without dyskinesias. There was improvement of 24.9% in "off" Schwab-England functional ability scores, 43.4% in time "off" and 16.1% decrease in levodopa requirement, but these were not statistically significant. There was minimal change in the "on" state aside from dyskinesias. PET improved at least 42% in at least 1 side in all patients. Two of the 6 patients died 18 mo after surgery of a pulmonary embolus and probable aspiration, which the authors felt was unrelated to the surgery.

(59)	5	15–36	Susp	Uni	4-C+P, 1-P	2–3/6–9	+63% in P, no change in C	As a group, patients showed significant improvement in measures of dexterity while off, and to a lesser degree while on. There was no significant improvement in gait. One patient became demented and became difficult to test. No group statistics for other features, such as time "off." There was no reduction in the need for levodopa, however other anti-Parkinson medications were reduced. The authors observed an increase in dyskinesias in 3 patients after grafting (possibly representing a recurrence of previously occurring dyskinesias). This may have negated improvement in motor functioning, which the authors describe as moderate.
(51)	10	60	Susp	Uni	C	1/6-8	NR	At 60 mo, patients in the "off" state had a mean improvement of 34% in total UPDRS, 39% in UPDRS motor scores, 63% in the Northwestern University Disability scale, with comparable improvements in the "on" state. There was a mean 85% increase in "on" time, with a decrease in the time "on" with dyskinesias. There was a 64% decrease in levodopa requirement.
(50)	22	6–24	Solid	Uni-9, Bi-13	11-C+P 11-P	1->4/6–10	NR	Patients had significant improvements in "on" and "off" UPDRS, "on" and "off" ADL, dyskinesias and timed motor tests. There was a significant reduction in time "off" per day and an average 54% reduction in amount of levodopa required 24 mo after surgery.
(51)	13	6	Solid	Bi	P	1->4/6–10	NR	Patients were randomly assigned to receive 1–2 donors or 3–4 donors. Those receiving larger grafts had more improvement: UPDRS "off" motor scores improved from 13 to 48% depending on graft volume; UPDRS "on" motor scores improved from 20 to 60%, "on" ADL improved from 3 to 49%, "off" ADL from 23 to 37%. Timed motor tests improved to a similar degree.

Bi, Bilateral; C, Caudate nucleus; NR, Not reported; Uni, Unilateral; P, Putamen.

Table 9
Autopsy after Fetal Mesencephalic Grafting for Parkinson's Disease

# Pts	Duration of benefit	Benefit	Description	Ref.
1	4 mo	No	Surviving neurons formed synapses with host brain, but no TH positivity; some neuromelanin in graft neurons. Patient had striatonigral degeneration	*(70)*
5	18–40 mo	?	TH positive neurons in 3/5, neuromelanin in some grafted neurons	*(71)*
1	8 mo	?	TH positive neurons in 3/5, neuromelanin in some grafted neurons	*(72)*
2	18–19 mo	Yes	Many surviving neurons, TH positive immunoreactivity, multiple processes extending into host tissue, evidence of synapses from graft to host and host to graft	*(73)*

bone, and squamous epithelium causing hydrocephalus and death *(67)*. In another case, transplanted choroid plexus tissue caused cyst formation leading to herniation *(68)*. The University of Colorado-Columbia University-North Shore University double-blind study *(52)*, which will be described later, included several patients who developed severe dyskinesias or dystonia in the absence of levodopa therapy as a late consequence of fetal grafting. There have been only several pathological reports after transplantation of fetal mesencephalic tissue for PD. Some of these are summarized in Table 9.

3.2.6. Double-Blind Studies

There have been only two prospective, placebo-controlled, double-blind studies of fetal tissue transplants for advanced PD. The University of South Florida-Mt. Sinai Hospital-University of British Columbia study is still in progress. The University of Colorado-Columbia Presbyterian-North Shore University Hospital study *(52)* has completed the double-blind phase and is currently collecting long-term followup data. In that study, 40 patients were recruited with PD of at least 7 yr duration and disabling motor symptoms despite optimal drug management. Patients were stratified in advance into two groups: patients over age 60 and patients age 60 or younger at the time of recruitment. At baseline, prior to implantation, and periodically throughout the year-long, double-blind phase of the study, patients underwent "off" and "on" inpatient UPDRS rating scales, timed motor tests, and other assessments. They filled out home diaries of their "off" and "on" states. Patients had fluorodopa PET scans at baseline and 1 yr after surgery. The blind was broken at 1 yr and patients who had received the sham procedure had the option of undergoing implantation immediately after the blind was broken. All patients who had fetal tissue implants continued home and hospital evaluations every 6 mo, and PET scans every 2 yr.

Embryonic dopamine cells from 45–55 d following conception according to Carnegie criteria were used. Fetal tissue was extruded into long strands 200 μm in diameter and placed in tissue culture. Two strands of tissue from 2 fetuses were placed in each putamen using MRI stereotactic guidance through two twist drill holes in the forehead on each side of the midline, one above the other. Patients scheduled for sham surgery underwent a similar procedure but buffer was used instead of tissue and the brain dura was not penetrated by twist drill.

There was no statistically significant difference between operated and sham groups in a subjective comparative global rating 1 yr after surgery. Placebo patients rated themselves improved by a mean +0.3 out of a possible +3, whereas operated patients rated themselves improved by a mean +0.6 out of +3 (the investigators considered a change of 1.5 out of 3 as clinically meaningful). There were no significant differences in any outcome measures in the "on" state for the group as a whole or for either younger or older patients. The total mean UPDRS "off" score improved more in the operated group (from 58 to 50) than in the sham group (from 66 to 63) and this was of borderline significance (p = .055). In addition, the total motor subscore of the UPDRS, bradykinesia, and rigidity subscores of the UPDRS and the Schwab & England disability scale were significantly more improved in the operated than the sham group (p ranging from .00001 to .017). However, this improvement occurred primarily in the group of younger patients, who improved markedly in the "off" UPDRS total score (from 60 to 45), UPDRS motor subscore (from 38 to 26), rigidity and bradykinesia subscores and S&E scales compared to placebo (p ranging from .0003 to .02). No age group had improved tremor in the "off" state. Walking did not improve significantly on examination or by history and walking and balance actually worsened in the group over 60 yr of age (p = .033). There were no significant differences between operated and sham patients in either age group in the amount of time "off," "on," or "on" without dyskinesias, or in the total daily dose of medication taken.

Twelve of 19 implanted patients had improvement ≥0.2 in PET striatal/occipital ratio (SOR) on at least one side of the brain. No sham operated patient had improvement in SOR of this magnitude. However, this improvement did not correlate with improvement in parkinson ratings in the "off" state because the older group had similar mean improvement in PET to the younger group but did not show a comparable improvement in UPDRS rating.

There were more serious adverse events in the operated group than in the sham group, although most of these seemed to be unrelated to the surgery (ischemic stroke, suicidal gesture, several cardiac events many months after the surgery, and accidental death). One subdural hematoma was detected 2 mo after surgery that was absent immediately after surgery. Of considerable greater concern are four patients who developed severe dyskinesias and/or dystonia after fetal tissue implantation. These continued in the absence of L-dopa in four patients and in the absence of all antiparkinson medications in two others. These patients had experienced among the most dramatic improvements in parkinsonism. So far these dyskinesias and dystonias have been unresponsive to medication.

Two patients have died since the beginning of the study. One woman died as a result of a motor vehicle accident 8 mo after implantation during the double-blind phase and one man died from a myocardial infarction 34 mo after implantation during the double-blind phase. Both had typical idiopathic PD with Lewy bodies in substantia nigra neurons and survival of tyrosine-hydroxylase positive transplanted neurons.

The results of the double-blind phase of this study indicate that fetal mesencephalic grafts using the techniques described and without immunosuppression can be done safely. The grafts survive in the majority of cases and produce dopamine as reflected in improvement in fluorodopa PET scans. The grafts were also associated with improved motor function while off medication in patients under but not over age 60. The disparity in older patients between improvement in PET scan but lack of improvement in motor functioning is unexplained. This is especially concerning since the majority of patients with PD are over 60 yr of age. However, even in patients with measurable improvement there was no improvement in motor fluctuations, which was a major motivation for patients to enroll in the trial. In addition, some patients, including those with the most dramatic improvement, have developed disabling dyskinesia and dystonia either because of or in spite of the fetal implant. Further follow-up will be required to understand the long-term implications of these problems. Overall, there appears to be a small group of younger patients with PD who might benefit from this procedure but this potential must be weighed against the possibility of serious long term complications.

3.2.7. Future Directions

As noted earlier, the maximum survival of dopaminergic neurons in fetal mesencephalic grafts is felt to be about 5–10%. Under most transplantation strategies, this leaves a substantial percentage of the striatum without dopaminergic replacement *(47)*. Most investigators believe that improved cell survival and more robust outgrowth of processes will improve clinical outcome. In addition, almost all studies to date have used human fetal mesencephalic tissue from elective abortions. However, it has been estimated that less than 0.01% of the tissue from all elective abortions is available for research use *(73)*. Because of limited availability and controversies concerning abortion and research use of aborted tissue, there has been growing interest in the use of other forms of tissue for transplantation. There has already been research into solving these problems.

3.2.7.1. Improving Graft Survival

Improving neuronal survival and increasing axonal outgrowth would allow for the use of less tissue and also possibly improve the magnitude of the response to grafting. Several trophic factors have been used in attempts to improve graft growth and survival. Glial-derived neurotrophic factor (GDNF) has been the most extensively studied of these factors. It has been shown to increase neuronal survival, neuronal size, and density of tyrosine hydoxylase positive fibers after ventral mesencephalic grafting in animal models *(74,75)*. Two patients with PD underwent grafting with GDNF-treated fetal ventral mesencephalon and seemed to show both clinical improvement and improvement in fluorodopa PET *(65)*. Other trophic factors that enhance survival of grafted dopaminergic neurons in animal models include brain-derived neurotrophic factor (BDNF) *(76)* and neurotrophin-3 *(77)*. Attempts have also been made to improve cell survival using antioxidants such as the lazaroid tirilazad *(78)* and flunarizine *(79)*.

3.2.7.2. Alternate Sources of Dopaminergic Tissue

Because of the limited availability of human tissue for transplantation, there has been an effort to develop animal sources of dopaminergic tissue. Pig mesencephalic tissue is currently available for human transplantation, and survival of pig dopaminergic neurons and improvement in symptoms in patients with PD has been demonstrated *(80,81)*. However, very few cells survived in an autopsied case *(81)*, immunosuppression is required, and there has been concern about the significance of porcine endogenous retrovirus commonly found in porcine tissue *(82)*. A double-blind, controlled study in 18 patients compared sham surgery and placebo immunosuppression vs implantation of porcine dopaminergic cells with cyclosporine and prednisone *(81a)*. The two groups showed equal improvement 18 mo after surgery in off state UPDRS motor scores, global evaluations, and percentage time spent in "off" state. It was concluded that porcine cell implants were not more effective than placebo. There were no serious adverse events or evidence for porcine retroviruses in the treated patients. Experimental attempts are now underway to use immortalized dopaminergic cells for transplantation or use viral vectors to insert dopamine producing enzymes into host cells *(83)*. In some paradigms, the tissue is encapsulated in micropore wrapping, which allows dopamine to pass out freely but prevents the exchange of immune factors and would keep transformed cells from leaving the graft *(84)*. More recently, attempts have been made to implant fetal stem cells into the adult nervous system *(85)*. Because there is serious concern about possible toxicity of a viral vector and the long-term consequences of implanting immortalized tissue, it is likely these techniques will require extensive preclinical testing before they are used in patients.

3.2.7.3. Alternate Targets

All current transplantation efforts have targeted the caudate and putamen because they are the natural targets of substantia nigra neurons. Previous attempts in animals to transplant fetal dopaminergic tissue into the substantia nigra itself have failed to produce reinnervation of the striatum. Reinnervation of the striatum does occur if fetal grafts are implanted in neonatal host animals *(86)* but this is unlikely to translate into a strategy for treating patients. Other strategies to induce long-distance axonal growth have included depositing fetal dopaminergic tissue along the nigrostriatal pathway or damaging the nigrostriatal pathway *(87,88)*, but these strategies are also unlikely to be applicable to patients. It has been demonstrated in animals that grafting of fetal dopaminergic tissue simultaneously into the striatum and the substantia nigra can induce axonal sprouting from the nigral graft that reaches the striatum *(89)*.

3.3. Conclusions

Most studies of fetal transplantation in PD have reported some lasting improvement after fetal mesencephalic grafting for PD with relatively modest short-term side effects. The data in animals are consistent with these results and suggest that establishment of functional dopaminergic connections between graft and host striatum underlies some of the clinical improvement. Pathological findings in humans also suggest survival of neurons and functional connections with host brain. The ideal tissue for implantation is still not identified. The use of autologous adrenal medulla tissue is highly unlikely to be revived unless the survival of this tissue can be greatly enhanced and morbidity and mortality greatly reduced. Porcine fetal tissue and genetically modified tissues are being actively investigated as alternatives to human fetal tissue but many obstacles remain before these techniques can achieve widespread use. The optimal preparation of tissue and surgical approach are also unknown. It is likely that future transplantation will be bilateral and performed under stereotactic control. Other aspects of the procedure, such as whether immunosuppression should be used, require definitive testing.

However, even in the most promising reports, the magnitude of clinical change after fetal grafting has been variable. In many studies, some patients have had no benefit, while only a small minority have experienced dramatic, functional improvement. Importantly, in two controlled trials *(52,81a)*, sham-operated patients showed substantial improvement in some measures of motor function, emphasizing the importance of carrying out sham-surgery-controlled studies. This variability characterizes most of the large studies and is probably not peculiar to one particular technique. This has also been reflected in variable PET scan results and a large variation in cell survival between different needle tracks in the same patient in autopsy studies. This variability will have to improve if transplantation is to become a routine treatment for PD.

In the only published double-blind study to date *(52)*, benefit in the "off" state often did not make a substantial difference in the lives of patients with complicated fluctuations. In addition, patients over age 60 with advanced PD did not significantly benefit from grafting. Moreover, delayed onset of severe dyskinesia and dystonia was a major problem in a small number of good responders. It is impossible to tell at this time whether these problems represent peculiarities of that technique, or whether these problems will also appear when other research groups attempt to increase the amount of dopamine delivery to the host brain with grafted tissue.

REFERENCES

1. Thompson, W. G. (1890) Successful brain grafting. *NY Med. J.* **51,** 701–702.
2. Dunn, E. H. (1917) Primary and secondary findings in a series of attempts to transplant cerebral cortex in the albino rat. *J. Comp. Neurol.* **27,** 565–582.
3. Halász, B., Pupp, L., and Uhlarik, S. (1962) Hypophysiotrophic area in the hypothalamus. *J. Endocr.* **25,** 147–159.
4. Stenevi, U., Björklund, A., and Svengaard, N. A. (1976) Transplantation of central and peripheral monamine neurons to the adult rat brain: techniques and conditions for survival. *Brain Res.* **114,** 1–20.
5. Björklund, A. and Stenevi, U. (1979) Reconstruction of the nigrostriatal pathway by intracerebral nigral transplants. *Brain Res.* **177,** 555–560.
6. Perlow, M. J., Freed, W. J., Hoffer, B. J., Seiger, Å., Olson, L., and Wyatt, R. J. (1979) Brain grafts reduce motor abnormalities produced by destruction of nigro-striatal dopamine system. *Science* **204,** 643–647.
7. Backlund, E.-O., Grandberg, P.-O., Hamberger, B., et al. (1985) Transplantation of adrenal medullary tissue to striatum in parkinsonism: first clinical trials. *J. Neurosurg.* **62,** 169–173.
8. Jiang, N., Jiang, C., Tang, Z., et al. (1987) Human foetal brain transplant trials in the treatment of Parkinsonism. *Acta Acad. Med. Shangai* **14,** 77.
9. Brundin, P., Duan, W. M., and Sauer, H. (1994) Functional effects of mesencephalic dopamine neurons and adrenal chromaffin cells grafted to the rodent striatum. In: *Functional Neural Transplantation* (Dunnett, S. B. and Björklund, A., eds.), Raven Press, New York, pp. 9–46.
10. Dunnett, S. B. (1998) Repair of the damaged brain. The Alfred Meyer memorial lecture 1998. *Neuropath. App. Neurobiol.* **25,** 351–362.
11. Björklund, A. (1992) Dopaminergic transplants in experimental parkinsonism: cellular mechanisms of graft-induced functional recovery. *Curr. Opin. Neurobiol.* **2,** 683–689.
12. Annett, L. E. (1994) Functional studies of neural grafts in parkinsonian primates. In: *Functional Neural Transplantation* (Dunnett, S. B. and Björklund, A., eds.), Raven Press, New York, pp. 71–101.

63. Iacono, R. P., Tang, Z. S., Mazziotta, J. C., Grafton, S., and Hoehn, M. (1992) Bilateral fetal grafts for Parkinson's disease: 22 months' results. *Stereotact. Funct. Neurosurg.* **58,** 84–87.
64. Levivier, M., Dethy, S., Rodesch, F., Peschanski, M., Vandesteene, A., David, P., et al. (1997) Intracerebral transplantation of fetal ventral mesencephalon for patients with advanced Parkinson's disease. *Stereotact. Funct. Neurosurg.* **69,** 99–111.
65. Mendez, I., Dagher, A., Hong, M., Hebb, A., Gaudet, P., Law, A., et al. (2000) Enhancement of survival of stored dopaminergic cells and promotion of graft survival by exposure of human fetal nigral tissue to glial cell line-derived neurotrophic factor in patients with Parkinson's disease. *J. Neurosurg.* **92,** 863–869.
66. Benabid, A. L., Pollak, P., Gao, D., Hoffmann, D., Limousin, P., Gay, E., et al. (1996) Chronic electrical stimulation of the ventralis intermedius nucleus of the thalamus as a treatment of movement disorders. *J. Neurosurg.* **84,** 203–214.
67. Folkerth, R. D. and Durso, R. (1996) Survival and proliferation of nonneural tissues, with obstruction of cerebral ventricles, in a parkinsonian patient treated with fetal allografts. *Neurology* **46,** 1219–1225.
68. Mamelak, A. N., Eggerding, F. A., Oh, D. S., Wilson, E., Davis, R. L., Spitzer, R., et al. (1998) Fatal cyst formation after fetal mesencephalic allograft transplant for Parkinson's disease. *J. Neurosurg.* **89,** 592–598.
69. Redmond, D. E. Jr., Leranth, C., Spencer, D. D., et al. (1990) Fetal neural graft survival. *Lancet* **336,** 820–822.
70. Hitchcock, E. H., Whitewell, H. L., Sofroniew, M. V., and Bankiewicz, K. S. (1994) Survival of TH-positive and neuromelanin-containing cells in patients with Parkinson's disease after intrastriatal grafting of fetal ventral mesencephalon (Abs). *Exp. Neurol.* **129,** 3.
71. Freed, C. R., Trojanowski, J. Z., Galvin, J. E., Rosenstein, J. M., Breeze, R. E., Greene, P. E., et al. (1997) Embryonic dopamine cells cultured as strands show long term survival without immunosuppression in a patient with advanced Parkinson's disease. *Soc. Neurosci. Abstr.* **23,** 1682.
72. Kordower, J. H., Freeman, T. B., and Olanow, C. W. (1998) Neuropathology of fetal nigral grafts in patients with Parkinson's disease. *Mov. Disord.* **13(Suppl. 1),** 88–95.
73. Lawson, H. W., Atrash, H. K., Saftlas, A. F., Koonin, L. M., Ramick, M., and Smith, J. C. (1988) Abortion surveillance, US 1984–1985. *Morbid. Mortal. Wkly Rep.* **38,** 11–42.
74. Rosenblad, C., Martinez-Serrano, A., and Bjorklund, A. (1996) Glial cell line-derived neurotrophic factor increases survival, growth and function of intrastriatal fetal nigral dopaminergic grafts. *Neuroscience* **75,** 979–985.
75. Granholm, A.-C., Mott, J. L., Bowenkamp, K., Eken, S., Henry, S., Hoffer, B. J., et al. (1997) Glial cell lin-derived neurotrophic factor improves survival of ventral mesencephalic grafts to the 6-hydroxydopamine lesioned striatum. *Exp. Brain Res.* **116,** 29–38.
76. Yurek, D. M., Lu, W., Hipkens, S., and Wiegand, S. J. (1996) BDNF enhances the functional reinnervation of the striatum by grafted fetal dopamine neurons. *Exp. Neurol.* **137,** 105–118.
77. Espejo, M., Cutillas, B., Arenas, E., and Ambrosio, S. (2000) Increased sruvival of dopaminergic neurons in striatal grafts of fetal ventral mesencephalic cells exposed to neurotrophin-3 or glial cell line-derived neurotrophic factor. *Cell Transplant.* **9,** 45–53.
78. Bjorklund, A., Spenger, C., and Stromberg, I. (1997) Tirilazad mesylate increases dopaminergic neuronal survival in the in Oculo grafting model. *Exp. Neurol.* **148,** 324–333.
79. Schierle, G. S. K., Hansson, O., and Brundin, P. (1999) Flunarizine improves the survival of grafted dopaminergic neurons. *Neuroscience* **94,** 17–20.
80. Deacon, T., Schumacher, J., Dinsmore, J., et al. (1997) Histological evidence of fetal pig neural cell survival after transplantation into a patient with Parkinson's disease. *Nature Med.* **3,** 350–353.
81. Schumacher, J. M., Ellias, S. A., Palmer, E. P., Kott, H. S., Dinsmore, J., Dempsey, P. K., et al. (2000) Transplantation of embryonic porcine mesencephalic tissue in patients with PD. *Neurology* **54,** 1042–1050.
81a. Watts, R. L., Freeman, T. L., Hauser, R. A., Bakay, R. A., Ellias, S. A., Stoessl, A. J., et al. (2001) A double-blind, randomized, controlled, multicenter clinical trial of the safety and efficacy of stereotaxic intrastriatal implantation of fetal porcine ventral mesencephalic tissue (Neurocell™-PD) vs. imitation surgery in patients with Parkinson's disease (PD). *Parkinsonism Rel. Disord.* **7(Suppl.),** S87.
82. Patience, C., Takenchi, Y., and Weiss, R. A. (1997) Infection of human cells by an endogenous retrovirus of pigs. *Nature Med.* **3,** 282–286.
83. Bankiewicz, K. S., Leff, S. E., Nagy, D., Jungles, S., Rokovich, J., Spratt, K., et al. (1997) Practical aspects of the development of ex vivo and in vivo gene therapy for Parkinson's disease. *Exp. Neurol.* **144,** 147–156.
84. Date, I. and Ohmoto, T. (1999) Neural transplantation for Parkinson's disease. *Cell Mol. Neurobiol.* **19,** 67–78.
85. Uchida, K., Roach, A. H., Kawaja, M. D., and Toya, S. (1999) Successful survival of grafted transgenic neural plate cells in adult central nervous system environment. *Cell Mol. Neurobiol.* **19,** 79–86.
86. Bentlage, C., Nikkhah, G., Cunningham, M. G., and Bjorklund, A. (1999) Reformation of the nigrostriatal pathway by fetal dopaminergic micrografts into the substantia nigra is critically dependent on the age of the host. *Exp. Neurol.* **159,** 177–190.
87. Dunnett, S. B., Rogers, D. C., and Richards, S.-J. (1989) Nigrostriatal reconstruction after 6-OHDA lesion in rats: combination of dopamine-rich nigral grafts and nigrostriatal "bridge" grafts. *Exp. Brain Res.* **75,** 523–535.
88. Zhou, F. C. and Chiang, Y. H. (1995) Excitochemical-induced trophic bridging directs axonal growth of transplanted neurons to distal target. *Cell Transplant.* **4,** 103–112.
89. Mendez, I., Sadi, D., and Hong, M. (1996) Reconstruction of the nigrostriatal pathway by simultancous intrastriatal and intranigral dopaminergic transplants. *J. Neurosci.* **16,** 7216–7227.

23
Future Surgical Therapies in Parkinson's Disease

Un Jung Kang, Nora Papasian,
Jin Woo Chang, and Won Yong Lee

1. RATIONALE FOR SURGICAL INTERVENTION

The resurgence of neurosurgical therapies in Parkinson's disease (PD), and movement disorders in general, is largely due to advances in transplant neurobiology and basal ganglia physiology. Developments in molecular biology, combined with growing insight into the pathogenesis of movement disorders, anticipate new rational treatments not only for PD but also for many other disorders unresponsive to traditional therapies. This chapter will focus on two of the most promising therapeutic approaches: gene therapy and cell-transplant therapy. Advances in gene-therapy methods over the past decades show promising vectors that are capable of long-term transgene expression without producing toxicity. Novel neuronal cell lines with desired phenotypes may circumvent many of the limitations of primary neuronal cell transplantation. The traditional concept of neural cells being terminally differentiated has been challenged by discoveries of multipotent and self-renewing neuronal stem cells. Using these approaches, one can not only enhance symptomatic therapy but also attempt neuroprotective therapy. The examples will be primarily illustrated in experimental studies of PD.

2. NOVEL SURGICAL APPROACHES

2.1. *Gene Therapy for the Nervous System*

Gene therapy delivers DNA and utilizes host machinery to create the desired product through transcription of the inserted DNA into messenger RNA, followed by translation of the mRNA into proteins and post-translational modifications of the proteins (Fig. 1). Delivering DNA can provide more efficient, sustained, and localized supply of product than delivering the product itself. An abnormal gene in genetic disorders could have a defective function, and the loss of function can be complemented by inserting normal genetic information. In cases where the genetic abnormality leads to a gain of new toxic function, a strategy to intervene and neutralize the toxic function is necessary (Fig. 1; Subheading 3.2.1.). In other cases, gene therapy provides biological minipumps for direct, site-specific delivery of pharmacological compounds that are therapeutic regardless of the etiology of the disorder (Subheadings 3.1. and 3.2.2.) *(1)*. This section will discuss the basic concepts and methodology of gene therapy, including current limitations and recent advances. Potential gene therapy for PD will be illustrated through animal models (Subheading 3).

From: Contemporary Clinical Neurology:
Surgical Treatment of Parkinson's Disease and Other Movement Disorders
Edited by: D. Tarsy, J. L. Vitek, and A. M. Lozano © Humana Press Inc., Totowa, NJ

The advantages of ex vivo gene transfer include the ability to control and monitor the gene-transfer process before transplantation. Thus the biochemical effect of the transgene product can be characterized, potential tumorigenesis assessed, and viral toxicity screened. Moreover, ex vivo grafted cells may provide useful functions beyond that provided by the transgene, such as serving as a substrate for axonal growth *(15,16)* or establishing synaptic connection with host neurons. The major shortcoming of current ex vivo gene transfer is the limited duration of transgene expression. This may be inherent in the nature of retroviral vectors used for ex vivo therapies, as discussed later.

2.1.2. *In Vivo Gene Transfer*

Though ex vivo therapy enjoys some advantages, certain situations require in vivo techniques. For example, whereas grafting genetically modified cells is suitable for delivery of secretable products, such as neurotransmitters and neurotrophic factors, delivery of intracellular proteins—such as protein kinases, receptors, and transporters—requires in vivo techniques. Moreover, long-term gene expression has been most consistently demonstrated in in vivo gene-transfer paradigms using adeno-associated virus (AAV) *(17)* or lentiviruses *(18)*. In addition, vector solutions seem to be less disruptive to normal brain physiology and architecture than are cell grafts. On the other hand, the consequences of delivering therapeutic molecules (e.g., dopamine) directly into host cells that do not normally express such molecules (e.g., striatal neurons) are not as predictable as the consequences of delivering them extracellularly by grafts serving as biological minipumps. Conceivably, intracellular expression of a foreign gene product could lead to untoward alteration of host-cell function.

2.1.3. *Vector Constructs*

The most efficient gene therapy vectors for both in vivo and ex vivo methods are derived from viruses *(19)*, although other methods of gene transfer *(20)* including liposomes *(21)* are also available. In choosing a gene-therapy approach, efficacy and safety factors must be evaluated for both the virus and the transgene. Virus vectors that have been most extensively applied to CNS gene transfer include the adenovirus, AAV, herpes simplex type I virus (HSV-1), retroviruses, and hybrid vectors. We will consider general vector parameters and then each virus in turn, keeping in mind that, in this rapidly moving field, there still exists no clear universal vector system of choice.

2.1.3.1. Parameters of Viral Vectors

The features of vector efficacy central to gene therapy are the ability to insert a large amount of foreign DNA within the vector, the titer of the virus particles, high efficiency of transduction, and controllable, long-term expression of the transgene at therapeutic levels. The major problem of gene therapy has been the inability to obtain long-term transgene expression in vivo *(22,23)*. Long-term expression is relatively easily achieved in culture; however once the cells are implanted in animals, transgene expression diminishes rapidly within days to weeks *(22)*. Although the mechanism for silencing of transgene expression is only partially understood, virus type seems to influence long-term in vivo expression. For example, AAV and lentivirus have been shown to achieve expression for several months both in rats *(17)* and monkeys *(18)* in vivo. Integration of transgenes into the chromosomes may be another factor for more stable expression *(24)*. In addition, the integration sites of vectors may play a significant role in the transcriptional activity of the transgene. For example, retroviruses integrate into chromosomes during active division, whereas lentivirus can enter the nucleus and integrate in quiescent, nondividing neurons *(24)*.

Promoter types may also significantly influence long-term expression. The effect of a promoter may vary with the vector and recipient cell type used *(25,26)*. Most gene-therapy vectors employ viral promoters for transgene expression. These promoters are often suppressed by various mechanisms including methylation of DNA, which inhibits transcription of the genes and negative regulatory elements that repress transcription. Nonviral promoters, such as constitutive housekeeping gene promoters *(27)* or cell type-specific promoters *(28)* have had some success, but most of these tissue-speci-

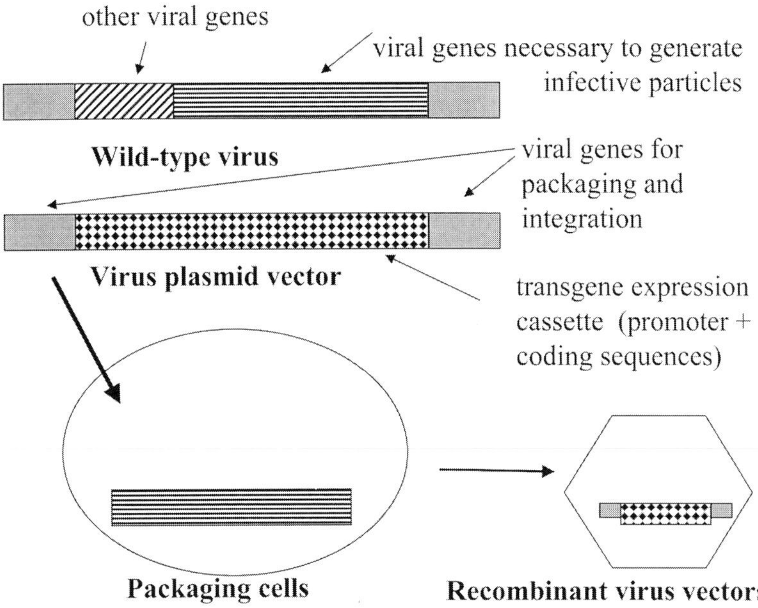

Fig. 3. A simplified general scheme for virus vectors. Wild-type viruses are genetically modified to engineer virus plasmid vector that has the minimum viral genes necessary for packaging the vector into the virus particles. The plasmid vector is then transfected into the packaging cells that incorporate the necessary components to generate infective viral particles.

fic promoters have low basal transcriptional activity. Recently, synthetic promoters engineered from a combination of operator elements have shown enhanced transcriptional activity *(29)*.

Once high and stable levels of transgene expression are achieved, the ability to regulate this expression becomes crucial. Excessive gene product levels increase the likelihood and severity of adverse effects, such as L-dopa-induced dyskinesias in PD. Therefore, levels for optimal physiological function must be maintained and regulated. Promoters that can be regulated externally or have a built-in feedback mechanism will be an important advance for the future. One such regulatable system was developed using promoters whose activities can be turned on or off by administration of tetracycline. Studies both in vitro *(10)* and in vivo *(30,31)* demonstrated regulatable transgene expression. Other combinations consisting of nontoxic substances and heterologous transcription factors that bind to regulatable promoters have also been developed *(32–34)*.

Safety issues concerning viral vectors include the risk of generating replication-competent virus, cytotoxicity, host immune response, and oncogenesis. A key feature of vector design is eliminating the components responsible for viral replication (Fig. 3). A viral plasmid vector is constructed from wild-type viruses with the minimum viral genes necessary for packaging the vector into virus particles. Viral components necessary to generate infective particles are incorporated into the packaging cells to complement the replication-defective virus plasmid vector. Thus, when the viral plasmid is transfected into packaging cells, infective virus particles containing the therapeutic transgene but minimal virus genes are produced. These viral vectors are capable of transducing cells, but they cannot replicate further. The chance of recombination events that could lead to wild-type virus is decreased by reducing the overlapping regions between vectors and viral sequences in the packaging cells *(35,36)*.

Viral protein immunogenicity and cytotoxicity limit safety as well as long-term expression of the transgenes. Eliminating as much of the viral genome as possible decreases production of viral proteins

(67,71) or basic fibroblast growth factor (bFGF, FGF-2) *(68,69)*. Neuronal stem cells can differentiate into glial or neuronal phenotypes not only in culture but also in both neurogenic and non-neurogenic sites of adult rat brain after transplantation *(69,72)*. They seem to respond to local cues to differentiate into site-specific neuronal phenotypes. The potential for neuronal stem cells to be differentiated into desired neuronal phenotypes has been recognized, suggesting an attractive combination of unlimited availability and therapeutically desired phenotypes.

The properties of neuronal stem cells are similar to those of the bone marrow stem cells in that stem cells differentiate sequentially into subtypes of neuronal or hematopoeitic cells, respectively *(73)*. In fact, there are hints of the existence of common neuro-hematopoeitic stem cells—hematopoetic cells can emerge after transplantation of neuronal stem cells *(74)* and bone marrow-derived cells can differentiate into glial cells in the brain *(75)*. Thus embryonic stem cells, which are even more primitive than neuronal or hematopoetic stem cells, may be even more versatile in their capacity to differentiate into therapeutically desirable phenotypes *(76)*. Derived from the inner cell mass of the developing blastocyst, these are clonal cell lines that can proliferate extensively in vitro and are capable of adopting all the cell fates in a developing embryo. Of course, the proper signals for differentiation must be elucidated before such applications can be explored.

When a specific differentiated phenotype is desired, such as dopaminergic cell features for treating PD, understanding the molecular signals for the differentiation pathway will be necessary. For example, an orphan nuclear receptor Nurr1 seems to be an important factor in generating the dopaminergic pheonotype. Mice lacking Nurr1 fail to develop dopaminergic neurons *(77)*. Nurr1 is essential both for survival and for final differentiation of ventral mesencephalic late dopaminergic precursor neurons into a complete dopaminergic phenotype *(78)*. Nurr1 alone *(79)* or in combination with factors derived from local type 1 astrocytes *(80)* induces dopaminergic phenotypes in neuronal stem cells. Other growth factors such as FGF have shown a similar effect on differentiation of stem cells into the dopaminergic phenotype *(81)*. Elaborate differentiating paradigms have been successfully employed to generate dopaminergic and serotonergic phenotypes from mouse *(13)* and human embryonic stem cells *(14)*.

These initial studies are very promising, and it is likely that further understanding of other differentiation signals for expressing the full complement of the dopaminergic phenotype, including dopamine processing and storage, will lead to even better cells for therapies. The various aspects of dopaminergic phenotypes will be discussed in detail in Subheading 3.1.1. In addition, partially differentiated neuronal stem cells could be genetically enhanced to achieve more desirable phenotypes, as outlined under ex vivo gene transfer *(82–84)*.

3. THERAPEUTIC GOALS

3.1. Symptomatic Therapy

The best example of symptomatic therapy is dopamine replacement for Parkinson's disease. However, long-term treatment with the precursor L-3,4-dihydroxyphenylalanine (L-dopa) produces motor response complications—consisting of wearing-off (short duration of response), on-off (sudden unpredictable loss of benefit), and dyskinesias—that limit its efficacy. These problems may be either prevented or ameliorated by continuous delivery of dopamine *(85,86)*. In addition, site-specific delivery into the striatum avoids central side effects, such as hallucinations. Cell therapy or gene therapy might provide such continuous, site-specific dopamine delivery.

3.1.1. Dopamine Replacement

To deliver L-dopa into the brain by gene therapy, early studies focused on introducing the tyrosine hydroxylase (TH) gene, which catalyzes the first and rate-limiting step of dopamine synthesis (Fig. 4). Established cell lines were first used, including rat fibroblast lines *(87)* and endocrine cell lines *(88)*. To overcome the problems of tumorigenesis inherent in cell lines, however, primary cells such as

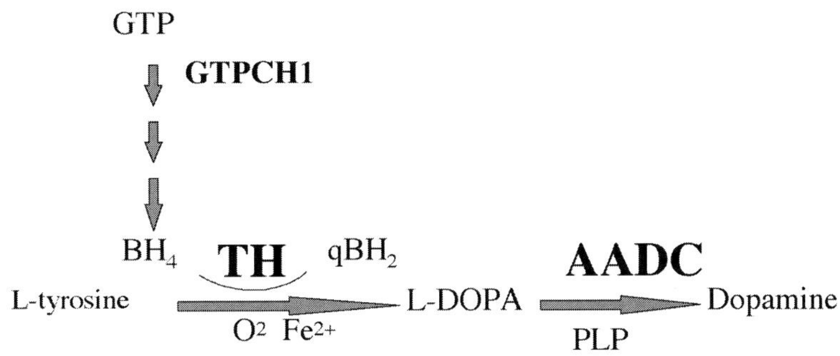

Fig. 4. Biosynthetic pathway of dopamine production. Dopamine is synthesized in a series of enzymatic steps starting from the precursor L-tyrosine, which is an essential amino acid present in all types of cells. The first and rate-limiting step is catalyzed by tyrosine hydroxylase (TH). TH requires the cofactors tetrahydrobiopterin (BH_4), iron, and oxygen for its function. BH_4 is in turn synthesized from GTP in a series of enzymatic steps, of which GTP cyclohydrolase 1 (GTPCH1) catalyzes the first and rate-limiting step. The second step is catalyzed by aromatic L-amino acid decarboxylase (AADC) with pyridoxal 5' phosphate (PLP) as the cofactor.

fibroblasts *(89)*, myoblasts *(90)*, and astrocytes *(7)* have been used and shown to produce long-term graft survival with neither tumor formation nor immunological rejection. More recently, neuronal precursor cells have been genetically modified to express the dopaminergic phenotype, but their efficacy in in vivo models is not yet clear. In vivo TH gene transfer into the brain using viral vectors has also been attempted *(91,92)*.

More refined L-dopa delivery has been achieved using the gene for GTP cyclohydrolase I (GCH1), which catalyzes the first and rate-limiting step in the biosynthesis of tetrahydrobiopterin, an essential cofactor for TH function *(93)*. Gene therapy studies have shown that double transduction with TH and GCH1, by either ex vivo *(3)* or in vivo *(46)* gene transfer, is necessary for restoration of L-dopa/dopamine levels in the denervated striatum of rat models of PD (Fig. 4). The importance of GCH1 has been underscored by the finding that mutations in GCH1 in L-dopa-responsive dystonia (DRD) patients are associated with a deficiency of tetrahydrobiopterin (BH_4) and parkinsonism in these patients *(94)*. Interestingly, symptoms of DRD patients can be greatly ameliorated by L-dopa therapy without development of the long-term complications commonly observed in PD patients. Such a strong response to L-dopa abrogates any need for gene therapy in DRD, but provides insight into the therapeutic importance of events downstream from L-dopa production.

Therefore, the approach of combining the oral administration of L-dopa with the genetic machinery to process L-dopa more efficiently may also be considered *(95)*. Providing the aromatic L-amino acid decarboxylase (AADC) gene, which decarboxylates L-dopa to dopamine, in the denervated striatum of animal models of PD resulted in higher levels of dopamine being produced from L-dopa *(17, 96,97)*. However, even more important than increasing the level of dopamine is prolonging the duration of elevation of and buffering the fluctuations in brain dopamine levels associated with oral L-dopa administration. The combined use of AADC for L-dopa decarboxylation and of vesicular monoamine transporter (VMAT) for efficient dopamine storage within cells produced significantly higher and more sustained levels of dopamine after oral L-dopa administration compared to using AADC alone *(98)*. One major advantage of this approach is the ability to regulate the level of dopamine delivery by controlling the amount of precursor, L-dopa administered, given that excessive dopamine may be detrimental to patients. In the aforementioned strategies of providing a source of L-dopa or dopamine, the precise control of the exact amount of L-dopa/dopamine provided by gene therapy will be critical and may be difficult to achieve with current vector technology.

Site-specific and sustained dopamine delivery as described earlier would provide a major advance in PD therapy, especially for the majority of motor symptoms. However, there are limitations to such nonsynaptic dopamine replacement. Synaptic restoration of neuronal connectivity and complex regulation, such as feedback interaction of dopaminergic neurons with striatal neurons, may be achieved, at least partially, by fetal dopaminergic neurons or dopaminergic neuronal cell lines. However, it is not clear whether even all these features of dopaminergic neurotransmission will be sufficient to normalize the entire symptom complex of PD. The role of nondopaminergic systems in PD needs to be explored further.

3.1.2. Nondopaminergic Approach

3.1.2.1. Downstream Pathways from Dopaminergic Neurons

The realization that the pathways downstream from dopaminergic neurons are significantly altered after dopaminergic deafferentation and contribute to the pathophysiology of Parkinson's disease has lead to novel therapeutic approaches. Excessive activity of output basal ganglia nuclei, such as the internal globus pallidus and the subthalamic nucleus, has been attenuated by surgical ablation or deep brain stimulation and shown to provide symptomatic amelioration *(99,100)*, as also described in previous chapters. Instead of surgical ablation, gene therapy or cell therapy might provide a means of biological inhibition. For example, combined transplantation of dopaminergic neurons into the striatum and gamma amino butyric acid (GABA)-rich striatal neurons into the SN produced additive effects of behavioral recovery in rat models of PD *(101)*. Gene therapy with glutamic acid decarboxylase could also be attempted to produce a local source of the inhibitory neurotransmitter GABA.

3.1.2.2. Other Neurotransmitter Systems Involved in PD

The degeneration of other neurotransmitter systems, such as those of serotonin and norepinephrine, has long been recognized in PD, and metabolites of serotonin and norepinephrine are significantly depleted *(102)*. However, therapy to restore these monoamines by precursor administration has not shown a major benefit in PD patients. Gene delivery of tryptophan hydroxylase or dopamine beta-hydroxylase might be a more effective therapy for replacing serotonin and norepinephrine in appropriate sites.

3.2. Neuroprotective Therapy

Although symptomatic therapy with dopamine replacement has been very successful in treating PD patients and improving their quality of life, intervention that slows or stops the progression of neuronal degeneration is even more desirable. Currently, no agent has been proven to slow the progression of PD, but neuroprotective therapy that alters the underlying disease process is being explored.

3.2.1. Intervention in Pathogenesis

Understanding the etiology of PD may allow us to intervene directly in the pathogenesis and either forestall the clinical manifestations or stop the disease progression. Although the precise etiology of PD is still unclear for sporadic cases, the role of oxidative stress and mitochondrial dysfunction has been implicated strongly *(103)*. Therefore, neuroprotective strategies involving antioxidants and mitochondrial enhancers could be contemplated. The major difficulties of this approach may be the access of potentially neuroprotective compounds to the degenerating dopaminergic neurons. One could envision therapy that introduces genes that produce antioxidants. Overexpression of a free-radical scavenging enzyme, such as superoxide dismutase (SOD), may protect dopaminergic neurons from degeneration. Experimental models show that SOD overexpression protects dopaminergic neurons from neurotoxicity of MPTP *(104)*. Moreover, SOD enhances survival of dopaminergic neurons grafted into parkinsonian rats *(105)*.

The recent discoveries of genetic mutations in PD, including the α-synuclein mutation in families with autosomal dominant inheritance of PD *(106)* and the parkin gene mutation in families with autosomal recessive juvenile parkinsonism *(107)*, may provide new avenues for therapy. Knowledge of the precise steps by which these mutations lead to dopaminergic neuronal death could allow us to apply these findings to understanding sporadic PD as well.

Although developing a precise strategy awaits further understanding of the mechanism of toxicity by these genetic mutations, general therapeutic approaches for a known genetic defect can be outlined (Fig. 1). These approaches could be applied to other neurodegenerative disorders, such as Huntington's disease, ataxias, and Alzheimer's disease. For autosomal recessive genetic disorders that commonly confer a "loss of function," augmentation of the missing genetic information may restore normal function. On the other hand, a dominant disorder may involve a "gain of toxic function" induced by the mutant protein. For these disorders, it is not possible to simply replace the defective function with a normal one. The toxic product itself must be neutralized. Techniques for specifically targeting the abnormal sequence and replacing it with a normal sequence exist and have been applied in the generation of transgenic animals with the "knock-out, knock-in" strategy *(108)*. However, these are not easily applicable to humans. Instead, the transcription of the genetic message to RNA could be attempted by using decoy promoter that will compete with the endogenous promoter (Fig. 1) *(109)*. Antisense RNA has been used to hamper transcription, processing, transport, and/or translation of mRNAs in a variety of cell types. It may also be possible to integrate viral or nonviral vectors carrying catalytic antisense RNAs or ribozymes that bind to, and irreversibly cleave, abnormal mRNAs *(110,111)*. Synthetic antibodies could be produced to neutralize the abnormal protein. Intervention further downstream of the abnormal protein will be possible once the biochemical consequences of the mutation are known. Blockade of these downstream effects may be envisioned by introducing genes that allow neutralization of the deleterious products/effects.

3.2.2. General Neuroprotection

Even without knowledge of the precise mechanisms of parkinsonian degeneration and regardless of what event initially triggers the neuronal degeneration, understanding the general process of cell death could direct other approaches in preventing disease progression. Namely, delivering neurotrophic factors or growth-promoting factors may prevent or slow the cell death cascade. For example, the genes preventing apoptosis, such as bcl-2, or other cell death cascade-blocking factors could be expressed in dopaminergic neurons to prevent their demise *(112)*. Among these are the caspase inhibitors and the peptidergic growth factors, which promote survival of neuronal populations.

Several growth factors possess trophic activity toward dopaminergic neurons. These include brain-derived neurotrophic factor (BDNF), neurotrophin-3 (NT-3), NT-4/5, basic fibroblast growth factor (bFGF), transforming growth factor-β (TGF-β), glial cell line-derived factor (GDNF), and Neurturin (NTN) *(113–119)*. These factors have been shown to enhance dopamine neuronal cell viability and to protect cells from experimental toxin lesions in vitro, although in some cases the effects of neurotrophic factors appear to be indirect, mediated by their effects on glial cells *(117,118,120)*.

One of the most potent growth factors for dopaminergic neurons is GDNF. In normal animals, GDNF increases both spontaneous and amphetamine-induced motor behavior. These motor effects occur in parallel with increased DA levels and DA cell turnover in the SN, and enhanced DA cell turnover and consequent reduction in striatal DA levels *(121)*. Infusion of GDNF into the striatum results in retrograde transport to the SN DA neurons *(122)*.

Given the promising results of these preclinical studies, clinical studies of intraventricular GDNF have been attempted in PD patients. No significant regeneration of nigrostriatal neurons or intraparenchymal diffusion of the intracerebroventricular GDNF to relevant brain regions was found. The problem with pharmacological delivery of the peptidergic growth factors is access to the target brain tissue. The parenteral delivery of these substances frequently requires methods that circumvent the blood-brain-barrier (BBB), for instance, by neurosurgical intraparenchymal or intraventricular infusions. These methods are site-specificic but invasive, and the effects are often unpredictable. Intraventricular administration of BDNF is limited due to its binding to truncated TrkB receptors in the ependymal lining of the ventricles as well as by limited diffusion within the brain parenchyma *(123)*.

As an alternative to direct infusion, methods for both ex vivo and in vivo gene delivery of these therapeutic proteins have been developed. Implants of BDNF-producing fibroblast cells have been protective against neurotoxins such as 6-hydroxydopamine (6-OHDA) *(124)* and 1-methyl-4-phenylpyridinium (MPP^+) *(125)*. In addition, sprouting of dopaminergic fibers has been demonstrated in BDNF-transduced fibroblasts implanted into the midbrain *(16)*. GDNF has also been delivered into rat substantia nigra neurons by adenovirus or AAV vectors and has protected these neurons from progressive degeneration induced by 6-OHDA lesion of the dopaminergic terminals in the striatum *(40, 126–128)*. GDNF expressing viruses in the striatum have also provided cellular and behavioral protection from striatal 6-OHDA lesions in rats *(126,129)* and from MPTP lesions in monkeys *(18)*.

In summary, gene and cell therapies have the potential to provide efficient delivery of various genes and products into a localized site. Along with advances in genetics and in the understanding of the pathogenesis of PD, these may prove to be the most efficient therapeutic interventions. The future looks bright for patients with various movement disorders, and we can anticipate close collaboration between neuroscientists, neurologists, and neurosurgeons in many novel endeavors in the coming decade.

REFERENCES

1. Gage, F. H. (1990) Intracerebral grafting of genetically modified cells acting as biological pumps. *Trends Pharmacol. Sci.* **11,** 437–439.
2. Kawaja, M. D., Fagan, A. M., Firestein, B. L., and Gage, F. H. (1991) Intracerebral grafting of cultured autologous skin fibroblasts into the rat striatum: an assessment of graft size and ultrastructure. *J. Comp. Neurol.* **307,** 695–706.
3. Bencsics, C., Wachtel, S. R., Milstien, S., et al. (1996) Double transduction with GTP cyclohydrolase I and tyrosine hydroxylase is necessary for spontaneous synthesis of L-DOPA by primary fibroblasts. *J. Neurosci.* **16,** 4449–4456.
4. Leff, S. E., Rendahl, K. G., Spratt, S. K., et al. (1998) In vivo L-DOPA production by genetically modified primary rat fibroblast or 9L gliosarcoma cell grafts via coexpression of GTP cyclohydrolase I with tyrosine hydroxylase. *Exp. Neurol.* **151,** 249–264.
5. Cunningham, L. A., Hansen, J. T., Short, M. P., et al. (1991) The use of genetically altered astrocytes to provide nerve growth factor to adrenal chromaffin cells grafted into the striatum. *Brain Res.* **561,** 192–202.
6. La Gamma, E. F., Weisinger, G., Lenn, N. J., et al. (1993) Genetically modified primary astrocytes as cellular vehicles for gene therapy in the brain. *Cell Transplant.* **2,** 207–214.
7. Lundberg, C., Horellou, P., Mallet, J., et al. (1996) Generation of DOPA-producing astrocytes by retroviral transduction of the human tyrosine hydroxylase gene: in vitro characterization and in vivo effects in the rat Parkinson model. *Exp. Neurol.* **139,** 39–53.
8. Renfranz, P. J., Cunningham, M. G., and McKay, D. G. (1991) Region-specific differentiation of the hippocampal stem cell line HiB5 upon implantation into the developing mammalian brain. *Cell* **66,** 713–729.
9. Snyder, E. Y., Deitcher, D. L., Walsh, C., et al. (1992) Multipotent neural cell lines can engraft and participate in development of mouse cerebellum. *Cell* **68,** 33–51.
10. Hoshimaru, M., Ray, J., Sah, D. W. Y., et al. (1996) Differentiation of the immortalized adult neuronal progenitor cell line HC2S2 into neurons by regulatable suppression of the v-myc oncogene. *Proc. Natl. Acad. Sci. USA* **93,** 1518–1523.
11. Svendsen, C. N. and Smith, A. G. (1999) New prospects for human stem-cell therapy in the nervous system. *Trends Neurosci.* **22(8),** 357–364.
12. Gage, F. H. (2000) Mammalian neural stem cells. *Science* **287(5457),** 1433–1438.
13. Lee, S. H., Lumelsky, N., Studer, L., et al. (2000) Efficient generation of midbrain and hindbrain neurons from mouse embryonic stem cells. *Nat. Biotechnol.* **18(6),** 675–679.
14. Sanchez-Pernaute, R., Studer, L., Bankiewicz, K. S., et al. (2001) In vitro generation and transplantation of precursor-derived human dopamine neurons. *J. Neurosci. Res.* **65(4),** 284–288.
15. Kawaja, M. D. and Gage, F. H. (1991) Reactive astrocytes are substrates for the growth of adult CNS axons in the presence of elevated levels of nerve growth factor. *Neuron* **7,** 1019–1030.
16. Lucidi-Phillipi, C. A., Gage, F. H., Shults, C. W., et al. (1995) BDNF-transduced fibroblasts: production of BDNF and effects of grafting to the adult rat brain. *J. Comp. Neurol.* **354,** 361–376.
17. Leff, S. E., Spratt, S. K., Snyder, R. O., et al. (1999) Long-term restoration of striatal L-aromatic amino acid decarboxylase activity using recombinant adeno-associated viral vector gene transfer in a rodent model of Parkinson's disease. *Neuroscience* **92(1),** 185–196.
18. Kordower, J. H., Emborg, M. E., Bloch, J., et al. (2000) Neurodegeneration prevented by lentiviral vector delivery of GDNF in primate models of Parkinson's disease. *Science* **290(5492),** 767–773.
19. Robbins, P. D. and Ghivizzani, S. C. (1998) Viral vectors for gene therapy. *Pharmacol. Ther.* **80(1),** 35–47.
20. Yang, N. S. and Sun, W. H. (1995) Gene gun and other non-viral approaches for cancer gene therapy. *Nature Med.* **1,** 481–483.
21. Felgner, J. H., Kumar, R., Sridhar, C. N., et al. (1994) Enhanced gene delivery and mechanism studies with a novel series of cationic lipid formulations. *J. Biol. Chem.* **269,** 2550–2561.

22. Palmer, T. D., Rosman, G. J., Osborne, W. R. A., et al. (1991) Genetically modified skin fibroblasts persist long after transplantation but gradually inactivate introduced genes. *Proc. Natl. Acad. Sci. USA* **88,** 1330–1334.
23. Mulligan, R. C. (1993) The basic science of gene therapy. *Science* **260,** 926–932.
24. Blomer, U., Naldini, L., Kafri, T., et al. (1997) Highly efficient and sustained gene transfer in adult neurons with a lentivirus vector. *J. Virol.* **71(9),** 6641–6649.
25. Roemer, K., Johnson, P. A., and Friedmann, T. (1991) Activity of the simian virus 40 early promoter-enhancer in herpes simplex virus type 1 vectors is dependent on its position, the infected cell type, and the presence of Vmw175. *J. Virol.* **65,** 6900–6912.
26. Blomer, U., Naldini, L., Verma, I. M., et al. (1996) Applications of gene therapy to the CNS. *Hum. Mol. Genet.* 1397–1404.
27. Scharfmann, R., Axelrod, J. H., and Verma, I. M. (1991) Long-term in vivo expression of retrovirus-mediated gene transfer in mouse fibroblast implants. *Proc. Natl. Acad. Sci. USA* **88,** 4626–4630.
28. Dai, Y., Roman, M., Naviaux, R. K., et al. (1992) Gene therapy via primary myoblasts: long-term expression of factor IX protein following transplantation in vivo. *Proc. Natl. Acad. Sci. USA* **89,** 10,892–10,895.
29. Li, X., Eastman, E. M., Schwartz, R. J., et al. (1999) Synthetic muscle promoters: activities exceeding naturally occurring regulatory sequences. *Nat. Biotechnol.* **17(3),** 241–245.
30. Dhawan, J., Rando, T. A., Elson, S. L., et al. (1995) Tetracycline-regulated gene expression following direct gene transfer into mouse skeletal muscle. *Somat. Cell Mol. Genet.* **21,** 233–240.
31. Corti, O., Horellou, P., Colin, P., et al. (1996) Intracerebral tetracycline-dependent regulation of gene expression in grafts of neural precursors. *Neuroreport* **7,** 1655–1659.
32. Suhr, S. T., Gil E. B., Senut, M. C., et al. (1998) High level transactivation by a modified Bombyx ecdysone receptor in mammalian cells without exogenous retinoid X receptor. *Proc. Natl. Acad. Sci. USA* **95(14),** 7999–8004.
33. Ye, X., Rivera, V. M., Zoltick, P., et al. (1999) Regulated delivery of therapeutic proteins after in vivo somatic cell gene transfer. *Science* **283(5398),** 88–91.
34. Burcin, M. M., Schiedner, G., Kochanek, S., et al. (1999) Adenovirus-mediated regulable target gene expression in vivo. *Proc. Natl. Acad. Sci. USA* **96(2),** 355–360.
35. Miller, A. D. and Rosman, G. J. (1989) Improved retroviral vectors for gene transfer and expression. *Biotechniques* **7,** 980–989.
36. Danos, O. and Mulligan, R. C. (1988) Safe and efficient generation of recombinant retroviruses with amphotropic and ecotropic host ranges. *Proc. Natl. Acad. Sci. USA* **85,** 6460–6464.
37. Neve, R. L. (1993) Adenovirus vectors enter the brain. *Trends Neurosci.* **16,** 251–253.
38. Davidson, B. L., Allen, E. D., Kozarsky, K. F., et al. (1993) A model system for in vivo gene transfer into the central nervous system using an adenoviral vector. *Nat. Genet.* **3,** 219–223.
39. Le Gal, L., Robert, J. J., Berrard, S., et al. (1993) An adenovirus vector for gene transfer into neurons and glia in the brain. *Science* **259,** 988–990.
40. Choi-Lundberg, D. L., Lin, Q., Changa, Y. N., et al. (1997) Dopaminergic neurons protected from degeneration by GDNF gene therapy. *Science* **275,** 838–841.
41. Byrnes, A. P., MacLaren, R. E., and Charlton, H. M. (1996) Immunological instability of persistent adenovirus vectors in the brain: peripheral exposure to vector leads to renewed inflammation, reduced gene expression, and demyelination. *J. Neurosci.* **16,** 3045–3055.
42. Kochanek, S., Clemens, P. R., Mitani, K., et al. (1996) A new adenoviral vector: replacement of all viral coding sequences with 28 kb of DNA independently expressing both full-length dystrophin and beta-galactosidase. *Proc. Natl. Acad. Sci. USA* **93(12),** 5731–5736.
43. Xiao, X., Li, J., and Samulski, R. J. (1998) Production of high-titer recombinant adeno-associated virus vectors in the absence of helper adenovirus. *J. Virol.* **72(3),** 2224–2232.
44. McCown, T. J., Xiao, X., Li, J., et al. (1996) Differential and persistent expression patterns of CNS gene transfer by an adeno-associated virus (AAV) vector. *Brain Res.* **713,** 99–107.
45. Samulski, R. J., During, M. J., Kaplitt, M. G., et al. (1997) Adeno-associated virus vectors yield long-term expression and delivery of potentially therapeutic genes into non-dividing neuronal cells. *J. Neurovirol.* **3(Suppl. 1),** S72.
46. Mandel, R. J., Rendahl, S. K., Spratt, S. K., et al. (1998) Characterization of intrastriatal recombinant adeno-associated virus-mediated gene transfer of human tyrosine hydroxylase and human GTP-cyclohydrolase 1 in a rat model of Parkinson's Disease. *J. Neurosci.* **18,** 4271–4284.
47. Johnson, P. A., Miyanohara, A., Levine, F., et al. (1992) Cytotoxicity of a replication-defective mutant of herpes simplex virus type 1. *J. Virol.* **66,** 2952–2965.
48. Isacson, O. (1995) Behavioral effects and gene delivery in a rat model of Parkinson's disease. *Science* **269,** 856.
49. Kennedy, P. G. (1997) Potential use of herpes simplex virus (HSV) vectors for gene therapy of neurological disorders. *Brain* **120(Pt 7),** 1245–1259.
50. Kolberg, R. (1992) Gene-transfer virus contaminant linked to monkeys' cancer. *J. NIH Res.* **4,** 43–44.
51. Miller, A. D., Miller, D. G., Garcia, J. V., et al. (1993) Use of retroviral vectors for gene transfer and expression. *Methods Enzymol.* **217,** 581–599.
52. Miller, D. G., Adam, M. A., and Miller, A. D. (1990) Gene transfer by retrovirus vectors occurs only in cells that are actively replicating at the time of infection. *Mol. Cell. Biol.* **10,** 4239–4242.
53. Naldini, L., Blomer, U., Gage, F. H., et al. (1996) Efficient transfer, integration, and sustained long-term expression of the transgene in adult rat brains injected with a lentiviral vector. *Proc. Natl. Acad. Sci. USA* **93,** 11,382–11,388.

54. Naldini, L., Blomer, U., Gallay, P., et al. (1996) In vivo gene delivery and stable transduction of nondividing cells by a lentiviral vector. *Science* **272,** 263–267.
55. Zufferey, R., Nagy, D., Mandel, R. J., et al. (1997) Multiply attenuated lentiviral vector achieves efficient gene delivery in vivo. *Nat. Biotechnol.* **15(9),** 871–875.
56. Jacoby, D. R., Fraefel, C., and Breakefield, X. O. (1997) Hybrid vectors: a new generation of virus-based vectors designed to control the cellular fate of delivered genes [editorial]. *Gene Ther.* **4(12),** 1281–1283.
57. Johnston, K. M., Jacoby, D., Pechan, P. A., et al. (1997) HSV/AAV hybrid amplicon vectors extend transgene expression in human glioma cells. *Hum. Gene Ther.* **8(3),** 359–370.
58. Feng, M., Jackson, W. H. Jr., Goldman, C. K., et al. (1997) Stable in vivo gene transduction via a novel adenoviral/retroviral chimeric vector. *Nat. Biotechnol.* **9,** 866–870.
59. Lindvall, O., Sawle, G., Widner, H., et al. (1994) Evidence for long-term survival and function of dopaminergic grafts in progressive Parkinson's disease. *Ann. Neurol.* **35,** 172–180.
60. Olanow, C. W., Kordower, J. H., and Freeman, T. B. (1996) Fetal nigral transplantation as a therapy for Parkinson's disease. *Trends Neurosci.* **19,** 102–109.
61. Freed, C. R., Greene, P. E., Breeze, R. E., et al. (2001) Transplantation of embryonic dopamine neurons for severe Parkinson's disease. *N. Engl. J. Med.* **344(10),** 710–719.
62. Emgard, M., Karlsson, J., Hansson, O., et al. (1999) Patterns of cell death and dopaminergic neuron survival in intrastriatal nigral grafts. *Exp. Neurol.* **160(1),** 279–288.
63. Barkats, M., Nakao, N., Grasbon-Frodl, E. M., et al. (1997) Intrastriatal grafts of embryonic mesencephalic rat neurons genetically modified using an adenovirus encoding human Cu/Zn superoxide dismutase. *Neuroscience* **78,** 703–713.
64. Yurek, D. M. (1998) Glial cell line-derived neurotrophic factor improves survival of dopaminergic neurons in transplants of fetal ventral mesencephalic tissue. *Exp. Neurol.* **153(2),** 195–202.
65. Luquin, M. R., Montoro, R. J., Guillen, J., et al. (1999) Recovery of chronic parkinsonian monkeys by autotransplants of carotid body cell aggregates into putamen. *Neuron* **22(4),** 743–750.
66. Deacon, T., Schumacher, J., Dinsmore, J., et al. (1997) Histological evidence of fetal pig neural cell survival after transplantation into a patient with Parkinson's disease. *Nat. Med.* **3(3),** 350–353.
67. Reynolds, B. A. and Weiss, S. (1992) Generation of neurons and astrocytes from isolated cells of the adult mammalian central nervous system. *Science* **255,** 1707–1710.
68. Tropepe, V., Sibilia, M., Ciruna, B. G., et al. (1999) Distinct neural stem cells proliferate in response to EGF and FGF in the developing mouse telencephalon. *Dev. Biol.* **208(1),** 166–188.
69. Gage, F. H., Coates, P. W., Palmer, T. D., et al. (1995) Survival and differentiation of adult neuronal progenitor cells transplanted to the adult brain. *Proc. Natl. Acad. Sci. USA* **92,** 11,879–11,883.
70. Palmer, T. D., Ray, J., and Gage, F. H. (1995) FGF-2-responsive neuronal progenitors reside in proliferative and quiescent regions of the adult rodent brain. *Mol. Cell. Neurosci.* **6,** 474–486.
71. Reynolds, B. A., Tetzlaff, W., and Weiss, S. (1992) A multipotent EGF-responsive striatal embryonic progenitor cell produces neurons and astrocytes. *J. Neurosci.* **12,** 4565–4574.
72. Winkler, C., Fricker, R. A., Gates, M. A., et al. (1998) Incorporation and glial differentiation of mouse EGF-responsive neural progenitor cells after transplantation into the embryonic rat brain. *Mol. Cell Neurosci.* **11(3),** 99–116.
73. Scheffler, B., Horn, M., Blumcke, I., et al. (1999) Marrow-mindedness: a perspective on neuropoiesis. *Trends Neurosci.* **22(8),** 348–357.
74. Bjornson, C. R., Rietze, R. L., Reynolds, B. A., et al. (1999) Turning brain into blood: a hematopoietic fate adopted by adult neural stem cells in vivo. *Science* **283(5401),** 534–537.
75. Eglitis, M. A. and Mezey, E. (1997) Hematopoietic cells differentiate into both microglia and macroglia in the brains of adult mice. *Proc. Natl. Acad. Sci. USA* **94(8),** 4080–4085.
76. Vogel, G. (2000) Cell biology: stem cells: new excitement, persistent questions. *Science* **290(5497),** 1672–1674.
77. Zetterstrom, R. H., Solomin, L., Jansson, L., et al. (1997) Dopamine neuron agenesis in Nurr1-deficient mice. *Science* **276(5310),** 248–250.
78. Saucedo-Cardenas, O., Quintana-Hau, J. D., Le, W. D., et al. (1998) Nurr1 is essential for the induction of the dopaminergic phenotype and the survival of ventral mesencephalic late dopaminergic precursor neurons. *Proc. Natl. Acad. Sci. USA* **95(7),** 4013–4018.
79. Sakurada, K., Ohshima-Sakurada, M., Palmer, T. D., et al. (1999) Nurr1, an orphan nuclear receptor, is a transcriptional activator of endogenous tyrosine hydroxylase in neural progenitor cells derived from the adult brain. *Development* **126(18),** 4017–4026.
80. Wagner, J., Akerud, P., Castro, D.S., et al. (1999) Induction of a midbrain dopaminergic phenotype in Nurr1-overexpressing neural stem cells by type 1 astrocytes. *Nat. Biotechnol.* **17(7),** 653–659.
81. Daadi, M. M. and Weiss, S. (1999) Generation of tyrosine hydroxylase-producing neurons from precursors of the embryonic and adult forebrain. *J. Neurosci.* **19(11),** 4484–4497.
82. Anton, R., Kordower, J. H., Maidment, N. T., et al. (1994) Neural-targeted gene therapy for rodent and primate hemiparkinsonism. *Exp. Neurol.* **127,** 207–218.
83. Martinez-Serrano, A., Lundberg, C., Horellou, P., et al. (1995) CNS-derived neural progenitor cells for gene transfer of nerve growth factor to the adult rat brain: complete rescue of axotomized cholinergic neurons after transplantation into the septum. *J. Neurosci.* **15,** 5668–5680.
84. Sabate, O., Horellou, P., Vigne, E., et al. (1995) Transplantation to the rat brain of human neural progenitors that were genetically modified using adenoviruses. *Nat. Genet.* **9,** 256–260.

85. Chase, T. N., Engber, T. M., and Mouradian, M. M. (1994) Palliative and prophylactic benefits of continuously administered dopaminomimetics in Parkinson's disease. *Neurology* **44,** S15–S18.
86. Mouradian, M. M., Heuser, I. J., Baronti, F., et al. (1990) Modification of central dopaminergic mechanisms by continuous levodopa therapy for advanced Parkinson's disease. *Ann. Neurol.* **27,** 18–23.
87. Wolff, J. A., Fisher, L. J., Jinnah, H. A., et al. (1989) Grafting fibroblasts genetically modified to produce L-dopa in a rat model of Parkinson disease. *Proc. Natl. Acad. Sci. USA* **86,** 9011–9014.
88. Horellou, P., Brundin, P., Kalen, P., et al. (1990) In vivo release of DOPA and dopamine from genetically engineered cells grafted to the denervated rat striatum. *Neuron* **5,** 393–402.
89. Fisher, L. J., Jinnah, H. A., Kale, L. C., et al. (1991) Survival and function of intrastriatally grafted primary fibroblasts genetically modified to produce L-DOPA. *Neuron* **6,** 371–380.
90. Jiao, S., Gurevich, V., and Wolff, J. A. (1993) Long-term correction of rat model of Parkinson's disease by gene therapy. *Nature* **362,** 450–453.
91. During, M. J., Naegele, J. R., O'Malley, K. L., et al. (1994) Long-term behavioral recovery in parkinsonian rats by an HSV vector expressing tyrosine hydroxylase. *Science* **266,** 1399–1403.
92. Kaplitt, M. G., Leone, P., Samulski, R. J., et al. (1994) Long-term gene expression and phenotypic correction using adeno-associated virus vectors in the mammalian brain. *Nat. Genet.* **8,** 148–154.
93. Nagatsu, T. (1983) Biopterin cofactor and monoamine-synthesizing monooxygenases. *Neurochem. Int.* **5,** 27–38.
94. Ichinose, H., Ohye, T., Takahashi, E., et al. (1994) Hereditary progressive dystonia with marked diurnal fluctuation caused by mutations in the GTP cyclohydrolase 1 gene. *Nat. Genet.* **8,** 236–242.
95. Kang, U. J., Fisher, L. J., Joh, T. H., et al. (1993) Regulation of dopamine production by genetically modified primary fibroblasts. *J. Neurosci.* **13,** 5203–5211.
96. Kaddis, F. G., Clarkson, E. D., Weber, M. J., et al. (1997) Intrastriatal grafting of Cos cells stably expressing human aromatic L-amino acid decarboxylase: neurochemical effects. *J. Neurochem.* **68,** 1520–1526.
97. Bankiewicz, K. S., Eberling, J. L., Kohutnicka, M., et al. (2000) Convection-enhanced delivery of AAV vector in parkinsonian monkeys; in vivo detection of gene expression and restoration of dopaminergic function using prodrug approach. *Exp. Neurol.* **164(1),** 2–14.
98. Lee, W. Y., Chang, J. W., Nemeth, N. L., et al. (1999) Vesicular monoamine transporter-2 and aromatic L-amino acid decarboxylase enhance dopamine delivery after L-3, 4- dihydroxyphenylalanine administration in Parkinsonian rats. *J. Neurosci.* **19(8),** 3266–3274.
99. Burchiel, K. J., Anderson, V. C., Favre, J., et al. (1999) Comparison of pallidal and subthalamic nucleus deep brain stimulation for advanced Parkinson's disease: results of a randomized, blinded pilot study. *Neurosurgery* **45(6),** 1375–1382; discussion 1382–1384.
100. Lang, A. E. (2000) Surgery for Parkinson disease: a critical evaluation of the state of the art. *Arch. Neurol.* **57(8),** 1118–1125.
101. Winkler, C., Bentlage, C., Nikkhah, G., et al. (1999) Intranigral transplants of GABA-rich striatal tissue induce behavioral recovery in the rat Parkinson model and promote the effects obtained by intrastriatal dopaminergic transplants. *Exp. Neurol.* **155(2),** 165–186.
102. Hornykiewicz, O. (1998) Biochemical aspects of Parkinson's disease. *Neurology.* **51(2 Suppl. 2),** S2–S9.
103. Jenner, P. and Olanow, C. W. (1998) Understanding cell death in Parkinson's disease. *Ann. Neurol.* **44,** S72–S84.
104. Przedborski, S., Kostic, V., Jackson-Lewis, V., et al. (1992) Transgenic mice with increased Cu/Zn-superoxide dismutase activity are resistant to N-methyl-4-phenyl-1,2,3,6-tetrahydropyridine-induced neurotoxicity. *J. Neurosci.* **12,** 1658–1667.
105. Nakao, N., Frodl, E. M., Widner, H., et al. (1995) Overexpressing Cu/Zn superoxide dismutase enhances survival of transplanted neurons in a rat model of Parkinson's disease. *Nature Med.* **1,** 226–231.
106. Polymeropoulos, M. H., Lavedan, C., Leroy, E., et al. (1997) Mutation in the a-synuclein gene identified in families with Parkinson's disease. *Science* **276,** 2045–2047.
107. Kitada, T., Asakawa, S., Hattori, N., et al. (1998) Mutations in the parkin gene cause autosomal recessive juvenile parkinsonism. *Nature* **392,** 605–608.
108. Westphal, C. H. and Leder, P. (1997) Transposon-generated 'knock-out' and 'knock-in' gene-targeting constructs for use in mice. *Curr. Biol.* **7,** 530–533.
109. Kawamura, I., Morishita, R., Tomita, N., et al. (1999) Intratumoral injection of oligonucleotides to the NF kappa B binding site inhibits cachexia in a mouse tumor model. *Gene Ther.* **6(1),** 91–97.
110. Blaese, R. M. (1997) Gene therapy for cancer. *Sci. Am.* **276(6),** 111–115.
111. Phylactou, L. A., Kilpatrick, M. W., and Wood, M. J. (1998) Ribozymes as therapeutic tools for genetic disease. *Hum. Mol. Genet.* **7(10),** 1649–1653.
112. Linnik, M. D., Zahos, P., Geschwind, M. D., et al. (1995) Expression of bcl-2 from a defective herpes simplex virus-1 vector limits neuronal death in focal cerebral ischemia. *Stroke* **26,** 1670–1674.
113. Hyman, C., Hofer, M., Barde, Y. A., et al. (1991) BDNF is a neurotrophic factor for dopaminergic neurons of the substantia nigra. *Nature* **350,** 230–232.
114. Hyman, C., Juhasz, M., Jackson, C., et al. (1994) Overlapping and distinct actions of the neurotrophins BDNF, NT-3, and NT-4/5 on cultured dopaminergic and GABAergic neurons of the ventral mesencephalon. *J. Neurosci.* **14,** 335–347.
115. Hynes, M. A., Poulsen, K., Armanini, M., et al. (1994) Neurotrophin-4/5 is a survival factor for embryonic midbrain dopaminergic neurons in enriched cultures. *J. Neurosci. Res.* **37,** 144–154.
116. Lin, L. F. H., Doherty, D. H., Lile, J. D., et al. (1993) GDNF: a glial cell line-derived neurotrophic factor for midbrain dopaminergic neurons. *Science* **260,** 1130–1132.

117. Knusel, B., Michel, P. P., Schwaber, J. S., et al. (1990) Selective and nonselective stimulation of central cholinergic and dopaminergic development in vitro by nerve growth factor, basic fibroblast growth factor, epidermal growth factor, insulin and the insulin-like growth factors I and II. *J. Neurosci.* **10,** 558–570.
118. Mayer, E., Fawcett, J. W., and Dunnett, S. B. (1993) Basic fibroblast growth factor promotes the survival of embryonic ventral mesencephalic dopaminergic neurons-II. Effects on nigral transplants in vivo. *Neuroscience* **56,** 389–398.
119. Poulsen, K. T., Armanini, M. P., Klein, R. D., et al. (1994) TGFb2 and TGFb3 are potent survival factors for midbrain dopaminergic neurons. *Neuron* **13,** 1245–1252.
120. Engele, J. and Bohn, M. C. (1991) The neurotrophic effects of fibroblast growth factors on dopaminergic neurons in vitro are mediated by mesencephalic glia. *J. Neurosci.* **11,** 3070–3078.
121. Hudson, J., Granholm, A. C., Gerhardt, G. A., et al. (1995) Glial cell line-derived neurotrophic factor augments midbrain dopaminergic circuits in vivo. *Brain Res. Bull.* **36(5),** 425–432.
122. Tomac, A., Widenfalk, J., Lin, L. F. H., et al. (1995) Retrograde axonal transport of glial cell line-derived neurotrophic factor in the adult nigrostriatal system suggests a trophic role in the adult. *Proc. Natl. Acad. Sci. USA* **92,** 8274–8278.
123. Morse, J. K., Wiegand, S. J., Anderson, K., et al. (1993) Brain-derived neurotrophic factor (BDNF) prevents the degeneration of medial septal cholinergic neurons following fimbria transection. *J. Neurosci.* **13,** 4146–4156.
124. Levivier, M., Przedborski, S., Bencsics, C., et al. (1995) Intrastriatal implantation of fibroblasts genetically engineered to produce brain-derived neurotrophic factor prevents degeneration of dopaminergic neurons in a rat model of Parkinson's disease. *J. Neurosci.* **15,** 7810–7820.
125. Frim, D. M., Uhler, T. A., Galpern, W. R., et al. (1994) Implanted fibroblasts genetically engineered to produce brain-derived neurotrophic factor prevent 1-methyl-4-phenylpyridinium toxicity to dopaminergic neurons in the rat. *Proc. Natl. Acad. Sci. USA* **91,** 5104–5108.
126. Bilang-Bleuel, A., Revah, F., Colin, P., et al. (1997) Intrastriatal injection of an adenoviral vector expressing glial-cell- line-derived neurotrophic factor prevents dopaminergic neuron degeneration and behavioral impairment in a rat model of Parkinson disease. *Proc. Natl. Acad. Sci. USA* **94(16),** 8818–8823.
127. Lapchak, P. A., Araujo, D. M., Hilt, D. C., et al. (1997) Adenoviral vector-mediated GDNF gene therapy in a rodent lesion model of late stage Parkinson's disease. *Brain Res.* **777(1–2),** 153–160.
128. Mandel, R. J., Spratt, S. K., Snyder, R. O., et al. (1997) Midbrain injection of recombinant adeno-associated virus encoding rat glial cell line-derived neurotrophic factor protects nigral neurons in a progressive 6-hydroxydopamine-induced degeneration model of Parkinson's disease in rats. *Proc. Natl. Acad. Sci. USA* **94(25),** 14,083–14,088.
129. Choi-Lundberg, D. L., Lin, Q., Schallert, T., et al. (1998) Behavioral and cellular protection of rat dopaminergic neurons by an adenoviral vector encoding glial cell line-derived neurotrophic factor. *Exp. Neurol.* **54(2),** 261–275.

Index

About the Editors

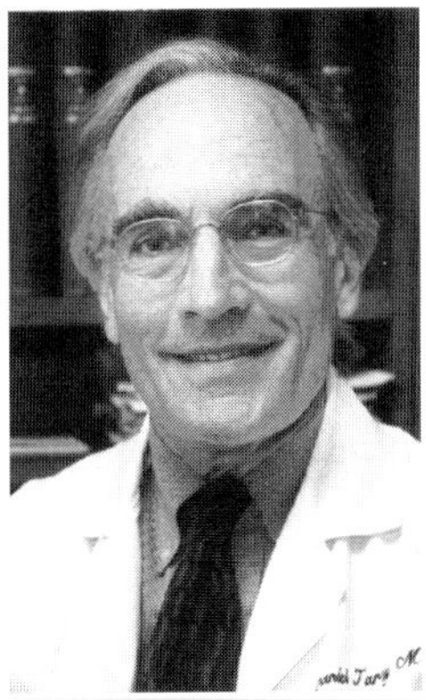

Daniel Tarsy, MD is an Associate Professor of Neurology at Harvard Medical School and Vice Chairman of the department of neurology and director of the Movement Disorders Center at Beth Israel Deaconess Medical Center in Boston. He received his undergraduate degree at Cornell University and MD degree at New York University School of Medicine. He received neurology training at Boston University School of Medicine and fellowship training in neuropharmacology at Massachusetts General Hospital and at the Institute of Psychiatry, London. He has carried out studies in behavioral and biochemical pharmacology of brain neurotransmitters, clinical studies in dystonia, and clinical trials of new treatments for Parkinson's disease, dystonia, tardive dyskinesia, and related movement disorders. Together with his neurosurgical colleagues, Dr. Tarsy directs the stereotactic neurosurgical program for the treatment of Parkinson's disease and tremor at Beth Israel Deaconess Medical Center. He is a member of the editorial board of the journal *Movement Disorders* and is on the boards of the Movement Disorders Society and the Movement Disorders section of the American Academy of Neurology.

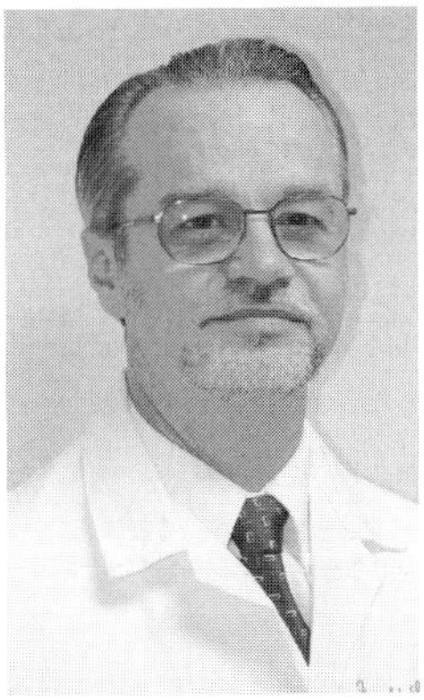

Jerrold L. Vitek, MD, PhD is a Professor of Neurology and Director of the Program for Functional and Stereotaxic Neurology, at Emory University School of Medicine in Atlanta, Georgia. He also serves as a senior member of the Neurology Clinic Section of The Emory Clinic. Dr. Vitek earned his medical and doctorate degrees from the University of Minnesota in Duluth. He received his postgraduate training in internal medicine at Mary Imogene Bassett Hospital in Cooperstown, New York. He later served his residency in neurology at The Johns Hopkins Hospital in Baltimore, Maryland. Dr. Vitek's research is directed towards understanding the pathophysiologic basis of and surgical treatment of movement disorders. He conducts basic electrophysiologic studies of the basal ganglia and thalamus in laboratory models of movement disorders and clinical trials of surgical therapy for Parkinson's disease, dystonia, and tremor. He is a member of the American Academy of Neurology, Movement Disorders Society, and The Society for Neuroscience.

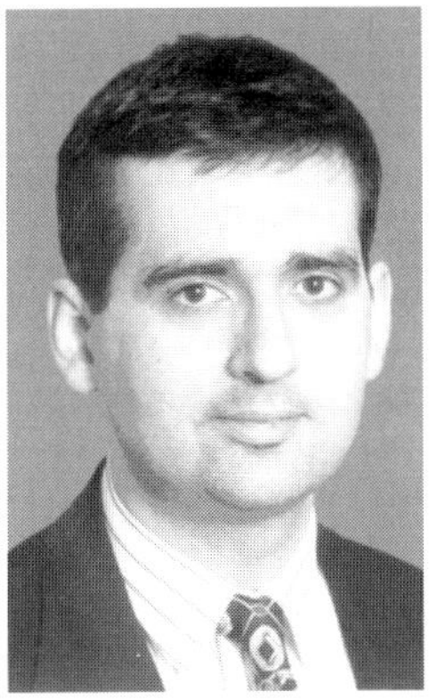

Andres M. Lozano, MD, PhD is Professor and RR Tasker Chair in Functional Neurosurgery at The Toronto Western Hospital and The University of Toronto. Dr. Lozano received his MD degree at the University of Ottawa and his PhD degree in neurobiology and his neurosurgical training at McGill University. He received post-doctoral training in movement disorders at Queens Square, London, and in cell and molecular biology in Toronto. Dr. Lozano is a Canadian Institute of Health Research Clinician-Scientist. Dr Lozano's research focuses on understanding the cellular pathogenesis and developing novel treatments particularly surgery, for movement disorders such as Parkinson's disease and dystonia. He serves on the board and executive of several international organizations including the World Society for Stereotactic and Functional Neurosurgery, the American Association of Neurological Surgeons and Congress of Neurological Surgeons section on Functional Neurosurgery, The Michael J. Fox Foundation for Parkinson's Research, and the Movement Disorders Society.

About the Editors